COMMUNITY HEALTH

COMMUNITY HEALTH

SEVENTH EDITION

Lawrence W. Green, B.S., M.P.H., Dr. P.H.
Professor and Head
Division of Preventive Medicine and Health Promotion
Department of Health Care and
Epidemiology;
Director,
Institute of Health Promotion Research
University of British Columbia
Vancouver, British Columbia

Judith M. Ottoson, B.S.N., M.P.H., Ed.D.
Assistant Professor
Adult Education Research Centre
Faculty of Education
University of British Columbia
Vancouver, British Columbia

with illustrations

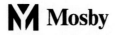
Mosby

St. Louis Baltimore Boston Chicago London Madrid Philadelphia Sydney Toronto

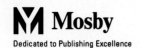
Mosby

Dedicated to Publishing Excellence

Editor-in-Chief: James M. Smith
Acquisitions Editor: Vicki Malinee
Developmental Editor: Catherine Schwent
Project Manager: Barbara Bowes Merritt
Editing and Production: University Graphics, Inc.
Design: University Graphics, Inc.
Manufacturing Supervisor: Karen Lewis

SEVENTH EDITION

Printed in the United States of America
Composition by University Graphics, Inc.
Printing/binding by R.R. Donnelley & Sons

Library of Congress Cataloging in Publication Data

Green, Lawrence W.
    Community health.—7th ed. / Lawrence W. Green and Judith M.
Ottoson.
          p.   cm.
    Includes bibliographical references and index.
    ISBN 0-8016-7898-6 ✓
    1. Public Health.   2. Public health—United States.   I. Ottoson,
Judith M.   II. Title.
    [DNLM: 1. Community Health Services.   2. Public Health.   WA 546.1
G796c 1994]
    RA425.G73   1994
    362.1—dc20
    DNLM/DLC
for Library of Congress   93-46815
                                                                CIP

Coming together is a beginning,
Staying together is progress,
Working together is success,
Laughing together makes it all worthwhile

Preface

Purpose

The seventh edition of *Community Health* remains a general textbook for use in undergraduate and introductory graduate courses in community health. Broader than any single profession or discipline, community health represents the intersection of many disciplines and sectors with public health, school health, occupational health, social and recreational services, and self-care. The book offers a synthesis of the perspectives and content of these spheres of health action.

Recent Developments

The sixth edition appeared in 1990 as a new era in disease prevention and health promotion was under way in several Western nations. Conservative governments were asserting political control in most of these countries, leaving the fate of earlier national health initiatives uncertain. Since then events have vindicated the proponents and architects of disease prevention and health promotion. Their vision was correct, their advice timely, and their plans viable. In Australia, Canada, New Zealand, some European countries, the United Kingdom, and the United States, new governments have endorsed and put their own stamp on disease prevention and health promotion. Some emphasized greater participation of private and voluntary sectors, decentralization, and deregulation. Others emphasized greater equity in the distribution of health resources, greater government responsibility, or greater coverage of preventive and primary care services within medical care plans.

The emphasis on private and voluntary participation has diversified the involvement of agencies, organizations, foundations, and professions in community health matters that were once the exclusive domains of traditional medical and public health agencies. The emphasis on decentralization has shifted health responsibilities from federal to state or provincial and community organizations. The deregulatory thrust of conservative governments put additional pressures on communities to monitor and enforce environmental protections that were previously the province of federal agencies.

Recession and deficit budgets have put pressures on financing traditional medical care and delivery systems. This has produced community innovations in health services and programs. Employers, who have borne a large share of the increased medical costs, have sponsored a myriad of new employee health insurance and health promotion programs with the hope of containing medical care costs.

Chemical and oil spills and the discovery of wastes polluting beaches, water systems, and food chains have brought the importance of environmental health protection measures more sharply into focus. Lung cancer has now surpassed breast cancer as the leading cause of cancer deaths among women, dramatizing the grim harvest of life-styles developed decades ago and the need to invest now in health promotion to prevent chronic diseases in the future.

Advocacy organizations and community action groups, such as Mothers Against Drunk Driving (MADD) and Action on Smoking and Health (ASH), have made great inroads on local and state ordinances to protect victims of drunk driving and passive smoking in public places. Highway traffic deaths have declined significantly. Dramatic reductions in hypertension and deaths from cardiovascular disease and stroke have demonstrated the effectiveness of community high blood pressure control programs and nutrition, exercise, and antismoking campaigns. In communicable disease control the success of the global eradication of smallpox has been forgotten in the face of the growing threat of acquired immunodeficiency syndrome (AIDS).

The World Health Organization's commitment to a global strategy of ''Health for all by the year 2000'' has placed renewed emphasis on community involvement in setting objectives and adopting appropriate technologies to meet their own health needs and to develop self-sufficiency in providing their own primary health care. The U.S. *Healthy People 2000* and *Healthy Communities 2000* documents have replaced the 1990 objectives for the nation in disease prevention and health promotion.

These and other late-breaking developments of 1990 through late 1993 are chronicled and examined in this edition in the context of the history and principles of community health.

Basis for Revision

We are very proud that the sixth edition of this text received a Book-of-the-Year award from the *American Journal of Nursing*. Other published reviews and feedback from both users and readers of the

sixth edition, interviews with dozens of instructors, and commissioned reviews by five professors representing various college and university programs teaching a community health course all helped with this revision. We have rewritten extensively to make the seventh edition more readable, more manageable within a trimester or semester course, more lively and contemporary, and more helpful. Each chapter includes objectives, boxed issues, summaries, annotated readings, and new and current bibliographies. The end-of-text glossary has been expanded in this edition. Glossary terms are in bold letters where they first appear in the text.

Increased utility. Now class-tested by thousands of students, this text has been repeatedly honed to include the material deemed useful and comprehensible to students. The text responds to student interests and difficulties experienced with the sixth edition. Content that instructors judged least useful has been eliminated. Most of the deletions have been sentences and paragraphs within sections, rather than whole sections. This makes the headings and subheadings more evenly spaced and the text under each subheading more efficiently presented.

Major Features

The book adapts to or anticipates the emerging shape and new content of the field. We have endeavored to reflect community health as it is today, but also to anticipate the directions in which it is heading and should head. Students today are preparing for community leadership in the years ahead. The task of this book is to build a set of concepts and skills for students that will enable them to ask the right questions and to tackle community health problems in the future. The text has undergone a metamorphosis in the last four editions from a primarily descriptive text to an inquiry and problem-solving guide.

Format of the chapters. Besides updated comparative and descriptive data, we have also suggested how these facts provide a social or epidemiological diagnosis. We then further suggest how the social and epidemiological data on the age group or problem addressed in that chapter can be understood in the context of change or prevention of change. Most chapters offer an inventory of educational, technological, economic, organizational, legal, regulatory, and service measures that can be taken to avert or solve potential health problems. Also indicated are selected objectives appropriate for most communities, based on U.S. national objectives for the year 2000 in disease prevention and health promotion. We have been highly selective in grouping and placing appropriate objectives within the chapters, after eliminating many of the 1990 objectives from the long lists in previous editions.

Part openings. One or two paragraphs at the beginning of each section of the book provide organization and continuity to the chapters in relation to each other. These build on the themes of the book, which cover national policy in community health in both Canada and the United States.

Chapter objectives. A set of objectives at the beginning of each chapter indicates what the reader can expect to learn and to be able to do after completing the chapter.

Case studies and contemporary issues. At least one boxed issue or case study appears in each chapter, bringing the history, organization, and challenges of community health into focus for today's students. Questions are asked in most of the boxed issues to motivate the student to reflect and apply the issue to his or her own community or future.

Photographs and graphs. Most photographs in this edition are new. Line drawings offering conceptual or schematic models are interspersed with the photographs to illustrate the more complex or abstract material. We use some photographs from Third World nations for contrast to build the student's comparative understanding and to illustrate conditions he or she is unlikely to encounter in the more developed world. This is an appeal in part to the inherent interest in the exotic, but it also represents an attempt to broaden perspectives and to emphasize the interdependence of nations for the health of their own citizens and the responsibility of everyone for the health of all. This is the spirit and the essence of community health.

Updated facts and figures. Data presented in this edition have been updated to the 1990s. Delay in publishing official vital statistics by the federal governments of Canada and the United States means that the 1992 or 1993 sources used for each chapter often contained data only through 1990, sometimes through 1991. Unpublished sources were used when permissible to provide the latest data. Most of the specific figures that could not be updated were eliminated for the sake of simplifying the text, making it more readable, and avoiding a cumbersome facts-and-figures memory approach. Epidemiological and vital statistics *concepts* were emphasized rather than *numbers*.

Readability and student interest. In addition to the boxed issues and illustrations, we have inspected every sentence for its utility, clarity, and contemporary tone. Sexist, ageist, or ethnocentric references have been purged. Active verbs rather than passive ones make the reading livelier; complex sentences broken into two or more sentences make the text more straightforward. Rhetorical and review questions and exclamations breathe life into some of the more descriptive material. Transition sentences aid the flow, and additional subheadings make the organization of ideas clearer.

Chapter summaries. At the end of each chapter, a summary highlights the essential concepts and facts and reinforces the objectives of the chapter.

Questions for review. Questions at the end of each chapter elicit application of what has been studied and encourage dialogue among students and class discussions.

Annotated readings. Selected resources are annotated to enhance the learning process.

Bibliographies. Each chapter provides the most complete and up-to-date resources for further study of the material covered.

Glossary. Important terms are defined in the comprehensive glossary and are printed in boldface type when they first appear in the text.

Appendixes. Three appendixes supplement the content by summarizing areas of community health specialization, common job titles, and graduate degree programs for public and community health accredited by the Council on Education for Public Health.

Supplements. An expanded *Instructor's Manual* and *Test Bank* are available to those who adopt the text. The *Manual* includes 1100 true-false, multiple choice, and matching test questions in the *Test Bank.*

The following elements enhance the *Manual*'s practicality: chapter overviews, additional objectives, student assignments, late-breaking headlines, additional resources, easy test questions, and 22 transparency masters of important illustrations, diagrams, tables, and charts. These transparencies were chosen to help the instructor explain difficult concepts and to illustrate key points.

Acknowledgments

To the students and instructors who classroom tested the previous editions, we express sincere thanks again. We also thank the following reviewers whose contributions are reflected throughout this revision:

Mary Barnwell
York College/CUNY

David Sleet
San Diego State University

Don Haynes
University of Minnesota-Duluth

Kelli McCormick Brown
Western Illinois University

Patricia Tyra
University of Massachusetts-Lowell

Finally, we wish to thank our family and friends, who have promoted our health along the way. A special thanks to patient Sophe. We are grateful to Cliff, Betty, Harry, and Helga for strong foundations. We hope to have honored those foundations in this book and in our anticipated future with Beth, Doug, and Jenny.

Since completing the previous edition, we have moved from California to the University of British Columbia in Vancouver, British Columbia, Canada. The opportunity here to start a new Institute of Health Promotion Research with an emphasis on evaluation of community health promotion has tested some of the assumptions and concepts written into previous editions. The Adult Education Research Centre in the Department of Administrative, Adult and Higher Education, Faculty of Education, has proved a hospitable home to study health from a community perspective. The importance of engaging adults in their own health and that of their communities reveals itself in the coming chapters. Helping adults move from understanding to acting on health is a shared commitment of the authors. Previous positions put us face-to-face with the many disciplines, professions, and organizations in communities across the United States that seek to develop their community health resources and programs. Now in British Columbia we have an opportunity to develop an understanding of how these issues and responses differ in Canadian communities.

A Visiting Professorship at the University of Limburg in the Netherlands afforded another opportunity to work for a concentrated period on the book and to draw comparisons of community health between North America and Europe, as previous editions did between the United States, Australia, Canada, and Singapore. These cross-national comparisons have enriched our understanding of the history, structure, and dynamics of community health. We hope the book reflects this deeper understanding. We are indebted to Professor Gerjo Kok at the University of Limburg for his support of the Visiting Professorship in Maastricht; Professor Rob Sanson-Fisher at the Newcastle University and the Cancer Council of New South Wales for the more recent opportunity to review developments in Australia; UNICEF for an opportunity for both of us to spend two weeks in the People's Republic of China on community health issues; the British Columbia and Canadian Ministries of Health for their support of the Institute, which has made possible our work on this revision; the Center for Substance Abuse Prevention, the BC Health Research Foundation, and the Social Sciences and Humanities Research Council of Canada for opportunities to carry out research on community partnerships, coalitions, and participation in health.

LAWRENCE W. GREEN
JUDITH M. OTTOSON

Contents

PART ONE

. . . .

Foundations

This journey into community health begins with a look at our past and at the foundations on which the structure of community health rests. The foundations are set among our historical roots—not just the happenings of the past but the ideas from primitive to modern that linger in our collective psyche. The essence of the primitive ideas is expressed by the opening quotation from St. Augustine, speaking to us from the fifth century AD, the beginning of the "Dark Ages" of history. The scientific foundations of community health, resting sometimes tenuously among these historical roots, are represented by the four components of the health field concept: *human biology* and *environment* represented in community health by human ecology, demography, and epidemiology; *life-style* and *health care organization* represented in community health by the social and behavioral sciences, including political science, economics, and health education.

Chapter 1

Through the Centuries

---❖---

All diseases are to be ascribed to demons.
SAINT AUGUSTINE

The history of public health might well be written as a record of successive redefinings of the unacceptable.
SIR GODFREY VICKERS

OBJECTIVES

When you finish this chapter, you should be able to:

- Identify the three essential elements of community health promotion (educational, social, and environmental interventions)
- Describe examples of how they have been reflected in the customs, beliefs, codes, laws, and programs of the major historical eras
- Relate current issues in community health to their historical precedents

Health has been defined by the World Health Organization as a state of complete physical, mental, and social well-being, not the mere absence of disease or infirmity. **Well-being,** especially social well-being, requires for its meaning an understanding of the historical circumstances that have caused a particular population or community to accept some conditions that another community would define as unacceptable. **Community health** reflects the philosophy, religion, economics, form of government, education, science, aspirations, and folklore of any given period. The history of community health chronicles the advances and declines of societies and human conditions. Consider your own community's history over the past few years, with population and industrial growth or decline, with economic improvements or recessions. Consider the health-related headlines in your local newspapers: abortion, acquired immunodeficiency syndrome (AIDS), teenage pregnancy, drug abuse, drunk-driving laws, toxic waste dumps, fitness, the aging population, seat belt legislation, air pollution controls, computer invasions of medical and vital registration records, and control of nuclear wastes.

Such controversies reflect community responses to historical trends in health and attempts to shape the history of health and community development.

Recent collapses of social order in Somalia and the former Yugoslavia illustrate how civilization depends on the quality and distribution of health in the general population. Health in turn depends on human advancement and community development in various spheres. Cast in a historical framework, community health is a result of life-styles as well as a barometer of conditions that shape life-styles, including human relationships.

These observations describe community health, but they risk characterizing it as only a passive consequence of historical circumstances. Community health also represents a dynamic human enterprise that shapes history. People devote their careers and organizations devote their missions to the promotion of community health.

WHAT IS COMMUNITY HEALTH PROMOTION?

C.-E.A. Winslow characterized public health practice as the science and art of preventing disease, prolonging life, and promoting health and well-being through organized community effort for the sanitation of the environment, the control of communicable infections, the organization of medical and nursing services for the early diagnosis and prevention of disease, the education of the individual in personal health, and the development of the social machinery to assure everyone a standard of living adequate for the maintenance or improvement of health.

By this definition public health practice overlaps some aspects of medicine, nursing, school health, and personal health, and overlaps most aspects of environmental health, disease prevention, and health promotion. Public health tends to be associated with the work of official governmental health agencies, so the term **community health promotion** has

come into increasing use to emphasize the more local, collaborative efforts of various public and private sectors. The spheres of action in community health include aspects of public health practice; school health practice; the professional practices of medical, dental, nursing, and allied health personnel; and the personal health practices of individuals and families. Community health lies in the areas in which these spheres overlap, as shown in Figure 1-1. Additional spheres of action overlap with these and contribute to community health, but usually as a by-product of their primary purposes. Such additional spheres include the worksite, in which employee health promotion, safety, and screening programs address adult health much as school health programs do for children. Likewise, the recreational system and the legal system contribute to community health in performing their primary functions. The coordination and integration of these spheres of action make up the practice of community health promotion.

Community health promotion, as described in this book, *is any combination of educational, social, and environmental actions conducive to the health of a population of a geographically defined area. Educational* interventions may be directed at high-risk individuals, families, or groups, at decision makers, or at whole communities by the mass media, schools, industry, and other organizations. *Social* interventions may take the form of economic, political, legal, and organizational changes, including the organization of health care services designed to support actions conducive to health. *Environmental* supports include the structure and distribution of physical, chemical, and biological resources, facilities, and substances required for people to protect their health. The health behavior of a community includes the actions of the people whose health is in question and the actions of community decision makers, professionals, peers, teachers, employers, parents, and others who may influence health behaviors, resources, or services in the community.

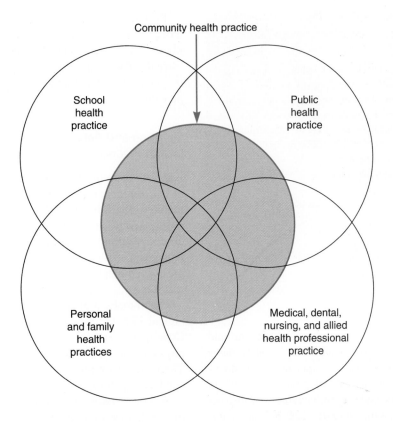

FIGURE 1-1
Overlapping spheres of health action. This book concentrates on the shaded areas of community health.

Organized community effort defines community health. Some things the individual can do entirely alone, but many health benefits can be obtained only through collective action or united community effort. Community health promotion seeks to make the fruits of health science available to all citizens.

HISTORY OF COMMUNITY HEALTH

Apart from carvings and drawings, such as the murals on cave walls in Spain recording physical de-

formities around 25,000 BC, the earliest records of community health practices were those of the Chinese, Egyptians, and Babylonians.

Chinese Health Practices

The Yellow River region of China, one of the world's most ancient cultural centers, gave rise to Chinese history and health practices. Ancient inscriptions on tortoise shells, and later evidence in books and historical relics, indicate that wells for drinking water were dug as early as the Xia and Shang Dynasties (twenty-first to eleventh centuries

---

The Sayings of Confucius on Life-style and the Pulse

The Master said, ''There are three things against which a gentleman should be on his guard. In youth, before his pulse has settled down, he is on his guard against lust. Having reached his prime, when his pulse has become strong, he is on his guard against strife. Having reached old age, when his pulse declines, he is on his guard against avarice.''

How did Confucius know about variations of the pulse with age in the fifth century BC when the concept of feeling the pulse did not appear in Western medical books until the seventeenth century AD? How did he use the concept to relate his advice on life-cycle, life-style, and self-discipline?

BC). Ruins of the Yin Dynasty reveal ditches around houses for draining rain water. The Zhou Dynasty of the eleventh to seventh century BC yields documents mentioning methods of protecting drinking water, killing rats, and preventing rabies. By the second century BC, Qin Dynasty (221-207 BC) communities had sewers, water spray carts, and latrines.

Accompanying these early environmental health references in Chinese history, many writings from 770 BC to the present mention personal hygiene, life-style, and preventive medical practices. Confucius (541-479 BC) said in the *Anelects: Xiang Dang,* ''Putrid fish . . . food with unusual colors . . . food with odd tastes . . . food not well cooked is not to be eaten.'' Similar wisdom from other sages advised Chinese people to eat, sleep, drink, and work in moderation and with regularity rather than with excess. The Chinese made their tea with boiling water as early as the Tang Dynasty (AD 618-907), thereby protecting themselves from some of the infectious intestinal diseases that plagued earlier generations and remain leading causes of death in some areas of the world today.

Besides the widespread influence of Confucian thought, especially on the rest of Asia, Chinese explorers and traders opened routes to the West and carried herbal medicines and diagnostic and preventive concepts, including feeling the pulse and acupuncture.

Egyptian and Babylonian Health Practices

Excavations in the Nile region, another river cradle of civilization, reveal that the Egyptians had community systems for collecting rain water and for disposing of sewage. Herodotus, in the fifth century BC, described the hygienic customs of the Egyptians. Personal cleanliness, frequent baths, and simple dress were emphasized. Earth closets were in general use.

Hammurabi, a great king of Babylon who lived around 1900 BC, formulated a set of laws called the Code of Hammurabi that governed the conduct of physicians and provided for good health practices. The code also regulated and defined unacceptable conduct in general.

Although highly spiritual and astrological in their interpretations of cause and effect, the Egyptians were practical in their application of knowledge for the community's protection. They believed that alcoholic intoxication, for example, was caused by the spirits inhabiting the fruit used to make the beverage. They regarded the consequences of using alcohol as beneficial in moderation but socially troublesome in excess. One of the oldest temperance tracts, advocating moderation, was written in Egypt about 1000 BC, with the text translated as follows: ''Don't drink yourself helpless in the beer garden. You speak, and you don't know what you are saying. If you fall down and break your limbs, no one will help you. And your drinking companions will get up and say 'Away with this drunkard.' ''

Similar sentiments appeared later in Chinese, Greek, Roman, Indian, and Japanese writings, and in the Old and New Testaments, tolerating alcohol but denouncing excessive drinking and drunkenness.

Hebrew Mosaic Law

Early Hebrew society extended Egyptian concepts of disease and the community promotion of health through the regulation of human conduct by the Mosaic law or code. Human behavior is fundamental in all health—community as well as personal. With the Hebrews, a weekly day of rest was a health measure as well as a religious measure. Family relations and sexual conduct were directed to the best interests of personal, family, and community health. While the Hebrews had rather crude concepts of the spread of disease, they did make concerted efforts at prevention. The first practice of preventive medicine was the segregation of lepers, as recorded in Leviticus. Recognition that eating pork sometimes resulted in illness led the Hebrews to regard pork as unclean and later to forbid it in the Jewish diet.

The Mosaic law or code provided for (1) personal and community responsibility for health, (2) maternal health, (3) control of communicable diseases, (4) segregation of lepers, (5) fumigation, (6) decontamination of buildings, (7) protection of water supplies, (8) disposal of wastes, (9) protection of food, and (10) sanitation of campsites. Without the aid of fundamental knowledge of the nature of infectious disease, the Hebrews nevertheless defined conditions unacceptable for health and mobilized community forces against them.

The Glory of Greece

The Greek era extended over many centuries, but the Classic period was the years 460 to 136 BC. The Greeks excelled in physical aspects of personal health. Games, gymnastics, and other exercises were directed toward their ideal of physical strength, endurance, dexterity, and grace. Harmonious development of all faculties was the guiding philosophy. Exercise was supplemented by measures in personal

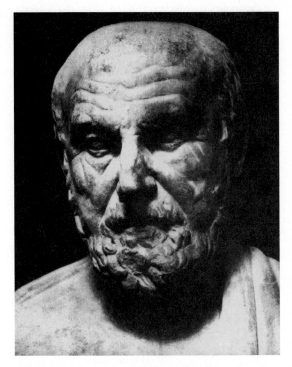

FIGURE 1-2
A Roman portrait of the Greek physician, Hippocrates, 460-370 BC, who has been credited with separating medicine and health science from superstition.
Courtesy World Health Organization.

cleanliness. Hippocrates (Figure 1-2) wrote of the relationship of diet to health around 400 BC. The Classic Period emphasized the individual, as reflected in the Hippocratic Oath. As a consequence, very little attention was given to environmental sanitation. Yet Hippocrates also wrote the definitive treatise on environment and health with his trilogy, *Airs, Waters,* and *Places* (see box on page 8).

The Greeks did not borrow health practices from other nations. The Hindus of ancient India had practiced surgery for at least a century, but there is no evidence that the Greeks used the Hindu methods of surgery, despite Alexander's conquests on the Indian subcontinent.

Hippocrates on Community Health Issues

Reflecting 25 centuries ago, in an epidemiological perspective in his advice to physicians, Hippocrates of Cos stressed the importance of studying the community and life-style contexts of place, time, and conditions of living:

"Whoever would study medicine aright . . . must consider the effect of each of the seasons of the year and the differences between them. . . . The effect of water on the health must not be forgotten. . . . When a physician comes to a district previously unknown to him, he should consider both its situation and its aspect to the winds. . . . Then, think of the soil, whether it be bare and waterless or thickly covered with soil and well-watered. . . . Lastly consider the life of the inhabitants themselves: are they heavy drinkers and eaters and consequently unable to stand fatigue, or—being fond of work and exercise—eat wisely but drink sparingly? . . . A physician who understands these subjects well . . . would know what epidemics to expect, both in the summer and in the winter, and what particular disadvantages threatened an individual who changed his mode of life. . . . He would be very successful in the practice of medicine."

The Roman Empire

With the destruction of Corinth in 146 BC, the health knowledge and practices of the Greeks migrated to Rome and were welcomed by the rising Roman Empire. In the philosophy of the Romans, however, the state and not the individual was of primary importance. To the Romans, the individual existed merely to serve the state. With this extreme emphasis on the importance of the state, the influence of Greek hygiene soon **atrophied.**

The Romans' advanced military, administrative, and engineering sciences all were reflected in their many community health projects. The registration of citizens and slaves and the taking of a periodic census served to help in planning community health measures, although their primary purpose was

doubtless mercenary. Regulation of building construction, the prevention of sewage in the streets and other nuisances, and the destruction of decaying goods and buildings were measures that are still practiced in the modern state. Building regulations provided for ventilation and even for central heating. Town planning served sanitation through the construction of paved streets with gutters. Street cleaning and repair were standard procedures in the interest of sanitation, although modern health officials regard such measures as being of esthetic rather than of direct health importance. Drainage networks to carry off rain and other water, removal of garbage and rubbish, and public baths were promoted as community health measures. Although street cleaning, garbage removal, and public baths were of less health value than the Romans contended, several other measures promoted by the Romans contributed significantly to the health as well as to the growth of civilization.

Roman officials had sufficient understanding of health to provide a protected water supply for their cities. Water was brought to Rome from great distances via aqueducts, some of which are still incorporated into the water system of Rome. City sewer systems were built, and some of these drains are still part of the sewer system of the city. This ability of the Romans to design and construct public water and sewer systems enabled Rome to grow to a city of 800,000 during the reign of Julius Caesar. The Greeks, who depended on family wells and private refuse disposal, were more limited in the size to which their cities could grow. Corinth at the pinnacle of its greatness had a population of only 35,000.

The downfall of the Western empire was related to social degeneration. The term *Byzantine,* which refers to the Eastern Roman Empire, connotes bureaucracy, luxury, and sloth. Even in this atmosphere, Galen (AD 130-201) did some experimentation relating to health, but his dogmatism limited the value of his work. In contrast to the attempt of Galen to understand disease is the statement of Saint

Augustine (AD 354-430): ''All diseases are to be ascribed to demons.''

Dark Ages

The early centuries (AD 476-1000) of the medieval period of history are usually referred to as the Dark Ages. Western civilization was in a chaotic, almost formless, state. The only existing science fostered by the state was but a trifle. Because the clergy were the only educated class, virtually the entire emphasis of the time was on the spiritual aspects of life. Rejection of the body and glorification of the spirit became the accepted pattern of behavior. It was regarded as immoral to see one's naked body. People seldom bathed, and they wore dirty garments. The use of perfumes appears to have stemmed from the attempt to conceal body and other unpleasant odors about the person. The more one could neglect and abuse one's body, the more esteemed one was. A legendary example of body neglect is that of Saint Stylites, who sat on top of a pole for 16 years to expose his body to the abuse of the elements. It was as though health itself had been defined as unacceptable. The poor diets of the time resulted in the use of spices to overcome the bad odor and the foul taste of the food. Masking the symptoms rather than removing the cause of the problems has always retarded the development of community health.

During the sixth and seventh centuries, Islam rose to prominence. After the death of Mohammed, a series of pilgrimages to Mecca began. Each pilgrimage was followed by a cholera epidemic. All through history migrations have been a vehicle for the spread of disease.

Leprosy spread from Egypt to Asia Minor and then to Europe. Most nations decreed lepers unacceptable and ''civilly dead,'' stripping them of their civil rights. Lepers were required to wear identifying clothing and to warn of their presence by a bell or a horn. This isolation, however, together with the early death of lepers, virtually eliminated leprosy in Europe.

Lead Poisoning in History

It was the common practice of medieval scribes to ''tip'' their quills on their tongues after dipping them into their metallic ink solutions. The scribes suffered lead poisoning as a result of this practice. Today lead poisoning is common in children who live in houses with old, chipping paint, because of the habit of children of putting the lead-based paint chips in their mouths. Lead poisoning also occurs frequently in children who live and play near heavily trafficked highways and intersections because of the lead still used in gasoline in older cars. Have we progressed in ''common practices'' or in community protections against lead poisoning?

Medieval Pandemics

The later medieval period, from AD 1000 to about 1453, is of special interest because of the severe **pandemics** of the time and the attempts to deal with the spread of disease. (*Pandemics* are widespread epidemics, usually affecting more than one country. **Epidemics** are outbreaks of disease that has spread through a population.) Between the years 1096 and 1248, the six great crusades to the Holy Land were of health significance. To provide crusaders who were fit for the long journey, attention was given to building up the best possible level of health. While the approach was similar to that of the ancient Greeks in building up physical prowess, the general result was to improve well-being in only one segment of the population. However, in their journeys the crusaders picked up cholera and spread it; their death rate from it was high.

In 1348 bubonic plague, or the **Black Death,** followed a devastating path from Asia to Africa, the Crimea, Turkey, Greece, Italy, and up through Europe. From 1348 to 1350, 20% of the population of Europe died from some combination of bubonic plague and pulmonary anthrax. Some idea of the devastation of the pandemic can be gathered by noting the deaths in several of the large cities in Europe:

Paris, 50,000; Seine, 70,000; Marseilles, 16,000 in 1 month; Vienna, 1200 daily. The Italian writer Boccaccio reported that in the terrible outbreak of plague in Florence in 1348, pity and humanity were forgotten. Families deserted their sick. In England 2 million died, representing approximately half the population of the country. London had 100,000 deaths. Over a number of years London's deaths exceeded its births. Had it not been for the influx of people from the rural areas, London's population would have declined steadily. Estimates that approximately 25 million people died of the Black Death in Europe attest to the virulence of the bubonic plague.

Control measures. Some attributed pandemics to storms, comets, famines, drought, crop failures, insects, and poisoning of wells by the Jews, but discerning officials of various communities recognized the possible relationship of crowding, poor sanitation, and migrations to the outbreak and spread of disease. Some communities took steps to establish control measures. In 1377 at Rogusa it was ruled that travelers from plague areas should stop at designated places and remain there free of disease for 2 months before being allowed to enter the city. Technically, this is the first official **quarantine** method on record. In 1383 Marseilles passed the first quarantine law and erected the first official quarantine station. In Venice the government appointed three guardians of public health and in 1374 denied entry to the city of infected or suspected travelers, ships, or freight. In 1403 a quarantine of 40 days was imposed on anyone suspected of having the disease.

Measures to control the spread of disease were not highly effective. The need was for a scientific understanding of the cause and nature of disease and its spread. Scholars of the time who turned to the scientific approach to pestilence suffered public persecution. As a consequence of such resistance, there was little progress in the understanding of disease control or health promotion.

Epidemics in Historical Perspective

Epidemics and pandemics of dreaded diseases have always aroused irrational fears and prejudices. Victims of the disease will be ostracized by society, shunned by some members of the medical community, abandoned by some family and friends. Religious fundamentalists will attribute the victims' suffering to God's wrath and just punishment for perversion and sin. As early as 4000 BC in Egypt, leprosy evoked the same response; as did the Antonine plague (probably measles) in classical Rome, syphilis and bubonic plague in medieval Europe, cholera and tuberculosis in eighteenth and nineteenth century Europe and North America, and influenza, polio, and Legionnaire's disease in twentieth century North America.

With each epidemic, hysteria develops as a second epidemic. People first deny the reality of the disease, then they search for scapegoats, then they rush to magical and commercially exploitative cures and protectors. Finally, they isolate the victims and suspected carriers of the disease until society becomes sufficiently educated about the modes of transmission of the disease to treat the victims with greater understanding and compassion.

Epidemics also influence the course of history. Bubonic plague contributed to the collapse of the European economic system, including the bonds of feudalism. Syphilis ushered in dramatic changes in puritanical life-styles of the Victorian Era.

When it first began to be reported in 1981, AIDS, still without a name, was thought not be contagious (denial), then dubbed a gay disease, later a Haitian disease, and still later an intravenous drug user's disease (scapegoating). Eventually people began turning to commercial and religious sources for help or protection (exploitation) when the medical profession offered little comfort. Victims became ''untouchables,'' children were barred from school, and the bodies of dead AIDS victims were shunned by undertakers (social isolation). How will AIDS influence modern history? How can communities ensure greater compassion for the victims of AIDS and the carriers of the HIV virus?

Occupational Health in History

Grinders in the sixteenth century inhaled the silica dust from their grinding and contracted silicosis, or ''grinder's disease'' as it was known then. Silicosis is common today among U.S. sandblasters in shipbuilding and other industries. For more than 30 years, the United States failed to follow the lead of Great Britain in banning the use of silica in sandblasting operations.

What progress does the law in Great Britain represent for community health? What is the process of the diffusion or spread of problems and progress from one country to another?

Renaissance

The **Renaissance** represented a revival of learning that germinated in Italy, stimulated by the fall of Constantinople in 1453. For many historians the Renaissance, as the term applies to western and northern Europe, encompasses the period from AD 1453 to 1600.

From the standpoint of community health, the Renaissance was particularly important because of its movement away from **scholasticism** and toward realism. An age of individual scientific endeavor, it ushered in a spirit of inquiry that would lead to the understanding of the cause and nature of infectious disease. The fifteenth and sixteenth centuries produced such distinguished figures as Copernicus, da Vinci, Vesalius, Galileo, and Gilbert. By the middle of the sixteenth century, scholars had differentiated influenza, smallpox, tuberculosis, bubonic plague, leprosy, impetigo, scabies, erysipelas, anthrax, and trachoma. Diphtheria and scarlet fever were not recognized as separate diseases but were recognized as being different from all other diseases. Fracastoro (1478-1553), a physician of Verona, theorized in 1546 that microorganisms caused disease. He also recognized that syphilis was transmitted from person to person during sexual relations. Learning advanced, but increasing social concentration, expand-

ing trade, and movement of populations tended to spread disease. Knowledge of communicable disease control lagged behind disease spread, and great plagues still harassed Europe.

Colonial Period

As Europeans colonized the rest of the world from 1600 to 1800, community health in North America, Australia, Africa, Asia, and South America responded to health problems in Europe and the contributions that European scholars made to health.

Community health in Europe. Between 1600 and 1665 Europe suffered three severe pandemics of bubonic plague. The plight of London indicates the severity of the outbreaks. In 1603 a sixth of London's population died of the plague. In 1625 another sixth of the population was destroyed by the plague, and in 1665 one out of five of London's residents died from the same disease.

This same era produced Descartes (1596-1650), Voltaire (1694-1778), and Boyle (1627-1691). The latter, an Englishman, made a prophetic pronouncement: ''He that totally understands the nature of ferments and the fermentation shall probably be much better able than he who ignores them to give a fair account of certain diseases (fevers as well as others) which will perhaps be never properly understood without an insight into the doctrine of fermentation.'' William Harvey (1578-1657) fairly accurately described the circulation of human blood. In 1661 Captain John Graunt completed the first study on vital statistics. In 1658 an English investigator, Thomas Sydenham, made a differential diagnosis of scarlet fever, malaria, dysentery, and cholera. Some historians contend that most of Sydenham's discoveries were accidental, but chance favors the disciplined mind. Sydenham is generally regarded as the first distinguished epidemiologist.

Athanasius Kircher (1602-1680) examined the blood of victims of plague, using a microscope with a magnification of 33 diameters, and thereby instituted a new method of study. In 1676 a Dutch draper and city hall janitor, Anton van Leeuwenhoek (1632-1723), using a microscope with a magnification of 200 diameters, succeeded in seeing bacteria in scrapings from his teeth. He found they could be killed with vinegar, but he never connected this fact with disease.

In 1693 an astronomer, Edmund Halley (1656-1742), complied the Breslau Table of births and funerals, which represented a contribution to the growth of vital statistics. In 1762 M.A. Plenciz, a physician of Vienna, studied scarlet fever and other infectious diseases and concluded that each infectious disease was caused by a specific kind of thing. While he did not identify ''thing'' factually, his theory predated the discoveries of Louis Pasteur and Robert Koch by a century.

Edward Jenner (1749-1823), a British physician and son of a Gloucestershire clergyman, scientifically demonstrated the effectiveness of smallpox vaccination. In 1796, using matter from pustules on the arm of a milkmaid who had contracted cowpox, Dr. Jenner vaccinated a young boy. Six weeks later he inoculated the boy with smallpox virus and demonstrated that the boy was immune to smallpox. Dr. Jenner showed scientifically that inoculation with cowpox virus can produce immunity to the smallpox virus. He derived his idea of inoculating with cowpox vaccine to prevent smallpox from the practice of English peasants of allowing themselves to contract cowpox in the knowledge that they would then be safe from smallpox. Some form of smallpox vaccination had been practiced in Turkey previous to Dr. Jenner's time, but he generally gets credit for the first scientific vaccination against smallpox.

Health in the colonies. Community health action was taken only during epidemics in the British, French, Dutch, and Spanish colonies and consisted essentially of isolation and quarantine. Sanitation consisted of community tidiness or general housecleaning.

Ironically, smallpox, measles, typhus, and scarlet fever aided the European settlers of the Americas. Introduced to the east coast by the Cabot and Gosnold expeditions, smallpox alone eliminated 50% to 90% of the Indians so that the new settlers were able to colonize with little or no opposition (Roberts, 1989). Yet smallpox took its toll among the whites as well and obliterated some of the early settlements. Some notable pandemics were those of the Massachusetts Bay colonies in 1633, New Netherlands (New York) in 1663, and Boston in 1752. Of Boston's 1752 population of 15,684, only 174 completely escaped the smallpox pandemic. During the life of George Washington, 90% of the people who attained the age of 21 had had smallpox, and 25% of those infected by smallpox died. Consider the significance of these statistics in the context of the 1979 declaration of the World Health Organization (WHO) that smallpox had been totally eradicated from the earth.

Yellow fever became a bigger scourge than plague or smallpox during the eighteenth and nineteenth centuries. In 1793 Philadelphia had the greatest single epidemic in America. Of a population of about 37,000, more than 23,000 had the disease and over 4000 of these died. A citizen's committee appointed to deal with the problem drew up the following set of regulations:

1. Avoid contact with a case.
2. Placard all infected houses.
3. Clean and air the sickroom.
4. Provide hospital accommodations for the poor.
5. Keep streets and wharves clean.
6. Encourage general hygienic measures such as quick private burials, avoidance of fatigue of mind and body, avoidance of intemperance, and adaptation of clothing to the weather.

Vinegar and camphor were used on handkerchiefs to prevent infection. Gunpowder was burned in the streets to combat the disease. Simple and perhaps ineffective as these measures may have been, they represented a sincere attempt of communities to combat the disease based on the fragmentary knowl-

Colonial North America	
C. 1000	Leif Ericsson and other Vikings visit Labrador and Newfoundland
1492	Christopher Columbus claims the ''New World'' for Spain
1497	John Cabot claims Cape Breton Island for England
1541	First French settlement in Americas
1625	Jesuits arrive in Quebec to begin missionary work among the Indians
1640	The Huron nation reduced by half from European diseases
1667	Canada's first census counts 3215 non-native inhabitants in 668 families
1754	Beginning of French and Indian War in America; first phase of struggle between France and Britain in North America
1763	France cedes its North American possessions to Britain by the Treaty of Paris
1783	American Revolutionary War ends; border between Canada and the United States accepted from Atlantic to Lake of the Woods
1812	The United States declares war on Britain, invades Canada from Detroit
1814	Treaty of Ghent ends the War of 1812
1818	The 49th Parallel accepted as U.S.-Canada border from Lake of the Woods to Rocky Mountains
1849	Border extended to Pacific; Gold Rush in California
1870	Louis Riel leads the Metis Indians in resisting Canadian authority in Canada's northwest
1885	Metis defeated in same year as last spike of transcontinental railway is driven in British Columbia
1897	Gold Rush in Klondike, stretching European influence and diseases into Eskimo and Inuit populations of last frontiers (Alaska and Yukon)

edge people had of yellow fever. Frosty nights on October 17 and 18 ended the epidemic. Citizens of Philadelphia did not understand the ''miracle,'' but from the vantage point of today we know that the frost killed the *Aedes aegypti* mosquito, the temporary host or vector for yellow fever. We owe a debt today to Dr. Benjamin Rush for a magnificent report of the Philadelphia epidemic published in 1815.

Health science advanced in the colonial period mostly during the eighteenth century. Occupational hygiene and the safety and well-being of the worker were addressed. Infant hygiene was not founded on any scientific basis but was represented in a humane attempt to give better care to the child. Mental hygiene was limited to a sympathetic understanding and care of the mentally disordered.

In 1639 the Massachusetts colony passed an act stating that each birth and death must be recorded, and the Plymouth colony did likewise. In 1746 the Massachusetts Bay colonies passed regulations to prevent the pollution of Boston Harbor. Between the years 1692 and 1708 Boston, Salem, and Jamestown passed laws dealing with nuisances and offensive trades. In 1701 Massachusetts enacted legislation providing for isolation of smallpox cases and for ship quarantine.

The superstitions expressed in witchcraft and other practices of the time indicate that the colonial period was hardly one in which to expect any great advances in health science. In America during George Washington's time the average duration of life was about 29 years. Measured by today's standards, the men who wrote the American Declaration of Independence and drew up the U.S. Constitution were extremely young. Decidedly few of them were over the age of 40.

Boards of health were established in New York and Massachusetts in 1797 as a result of the yellow fever **outbreaks.** Local boards of health were established in Petersburg, Virginia (1780), in Baltimore (1793), in Philadelphia (1794), in New York (1796), and in Boston (1799). Paul Revere served as chairman of the Boston Board of Health. All of these were formally organized boards, but none of them functioned as boards of health function today.

Early Nineteenth Century

From 1800 to 1850 North America experienced rapid industrial expansion. As remarkable as this expansion was, public health activities were stymied, and many epidemics occurred. The rapid growth of cities outstripped other developments. Community health could hardly flourish under such conditions, and organized health measures were almost nonexistent.

Community health promotion in England. Developments in England in the first half of the nineteenth century were important for several reasons. Public health was officially recognized in England in 1837 when legislation relating to community sanitation was enacted. This indication of an awakening interest in community health led to the appointment of a Factory Commission to study the health conditions of the laboring population of the nation. Particular emphasis was placed on the study of child employment conditions. Edwin Chadwick, a civilian who had a special interest in social problems, was made secretary of the Factory Commission. In 1842 his ''Report on the Inquiry into the Sanitary Condition of the Laboring Population of Great Britain'' appeared. Chadwick's colorful descriptions of the deplorable conditions of the time had more than just a popular appeal. They aroused the determination of well-meaning people to improve the conditions of the laboring class, particularly the child employment conditions. Chadwick's report pointed out that half the children of the working classes died before their fifth birthday. Although the death rate and infant mortality do not indicate the complete picture of a community's health, the length of life and the infant death rates reported by Chadwick indicate health conditions in which mere survival could be the sole health goal (Table 1-1).

TABLE 1-1

Mean age of death and infant death rates, England, 1842

| Class | Mean age of death | | Infant deaths per 1000 births (England) |
	London	England	
Gentry, professional persons, and their families	44	35	100
Tradesmen, shopkeepers, and their families	23	22	167
Wage classes, artisans, laborers, and their families	22	15	250

Based on Chadwick. See Richardson BW: *The health of nations: a review of the works of Edwin Chadwick,* vol 2, London, 1887, Longmans Green.

The price of such appalling health conditions was paid by some of England's outstanding literary figures of the time. Shelley died at the age of 30, Keats at 25, Byron at 36, Robert Burns at 37, Charlotte Brontë at 39, Emily Brontë at 30, and Anne Brontë at 29. On the continent, Chopin died at 40, Mendelssohn at 38, and Schubert at 31. Consider what these master artists might have produced for humankind if today's knowledge of health could have been applied during their time (Figure 1-3).

Chadwick's report led to the establishment of a board of health in 1848. John Simon was appointed first medical health officer of London. England was not yet ready for the reforms that Chadwick's report pointed out, for the general board of health lasted but 4 years. Perhaps his enthusiasm led to overpromotion. Nevertheless, his report stands as a landmark in the history of public health.

During the early nineteenth century wars were rampant on both the American and European continents. Direct loss of life was limited in comparison with the losses from epidemics or in contrast to the

SOUVENIRS DU CHOLERA-MORBUS.

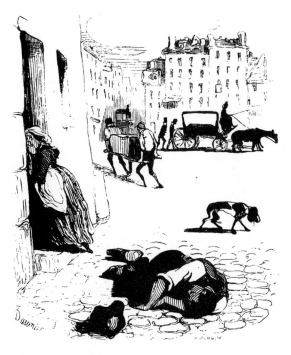

FIGURE 1-3
This engraving by Honore Daumier depicts a street scene in Paris during a cholera epidemic. In the course of the Paris epidemic of 1832, the registered number of deaths from cholera was 18,402 in 6 months. This was about 2.3% of the city's population.
Courtesy World Health Organization.

destructive potential of modern wars, but the death rate among those in battle, especially among those wounded, was high. Ironically, however, these wars contributed to medical and community health advances. In 1815, during the Napoleonic wars, Delpech first understood the cause of the infection of wounds. Many of the hundreds of casualties in the hospitals developed gangrene. Delpech noticed the patterns of development of gangrene in connection with dressings on the wounds. He theorized, 50 years before Lister developed antiseptic methods,

that "animal-like matter jumps from one object to another."

In the mid-nineteenth century the Crimean War led to such high casualties that nursing had to invent the method of triage to sort the injuries of battleground victims into three categories of severity and urgency so that valuable time and resources would not be lost on those who could wait or on those who were certain to die. The method of triage persists in emergency room and community disaster procedures today.

Health developments in North America. Not until the close of the first half of the nineteenth century was there a significant North American development in community health promotion. Lemuel Shattuck (1793-1859) drew up a health report that was to serve as a guide in the field of health for the next century. Shattuck was successively a teacher, historian, sociologist, statistician, and state legislator. From the health standpoint he was a layman, but one with an intense and intelligent interest in sanitation. He was appointed chair of a legislative committee to study sanitation and health problems in the Commonwealth of Massachusetts. Its report, written by Shattuck and published in 1850, revealed Shattuck's insight and foresight. It charted health pathways for generations to come, and many of its provisions have not yet been fully attained. The importance of this remarkable document can be appreciated by reviewing its various recommendations:

1. Establish state and local boards of health.
2. Collect and analyze vital statistics.
3. Exchange health information.
4. Initiate sanitation programs for towns and buildings.
5. Maintain a system of sanitary inspections.
6. Study the health of schoolchildren.
7. Conduct research on tuberculosis.
8. Study and supervise health conditions of immigrants.
9. Supervise mental disease.
10. Control alcoholism.

11. Control food adulteration.
12. Control exposure to nostrums.
13. Control smoke nuisances.
14. Construct model tenements.
15. Construct standard public bathing and wash houses.
16. Preach health from the pulpit.
17. Teach the science of sanitation in medical schools.
18. Introduce prevention as a phase of all medical practice.
19. Sponsor routine health examinations.

The wisdom of Shattuck's report stands as a valued guidepost in the history of public health. Shattuck was considerably in advance of his time. Perhaps because he did not have the flair for writing that Chadwick possessed, and he did not depend on vivid descriptions of appalling conditions, the report produced no results until 1869. Then a Massachusetts state board of health was established. Its membership included both laymen and physicians. The Shattuck report served as the guide for the board in its early years of activity.

Modern Era of Health

Shattuck's report signaled the modern era of health, dated from 1850 to the present. An organized, disciplined attack on problems of health and disease grew out of a general recognition, initially in Western societies and later in the Third World, of the importance of a united public approach to health protection.

The modern era of health can be divided into five phases. The first phase (1850-1880) was the *miasma* phase; the second phase (1880-1910), the *bacteriology* phase or health protection era; the third phase (1910-1960), the *health resources* or medical phase; and the fourth phase (1960-1975), the *social engineering* phase. The fifth phase began in the late 1970s with the *health promotion* period, sometimes referred to as the "second epidemiological revolution," in which the behavior and life-styles of in-

dividuals, communities and societies were recognized as the major causes of illness, disability, and death. These became the targets for improved health and quality of life.

Miasma phase (1850-1880). The term *miasma* means noxious air or vapor. During the **miasma phase,** the approach to disease control was based on the misconception that disease was caused by noxious odors (Figure 1-4). For example, diphtheria was thought to be caused by gases associated with putrefaction. Because it was observed even as early as Hippocrates that people who ventured about at dusk were those who invariably contracted malaria, the common belief persisted into the late nineteenth century that this disease was a result of the particular air existing at dusk. Indeed, the term *malaria* literally means "bad air." Here is an illustrious example of the interpretation of mere coincidence as a cause-and-effect relationship. Disease control efforts were directed entirely toward general cleanliness. Garbage and refuse collection became important to communities. Street cleaning was pursued relentlessly. These general cleanliness measures were not directed at the specific causes of disease and consequently were of little value in control of disease.

The topics discussed at the first quarantine convention in Philadelphia in 1857 indicate the interests of the time: prevention of typhus, cholera, and yellow fever; port quarantine; stagnant and putrid bilge waters, droppings, or drainage from putrescible matter; and filthy bedding, baggage, and clothing of immigrant passengers where they had been confined. The convention recommended the vaccination of all incoming immigrants.

The first state health department was organized in Massachusetts in 1869, with Dr. Henry I. Bowdich as the first head. The department's program was directed to the following six areas:

1. Professional and public education in hygiene
2. Housing
3. Investigation of certain diseases
4. Slaughtering

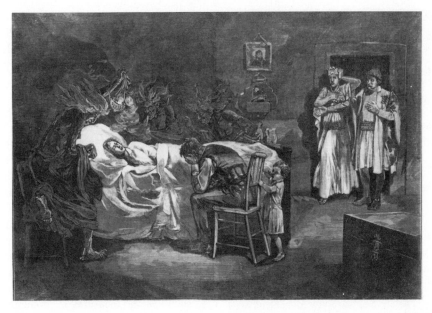

FIGURE 1-4
Depiction of the belief in foul odors as cause of illness at the end of the miasma phase.
Line lithograph after W.A. Rogers, from *Harper's Weekly* 25:565, Aug. 20, 1881; courtesy National Library of Medicine.

5. Sale of poisons
6. Conditions of the poor

Against today's standards in public health, the program of the first state health department would rate rather poorly.

The American Public Health Association, founded in 1872 at Long Beach, New Jersey, elected Dr. Stephen Smith as its first president. The new association proposed to go considerably beyond the thinking of the quarantine conventions in dealing with sanitation, prevention and transmission of disease, longevity, hospital hygiene, and all other health problems of interest and of concern to the public.

Public health teaching began during this period. An English manual of hygiene edited by E.A. Parkes, professor of military hygiene in the army medical school of England, was published in 1859. The first as well as subsequent editions were used in the United States. In 1879 A.H. Buck edited his pioneering text, *Hygiene and Public Health*. This volume dealt with environmental sanitation, housing, personal hygiene, child hygiene, school hygiene, industrial hygiene, food sanitation, communicable disease control, disinfection, quarantine, infant mortality, and vital statistics. Several distinguished men contributed to the volume. Dr. J.S. Billings wrote the introduction with foresight regarding the jurisprudence of public health. His concepts, such as the following, reflect the growing influence of medicine in public health:

1. County lines are not natural boundaries and have no relation to causes of disease.
2. Administrative health areas should be large enough and populous enough to require full-time sanitary and executive forces.
3. There should be nonpracticing full-time health officers with medical education.

John Snow and the Broad Street Pump

In 1854, as England entered the Crimean War, a cholera epidemic in the Soho district of London killed dozens of people in a brief period. Dr. John Snow, an anesthetist, lived close to the area and began mapping the sources of drinking water of those who died. He traced a cluster to the Broad Street pump. Because the prevailing notion at that time was that bad air caused cholera, Snow encountered opposition to his suggestion that the pump be closed. He persevered in having the pump handle removed. The outbreak ended soon after that.

This event illustrates two public health principles: First, action often must be taken before conclusive evidence is in hand. Snow constructed epidemiological evidence of the source of the problem, but this was some 30 years before Koch isolated the cholera vibrio, so he could not prove that it was the water and not the air causing the cholera. Second, Snow sought a means to prevent the problem by going to its source rather than merely treating its victims.

In 1992 the Westminister City Council of London unveiled a monument to Dr. Snow: a pump that stands in an open paved area near the site of the original. A plaque tells the story. Nearby, the ''John Snow Public House'' is frequented by epidemiologists over the world as a place to celebrate their profession and Snow's contribution to their method of research. The pub's management keeps a guest book under the bar for researchers worldwide to sign.

A short distance across the river Thames is the Florence Nightingale Museum, a monument to the pioneer of another health profession. Nightingale's contributions were not only to nursing but also to epidemiology during her service in the Crimean War (1854-1856).

charged with the supervision of all medical charities such as hospitals and dispensaries. The seeds of professional public health preparation were being planted before the next phase of the modern health era was reached.

Bacteriology phase (1880-1910). The *bacteriology phase* was initiated by the work of Louis Pasteur, Robert Koch, and other bacteriologists who demonstrated that a specific organism causes a specific disease. The knowledge that an organism causes a certain disease made it possible to change from general measures in attempting to control diseases to specific measures in protecting health by blocking the routes over which the causative agents would travel. As it became apparent that certain vehicles served as the means for the transmission of disease-producing organisms, attention was directed to such specific measures as protecting water supplies, milk, and other foods, eliminating insects, and properly disposing of sewage (Figure 1-5). A natural further advance was the development of laboratory procedures.

The scientific productivity of the bacteriologists of this period is legendary. The French bacteriologist Louis Pasteur (1822-1895), in addition to demonstrating that a specific organism causes a specific disease, made other outstanding contributions to bacteriology. He discovered the fowl cholera bacillus and developed a method of inoculation against rabies. Robert Koch (1843-1910) discovered the tubercle bacillus and the streptococcus; he also discovered the cholera vibrio, which he demonstrated was transmitted by water, food, and clothing.

During this same period Lord Joseph Lister (1827-1912) developed the practical use of phenol (carbolic acid) as an effective antiseptic.

Official public health departments were staffed with bacteriologists, laboratory technicians, sanitarians, sanitation inspectors, sanitary engineers, quarantine officers, and others who specialized in communicable disease control measures. With the extreme emphasis placed on isolation and quaran-

4. The health officer should be specially trained for his job.
5. If a municipal board of health is properly constituted so that its relationship to the medical profession is harmonious, it should be

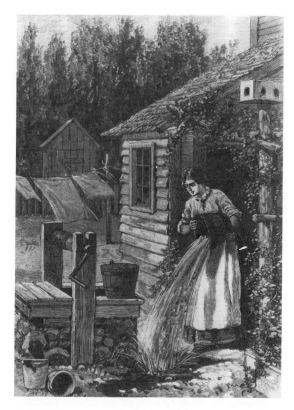

FIGURE 1-5
The beginning of the bacteriological phase recognizes danger to the water supply as a woman is depicted throwing slops out her door, beside a well. The caption reads "Sowing for diphtheria."

Wood engraving after Gaston Fay, from *Harper's Weekly* 25:36, Jan. 15, 1881; courtesy National Library of Medicine.

Milestones of the Bacteriology Phase	
1880	Typhoid bacillus discovered
	Pneumococcus identified
	Malaria plasmodium discovered
1882	Tubercle bacillus discovered
1883	Rabies treatment successful (Pasteur)
	Cholera vibrio discovered (Koch)
1884	Diphtheria bacillus identified
	Federal research laboratory established at Staten Island later named National Institute of Health
1889	Massachusetts Public Health Laboratory and Johns Hopkins Hospital opened with new emphasis on scientific health care
1893	Lawrence, Massachusetts, water treatment plant completed
	Transmission of Texas fever from ticks to cattle demonstrated (Theobald Smith, U.S. Department of Agriculture)
1894	Diphtheria antitoxin successfully demonstrated (Emil von Behring)
	Pasteurella pestis, cause of plague, discovered
1895	Cause of hookworm discovered
1896	African sleeping sickness traced to the tsetse fly
1898	Relation of *Anopheles* mosquito to malaria established (Ronald Ross)
1990	Relation of *Aedes aegypti* mosquito to yellow fever demonstrated (Walter Reed)
1901	Infectious nature of yellow fever established
1902	U.S. Public Health Service established
	International Sanitary Bureau created
	First health instruction in schools in New York City
1904	Typhoid fever immunization successful
1905	Spirochete of syphilis identified
1906	Pure Food and Drug Act passed;
	Standard methods of water analysis adopted
1908	Chlorination of Jersey City water supply
	Syphilis successfully treated using arsphenamine
	Haemophilus pertussis identified

tine during the first two decades of the twentieth century, one might with justification refer to these 20 years as the "tackhammer" period in public health history. To the public of that time, ubiquitous quarantine officers with their hideous placards were the identifying symbol of public health.

Limited as the health protection programs of this period were, they had an apparent effect in reducing the death rate. A comparison of the death rate for 1920 with the average death rate for the years 1881 to 1885 indicates a pronounced reduction in deaths in western Europe and in North America.

Health resources phase (1910-1960). The first broad-scale measure of the health status of the people of the United States came with the medical examination of men being inducted into the U.S. armed services during World War I. Even using health standards for induction lower than usual, the armed services found it necessary to reject 34% of the men examined because of physical and mental disabilities. The nation was appalled to learn that one third of its youth were unfit for military service. Professional health personnel analyzed the data obtained in the medical examination of draftees and arrived at a conclusion that was to change the course of public health in the United States.

Public health experts learned from these data that while communicable diseases had been controlled quite well, other health hazards and problems had been neglected. Many of the defects reported could have been prevented, and most of the defects could have been corrected. It was clear that public health programs had neglected the citizen as an individual and that it was necessary to build up and maintain the highest possible level of health resources for each individual citizen. The prevention and control of communicable disease was not enough.

State health departments began expanding their programs and directing their efforts toward personal health services as well as toward community disease control. This development required administrative reorganization within the state health departments and the inclusion of many new specialties in the health services field.

In 1911 Guilford County, North Carolina, and Yakima County, Washington, organized the first full-time county health departments. The organization of official health departments on a county basis was slow in developing until the second decade of the health resources phase. Then, under the stimulus of financial support from such organizations as the Rockefeller Foundation, the Children's Fund of Michigan, the Kellogg Foundation, and the U.S. Public Health Service, county health departments became recognized as the desirable health unit in the age of modern transportation. County health departments with full-time professional personnel gradually displaced city health departments with part-time health officers and nonprofessional personnel. Only a few large cities with full-time professionally prepared personnel still continue to function apart from the 3102 counties in the United States.

The largest investments during this era, however, were not in public health services or even in personal health services for mothers, infants, and children, but rather in three other resources: hospitals, health manpower, and biomedical knowledge from research. The Hill-Burton Act passed by the U.S. Congress in 1946 provided for the construction of massive facilities for medical care. Medical, nursing, and dental schools proliferated to train the personnel required to staff the new hospitals. The National Institutes of Health were established to generate the research and strengthen the knowledge resource from which scientific medicine and public health could draw new methods, drugs, vaccines, and diagnostic tests.

Voluntary health agencies played an increasingly important role in the promotion of health in the United States, particularly through health education, bringing to public attention the importance of certain health problems. Unfortunately, some of them oversold the importance of relatively rare diseases, causing the public to contribute unnecessary services or resources at the expense of more urgent or pervasive problems. The burden of being solicited for contributions repeatedly by too many voluntary agencies led many communities to establish joint fund-raising through ''community chests'' and ''united campaigns.'' The voluntary agencies also tended to be drawn into the aura of medical research and medical services, usually at the expense of their public health education function. Thus even in the private sector the resources for community health during this era were concentrated in medical rather than health activities and development.

Social engineering phase (1960-1975). By 1960 it had become apparent that technical health advances and personal health resources were not equally available to all people. Indeed, large segments of the world and of each community were completely isolated from developments in health. The husbanding of human resources required that the products of technological developments be made available to every world citizen. The social equity aspects of health were given a new priority in legislation and policy.

Making the advances of health science available to all people posed a pyramid of problems because of the various individuals and groups unable to acquire health knowledge or to obtain health services. The poor—economically, educationally, and socially—often missed the benefits of community health programs. The economic barriers were considered the most urgent, so Medicare and Medicaid legislation was passed in the United States to put purchasing power in the hands of the poor and medically indigent to enable them to receive needed health services.

The educational and social isolation of the poor necessitated carrying health resources and services to those who apparently were not receiving the benefits of health programs. The ''outreach'' services of public health nurses and indigenous community health workers thus became a mainstay of local health departments.

The Peace Corps also attempted to address this need by placing young Americans with training in health and other professional disciplines in developing countries. The concept was later expanded to include a domestic Peace Corps and all age groups. The Peace Corps continues to recruit from all age and professional groups (Figure 1-6). Canada developed a similar corps called CUSO.

The trend in community health programs during the late 1960s was the funneling of federal funds

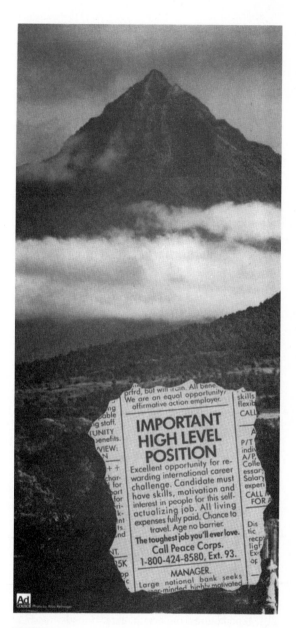

FIGURE 1-6

The social engineering phase in the history of community health was signaled by the launching in 1962 of the Peace Corps by President Kennedy. A thirtieth anniversary Peace Corps recruitment campaign featured this magazine appeal to all age groups.
Courtesy Advertising Council, New York, 1992.

through state and county agencies to provide medical and hospital services for medically deprived groups in the community. Certain guidelines were laid down by the federal agencies, but within these stipulations health departments had considerable leeway in the use of these funds. Most of the funds went to practicing physicians for professional services rendered to citizens who otherwise would not have had the medical care they needed. The tendency to channel some of the funds for medical services through county health departments cast an additional burden on the staffs of these local health departments because provisions for additional personnel were seldom made.

By the late 1960s the resources of health facilities, manpower, and research developed in earlier decades had been more equitably distributed to the poor and the medically indigent. This equalization had occurred in the United States as a result of the "New Frontier" legislation of the Kennedy years and the "War on Poverty" legislation of the Johnson years. In Europe, Canada, Australia, Asia, and Africa even more sweeping social and medical reforms were made. Citizens in most communities had a growing voice in allocating health resources at the local level. The "maximum feasible participation" provision in most of the U.S. legislative acts required policy and planning bodies for neighborhood health centers and other new entities to include 51% lay membership. The 1960s had achieved a closing of much of the gap between high-income and low-income people in their use of medical services.

These accomplishments, however, were not universally reflected in the mortality and morbidity statistics. The differences between the death and disease rates of rich and poor, white and black, urban and rural populations persisted. Indeed, the increasing expenditures on health care (mostly medical care) were not yielding proportionate improvements in the health of nations in general. The rapidly escalating costs of medical care were attributed to the expensive medical technology and facilities created by the earlier investments in medical resources, now

made more universally accessible by new health insurance coverage and related programs of distribution. The 1970s, then, were devoted heavily to the search for ways to contain the costs of medical care and hospital care.

The search for cost-containment strategies in the United States led first to the "health planning" acts of the late 1960s and early 1970s; then to "peer review" requirements to encourage medical practitioners to restrain themselves in the use of unnecessary medical procedures; then to new forms of delivery, such as "health maintenance organizations," designed to encourage physicians to keep their patients out of hospitals rather than to admit them unnecessarily. During this period of concentrated tinkering with the *medical* care system, the *health* care system was almost forgotten. State and local health departments lost much of their financial base to medical institutions and much of their political force to health planning agencies.

Health promotion phase (1974-present). By the mid-1970s a renewed interest in disease prevention and health promotion had occurred almost simultaneously in several English-speaking countries. The milestones of this era are marked by a series of influential documents. The United States began the decade with the report of *The President's Committee on Health Education,* but the Canadians followed soon after with a more comprehensive and influential report by the Minister of National Health and Welfare, *A New Perspective on the Health of Canadians* (Lalonde, 1974), and later *Achieving Health for All: A Framework for Health Promotion* (Epp, 1986). In Great Britain the famous "red book" was issued by the government with the title *Prevention and Health: Everybody's Business, 1976* and more recently the *Health of the Nation* White Paper (1992), outlining priority objectives for the year 2000 and plans for monitoring progress.

The Americans continued their refocusing with a series of official and still living documents and legislative acts, including the National Health Infor-

	Milestones of the Social Engineering Phase		

| 1961 | Peace Corps and Food Stamp programs established by President Kennedy | 1971 | White House Conference on Aging held |

1961 Peace Corps and Food Stamp programs established by President Kennedy
1962 Saskatchewan introduces the first Canadian Medicare plan
1963 Measles vaccine demonstrated successfully
1964 Mumps vaccine developed
       Canadians get Social Insurance cards
       Economic Opportunity Act launches President Johnson's "War on Poverty"
       First Surgeon General's Report on Smoking and Health released
1965 Medicare and Medicaid legislation passed
1966 Rubella vaccine trial-tested
       Canadian Pension Plan established
       Fair Packaging and Labelling Act passed
       Model Cities program launched in United States
1967 Medicare and Medicaid begin coverage
1968 U.S. Senate Select Committee on Nutrition and Human Needs established
1969 Rubella vaccine introduced
       Canadian abortion law liberalized
1970 National high blood pressure education and screening programs initiated
       Family Planning and Population Act signed in United States
       Occupational Health and Safety Act signed in United States

1971 White House Conference on Aging held
       Sickle Cell Disease Program initiated in United States
       President's Committee on Health Education established
1972 Special Supplementary Food Program for Women, Infants, and Children (WIC) initiated in United States
1973 Health Maintenance Organization Assistance Act passed in United States
       World Health Assembly, noting widespread dissatisfaction with health service, decides that WHO should collaborate with, not just advise, its Member States in developing national health care systems
1974 National Institute on Aging established in United States
       National Health Planning and Resources Development Act replaced Comprehensive Health Planning and Regional Medical Programs in United States
       Safe Drinking Water Act passed in United States

mation and Health Promotion Act of 1976; the task-force report *Preventive Medicine USA* (1976); the two-volume Surgeon General's report on health promotion and disease prevention. *Healthy People* (1979); *Promoting Health, Preventing Disease: Objectives for the Nation* (1980); and *Healthy People 2000* and its companion document *Healthy Communities 2000* (1990). The Australian-Commonwealth Department of Health published *Health Promotion in Australia 1978-79* (Davidson, Chapman, and Hull, 1979) and the *Better Health Commission Report* (1986).

The global health promotion movement was spurred by the World Health Organization (WHO) with its several initiatives under the banner of Health for All by the Year 2000. In September 1978 representatives of 134 nations met at Alma-Ata in what was still then the USSR, now Russia. The national representatives pledged their support for a worldwide effort to bring about a new emphasis on primary health care emphasizing community participation and more equitable access to health for all than has been achieved by the emphasis on hospitals in the past. In 1986 WHO and the Canadian gov-

	Milestones of the Health Promotion Phase		
1974	*A New Perspective on the Health of Canadians* published (Lalonde Report)	1984	New federal reimbursement policies force many community hospitals to close
1975	National Center for Health Education established in San Francisco		U.S. Congress passes laws authorizing new system of labels on cigarettes warning of emphysema, fetal damage, and cancer
1976	U.S. Health Information and Health Promotion Act signed		Legislation authorizes federal support for university research centers for disease prevention and health promotion
1977	WHO announces the eradication of smallpox in Asia and adopts health for all by the year 2000 as target.	1986	Reports by Australia, Canada, U.S., and WHO indicate progress and plans toward objectives in health promotion and health for all
1978	National initiatives in childhood immunization, adolescent pregnancy, smoking, and nutrition announced		Ottawa Charter for Health Promotion published by Canadian Public Health Association
1979	U.S. and Australian national reports on health promotion released	1988	Surgeon General's Report on Nutrition and Health
	Smallpox officially declared eradicated worldwide	1989	U.S. Preventive Services Task Force presents assessment of 169 clinical interventions for health promotion and disease prevention
1980	Department of Education created, leaving Public Health Service and Health Care Finance Administration in Department of Health and Human Services	1990	*Healthy People 2000* published by the U.S. Department of Health and Human Services
1981	Public Health Services' *Objectives for the Nation* in disease prevention and health promotion adopted as policy in United States	1991	*Healthy Communities 2000* published by American Public Health Association
1982	Block grants to states replace categorical funding of community health programs	1992	*Health of the Nation* White Paper published by the Government of Great Britain

ernment co-sponsored the first international conference on health promotion and issued *The Ottawa Charter.* This document went beyond the Alma-Ata declaration in playing down the importance of the *medical* care system in contributing to *health* care. It emphasized, as had the Lalonde Report in 1974 and the U.S. Surgeon General's Report in 1979, that life-style and conditions of living contribute more to health or the avoidance of disease and disability than medical care do, even though most countries spend much more on medical and hospital care than on disease prevention and health promotion.

The Ottawa Charter's message went still further, departing from the apparent emphasis in the Lalonde Report and the U.S. Surgeon General's Report on the personal responsibility aspects of life-style. The Ottawa Charter emphasized the social and economic aspects of life-style, stressing the importance of community or collective action to ensure greater opportunities for people to practice healthful lifestyles.

Subsequent Australian, European, and North American health policy documents have attempted to live up to the Ottawa Charter's ideals for health promotion. But the Health Promotion Phase has been both fueled by and retarded by the conservatism of the 1980s and the global recession extending into the 1990s. National governments sought to reduce federal involvement in states' rights and to encourage local autonomy and initiative. This has re-

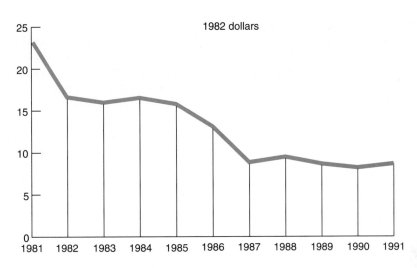

FIGURE 1-7
The health promotion era and its emphasis on community health owe their origins and their slow pace to the international recession, which has produced a steady decline in support from national to local governments, shown here for U.S. direct federal aid to cities in billions of dollars.
Source: National League of Cities.

sulted in a relentless decline in federal direct funding to states, provinces, or communities (see Fig. 1-7). When viewed in the longer historical perspective, however, this decline began during the earlier social engineering phase after a continuous build-up of national investments in local development during the health resources phase. Whether communities can rise to the challenges and opportunities to take control of their health in the face of dwindling resources from higher levels of government remains to be seen. This book will chronicle some of the principles and examples that have emerged from the past and from recent experiences of communities in controlling their own health.

Lessons from the Past, Challenges for the Future

AIDS, cost containment, and competition took over as the hallmarks of national health policy and medical practice in the 1980s, but they did not displace community interest in health promotion. One key lesson from the past is that communities sometimes innovate and initiate concepts, methods, strategies, and programs that subsequently become national policy. Indeed, we have seen that most national health-related policies originated in ideas developed in local communities.

Of particular concern with the current emphasis on cost containment and market competition in health services is that disadvantaged populations have been left out of the marketing strategies. Some 34 million Americans were left without health insurance. Their limited income or education make them unattractive, hard-to-reach markets, and the constricted budgets of official health agencies leave them to fend for themselves. Self-care education is only a partial solution. Once again, local health agencies must pick up the responsibility for outreach to the economically disadvantaged or socially isolated.

Migrant workers, mothers, infants, children, adolescents, the chronically ill, and the elderly all need more than health services; opportunities must be provided at the community level for these people to gain control over the determinants of their health. This effort calls for the enlistment of many community resources, voluntary and official agencies, in many categories of human services besides health.

Creating a favorable environment and favorable living conditions for these people means creating opportunities for self-improvement, calling for a form of social engineering that was tried in the 1960s in the United States but later was abandoned by the federal government. This approach has been criticized as being paternalistic. Yet to offer people more healthful channels of living and to help them develop the ability to guide their own mode of life is no more paternalistic than to award people state scholarships for a college education.

The modern community health program covers all citizens of all ages, but of necessity it must give a proportionately higher degree of attention to the people at greatest risk, who are usually of the least advantaged social, economic, and educational strata. The human ecology involved is apparent. The health of these people affects the dignity, health, and economy of the entire community. Abandoned to their own resources, many people would decline in health and consequently in their social condition.

Community health programs must give highest priority to the allocation of resources to those least able to provide for their own health needs. These people are entitled to a better quality of health, the capacity for a productive life, and a greater life expectancy—the objectives of community health programs.

Increasingly, these objectives will be met outside the traditional medical and public health settings of the past. As the challenges of the future entail more complex life-style issues related to risk factors for injury and chronic diseases, which now account for the leading causes of death and disability, community health practice must be centered increasingly in schools, worksites, recreational settings, and homes.

SUMMARY

This chapter has defined community health promotion and has addressed the historical context of community health. Some of the social, cultural, and economic forces that shape history also shape behavior and health simultaneously. Later chapters will draw on history to help show more clearly how social, behavioral, environmental, and technological forces can be harnessed and directed in the planning and development of community health. Finally, to understand and apply these several forces you should draw back from the parochial perspective of your own community to place the historical, social, behavioral, environmental, and technological aspects of health trends in a national or international perspective.

Health promotion will gain momentum in the 1990s as more professionals and decision makers recognize the growing importance of behavior and social conditions as the key to preventing or controlling the leading causes of death and disability. Heart disease, cancer, stroke, and injuries account for the majority of deaths in Western countries today. All of these have as their principal causes one or more behavioral or life-style problems. The voluntary adoption of behavior conducive to health is the goal of **health education.** In concert with social and environmental supports for such behavior, health education becomes health promotion. In emphasizing behavior one must never lose sight of its historical, social, and environmental origins and constraints. Community health promotion addresses educational, social, and environmental interventions in combination with each other.

The chapters that follow will reflect largely on the latest historical landmarks. The foregoing historical background can be understood as the repeated redefining of the primary or prevalent causes of illness and death, from supernatural causes in the earliest Egyptian through medieval times, to natural causes in the Greco-Roman and modern eras, to social causes in the mid-twentieth century, to personal or behavioral causes in the present health promotion period. The personal or behavioral causes of current health problems, however, must be understood and addressed in their historical, cultural, social, economic, and community contexts.

QUESTIONS FOR REVIEW

1. Why and how does a knowledge of the past in any field of human endeavor benefit those who now work in that field?

2. How has disease altered the course of history?

3. Why should people in the parahealth professions have a broad knowledge of community health?

4. Why was the Mosaic law or code of special importance to the advancement of the community health movement?

5. How does the political philosophy of a nation affect its health program?

6. What specific lesson in health can the present generation gain from a study of health conditions during the Dark Ages?

7. To what extent did the Renaissance influence the direction of community health?

8. What, in your judgment, was the most important health discovery in Europe during the period of American colonization between 1600 and 1800?

9. How would you evaluate this statement: "Colorful reporting can get more public action than can scientific fact"?

10. How would you evaluate this assertion: "Lowering the death rate among laborers and their families does not improve their lot because it results in a surplus of laborers"?

11. What questionable health practices in the miasma phase of health are still regarded by the general public as important to health?

12. What is the basis for the contention that scientific public health should be dated from 1880?

13. Why did the application of scientific methods have such a profound effect on the death rate in Europe and North America?

14. Why is the postponement of death not sufficient as the objective of a community health program?

15. What is meant by the expression, "Public health is social engineering"?

READINGS

Epstein PR: Commentary: pestilence and poverty—historical transitions and the great pandemics, *Am J Prev Med* 8:263, 1992.
  Reviews changing historical circumstances in the populations and environments that would account for the spread and impact of epidemics that reached pandemic proportions from the bubonic plagues to current HIV infections.

Guinta MA, Allegrante JP: The President's Committee on Health Education: a 20-year retrospective on its politics and policy impact, *Am J Public Health* 82:1033, 1992.
  Analyzes the Committee's origins, methods, and impact on subsequent developments in the health promotion era of national health policy.

Hamlin C: *The science of impurity: water analysis in nineteenth century Britain,* Berkeley, 1991, University of California Press.
  A history of the various branches of nineteenth-century water science, this book also places the sanitation issues of Great Britain during that formative period of public health in historical, philosophical, and social science perspective.

Henig RM: *A dancing matrix: voyages along the viral frontier,* New York, 1993, Knopf; also adapted as "Flu pandemic," *New York Times Magazine,* Nov. 29, 1992.
  Traces the history and impact of influenza from the 1918 Spanish flu pandemic that killed 20 million people, more in a single year than any war, famine, or epidemic, including the 4-year bubonic plague in Europe from 1347-1351. Predicts another pandemic in the near future, one that will be difficult to control.

Kass LR: Thinking about the body, *Aspen Inst Quar* 3: 117, 1991.
  This essay examines the cross-cultural and historical variations in perspectives on the human body as evidenced in rituals, worship, funeral preparations, burial procedures, hygienic practices, body building, surgery, and medical practices.

Smolan R, Moffit P: *Medicine's great journey: one hundred years of healing,* Boston, 1992, Bulfinch.
Documents through photography the progress of medicine and community health over the past century, from Florence Nightingale through the laboratory pioneers to today's technological heros.

BIBLIOGRAPHY

Ackerman EB: *Health care in the Parisian countryside, 1800-1914,* New Brunswick and London, 1990, Rutgers University Press.

Anderson OW: *The evolution of health services research,* San Francisco, 1991, Jossey-Bass.

Breslow L: The future of public health: prospects in the United States for the 1990s, *Annu Rev Public Health,* 11:1, 1990.

Buck AH: *Hygiene and public health,* Philadelphia, 1879, William Wood.

Bullough B, Rosen G: *Preventive medicine in the United States, 1900-1990: trends and interpretations,* Canton, Mass, 1992, Science History.

Callahan D: *What kind of life: the limits of medical progress,* New York, 1990, Simon & Schuster.

Chadwick E: *The sanitary condition of the labouring population of Great Britain,* Edinburgh, 1965, Edinburgh University Press.

Chenglie L et al: *A collection of Confucius' sayings,* Ji Nan, 1988, Qi Lu Press.

Curtain PD: *Death by migration: Europe's encounter with the tropical world in the nineteenth century,* New York, 1989, Cambridge University Press.

Davidson L, Chapman S, Hull C: *Health promotion in Australia 1978-79,* Canberra, 1979, Commonwealth of Australia.

DeFries RD, editor: *The development of public health in Canada,* Ottawa, 1940, Canadian Public Health Association.

Derickson A: Making human junk: child labor as a health issue in the progressive era, *Am J Public Health* 82: 1280, 1992.

Epp J: *Achieving health for all: a framework for health promotion,* Ottawa, 1986, Minister of Supply and Services Canada, H 39-102/1986 E.

Fee E, Acheson RM, editors: *A history of education in public health: health that mocks the doctors' rules,* New York, 1991, Oxford University Press.

Great Britain Expenditures Committee: First report from the Expenditures Committee, Session 1976-77, Preventive Medicine, London, 1977, HMSO.

Green LW, Kreuter MW: Health promotion as a public health strategy for the 1990s, *Annu Rev Public Health* 11:319, 1990.

Haifeng, C: Brief history of public health in China. In Haifeng C, editor, *Chinese health care,* vol 3, Boston, 1984, MTP Press.

Health of the nation: white paper, London, 1992, HMSO.

Healthy communities 2000: model standards, ed 3, Washington, DC, 1991, American Public Health Association.

Healthy people, the Surgeon General's report on health promotion and disease prevention, 2 vols, Washington, DC, 1979, DHEW (PHS) Pub. No. 79-55071A.

Lalonde M: *A new perspective on the health of Canadians: a working document,* Ottawa, 1974, Government of Canada.

Ling GN: *A revolution in the physiology of the living cell,* Melbourne, Fla, 1992, Krieger.

Lochhead AG: *A history of the Bacteriology Division of the Canada Department of Agriculture, 1923-1955,* Ottawa, 1968, Canada Department of Agriculture.

MacDougall H: *Activists and advocates: Toronto's health department, 1883-1983,* Toronto and Oxford, 1990, Dundurn.

McLachlan G, editor: *The planning of health services: studies in eight European countries,* Copenhagen, 1980, Regional Office for Europe, World Health Organization.

Ottawa charter for health promotion, Ottawa, 1986, Canadian Public Health Association.

Preventive medicine USA: a task force report, New York, 1976, Prodist.

Promoting health, preventing disease: objectives for the nation, Washington, DC, 1980, Public Health Service.

Rapoport A: *History and precedent in environmental design,* New York, 1990, Plenum.

Read JH: The Canadian Association of Teachers of Social and Preventive Medicine accord: history in the making, *Ann Royal Coll Physicians and Surgeons of Canada* 24:399, 1991.

Richardson BW: *The health of nations, vol 2, A review of the works of Edwin Chadwick,* London, 1887, Longmans Green.

Roberts L: Disease and death in the new world, *Science* 246:1245, 1989.

Rosenberg CE, Golden J, editors: *Framing disease: studies in cultural history,* New Brunswick, 1992, Rutgers University Press.

Scherl DJ, Noren J, Osterweis M, editors: *Promoting health and preventing disease,* Washington, DC, 1992, Association of Academic Health Centers, Health Policy Annual II.

Shattuck L et al: *Report of the Sanitary Commission of Massachusetts, 1850,* New York, 1948, Cambridge University Press.

Stachenko S, Jenicek M: Conceptual differences between prevention and health promotion: research implications for community health programs, *Canadian J Public Health* 81:53, 1990.

U.S. Preventive Services Task Force: *Guide to clinical preventive services: an assessment of the effectiveness of 169 interventions,* Baltimore, 1989, Williams & Wilkins.

Vertinsky P: Sport and exercise for old women: images of the elderly in the medical and popular literature at the turn of the century, *Int J Hist Sport* 9:83, 1992.

Winslow C-EA: The untilled fields of public health, *Science* 51:23, 1920.

World Health Organization: *Alma-Ata 1978, Primary health care,* Geneva, 1978, World Health Organization Health for All series no. 1.

World Health Organization: *Facts about WHO,* Geneva, 1990, World Health Organization.

● ●

Chapter 2

Community Ecology, Organization, and Health

❖

Sense of community is a feeling that members have of belonging, a feeling that members matter to one another and to the group, and a shared faith that members' needs will be met through their commitment to be together.

    DAVID W. MCMILLAN

OBJECTIVES

When you finish this chapter, you should be able to:

- Identify and describe elements of ecology that apply to community health
- Identify the four factors influencing health
- Describe ways in which these factors occur and change in populations and communities
- Distinguish between the natural history of health and the social history of health

The concept of community implies an interdependence of many elements. As one element changes it sets up a chain reaction of adaptations or adjustments in at least some individuals and often in whole populations, organizations, and environments. As described in Chapter 1, the history of health reflects the **adaptation** of the human species to its physical and biological environment. Human **ecology** is the study of that relationship as it works in both directions—from human adaptation to the environment and from environmental adaptation to human behavior and organization. Your own survival depends on the psychophysical impulses programmed into your inherent responses to the environment by centuries of evolution. As this chapter will reveal, the environment has changed over the centuries too, partly in response to human behavior. Both have consequences for health.

Besides your genetically endowed drive for survival, you have inherited a culture and a society in which communities of people have organized human resources and technology to further the goals of survival and quality of life. To understand community health, you need to understand the ecology and organization of communities.

HUMAN ECOLOGY

In striving to organize resources, develop technology, control behavior, and regulate the environment society creates new problems, some of them harmful to health. The production of nuclear energy produces a Chernobyl incident; coal mining strips mountains of protective foliage, causing erosion and flooding; transporting oil and toxic material by ships, trucks, and trains pollutes the environment when a spill occurs; computers produce ''techno-stress'' for many people. And each of the past methods of meeting society's energy needs has produced other problems. Social history, then, imposes both help and hazard on the natural history of health. The help can be great when organized on a national level, because resources and authority of the greatest magnitudes can be pooled and deployed at that level. Yet the hazards are greater when authorities who make highly centralized decisions fail to take into account the special needs and delicate balance of human and other resources at the local community level. For this reason, community health planning and community-based health services are essential to an ecologically sound, culturally sensitive, socially responsive health system. Sustainable development of health depends on sustainable development and conservation of other resources including air, water, soil, trees, and other species of flora and fauna.

The human species is widely dispersed over the planet. Of all forms of life, it possesses the greatest degree of adaptability, being able to adjust to a greater variety of conditions than any other living form. In the Arctic regions as well as in the tropics human communities have the great ability to bend nature to will and to solve problems of survival created by environmental conditions. *In solving one problem relating to survival, however, society frequently creates another problem.* Survival and health are constant challenges in which human beings must look for other problems as soon as they have solved one. This search is short because often a new problem is created by the solution to the last.

Community health programs must be planned with this lesson of ecology in mind. Besides the concepts of ecology, the analytical tools of demography and epidemiology in Chapter 3 will enable you to assess a community's health problems, trends, and potentials.

Components of Ecology

Human ecology is the study of the relationship between human beings and their environment. **Society** deals with an environment that is physical, chemical, biological, social, and behavioral (Table 2-1). The community lives in an organic relationship with its environment. The community strives to alter the environment to its advantage, but there are times when alteration of the environment may work to the disadvantage of specific communities, populations, or individuals. This chapter will deal with those factors relating to the conservation of human resources and will leave discussions of other factors to subsequent chapters.

Adaptation and Conservation

Society has not conquered nature and doubtless never will, for biological and physical laws are always at work. Society can, however, modify the course of nature, adapt to nature, and alter conditions to aid in survival. Society even makes it possible for the biologically weak to survive. A com-

TABLE 2-1
Three dimensions of ecology

Physical-chemical factors	
Climate	Debris
Chemical pollution of water	Soil
Air pollution	Fuel
Radiation	
Noise	

Biological factors	
Food production	Poisons and toxic agents
Food conservation	Pathogens
Growth and development	Other parasites
Nutrition	Vectors
Physiological effects	Organic pollution of water

Social, organizational, and behavioral factors	
Social structure	Mobility
Communication	Leisure
Consumption	Stress
Learning	Population imbalance
Economics	Culture

mon misconception is that this ''artificial selection'' is dysgenic because it enables the ''poorest'' segments of our species to survive. Biologists reject the notion of artificial selection. It is just as much natural selection when the brain is used to aid survival as when legs and wings are used.

The human species today is neither biologically inferior nor superior to its ancestors of previous centuries. By definition the survivors of any generation were the ones best suited for adaptation and survival in their time. All who survive may be considered fit to survive, even if their survival was made possible by technological means. Civilization recognizes values other than health and biological endowment. Why should not people with chronic diseases have the right to life? By making it possible for these people to survive, society in return has received the intellectual, artistic, technological, and other benefits that the special gifts of many of these people have made possible. In short, adaptation and survival have become more than biological phenomena; they have become social and organizational enterprises as well.

Conservation is not the hoarding of resources but the wise use of them. Conservation of human resources means the most effective use of the environmental factors essential to survival, quality of well-being, and extension of the prime of life. It entails balancing future needs as well as present requirements. Conservation of human resources means giving consideration to climatic conditions, food supply, productive and recreational use of land, fuel, and water, the birthrate, other living forms, technological developments, and other factors fundamental to the existence and quality of life of the human species.

Climatic and Seasonal Effects on Health

The temperate zones appear to produce a longer life expectancy than the tropics. This holds true for people who normally live in temperate zones but who migrate to the tropics and live there. In conditions of excessive heat and ultraviolet rays from the sun, physical functioning tends to become reduced. Resistance to infection is apparently less than under cooler temperatures. Standard aptitude and intelligence tests administered to college students reveal lower performances in the heat of summer than in the cool days of the winter months. Experiments with rats indicate reduced performance when the ambient temperature is increased.

With animal husbandry it has been observed in the United States that twice as much time is required to grow a steer to a 1000-pound weight in Louisiana as is required in the northern states. The animal's maximum weight in Louisiana is considerably less than that of the animal raised in the northern states.

Temperature cycles of the world have had a significant influence not only on the health of the human species but also on the economy and culture of nations. During the glory of Greece and the height of Rome, Europe was in the throes of a cold cycle that provided ideal temperatures for agriculture in the Mediterranean area. Culture flourished in those nations that enjoyed a thriving agriculture, but the nations in northern Europe that had prevailing temperatures too low for growing crops declined culturally as well as in other respects. During the period of low temperatures, the population of Ireland consisted of sheep, goat, and cattle herders and their families. Vegetable crops were almost nonexistent. Ireland's general culture declined with its economy.

During the Dark Ages, the thermometer swung to the other extreme and reached its peak about AD 850. Grapes and other crops usually associated with the Mediterranean area grew abundantly in England. This was the period when the Vikings were making their explorations of the North American continent and elsewhere. During this hot era, Greece experienced a steady decline as her agriculture and general economy faded. Ireland flourished and probably was the most culturally advanced nation in Europe. This hot period was followed by a cooling period. Ice that formed in some of the northern nations during the year AD 1000 did not begin to melt until the onset of the present upward trend in temperature.

The most recent rising phase of the temperature cycle appears to have begun around 1880, but the rise in temperature was not appreciable until the period beginning in 1930. Since that time there seems to have been a gradual, somewhat irregular, but nonetheless measurable increase in the world's temperature. Glaciers are receding, and objects and forms of life frozen in ice 1000 years ago are being exposed. How long this upward cycle will continue is unknown, but the continuing increase in carbon dioxide is accumulating an atmospheric blanket that holds heat next to the earth, creating a "**greenhouse effect.**"

THE HEALTH FIELD CONCEPT

The hundreds of things thought to exert some influence on health can be subsumed under four general categories or factors. These four factors—human biology, environment, behavior, and health care organization—make up the health field. The **health field concept** was used by governments in shifting their national health policies at the beginning of the current health promotion era. Earlier emphasis in health policy was on health care organization and environmental controls of communicable diseases. The United States, Canadian, Australian, New Zealand, and some European governments now have come to a new emphasis on behavior or life-style and on the environment. These new emphases are now related to the new leading causes of death and disability: chronic diseases—particularly heart disease, cancer and stroke—and violent deaths and injuries. Both of these sets of leading causes of death and disability are associated with some combination of life-style and environmental causes (see Figure 2-1).

Human Biology

Human biology encompasses the health outcomes that directly derive from the genetics of the individual, natural growth, and aging. Human biology is a necessary substrate for the remaining three categories, but there is little that individuals or communities can do to alter it except through genetic counseling for the sake of future generations.

At the turn of the century only 3% of infant deaths were from genetic causes. With the reductions in environmental causes of infant mortality and the control of infectious diseases, now nearly 33% of infant deaths are attributable to gene-related causes. About 50% of spontaneous abortions and 5% to 7% of stillbirths are caused by chromosomal abnormalities. Major malformations such as cleft palate and neural tube defects amount to 3% in newborns. Minor malformations from genetic causes range from 10% to 12% of all children at 1 year of

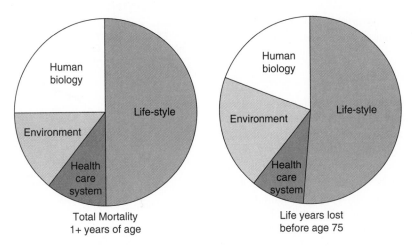

FIGURE 2-1
Estimated proportions of North American total mortality after infancy and total life years lost before age 75 influenced by each of the four factors in the health field.
Courtesy Centers for Disease Control.

age. Nearly one third of all hospitalized children ages 1 to 4 are admitted because of genetically determined or influenced disorders. Recent technological advances permit the early detection of many genetic disorders before birth or in newborns. The early diagnosis and treatment or prevention possibilities for many of these problems can guide reproductive decisions and can offer lifelong emotional savings to families and real economic savings to communities and society.

Environment

Environment includes all those factors related to health that are external to the human body. The individual has limited control over these. The community may have a larger degree of control. Examples include safe, uncontaminated food, air, water, and drugs; control of air, water, and noise pollution; effective garbage and sewage disposal; and prevention of spread of communicable diseases. Providing a safe social environment by accident and fire prevention, gun control, and television programs

that do not glorify and exploit violence are further examples. Urbanization, with resultant crowding and poor housing, is another environmental influence on community health. Isolated rural living also can be detrimental to health under some circumstances.

Rapid social change or population growth with disintegration of established community values and their replacement by newer, untested mores may cause alienation and stress. Pursuit of private profit at the cost of common good may result in deterioration of the community environment and health.

Life-style and Behavior

Life-style, the third category, covers decisions, actions and living conditions of individuals that affect their health. These include self-imposed risks such as cigarette smoking, overeating, drug misuse, alcoholism, promiscuity, careless driving, unsafe sex, and failure to wear seat belts. Lack of exercise, recreation, or relief from pressure of work or other stressors are further examples of self-imposed risks that produce health hazards, but some of these are imposed also by socioeconomic conditions.

Health Care Organization

Health care organization, the fourth category in the health field concept, is the one that has received the most attention and money. Its elements are medical practice, nursing, hospitals, nursing homes, dental services, drugs, mental health care, and other community health services. These services use an array of interventional methods, such as bedside nursing and surgery. These are usually applied late in the natural history of disease, when little in the way of cure can be expected but much in the way of effort and cost can be expended. Society has developed a dependence on this fourth category while overlooking the benefits to be derived from health-related changes in environment and life-style.

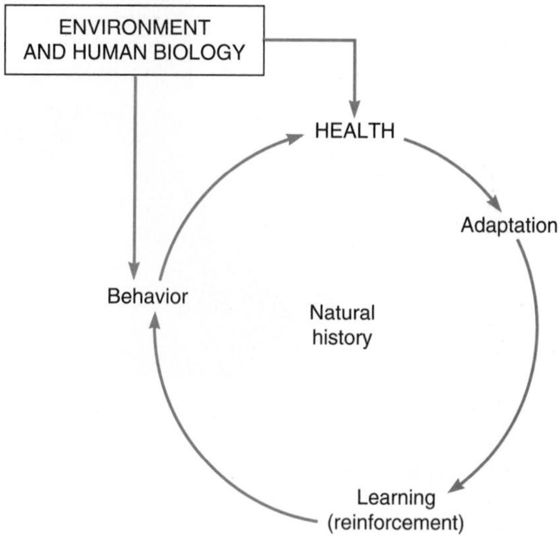

A MODEL OF COMMUNITY HEALTH

Community health programs must combine the four health field elements of environmental, biomedical, organizational, and behavioral interventions. A clinical procedure or research study on disease might be able to limit its focus to one or two of these elements, but community health practice must keep all four in view.

The **natural history of health** can be represented by the cycle shown in Figure 2-2. Human biology and the environment combine to influence both behavior and health. Behavior, in turn, influences health, and healthy people are better able to adapt to the challenges of life. Some scholars have even defined health as the capability to adapt to life's circumstances.

With rewarding or successful adaptation comes learning the skills and actions that led to the success. This learning reinforces or strengthens those health-promoting or health-protecting behaviors that were most successful. Over a lifetime, many health-

FIGURE 2-2
The natural history of health before social organization.

Before Organization

Consider the "natural" process of health in a prehistoric time when people wandered as nomads without communities. Having little or no organization, they depended on their inherited biological strength and protective capacities to contend with the environment. They lived "in harmony" with nature, meaning that they adapted to their genetic endowment and their environment rather than trying to control these factors. Adaptation was made with a minimum of help from other people. Those who survived were the best learners, and their reward (reinforcement) for successful adaptation was survival itself. In this "natural" state, only three factors directly influenced health—human biology, the environment, and behavior. There was little organization, and no health care technology to organize. How has the organization of people into clans, then communities, then governments and nations, influenced the natural history of health?

promoting and health-protecting behavioral patterns are learned. Over several lifetimes and generations in primitive conditions the healthiest practices tend to survive to be passed on to succeeding generations. All this can occur, however inefficiently, with little or no social organization.

As communities form, however, people impose another cycle on the natural history of health. They add a social history. They do this by passing information and social influence from parents to children, from neighbor to neighbor, and from elders and other leaders to followers. By this means, behavior becomes more and more organized or ''civilized'' by means of expectations and social influence. Figure 2-3 shows how these socializing influences lead to what sociologists call ''**norms**'' or ''**social norms.**'' The norms of one generation are transmitted to the next in the form of cultural values, which shape the purposes and methods of social organizations. Some social organizations, such as

churches, include in their mission the control of behavior. Others, such as sanitation and conservation organizations, attempt to control the environment.

Thus the community cycle closes on the **social history of health.** The behavioral and environmental controls exercised by community organizations include behavior related to health and environmental factors related to health. The social history of communities thereby imposes human organization as a fourth influence, for better or for worse, on the natural history of health. Two types of social organization that pertain to community health are consumer health and the organization of health services.

Consumer Health, Economics, and Competition

Another way of constructing the social cycle in Figure 2-3 is to replace norms with **supply and demand.** A widely practiced or ''normative'' behavior

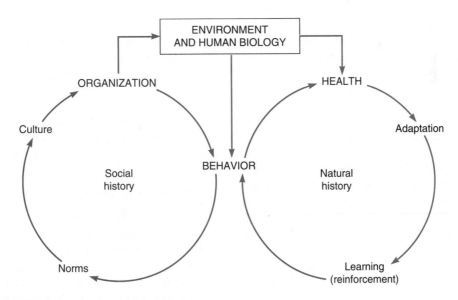

FIGURE 2-3
The social history of health has imposed both positive and negative influences on health through community organization of behavior, environment, and health care, three of the four elements of the health field.

in relation to goods and services available in the community expresses itself economically as demand. For example, people who shift their purchasing behavior in large numbers from butter to margarine establish a norm and create a demand for more margarine. Demand, in turn, influences supply; or if supply is limited, demand influences price. These three economic factors—demand, supply, and price—produce a social cycle similar to the behavior-norms-values cycle. Prices equate with values. Prices apply especially well to consumable goods and services. Values apply to consumables as well as to abstract goods such as loyalty, faith, love, and responsibility to care for children.

How does health come into the *Price = Value* equation? Is health a consumable good or an abstract value? How much are people willing to pay for health? If health is a right, rather than a privilege, then the community (or government at some level) has a responsibility to ensure that those who cannot afford the prices attached to health promotion, health protection, and health services still have access to these goods and services. **Accessibility** requires organization.

Even to those who can afford to pay for health products and services, the community has some responsibility to ensure the quality and safety of those products and services. This responsibility is exercised through governmental rules and regulations for consumer health protection. Administering and enforcing consumer protection laws requires organization. In addition, consumers themselves organize for collective action or advocacy to pass new laws or to educate the public to protect themselves through selective purchasing. These forces put pressure on the manufacturers, advertisers, and providers of health-related products and services—including foods, toys, and automobiles—to give greater attention to the health and safety implications of their practices, or else lose out in a competitive marketplace.

Nowhere has this "invisible hand" of the marketplace been more invisible than in medical care services. The medical profession in the United States, for example, is the only industry that has been legally exempted from most of the economic rules of monopoly and at the same time has avoided much of the government regulation applied to other social services. Laws restrict other professions from practicing medicine, hence the monopoly. Yet the medical profession enjoys the highest privilege of the professions: self-regulation. Listing of fees is not the custom of medical practitioners. Until recently, advertising by physicians was forbidden by most medical societies. Consumers had little economic information and little encouragement for doctor "shopping." One of the most powerful tools of the consumer in other marketplaces is shopping for the best prices. Without prior knowledge of fees, patients exert little influence on medicine.

The health insurance industry has further complicated the economic market forces as they apply to the medical marketplace by removing the consumer's awareness of the price being paid for health care services. This "third-party payer" arrangement transfers fees for services directly from the insurance company or the government to the medical service providers—hospitals or physicians. This means that the consumer or patient is often unaware of the costs of care, much less financially responsible for their payment. These conditions undermine the potential of competitive economic market forces to control the social history of health so that additional responsibilities fall on the community to organize to control the cost and distribution of health resources.

The Place of the Individual in Community Health

An ecological view of community health insists on looking at the interaction of populations or species and their environments, but the cumulative behavior of individuals is at the center of the ecological relationship of populations to their environment. Individual behavior is motivated by a lifetime of experience, which shapes beliefs, as shown in Figure

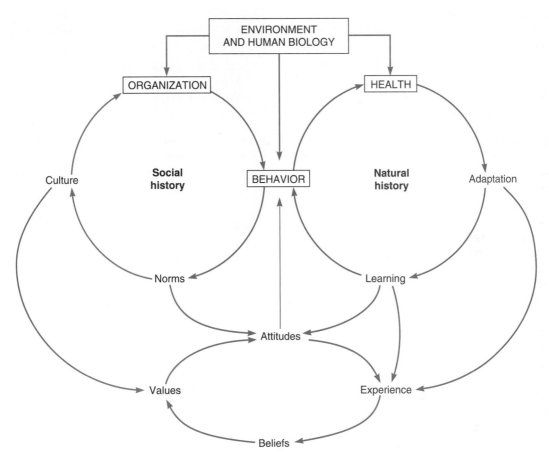

FIGURE 2-4
The place of personal histories and motivation in the development of life-style (behavior) and health shows the interaction of environmental, social, and individual determinants of community health.

2-4. Beliefs, in turn, combine with cultural influences to shape each individual's values. Values are deep-seated, enduring orientations toward social goods and evils, right and wrong, and ethical and unethical behavior. These combine with the perceived norms of behavior, and with current social learning about the desirability and efficacy of specific actions, to produce in the individual an attitude toward a specific behavior.

Note that Figure 2-4 shows four sources of influence on behavior as it relates to health. One is the immediate attitude or intention of the individual that *predisposes* him or her to take an action. Organizational and environmental factors combine with innate capacities endowed by human biology to *enable* the individual to take a desired action to promote or protect his or her health. Learning from past experiences *reinforces* the behavior by recalling previous successes and satisfactions associated with a type of behavior, which translates as anticipated rewards for repeating or generalizing the behavior. How community health programs can predispose, enable, and reinforce behavior conducive to health will be the subject of Chapter 4. Here we are concerned with the ecology and organization of communities as these relate to health. The natural history of health converges with social history and personal histories to influence health through the behavior of individuals and the organization of the environment. The three cycles of Figure 2-4 are continuous rather than static. They connect with each other in such a way that everything influences and is influenced by everything else, however indirectly or remotely. This is the lesson of human ecology.

The pivotal factor linking personal and social histories to health is behavior. According to the arrows representing causation in Figure 2-4, personal history can influence health only through behavior. The behavior may be individual action (self-care, lifestyle, or use of health services), or it may be collective action (organizing community groups for health, family decisions, neighborhood petition, voter recruitment, or other social process). Collective action results in some change in the organization of health resources or the environment to influence health.

The Organization of Health Services and Technology

Communities recognize the need to provide for the care of their sick, but the demand for and the cost of such care tend to exceed the community's resources. When that happens, the community's greater responsibility to protect the health of all of its citizens is compromised and its opportunities to promote and protect the health of those who are not sick slip away. Decisions between the best medical care for a few and the best health care for the masses confront those who must allocate community health resources.

Over 90% of the governmental budget allocations for health care in most nations are for tech-

Social Ethics in Organized Health Care

Some decisions must be made by the community concerning its own priorities in allocating its resources to social and health services, each with competing interest groups and competing value judgments. Is it more important to spend several million dollars providing for kidney dialysis for a single child who will die without it, or to spend half as much for each of two programs to ensure the improved nutrition and immunization of thousands of children in the same community? Few if any of the children would likely die without the nutrition and immunization programs, but hundreds might be healthier, more productive in school, and less likely to contract a disabling or disfiguring disease if the nutrition and immunization programs are maintained.

nologically advanced services that can be provided only by medical specialists and hospitals. Only 3% of the U.S. health budget is devoted to prevention. The high cost of maintaining the specialized medical services, equipment, and facilities, especially under the market conditions described in the preceding section, has caused the price for medical and nursing care to skyrocket in recent years, far beyond the resources of many families and even communities to pay. Medical costs have been soaring at an average increase of 20% per year.

These changing circumstances have caused most families to become reliant on insurance or welfare systems to provide for their medical care. "Catastrophic" care has come to mean anything requiring more than a few days in the hospital. The insurance system, in turn, has had to reorganize its premium structures to cover the outlays for claims made on behalf of the insured by their medical providers. Most families cannot afford these new "health insurance" policies, which are really medical and hospital insurance. They depend increasingly on employer contributions to pay at least a share of the premiums. As a result, labor unions have found more and more of their progress in collective bargaining taken up by health insurance benefits, leaving less for wages and other benefits. Similarly, employers have found larger and larger percentages of the price on their products being taken up by health insurance benefits to their employees. This means less profit and less investment in growth or modernization.

These trends in the competitive private sector have led many companies to seek new ways to control the costs of health care. They have supported government efforts to force more competition in the medical care field, while spawning their own versions of self-insurance, health maintenance organizations, and employee health and fitness programs at the worksite.

Policies to Achieve Better Distribution of Health Resources

Great Britain established its National Health Service, but this has not entirely solved the ethical and political problems relating to the equitable allocation of technology. More recently Canada initiated reforms in its health care system to address some of the problems of access to affordable care by the average citizen. The federal government in the United States has experimented with a series of adjustments in its policies governing health facility planning, purchasing power for the elderly under Medicare and for the poor under Medicaid, and more recently the market controls on pricing, reimbursements, and competition. These new policies will be the subject of Part Four of this book. They are mentioned here to contrast the predominant thrust of national policies to contain costs with the policies addressing the greater determinants of community health in lifestyle and the environment.

National policies to contain cost in medical care cannot be disparaged, given that more than 90% of the national expenditures for health go into this sector. The urgency for shifting the emphasis and resources to other sectors is compelling: the total contribution to mortality reduction or increased longevity that can be made by health care organization is less than 20% of the total contribution from all sectors (Figure 2-1). By this measure, the greatest potential for progress in community health clearly lies in programs addressing life-style and the environment.

A balanced model of community health, then, is one that recognizes all four elements of the health field. Communities in democratic societies can exert very little direct control over human biology other than through genetic counseling. This leaves three points for intervention, as shown in Figure 2-5. Following the terminology adopted in the federal policies for disease prevention and health promotion in the United States and Canada, the interventions directed at the environment are referred to broadly as *health protection,* those directed at life-style as *health promotion,* and those directed at the health care system as *preventive health services.* The three sections of this book following this introductory section are organized around these three broad strategies for community health.

Figure 2-5 shows that health education is the primary strategy in health promotion, but that it has a major contribution to make in health protection and health services as well. In addition to health education, health promotion requires organizational, economic, and environmental supports to *enable* people to change their life-styles and to *reinforce* positive health behavior. Health behavior in turn can support the environmental goals of health protection and the medical goals of health services, as indicated by the vertical arrows. Environmental factors and the organization and accessibility of health services also condition life-style.

For example, the use of health services by women when they detect an early warning sign for cancer, such as a lump in the breast, is a behavior that can make a great difference in the ability of these health services to reduce mortality from cancer. The accessibility of the health services, in turn, influences the likelihood that people will use them

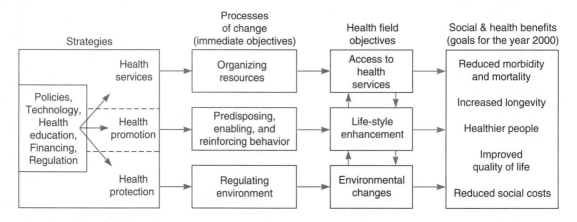

FIGURE 2-5

Relationships between the strategies in health services, health protection, and health promotion, the processes of change they seek to set into motion, the three modifiable elements of the health field they can influence, and the ultimate health and social benefits they are expected to yield.

Adapted from Green LW: Prevention and health education. In Last JM, Wallace RB, editors: *Maxcy-Roseneau-Last public health and preventive medicine,* ed 13, Norwalk, Conn, 1991, Appleton-Century-Crofts.

early enough to make a difference. Similarly, behavior or life-style determines the ways in which people expose themselves to environmental hazards and the actions they will take, individually and collectively, to alter environmental hazards. The environment, in turn, influences behavior by setting the conditions for work and play.

CONCEPT OF COMMUNITY

A community consists of interdependent social units that transact a common life among the people making up the units. As a social group, functioning with norms of behavior and organization of resources, the community regulates both the environment and behavior.

A community may exist in a limited territory, but increasingly the community is characterized by a constantly enlarging geographical expanse. Our concept of community has changed from the limited view that a city in its boundary constitutes a community to a consideration of the interaction of social norms, values, and organizations. A few decades ago a single large city was regarded as an independent community. Today we speak of a metropolitan area, implying that the entire area functions as a unified community. In the United States the Metropolitan Statistical Area (MSA) is a county or group of contiguous counties containing at least one city of 50,000 inhabitants or more and a total population of 100,000.

Areas outside the legal limits of a city are an integral part of the total community. Erecting hospitals, establishing clinics, and providing other medical services today require planning based on estimates of the health needs of the entire population served. Such planning is best accomplished by elected bodies that include consumers as well as health providers. By such planning it is possible to organize more efficiently for all people living within the area.

In addition to the geographic community, modern communications and transport have created more active and effective communities of interest (such as national advocacy groups), communities of need (such as minority associations), and communities of solution (such as national voluntary and professional health associations). A **community,** for most purposes in this book, is a group of inhabitants living in a somewhat localized area under the same general regulations and having common norms, values, and organizations.

Physical Factors

The organization of a community influences how the larger community deals with health problems. Varying environmental and social influences can identify subcommunities within the community. Such subcommunities are made up of towns within counties, or ethnic or neighborhood groupings within cities. Thus in some respects a large metropolitan area can be thought of as a group of villages. Environmental factors to be recognized in diagnosing community health problems include the physical environment; geography, topography, and climate; neighborhood organization; and industrial conditions.

Physical environment. The physical environment sometimes reflects the community's general health status. This applies to the mental, emotional, and social health of a community as well as to its physical health. The community that possesses a degree of orderliness, however old or simple its buildings, usually reflects an awareness and a pride in the well-being of its citizens. Clean air and water, however, are the critical environmental factors in health (see Figure 2-6).

Geography, topography, and climate. Geography refers to the surface of the earth. Topography indicates the features of a region or locality. Together with climate, these two phenomena may cause or contribute to special community health problems. Lowlands, marshy areas, and hot climates give rise

to health problems not of concern elsewhere. Tropical diseases are limited in most instances to such areas. Dry, dusty areas may create health conditions differing from those of more humid regions. The minerals of an area, the types of soil, and the functions of the rivers, canals, waterways, and harbors can be significant factors in determining the general health of the local population, depending on how the people use or abuse these natural resources.

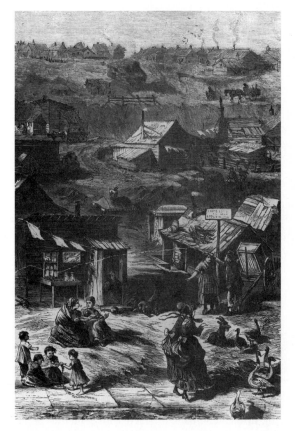

FIGURE 2-6

"The squatters of New York," settling in shacks near Central Park during the mid-nineteenth century, created a semblance of community despite meager support from the city.

Wood engraving after Wyand DE, *Harper's Weekly* 13:412, June 26, 1869, courtesy National Library of Medicine.

Community size. A neighborhood traditionally was thought of as an area that houses a population for which one elementary school is ordinarily required. Such a neighborhood ranges in size from 1000 to 3000 families. This usually means an entire population of about 5000. Areas deviating from this general pattern are increasingly common, but still can be designated as true neighborhood units. As the birthrate or death rate declines, more people live alone, and more elderly people live without children, the elementary school as a criterion of neighborhood becomes less relevant.

In many of the smaller villages of Western nations there is a tendency for the younger people to move away, so that today most of the small rural and even nonrural villages are populated by older people. (In developing countries the opposite condition arises, with high birthrates in rural areas.) With a proportionately high percentage of their citizens over 65 years old, these small communities find themselves faced with low birthrates, high death rates, and the special health problems of the elderly. Many of these communities are unable to keep their hospitals open or to provide the necessary health services for the health needs of their older citizens or children. Some communities are fortunate in being near or part of a large community in which complete health services are available. Health planning agencies are attempting to address the needs of these outlying communities by linking them with urban facilities and resources.

Neighborhood organization. Some of the older, long-established neighborhoods have an amazing unity and rapport. Some of the newer neighborhoods, particularly in the suburban areas, frequently are neighborhoods in area only. Speculative building in the suburbs, combined with a mobile population, tends to produce communities of individuals who are almost transients, with scant allegiance to a common health standard. Time is needed before the influence of schools, churches, and community

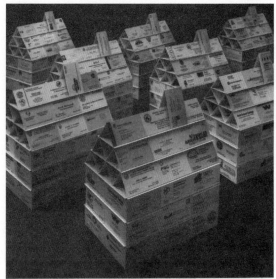

REBUILDING AMERICA'S NEIGHBORHOODS IS EVERYONE'S BUSINESS.

A community is like a house of cards. When one neighborhood starts to slip, the rest can easily collapse.

That's why a non-profit partnership called NeighborWorks is building a stronger community by rebuilding housing and restoring pride.

The support of the business community is key to NeighborWorks's success. So make it your business to get involved. Send us your card.

NeighborWorks
Reversing decline. Rebuilding pride.

P.O. Box 41406,
Baltimore, MD 21203-6406
1-800-243-6957

FIGURE 2-7
A national campaign to rebuild community pride in neighborhoods where housing stock has declined used this public service advertisement to recruit private business support for rebuilding.
Courtesy Advertising Council.

groups becomes established. Social unity in such neighborhoods is loose. The degree of neighborhood unity, past practices, leadership, and established standards all contribute to existing health conditions (see Figure 2-7). More revealing, however, is the nature of the neighborhood unity that exists when a particular health problem arises and must be dealt with on a cooperative basis. Where a long-established neighborhood cohesiveness already exists, the necessary leadership and united support will be mobilized quickly, and a program to solve the health problem will be initiated summarily. In a neighborhood with little cohesiveness, valuable time will be consumed in the effort to mobilize the neighborhood's resources to deal with the problem requiring attention. Such a neighborhood may require several years to cope with a health problem that a more cohesive neighborhood will have well in hand in a matter of days.

Industrial conditions. Health problems can sometimes be identified with particular industrial conditions that either prevail within the community or indirectly affect the community. A "garden city" or a residential community will not have some of the health problems that citizens in a highly industrialized community will encounter. An industry that causes a great deal of noise may create special problems of an emotional as well as of a physical nature. The social health of the community can be affected by chemical plants creating noxious odors. A mining community or a logging community living in the shadow of extreme occupational hazards is a community different from one in which industrial injuries are rare.

A particular industry will have direct environmental effects on the health of a community. Another will have effects on individual workers exposed to health hazards on the job.

Social and Cultural Factors

The essence of communities does not lie simply in the observable physical characteristics of the buildings, industries, size, and topography. Communities are identified by less visible social and cultural factors that distinguish them. The traditions of the community, its social stratification, its religious influences, its stability or tenure of residence, and other social and cultural processes operate to give the community a distinctive personality. These same factors directly and indirectly influence the health of

the community. The recognition of health problems, the promotion of community health, and the ability to deal with health emergencies will be affected by the cultural and organizational tendencies and capabilities that have evolved over years.

Traditions and prejudices. New health problems such as HIV and AIDS, new aspects of old health problems such as tuberculosis, different health requirements, and new discoveries call for new approaches to health. In some communities long-established conventions inhibit attempts to deal with evolving health needs. In some instances these orally transmitted notions are not readily identifiable but appear as norms of resistance in the form of "We have always done it this way." Sometimes obstacles to health advances in the community are preconceived judgments or values relating to health matters or health procedures. A health bias can be as deeply ingrained as a religious bias. Indeed, sometimes they are the same, as with abortion.

Socioeconomic status (SES). The population may be classified into strata on the basis of income, residence, occupation, or education. According to which of these four criteria are used, the resulting hierarchy of socioeconomic status (SES) is graduated into any number of upper, middle, and lower levels. SES influences life-style, which in turn governs environmental exposures, customs, and habits that affect health status. There is considerable overlap between income and residence, as well as between occupation and education. The latter is the most powerful determinant of the four criteria with regard to influence on health-related behavior. Persons of high educational attainment often enjoy the best health status. They respond readily to appeals from health professionals to modify their life-styles related to smoking cessation, weight control, exercise programs, dental care, and immunization. In contrast, persons of a low educational level often suffer the worst health and are more difficult to reach with persuasive health messages. A cultural barrier frequently exists between the efforts of health professionals to educate and the perceptions of people with less education.

Both chronic and communicable diseases cut across all strata of society, although the lower strata are most affected. Prevention and control of communicable diseases among the less privileged groups indirectly protect and thus benefit the entire population. Preventive health services and health promotion activities are most needed by low-income groups and those of less educational attainment, but all people in a community will benefit from an overall community health program.

Social norms. Customs and norms imbued with ethical significance can have the force of law. Usually the social norms of a community, such as the norms restraining sexual activity in teenagers, can serve as an asset in the promotion of community health. It is sometimes necessary, however, to change established customs in a community to obtain the necessary gains that modern health procedures can contribute. Tobacco, alcohol, and drug use have become customs or norms in some communities. Reversing the widespread use of such substances is as much a political process as an educational one. Modification of customs in a community usually represents a compromise. Attempts to eliminate or reverse a custom often generate hostile resistance to a health program. When norms are transmitted from one generation to the next, they become embedded in the culture of the community as values. Effective health programs more often adapt to the customs and values of a community than attempt to change them totally.

Religious influences. Communities composed of citizens of diverse religious faiths living in harmony permit no particular denomination or group of churches to dominate the community. The total effect is to enrich community life and provide a co-

operative spirit in which community health promotion can flourish. This effect is achieved if those who provide the community's health leadership properly seek the support of the many church groups in the community. Health leadership must be sensitive to possible conflicts, religious or otherwise, that may exist in a community.

Political influences. Some community health programs or factors are political in nature. Law enforcement is increasingly significant as a factor in modern community health protection and promotion. The caliber of officials a community has and the extent of social-mindedness in its officialdom directly and indirectly affect community health standards. The willingness of community officials to raise taxes for health services or health promotion and their interest in giving a high priority to matters of health are significant in the final determination of the kind of health the community's people will have. Even when official support of community health is inadequate, however, it is often possible through other avenues, through other agencies, and through other means to promote community health action.

Economy. The size of a trade area, the importance of farm people in a trade area, the diversity of industry, the fluctuations in the economy, and the extremes of rich and poor are of significance to community health. Different economic conditions mean differences in the amount of money available for food, clothing, housing, and other basic needs. They also mean differences in the amount of money available for health facilities, health services, schools, sanitary facilities, leisure-time activities, and general health promotion programs.

The family income that an economy provides appears to be directly related to the level of health enjoyed by the people in a community. Vital statistics indicate that people residing in prosperous cities live longer than people who reside in low-income cities. It must be recognized, however, that the average income may conceal homeless people and other groups that do not share in the community's wealth. Prosperous communities usually provide more and better medical facilities than impoverished communities, though this is a factor of overrated importance in community health.

Tenure of residence. Growth in population is sometimes a sign of a prosperous and healthy community, but population growth may cause certain temporary displacements within a community that may be adverse for health promotion. Additional schools may be required, and additional community services may be necessary. There may be some disorganization during the time between the occurrence of these new needs and their fulfillment. This is the experience of suburban communities adjacent to large metropolitan areas, especially during periods of heavy immigration and most dramatically with refugee settlements. In such communities the tenure of residence of many of the families is relatively short. Usually the newcomers are young couples with small children. In other communities where families are moving in and out constantly an unfavorable health situation usually exists. A high number of transient families tends to weaken the stability and social networks that support the health of a community.

Organizational Factors

Any community needs a diversity of agencies and individuals to provide services of direct and indirect health significance. Too little coordination or integration of services often leads to duplication and overlapping of functions. Despite the lack of efficient coordination, both tax-supported and non-tax-supported health services often cooperate and form **coalitions** to meet specific community health needs.

Tax-supported services. The official agencies that contribute to the health of a community usually touch the individual citizen directly. Some of the services given by these tax-supported agencies may be of an indirect nature, but the majority of their services directly affect individual citizens in their everyday living. Obviously, the most important of these tax-supported agencies is the county, city, or district health department. Other official agencies providing health services include the department of welfare, public hospitals, special boards and commissions, the department of public works, public schools, the local housing authority, agricultural agencies, recreational agencies, and the police department. Each of these, individually and collectively, has an important role in community health promotion or health protection.

Non-tax-supported services. Health promotion and health services available to communities through voluntary agencies or organizations represent the true spirit of community reflected in the quotation at the beginning of this chapter and in Figure 2-8. The giving of donations or of blood voluntarily and anonymously to help others less fortunate is an expression of community in its purest form. Civic clubs, church groups, parent-teacher associations, the Red Cross, visiting nurse associations, the United Way, and sometimes the community hospital are examples of non-tax-supported services. Special clinical services, as well as medical care and hospital service plans, may also be available.

National voluntary health organizations may have an indirect effect on the health of any given community and in some instances may play a direct role in the health of individual citizens. These national voluntary health organizations serve several functions, such as educating, conducting demonstrations, supplementing and supporting official health activities, and coordinating community health efforts. Some of these organizations are concerned with specific diseases. In the United States and Canada this group would include chapters of organizations such as the American or Canadian Cancer Society, American Heart Association or the Heart and

When you give blood
you give another birthday,
another anniversary,
another talk with a friend,
another laugh,
another hug,
another chance.

American Red Cross

Please give blood.

Ad
Council

FIGURE 2-8
Voluntary health organizations depend on the impulse of people to help others through charitable donations of time, money, and blood.
Courtesy Advertising Council, American Red Cross, and Cabot Communications.

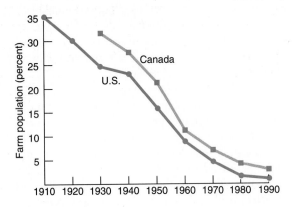

FIGURE 2-9
Farm population as a percentage of total U.S. and Canadian resident populations, 1910-1990.
Sources: U.S. Bureau of the Census and Statistics Canada.

Stroke Foundation of Canada, American or Canadian Lung Association, March of Dimes, and various self-help groups.

Non-tax-supported services in many communities also include practicing physicians, dentists, nurses, and other health specialists represented by the medical society, the dental society, and medical service plans.

AGRICULTURAL AND TECHNOLOGICAL FACTORS

The food supply of a nation determines not only the health of its people but also the nature of its population growth. America's farm situation is undergoing some changes that are of interest in terms of the nation's health and its population. According to the U.S. Bureau of the Census, the farm population declined from 35% of the total in 1910 to barely 2% of the total in 1990 (Figure 2-9), but total farm acreage increased.

Poverty and Hunger

Poverty is the primary cause of hunger. Nearly 40% of the people in the developing world live in such dire poverty that they cannot provide themselves with a minimally adequate diet. This impoverished two fifths of humanity lack the land to grow its own food or the money to buy it—even in years when local crops are good, world production is high, and storage bins are filled to overflowing. Even doubling food production on present patterns would not materially change the status of the great majority of those who are hungry and malnourished today. Children are more likely to be living in poverty and to suffer the health consequences of poverty than any other age group.

Sharp extremes of wealth and poverty persist between and within nations. Three major national factors give rise to most developing world poverty: inequitable distribution of resources and income, low productivity and slow economic growth, and excessive population increases. As recent events in Somalia and the former Yugoslavia demonstrate, war and civil disintegration of social order can lead to starvation conditions in even shorter time than the other three conditions combined. These major factors interact with one another and a number of subsidiary factors to perpetuate world poverty and thus hunger.

Measures for Overcoming World Hunger

Lasting solutions to the problem of world hunger can result only from rapid, equitable, and self-reliant economic growth. The industrialized nations can do their part by providing various forms of development assistance. The effort, however, to assure equitable economic growth cannot end with developmental assistance, no matter how generous and effective. Because hunger and poverty are deeply rooted in political and economic relations among nations, fundamental changes in global patterns of food production and trade (e.g., the General Agreement on Trade and Tariffs of 1993), are needed to improve the conditions for the developing countries themselves to break the cycle of stagnant agricultural productivity, hunger, poverty, high birthrates, unemployment, and disease.

The economic prospects of poor nations and poor people depend heavily on the evolution of the international economy as a whole. A number of related factors will govern the general direction of the world economy and the performance of individual communities and developing nations. In addition to the economic health of the industrialized nations, these factors include developments in world trade, private and public capital flows, and energy issues, among others. The rate at which the world economy grows during the next 20 years will make the major difference between the possibility of better conditions of life or continuing misery for millions of people. It is imperative that policymakers in every nation search for all possible ways to further economic growth as the most self-sustaining means of overcoming hunger.

Technology

The use of insecticides, weed killers, and fertilizers has reduced the amount of cultivation necessary on farms. Better strains of plants and animals and the addition of antibiotics to animal feeds have increased the productivity of farms. Improved methods of food processing, better refrigeration, improved packaging, and better methods of food preservation have reduced food wastes considerably and thus have contributed tangibly to the total food supply available.

But such technologies also bear less wholesome results. Fertilizers and chemicals used against weeds, insects, and funguses have accumulated in the soil, the water, and some food products to the point that new hazards to health have been introduced (Figure 2-10). Where environmental health was once concerned primarily with microorganisms, environmental and occupational health today are concerned chiefly with toxic agents of the chemical variety including refrigerants that escape to the upper atmosphere and threaten the global ozone layer.

Technology has had as much impact on the behavioral and organizational aspects of the health field as on the environmental aspects. The computer, for example, has revolutionized the ways we handle information and communication. Consequently, it has invaded human relationships, creating a newly emerging set of mental, emotional, and social health concerns referred to broadly as technostress, and ethical issues concerned with privacy and confidentiality of health information.

Tampering with Nature?

Gene-splicing, a technology made possible by the electron microscope (Figure 2-10), allows scientists to splice a minute bit of genetic material from one organism with another to obtain potentially valuable biological products. At first, great fear gripped the scientific community, then the public, that these techniques could unleash dangerous pathogens through biological warfare or by laboratory accidents. The fears subsided as government health agencies imposed rigorous guidelines for experimentation.

New fears have arisen over the release of commercially engineered organisms for agricultural purposes. The concern now is that genetically engineered plants or microbes used in agriculture might harm the ecology if they escaped from their agricultural niche and upset nature's balance. Ecologists point out that the European gypsy moth wreaked havoc in North America because there were no natural predators to keep it in check. Could the same happen with genetically altered agricultural products? Do the new technology's benefits outweigh its risks, assuming that gene-splicing should be able to improve the nutritional quality of crops and increase their resistance to pests, disease, and drought? Will gene therapy be allowed to alter the inherited characteristics of newborn children?

QUALITY OF HEALTH

Many people regarded as being well still do not have the quality of health that enables them to live effectively and enjoyably. They may be free from disabilities and overt symptoms and yet not possess an adequate level of well-being.

Community health seeks not only to minimize disabling defects and disorders, but also to enable the people of the community to be productive and to do the things they reasonably expect to do with enjoyment and gratification. Not perfect health but a high level of well-being in which an individual finds life productive and stimulating is a realistic goal for citizens of every community.

Despite the advances that have been made in lon-

gevity and in communicable disease control during this century, poor health, with its attendant human suffering and soaring social and economic costs, remains all too prevalent in most communities. In Western societies today most of the serious diseases and disabilities people can control are related to personal habits: drinking, smoking, drug misuse, overeating, poor nutrition, lack of exercise, and careless behavior. If people can be helped to change these habits, both health and the quality of life can be greatly improved for individuals and communities.

Not all solutions will be behavioral. Indeed, in

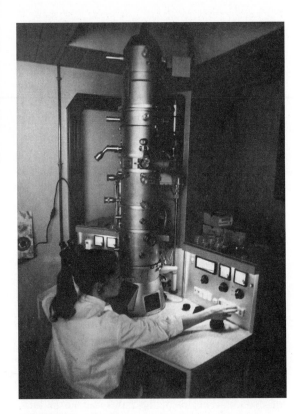

FIGURE 2-10
The electron microscope made possible some of the genetic studies that have led to the decoding of the gene and the ethical quandaries that follow.
Courtesy World Health Organization, photo by J Mohr.

the last years of the twentieth century, as in the first years, the results of basic research, technological development, and environmental modification may offer further control of health problems. Currently, however, knowledge to prevent or minimize many health problems is not being used to a satisfactory degree. After-the-fact medical care, unfortunately, still takes precedence over programs of disease prevention and health promotion.

The challenge, then, is to develop integrated community programs to support better health practices and health protection. Given the ever-increasing social and economic burden of health care costs resulting from negative community conditions and life-styles, how can governments, community organizations, and individuals work together to improve these conditions?

COMMUNITY ACTION AND INNOVATION

Integrated community programs—as distinct from replications of many school health programs, worksite programs, or patient care programs—require a distinct set of concepts, methods, and procedures. How are they different from the numerous applications of the same health programs or interventions used in various organizations within the community? What distinguishes integrated community health programs besides being bigger than their counterparts at the clinical, school, or worksite levels? Are community programs qualitatively different from their component interventions in medical and other institutional settings, or do they merely represent the sum of these parts? Besides coordinating the pieces, how do community programs function? Other than reaping the additive effects of small-scale programs, what makes large-scale community programs effective?

These questions are at the heart of a community approach to health. They defy simplistic answers that would merely distinguish community approaches from institutionally based programs in terms of greater magnitude, scope, or volume. Something more than size holds such community programs together over time. They are more than medical models enlarged; more than pedagogical methods transferred to the media; more than a step up the bureaucratic ladder from school to district, from neighborhood clinic to city or county health department.

Levels of Community Intervention and Change

One fact of community life that distinguishes integrated community health programs is that change must occur at several levels if the program is to penetrate the whole community (Figure 2-11). At the individual level change can be expected to occur among the more affluent citizens without much intervention, but the majority, and especially the poor and socially isolated, will require more intensive and coordinated effort to be reached and persuaded to make changes in their behavior or environment. At the organizational level supports for individual change can be mobilized through advocacy, consultation, professional networks, and training of agency leaders and staff.

At the governmental level local, state, or national government agencies and legislative bodies can be mobilized in support of community programs through advocacy groups such as Students Against Drunk Driving, who insist on better enforcement of existing regulations or the passage of more restrictive legislation. Individual health professionals and other citizens also can bring about change in governmental support for community health by giving testimony at city council, state, or national legislative hearings, or at public hearings of local government agencies contemplating revisions of rules, codes, or regulations. Health professionals and local groups also can support governmental action by preparing position papers analyzing the impact of proposed changes. Such papers can be presented to policy-making bodies, government agencies, and the

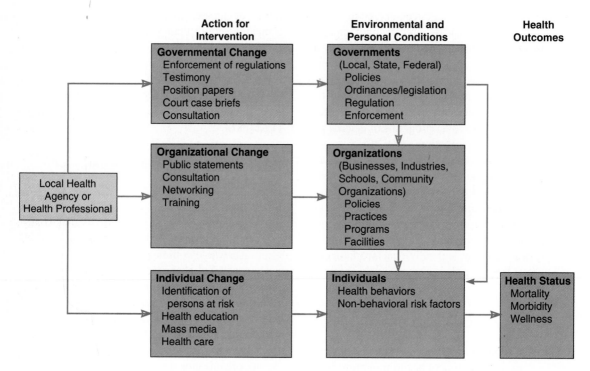

FIGURE 2-11

Levels of action for community health intervention suggest roles for various sectors, citizens, and professionals.

Adapted with permission from Brink SG et al: *Community intervention handbooks for comprehensive health promotion programming*, Atlanta, 1988, Centers for Disease Control.

press. Other actions and their targets are suggested by Figure 2-11.

One thesis of this book is that integrated community programs, as compared with the sum of numerous small-scale programs in a community, require a shift in perspective and the employment of a set of analytic and programmatic tools distinct from those used with individual patients, students, clients, or customers. The differences between small-scale and community programs reflect the distinctions between clinical and epidemiological methods of analysis, between psychological and sociological theories, between counseling and mass-media methods of communication, between accounting and economics, and between intraor-

ganizational and interorganizational levels of intervention and management.

THE MULTIPLE GOALS AND SECTORS OF COMMUNITY HEALTH

The 1990 Objectives for the Nation in disease prevention and health promotion described in Chapter 1 captured the imagination of many American health professionals and the commitment of some health organizations. The objectives for the year 2000 appear to be doing the same. If the enthusiasm and esprit de corps of health professionals were all that we needed to accomplish the objectives, the road to health for all by the year 2000 would indeed be smooth.

The reality of these health objectives is that most of them cannot and will not be accomplished by health professionals and health agencies alone. They require for their success the active participation of other sectors, other professionals, other institutions than those primarily identified with health (see Figures 1-1 and 2-11). Most of these nonhealth organizations operate at the community level. Schools, worksites, recreational facilities, social welfare agencies, restaurants, and supermarkets all have important roles to play in community health.

Not since the seventeenth century has the medical establishment—or for that matter the public health establishment—been more irrelevant to the task of improving the public's health. They possess the knowledge of what needs to be done, hence the ability to state achievable health objectives. But they are helpless by themselves to achieve most of those objectives. Success depends on reaching people where their daily decisions about the environment and life-style are influenced and made. This means reaching them in schools, in worksites, and in community settings other than medical.

Health professionals typically assume that their own coordinating ability will bring disparate interests into line. Such wishful thinking by the health professions is based on the mistaken impression that other sectors of human services are all too willing to set their own priorities aside if presented with a health problem or threat. Coordination was easier when epidemics were imminent enough to galvanize concerted community action. Not today.

A remarkable thing about the 1990 Objectives is that they drew any attention at all, considering their remote and sober character. They hardly had the siren appeal of the epidemics and scourges of the past. They scarcely competed even with matters of economics—the dismal science—much less with threats of war and nuclear holocaust. Little wonder then that other sectors and the public at large seem somewhat unresponsive when we call on them to

help achieve the disease prevention and health promotion objectives for the nation or for a community.

Building Coalitions on Mutual Interests

Why have nonhealth organizations shown even a glimmer of interest, considering all this? Two reasons seem to account for most of the interest shown by other sectors in community health promotion. One is the perceived demand of the public; the other is the possibility that it could contribute to other goals that they seek.

Perceiving a public demand for health promotion, better health protection, or health services, many organizations outside the health field have taken up health-related programs. Commercial interests, in particular, have risen to the challenge of consumer demand. Many organizations have begun to offer health promotion programs or facilities for their own employees. Some have justified these expenditures on the argument that they gain a competitive edge in attracting and holding the best employees.

The mutual interests of many public and private sectors in health issues has led to the development of community coalitions on specific health issues. Coalitions often include representation from recreation, business, media, and welfare sectors as well as medical and health sectors.

How did this consumer demand come about? Can we sustain it or even nurture it to gain even more support from other sectors? At least part of the answer to these questions lies in an enlightened public. Continuing health information and education programs will stimulate increased consumer discretion in matters of health. This in turn stimulates commercial and news media to provide yet more information, some of which strays from fact. This stimulates debate and controversy, further whetting the public's appetite for more health information and education.

The downside to this escalating market of health ideas is the consequent glutting of information and the withering crossfire of health information presented in the media. The "carcinogen of the week" race between agencies such as the National Cancer Institute, the Food and Drug Administration, the American Cancer Society, and between all of them and the tobacco and polluting chemical industries makes the legitimate messages of any of them lose credibility and impact. The public pleads for relief from this tumult. Nowhere does the cooperation of public and private organizations in various sectors promise greater relief for the public than in the development of consensus on selected health messages and the dissemination of joint communications such as the dietary guidelines for Americans or the Canadian Food Guidelines. The objectives for the nation in disease prevention and health promotion offer such consensus points among community service agencies and commercial organizations that can be presented to the public with one voice.

Planning and Implementing Community Programs

Community-wide programs require, above all, more planning and coordination than do small-scale programs. More participants in planning and execution means more meetings and telephone calls to achieve consensus, more letters and documents to convey concepts and procedures to more varied actors. The complexities grow exponentially with each organization added to the roster of participants. The point of efficiency in numbers comes only when added organizations can be matched or clustered into partnership according to their similarities and mutual interests. Typically, such a point is not reached until a large number of dissimilar organizations have been accumulated. In short, a truly orchestrated community program—as distinct from numerous replications of a small-scale program—requires additional planning and coordination for each unique unit added, because each new organization added to the program calls for its own functions and role in the larger community program.

The number of units (organizations, clinics, schools, persons) reaches a point where newcomers are more and more likely to be similar to some previous comers. At that point large-scale programs begin to realize an **economy of scale.** This means that for each newcomer the job of planning and coordination gets easier because it is more and more likely to be repetitious. The cost in time, effort, and resources per unit of production or service goes down as the number of organizations and people reached goes up. Some programs never reach this threshold, because their initial planning, production of materials, or coordination fail in the early stages to satisfy early participants and thereby fail to establish the program's reputation and to ensure its **diffusion.**

Diffusion of a new program or practice depends first on satisfying the early adopters and then on timing and placing interventions strategically according to stages in the natural history of the diffusion process. The natural history of the diffusion process across organizations follows a logistic curve similar to that of the diffusion of innovations or ideas in a population, as shown in Figure 2-12.

Theories associated with the diffusion curve can describe and explain important features of the diffusion process: (1) the characteristics and distribution of individuals or organizations according to their relative time of adoption; and (2) the forces pushing the diffusion process forward and those holding it back at each stage. This same curve describes the diffusion or rate of spread of an infection or epidemic in the community.

The classification and distribution of adopters. Figure 2-12 shows the normal distribution of adoption over time, with the curve divided into standard deviations from the theoretical midpoint of the program or diffusion process. This curve has a vertical axis of percentage of *new* people or organizations adopting an idea or program *at a given point in time.*

A community health program seldom enters at time zero on the adoption curve to stimulate or pre-

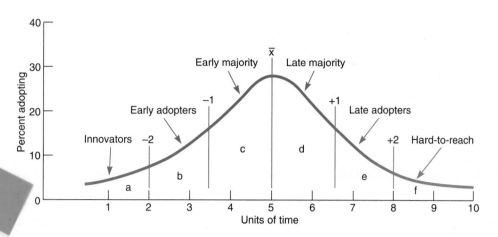

FIGURE 2-12

Over time the distribution of people adopting a new idea or innovation tends to follow the normal or bell-shaped curve. Classifying people by standard deviations of their time of adoption from the average time produces categories of adopters who differ also in their response to different communication channels.

From Green LW et al: Diffusion theory extended and applied. In Ward WB, Lewis FM, editors: *Advances in health education and promotion,* vol 3, London, 1991, Jessica Kingsley, pp 91-117.

vent the diffusion of a health practice. It is no criticism of government to say that in free-market economies with high literacy rates and extensive communication networks, the innovators and early adopters (indeed, often the majority of citizens) have been ''skimmed'' by commercial interests by the time government is called upon to take action. In fact, the relative deprivation of those who could not avail themselves of privately sponsored programs or services is often the very impetus for government initiative in health. The previous adoption by the affluent and the middle majority causes a health-related innovation to be perceived increasingly as a benefit, first negotiated in collective bargaining, then demanded as a right. Whether in the interest of equity or in the interest of health as a right, government agencies often undertake large-scale programs in public health when previously acceptable circumstances have been recast in the public's perception as unsatisfactory.

For example, when a new drug, vaccine, or medical procedure is approved by the Food and Drug Administration, it is immediately prescribed to or purchased over the counter by the more affluent segment of the community. Later, the health department may be directed to make the same product available to the poor at reduced cost.

The late point of entry on the diffusion curve has several implications for community health programs. Certain of these implications distinguish such government or voluntary agency programs from large-scale commercial marketing efforts. Some would like to imagine that all that is needed for the success of community health programs is to employ marketing principles and strategies. The implicit criticism that community health agencies have failed where commercial marketing has succeeded is an unfair oversimplification of the task community health faces. A percentage-point gain in the early-adopter phase when commercial interests prevail is much easier to obtain than a percentage-point gain in the late-adopter phase when nonprofit organizations pick up the responsibility to reach the poor or isolated segment of the population.

Innovators and **early adopters** in Figure 2-12 typically are more affluent and attuned to the national media. They are cosmopolitans who know the most about health, can afford the most in private purchase of health care products and services, and least need some of the products and services they buy. They are the ''upscale'' market of Madison Avenue and the social models for the majority. Mass media alone can suffice in reaching them.

The **middle majority** of people in the diffusion curve (the early majority and late majority in Figure 2-12) attend less to national media and more to local media, and respond less to the media in general than to interpersonal influence. This is why most of the programs in community health put so much emphasis on involving the local media and organizational channels of communication rather than depending on network broadcasts or national publications. This middle majority is the primary target of those public health programs addressing problems for which everybody has life-style concerns, such as fitness, stress, nutrition, and injury control programs. These problems and concerns relate to socially and culturally conditioned behaviors embedded in a complex web of life-style. This fact, in addition to the characteristics of people in this phase of the diffusion process, makes organizational and institutional channels essential to the health promotion strategies required to support changes in behavior. The media alone no longer suffice. The cooperation of institutions such as schools and of private organizations such as worksites, clubs, and churches is required to reach people effectively at this stage.

Finally, the **late adopters** and the ''hard-to-reach'' in Figure 2-12 are even more likely to be the primary targets of public health campaigns, especially in the preventive health services, which focus on such concerns as hypertension, immunization, maternal and child health, family planning, and occupational health and safety. The people and organizations in these late-adopter categories are typically disadvantaged in economic or status terms, they are socially more isolated or alienated, and they tend to be suspicious of organizations, including government agencies that purport to help them. Their use of the media is more exclusively for entertainment, and their membership in organizations or coalitions is sporadic and limited in comparison with that of the earlier adopters. Reaching these people and organizations requires more expensive and labor-intensive forms of community organization, communication, and outreach. Home visits, personal counseling and small group meetings require more effort and personnel. The payoff is often greater because of this group's high health risk, but the cost per unit of service effectively delivered is necessarily higher.

Communication channels need to adapt their messages to the forces operating variously at successive stages of community programs. Recognizing that many of the forces pushing or inhibiting the diffusion and adoption process are not strictly personal or motivational, community health promotion programs seek to mobilize organizational, economic, and environmental supports for the changes advocated.

Examples of organizational strategies that complement communications to the public may be found in high blood pressure programs and alcoholism detection programs. These give particular attention to the mobilization of community organizations. They also emphasize the channeling of communications through worksites and churches where interpersonal influence can complement the formal efforts of the media. In California a media campaign called ''Friends Are Good Medicine'' appealed to the public to seek out their friends when they felt depressed, bereaved, or under stress. This approach made the reduction of social isolation both a means and an end in itself. By encouraging the contact of people with their social support networks, the mental health goals of the program were served and the diffusion process was facilitated.

DECENTRALIZATION AND PARTICIPATION

One thing common to community programs and small-scale programs is the importance of the principle of participation. It applies equally to organizations and individuals, to highly educated and illiterate people. Involving people actively in identifying their own needs, setting their own priorities and goals, and planning their own programs of change is necessary at the individual, organizational, community, and national levels. The paradox for large-scale programs is that almost by definition they require a degree of centralization of authority and responsibility. Decentralization has occurred most commonly in the implementation of community programs, not in their planning or evaluation. As a result the concept of community participation has a bad reputation in some circles as a form of exploitation, co-optation, or cheap labor for central agencies. Large-scale programs ideally favor localized neighborhood planning, implementation, and evaluation.

Asking neighborhoods and organizations to implement programs planned elsewhere usually yields only limited local commitment to the goals and methods of the programs. People need to be consulted from the start in assessing their needs and setting priorities. Whether the outside ''help'' comes in the form of finances, technical consultation, or other resources, people in neighborhoods, organizations, or communities are more likely to accept and use those resources if they have participated actively in identifying their own needs and priorities.

The ideal decentralization of community programs is to place the planning and evaluation functions at the local level and the highly specialized resources, including expensive technology and facilities, at the central level. The effective delivery of such programs necessarily depends on local organizations, and it should not be expected to occur without the transfer of planning and evaluation functions to the local level as well.

The Community Development Model

How can communities take responsibility for their own health aspirations and the solution of their own health problems if they lack some of the resources needed? How can state and national organizations support community health without undermining the initiative and self-reliance that communities need to develop? How can the many sectors collaborate in community health if they each have state, provincial, or national headquarters that direct their priorities? For example, how can the local cancer society and a local manufacturing plant collaborate on the development of a worksite breast cancer education program for female employees if both organizations need support and approval from their parent organizations at the regional or corporate level?

The organizational model for community health promotion most likely to succeed if the concepts of decentralized, multisectoral, and participatory planning and implementation are fully expressed in policy and practice is the community development model. This model sequences and balances community (decentralized) functions and regional or national (centralized) functions as shown in Table 2-2.

This sequence and allocation of roles to local and centralized agencies assumes some form of grants to communities and a stimulus for coordinated planning at the community level. Such a complex process would not be needed if there were no prior existence of fragmented sectoral programs, no tradition of centralized planning and implementation of programs, and no barriers to coordination to be overcome.

Table 2-2 illustrates how the steps in the community development process ideally should play out at the community level with maximum participation and intersectoral involvement. The first step should be initiated locally by members of the community rather than by central planning agencies. Health professionals can aid the local assessment and priority-

TABLE 2-2

The ideal sequence of steps in the decentralization of planning, implementation, and evaluation, and the use of centralized resources.

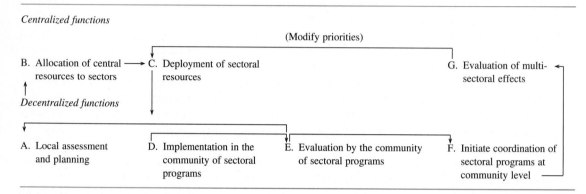

setting processes through health education and technical assistance in data collection and analysis.

At B the state, provincial, or national organization takes a more active role. Centralized agencies or corporate headquarters will be faced with competing demands and expectations from various local constituents, so they must make decisions on the allocation of centralized resources (funds, technical assistance, and materials). They do this through procedures such as review of grant applications and allocation by formulas based on need as estimated by the population size or wealth of local communities requesting support and on political considerations such as the influence of the local community on legislators or other decision makers.

At C the centralized organizations (state or national agencies, foundations, or corporate home offices) ideally would work out the coordination of resources with other centralized organizations in health and in other sectors to minimize the duplication of resources being channeled to the local community. The coordination among central offices also serves to reduce the bureaucratic inconsistencies in rules and regulations that accompany grants or other forms of assistance to local communities. If the American Heart Association and the American

Lung Association, for example, wish to cooperate in supporting a local smoking prevention project, they need to work out their conflicting rules on the use of their respective national resources for local projects.

In D the responsibility ideally falls to the local community to decide whether the forms of assistance, especially technological resources, are appropriate for their community needs. Too often in rural or underdeveloped communities the advanced technologies and written or video resources offered by central agencies are inappropriate for local application or maintenance. Some types of equipment, for example, will last only until it first needs repair; then it will rust in a storage room awaiting parts or technical repair skills unavailable in the local situation. Some educational materials produced by central agencies prove to be inappropriate for use in local populations because of the literacy level or specific cultural sensitivities.

Community Self-reliance

Starting with E, the community has the opportunity to develop increasing self-reliance. By documenting changes in the needs first identified in A, the com-

Case Study of Community Development

Andy Chelsea and his wife were the first tribal members to join Alcoholics Anonymous from the Alkali Lake Canadian Indian Reserve where they lived. Their personal histories led to Andy's election to Tribal Chairperson. In that office he was able not only to lead by example, but also to identify community needs and to organize for community reform around alcohol abuse issues. With the help of a growing number of community members, some in recovery themselves, he enacted regulations on bootlegging and importing of alcohol onto the reserve, revised rules on welfare payments for tribal members who refused to quit drinking to limit their payments to vouchers that could be redeemed only for food and clothing, he pressured the alcoholic priest to leave, he counseled and urged members to get treatment for their alcoholism, he started community development projects such as housing renovations for members who quit drinking, and he established community development programs in education and job training. The prevalence of alcohol abuse in the tribe dropped from 97% in the early 1970s to 5% in 1981 (Guillory, Willie, and Duran, 1988).

How did the personal histories of the Chelseas lead to community organizing and social change in Alkali Lake? How did the diffusion of the nondrinking norm support community development in Alkali Lake? How did centralized resources (like Alcoholics Anonymous and the government welfare agency) support local development in this community?

TABLE 2-3
Model standards for community participation and training in community organization

Objective 1

By _____ each community will utilize open participatory processes in developing community health policies and plans.

Objective 2

By _____ a mechanism will exist in the community to ensure that:
    a. Official health agency staff will be trained in facilitating open processes to obtain public advice and guidance.
    b. Members of health-oriented boards, committees, task forces, etc. will be provided an orientation and training.

Source: Healthy communities 2000: model standards, Washington, DC, 1991, American Public Health Association

at the central level to form new partnerships or strengthen old alliances among central organizations to fill gaps in services and resources needed by communities.

Table 2-3 shows the model standards for community participation and training in community organization that support these steps.

SUMMARY

Human ecology provides an understanding and appreciation of the interdependence of a human population and its physical and biological setting. This, together with an understanding of the social and economic processes of community organization, gives definition to the concept of community. Further understanding from the social and behavioral sciences concerning how people feel about belonging and cooperating gives meaning to the subjective ''sense of community'' that makes possible many of the collective efforts and sacrifices of individual pursuits necessary for the promotion and protection

munity obtains feedback and reinforcement on its progress in meeting those needs. This builds local confidence and a sense of hope in their ability to solve their own problems using indigenous resources and talents.

The community also should have the opportunity to participate in the evaluation of the community efforts supported by multiple sectors or centralized agencies. F shows this step leading to G, in which centralized agencies review the data from various communities and decide how they can work together

of the population's health. Enhancing the health and reducing the social and economic impact of premature death and disability of the entire community are the major goals of community health. Higher morale, greater productivity, and reduction in disease and costs of health care all represent the potential benefits of a community health program. Models to understand how these goals and benefits have been accomplished in the past and how they can be achieved in the future have been presented in this chapter. The epidemiological context of these and other problems and potentials for community health are the subjects of the following chapter.

QUESTIONS FOR REVIEW

1. What are the advantages and disadvantages of a high degree of mobility in a population?
2. What constitutes the community in which you live?
3. What favorable characteristics would you look for in a community?
4. How would you describe the social history of health in the neighborhood in which you live?
5. How can one dramatic incident unite a community in a common health cause?
6. How can one citizen provide the spark necessary to deal with a long-existing, unresolved health problem?
7. How does a particular industry attract a particular type of people with particular health problems?
8. What are some obstacles to community health progress?
9. Is this statement true: "It is impossible to eliminate community customs but not difficult to modify them"?
10. Why should churches have an interest in community health?
11. How does economics enter into community health promotion?
12. Evaluate this statement: "Transient families are community health liabilities."

READINGS

Committee on Fuel Economy of Automobiles and Light Trucks, Energy Engineering Board, National Academy of Sciences: *Automotive fuel economy: how far should we go?* Washington, DC, 1992, National Academy Press.

Illustrates the trade-offs between strategies to maximize fuel economy (including smaller cars) and strategies to minimize injuries and air pollution. In a given community, costs of transportation and jobs may also be at stake in fuel economy measures.

MacNeill J, Winsemius P, Yakushiji T: *Beyond interdependence: the meshing of the world's economy and the earth's ecology,* London, New York, Toronto, 1991, Oxford University Press.

Presents the key issues and options debated by the first United Nations Earth Summit in Rio de Janeiro in 1992. Recommends a worldwide monitoring system to track the impact of climate change. Suggests realistic steps to achieve sustainable development.

Robichaud J-B, Quiviger C: *Active communities,* Ottawa, 1991, Canadian Council on Social Development.

Examines the state of community health and social service centers in all ten provinces of Canada; notes differences between types of centers, between types of communities, and between sources of support for community programs.

Stokols D: Establishing and maintaining healthy environments: toward a social ecology of health promotion, *Am Psychol* 47:6, 1992.

Presents the advantages of integrating life-style modification, injury control, and environmental enhancement strategies of health promotion. Describes a multilevel approach to community health, including person-focused and environment-focused strategies such as urban planning, land use policy, ergonomic and organizational development.

Stryker J, Jonsen AR, editors: *The social impact of AIDS,* Washington, DC, 1992, National Academy Press.

Examines the social and political impact of AIDS on communities and society. Forecasts the effects over the next decade when a million or more Americans will likely die of the disease; the role of public agencies, churches, community-based organizations.

BIBLIOGRAPHY

Barringer F: Shift for urban renewal: nurture the grass roots, *New York Times,* Nov. 29, 1992.

Board on Science and Technology for International Development: *Saline agriculture: salt-tolerant plants for developing countries,* Washington, DC, 1990, National Academy Press.

Bracht N, editor: *Health promotion at the community level,* New York, 1990, Sage.

Brink SG, et al: Community intervention handbooks for comprehensive health promotion planning, *Fam Community Health* 11:28, 1988.

Brundtland GH, chair, World Commission on Environment and Development: *Our common future,* New York, 1987, Oxford University Press.

Daily G, Cobb J: *For the common good: redirecting the economy towards community, the environment, and a sustainable future,* Boston, 1989, Beacon Press.

Dean K, Hancock T: *Supportive environments for health: major policy and research issues in creating health promoting environments,* Copenhagen, 1992, World Health Organization Regional Office for Europe.

Dever GEA: *Community health analysis: global awareness at the local level,* Gaithersberg, Md, 1991, Aspen.

English JCB, Hicks BC: A systems-in-transition paradigm for healthy communities, *Can J Public Health* 38:61, 1992.

Giampietro M, Pimentel D: Energy analysis models to study the biophysical limits for human exploitation of natural process. In Rossi C and Tiezzi E: *Ecological physical chemistry,* Amsterdam, 1990, Elsevier.

Green LW: The revival of community and the obligation of academic health centers to the public. In Bulger RE, Reiser SJ, editors: *Integrity in health care institutions: humane environments for teaching, inquiry and practice,* Des Moines, 1990, University of Iowa Press.

Green LW, Gottlieb NH, Parcel G: Diffusion theory extended and applied. In Ward WB, Lewis FM, editors: *Advances in health education and promotion,* vol 3, London, 1991, Jessica Kingsley.

Guillory B, Willie E Jr, Duran E: Analysis of a community organizing case study: Alkali Lake, *J Rural Psychol* 9:27, 1988.

Healthy communities 2000: model standards, ed 3, Washington, DC, 1991, American Public Health Association.

Jacobs P: *The economics of health and medical care,* ed 3, Gaithersberg, MD, 1991, Aspen.

Johnson D: Forget the last picture show; in some towns the bank and the school are closing, too, *New York Times,* Aug. 18, 1991.

Jones RR, Wigley T: *Ozone depletion: health and environmental consequences,* New York, 1989, John Wiley.

Khassay HM: Wisdom and guidance from the community, *World Health,* May-June 1992.

Lawson JS: *Public health in Australia: an introduction,* Roseville & Auckland, 1991, McGraw-Hill.

Levin LS: Listen to the community, *World Health,* May-June 1992.

McMillan DW, Chavis DM: Sense of community: a definition and theory, *J Community Psychol* 14:6, 1986.

Minority health resources directory, Rockville, Md, 1991, ANROW.

O'Neill M: Community health projects in Quebec: can they participate significantly to promote the health of the population in the years to come? *Health Promotion* 4:189, 1989.

Patton RD, Cissell WB, editors: *Community organization: traditional principles and modern applications,* Johnson City, Tenn, 1989, Latchpins.

Perreault R, Roy D, Renaud L: Promotion de la santé: un exersice de mise en application de la Charte d'Ottawa, *Can J Public Health* 83:37, 1992.

Schmidheiny S, with the Business Council for Sustainable Development: *Changing course,* Cambridge, Mass, 1992, MIT Press.

Schneider SH: *Global warming,* New York, 1990, Random House.

Varilla J: Making things whole, *New York Times Mag,* Sept. 27, 1992.

Vega WA: Theoretical and pragmatic implications of cultural diversity for community research, *Am J Community Psychol* 20:375, 1992.

Weil DEC et al: *The impact of development policies on health: a review of the literature,* Geneva, 1990, World Health Organization.

World Resources Institute: *World resources 1992-93: a guide to the global environment,* Oxford and New York, 1992, Oxford University Press.

Chapter 3

Community Diversity, Demography, and Epidemiology

Each of us is responsible for everything, and to every human being.
    DOSTOEVSKI

OBJECTIVES

When you finish this chapter, you should be able to:

- Identify and describe elements of demography that apply to community diversity and change
- Compute some basic statistics for a community epidemiological analysis
- Distinguish between incidence and prevalence
- Distinguish between life span and life expectancy

Demography reflects population diversity and trends by studying population composition, growth, and movement. Birth, death, and migration data from demography combine with the study of disease transmission and development in populations to constitute **epidemiology.**

DEMOGRAPHY

Ecology leaves off with the study of the physical and biological interactions of human populations with their environments. Demography takes up the study of population trends as measured over time by vital indexes such as birth and death rates and population diversity measures such as density, rural-urban-suburban residential patterns, and migration, and socioeconomic indicators such as income, occupation, race, and ethnicity.

Seasonal variations in population movement and vital rates result partly from climate and partly from cultural and social conditions affecting employment and traditions associated with seasons and holidays. In North America, for example, the highest death rates tend to occur in the winter months, as shown in Figure 3-1. The holiday season of Christmas and New Year's contribute a large share of the increase through automobile crashes, suicides, and heart attacks. The relatively higher incidence of respiratory conditions and associated deaths in the winter attests to some climatic effect, but not just because of exposure to cold temperatures. Some of it is attributable to being more exposed to the transmission of communicable diseases among people confined indoors. The latter explanation suggests that social norms of adaptation to climatic conditions are important both in providing protection and in exposing the individual to additional risks.

The growing capacity to insulate, heat, and air-condition large indoor spaces brings more people together. Indoor air pollution is becoming as much an issue in community health as outdoor air pollution has been in the past. The ability of new populations to grow in regions previously considered uninhabitable has been made possible by these expansions of air-tight indoor space.

Seasonal adjustments on vital rates are made by averaging monthly rates for several consecutive months, as shown in Figure 3-2, *A*. Note that although North American and European marriage rates follow a predictable pattern of seasonal and monthly variation, fertility rates are much less predictable and less associated with marriage rates than one might expect. The pattern of births is more predictable in some primitive and traditional societies where cultural and social restrictions on birth control are greater. Society imposes both positive and negative influences on natural cycles and conditions.

Population Growth

From 1910 to 1991 the world population increased from 1.5 to 5.4 billion (Figure 3-3). The rate of increase is such that, if maintained, the population will double in 40 years. However, the world birthrate declined from 34 per 1000 in 1965 to below 30 per 1000 in recent years for the first time in recorded

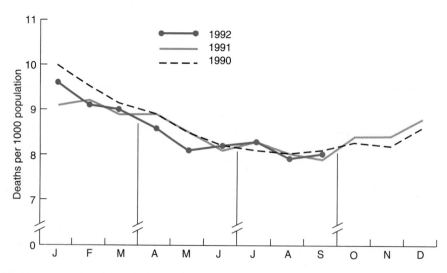

FIGURE 3-1
Seasonal variations can be seen in the consistent patterns of monthly mortality rates per 1000 population from year to year.

Source: National Center for Health Statistics, U.S. Department of Health and Human Services, 1993.

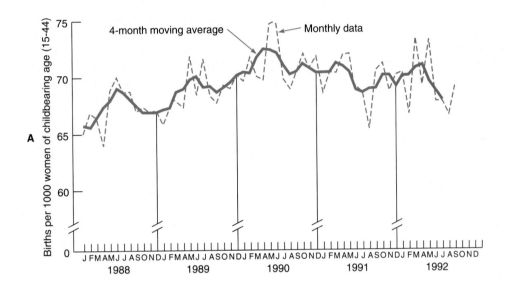

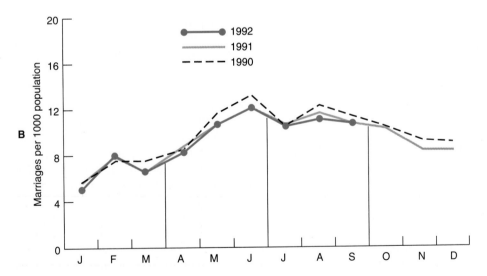

FIGURE 3-2
Seasonal variations in fertility rates (**A**), whether adjusted or unadjusted, do not follow the same variations seen in marriage rates (**B**) because people vary in their fecundity and birth control practices.
Source: National Center for Health Statistics, U.S. Department of Health and Human Services, 1993.

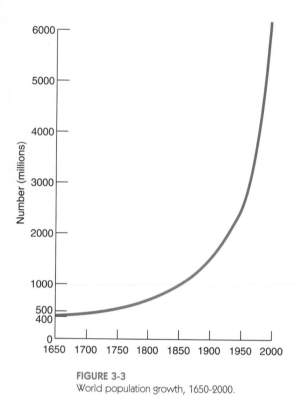

FIGURE 3-3
World population growth, 1650-2000.

Chapter 2 introduced diffusion theory with a curve that described the growth or spread of an innovation in a population. Exactly the same mathematical principle of growth or spread applies to human population growth and the spread of communicable disease. The essential underpinning of diffusion theory and of demography is the simple mathematical law of nature that defines any spreading or growing process as a logistic function. This means that each new cell, organism, person, or adopter has the possibility, respectively, of dividing, reproducing, or influencing at least one more of its kind. The progression is then geometric: 1 becomes 2, 2 becomes 4, 4 becomes 8, with each generation or unit of time realizing a doubling of the number from the previous generation or unit of time. You can see the shape of this accelerated growth curve by simply plotting the numbers, 1, 2, 4, 8, 16, and 32 on a sheet of graph paper as shown in Figure 3-5. If this same curve were plotted on logarithmic graph paper, it would take the form of a straight diagonal line, hence the name ''logistic function.''

The growth curve continues to increase the rate of growth in numbers until it reaches a natural limit. This is where the curve representing the diffusion or epidemic process differs from the reproductive growth curve. All three phenomena have a natural limit on accelerated growth, so the shapes of the curves ultimately are similar, as shown by the broken line forming the S-shaped curve in Figure 3-5, but the causes of the limits differ. Diffusion slows down when the number of new people available to adopt an innovation no longer exceeds the number of people who have already adopted it—that is, at the halfway point in the existing population. Population growth slows down when the size of the population exceeds the resources available to sustain continued growth. New offspring or their parents starve, cannibalize, or commit suicide, infanticide, or fratricide; or people voluntarily limit their reproduction before their population reaches such limits.

demography, bringing the world growth rate closer to that of Western countries such as the United States (Figure 3-4). The United Nations and the World Bank predict that world population will not stabilize until it reaches 10 or 11 billion people within the next 150 years. Technological, legislative, economic, climatic, and cultural influences on population growth make long-term predictions highly speculative.

Two thirds of the people of the world do not have sufficient food, with over 450 million severely malnourished. Where starvation exists, disease flourishes, because the malnourished are more susceptible to infection. Famines cause people to migrate and, by so doing, to spread infectious disease and to redistribute populations as seen recently in Somalia.

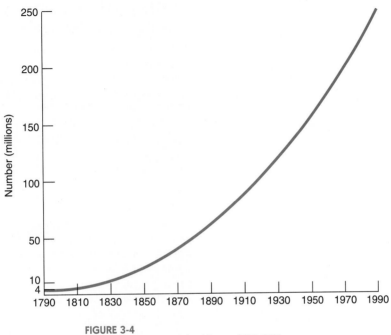

FIGURE 3-4
Resident population, United States, 1790-1990.

Biotic Potential

Population changes reflect the **biotic potential** of a nation as related to environmental resistance. Environmental resistance is expressed in terms of parasitism, food supply, floods, cold, heat, fuel supply, and other factors that may affect life adversely. The biotic potential of the human species is generally thought of as a **fecundity** level that would produce a birthrate of 50 per 1000 per year. This rate was attained in the Ukraine over a 5-year period and in Bengal over a 10-year period. During the 10-year period from 1930 to 1940, the Warm Springs Indians of Oregon had an average birthrate of 50 per 1000 per year. Scientific advances in the prevention and correction of human infertility and sterility could raise the present acknowledged maximum human birthrate, but declining family size preferences in most countries make it unlikely that the maxmimum will be tested.

Government Policy

A pronatal government policy incorporates inducements and rewards for large families; the reverse is true of antinatal policy. Canadian and U.S. policies have been inconsistent in this regard. Both the birthrate per 1000 population and the absolute number of births were falling between 1957 and 1977. A reversal in this trend seemed to correspond with the "pro-life" policy. The United States saw more babies born in 1991 than it will see again until the year 2080 (see Chapter 7). This so-called "baby-boomlet" yielded 4.1 million births in 1991, the largest number in 24 years, but still fewer than the 4.3 million births in 1957, the peak year of the postwar baby boom.

The total number of new births minus deaths in a given year make up the **natural increase.** The rate of natural increase is the difference between births per 1000 population and deaths per 1000 population.

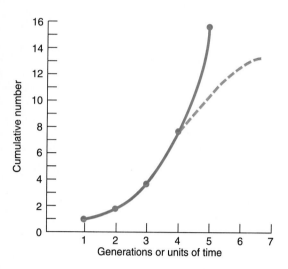

FIGURE 3-5

The geometric rate of growth or diffusion illustrates how quickly a population can grow or a disease can spread when unchecked. The dotted line reflects the usual S-shaped curve of diffusion, epidemic spread, or reproductive growth when natural limits take hold. Consider the implications for Figures 3-3 and 3-4.

The Tragedy of the Commons

Garrett Hardin (1968) revived a scenario first told in 1833 by a mathematical amateur named William Forster Lloyd. It was a rebuttal to the Malthusian doctrine of natural limits on population growth and Adam Smith's notion of "the invisible hand" in economic affairs. Malthus believed that populations would stop growing when resources became too limited to support further growth. Smith believed that individuals pursuing only their own gain would be "led by an invisible hand to promote ... the public interest." Lloyd created and Hardin popularized the analogy of individual farmers grazing ever-increasing numbers of cows on a common pasture, until each additional cow caused overgrazing to the detriment of all. They applied this analogy to illustrate the tragedy of individual procreation beyond the point of community resources to provide for the sustenance of all. The individual might gain in the short run, but both the individual and the community will suffer in the long run.

How might the same tragedy be seen in the short-term gratification of indulgent, sedentary, or reckless behavior of individuals relative to the long-term well-being of the community?

If the United States has a birthrate (Figure 3-6) of 16 per 1000 and a death rate (see Figure 3-1) of 8.5 per 1000, the rate of natural increase is 7.5. When a nation's rate of natural increase begins to approach 2, that nation's population is becoming stable. If deaths exceed births in a community, the community will have a negative rate of natural increase symptomatic of population decline, unless it also receives a large influx of immigrants. Nations with declining birth rates and declining death rates will tend to have high rates of growth in their older populations, as seen in Figure 3-7.

Food Limits

In the 1960s and 1970s food production increased at a faster pace in the developing countries than in the developed countries, yet because of much higher population growth rates in the developing countries, per capita food supplies are becoming smaller where the need is greatest. In Africa, in particular, food production per capita has declined dramatically in recent years, mainly because of population growth. If present trends continue, substantial portions of the developing world will encounter rapidly increasing grain shortages and increasing hunger and malnutrition as domestic demand outstrips the ability of nations to grow or purchase their own food (Figure 3-8).

The wealth and abundance of food in the developed nations still leaves pockets of poor, hungry people within their national borders. Readily identifiable groups with a high incidence of hunger in the United States are migrant and seasonal farm workers, native Alaskans, American Indians, the el-

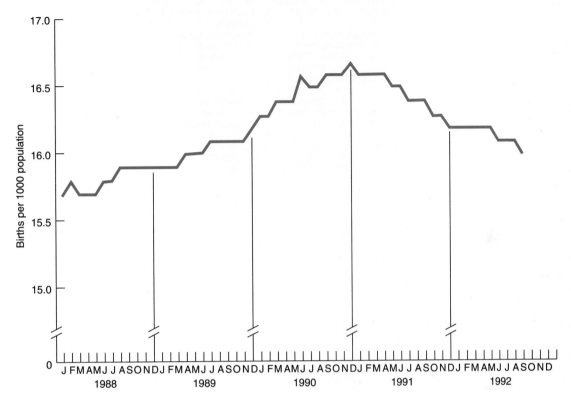

FIGURE 3-6
Birth rates per 1000 population for successive 12-month periods ending with month indicated, United States, 1988-1992.
Source: National Center for Health Statistics, *Monthly Vital Statistics Report,* vol 41, no 9, 1993.

derly, and those with incomes below the poverty level.

The U.S. Food Stamp, Meals on Wheels, and Women-Infants-Children (WIC) programs have made great improvements in the nutrition of the poor. The persistence of hunger and malnutrition in the United States can be attributed in part to the fact that only about 60% of the eligible poor persons participate. Budget cuts in these programs in the 1980s made this situation worse. Significant improvements in nutrition could be achieved by increasing participation in these programs without instituting new programs.

Most countries can produce sufficient food for their current populations. Distribution of food still poses a problem. The critical problems created by the present population increase and distribution are high prices and inflation, waste disposal, transportation, and fuel supply. These problems challenge economic means, technological creativity, and political will.

Fuel Limits

The Western world faced a major fuel crisis some 400 years ago when Europe ran out of wood. Since

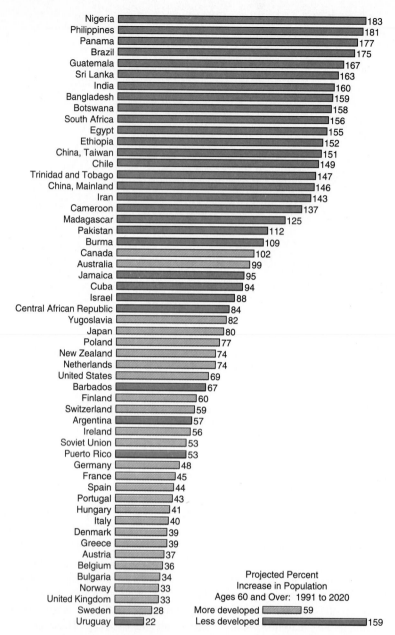

Nigeria 183
Philippines 181
Panama 177
Brazil 175
Guatemala 167
Sri Lanka 163
India 160
Bangladesh 159
Botswana 158
South Africa 156
Egypt 155
Ethiopia 152
China, Taiwan 151
Chile 149
Trinidad and Tobago 147
China, Mainland 146
Iran 143
Cameroon 137
Madagascar 125
Pakistan 112
Burma 109
Canada 102
Australia 99
Jamaica 95
Cuba 94
Israel 88
Central African Republic 84
Yugoslavia 82
Japan 80
Poland 77
New Zealand 74
Netherlands 74
United States 69
Barbados 67
Finland 60
Switzerland 59
Argentina 57
Ireland 56
Soviet Union 53
Puerto Rico 53
Germany 48
France 45
Spain 44
Portugal 43
Hungary 41
Italy 40
Denmark 39
Greece 39
Austria 37
Belgium 36
Bulgaria 34
Norway 33
United Kingdom 33
Sweden 28
Uruguay 22

Projected Percent
Increase in Population
Ages 60 and Over: 1991 to 2020

More developed 59
Less developed 159

According to the classification used by the United Nations, more-developed countries
include all nations in Europe and North America, plus Japan, Australia, and New Zealand.
The remaining nations of the world comprise the less-developed category.

FIGURE 3-7
Percentage increases in older populations (ages 60 and over) of selected countries projected from 1991 to
2020.

Source: Economics and Statistics Administration: *Global aging—comparative indicators and future trends,* Washington, DC,
1991, U.S. Department of Commerce.

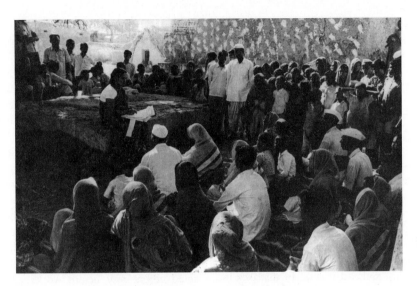

FIGURE 3-8
Treating malnutrition is feasible but inefficient compared with the possibility of prevention through nutrition education, agricultural development, and family planning programs. Here a government worker in India provides nutrition education in a village.

Photo courtesy World Health Organization.

time immemorial wood had provided heat and shelter. The dense forests that covered the continent and the British Isles seemed inexhaustible, and no thought was given to conservation or management. As long as the population remained relatively sparse and stable, the consequences were not serious. But in the sixteenth century prices for firewood and lumber suddenly began to skyrocket.

The shortage was particularly acute in England and Wales, whose collective population had doubled within a century and a half—from about 3 million in 1550 to twice that figure by 1690. At the same time the mass movement from country to city got under way, creating excessive demands for building material. London alone grew from 60,000 inhabitants in 1534 to some 530,000 in 1696, making it the largest city in Europe and perhaps in the world.

Similar trends marked the population explosion throughout much of Europe, but other pressures contributed to depleting its forest reserves: the shipbuilding boom in the age of exploration, the soaring production of metal ore mines with their wood-burning smelteries, and the rising consumption of wood pulp—used in the manufacture of paper—following the invention of printing.

Eventually coal came to the rescue. A massive shift from wood to coal, along with the discovery of vast new forest reserves in the New World, helped to overcome the crisis. Coal, however, turned out to be much more than a mere substitute; compact and efficient as a fuel, it made possible a whole new technology that led to the industrial revolution and ultimately to many of our current worldwide difficulties. It also now contributes much of the carbon dioxide to the atmosphere, which is producing the "greenhouse effect" discussed in Chapter 2.

One lesson of this earlier near-disaster is that

there are few final answers. But if each solution engenders new problems, facing up to them is what led society out of the Stone Age—reason enough to hope that the latest oil and nuclear fuel challenges will again be met.

EPIDEMIOLOGY

A companion science to ecology and demography in community health is epidemiology. All three represent perspectives on health that go beyond the individual. Whereas ecology views the individual in the context of environment, demography and epidemiology view the individual in the context of a population. Epidemiology is the science of the causes, frequencies, and distribution of diseases in a population.

Epidemiology differs in two essential respects from the study of medicine. First, epidemiology studies populations or groups rather than individuals; second, in studying whole populations, epidemiology measures health as well as disease, injury, and disability patterns. Its objective is to find causes (**etiologies**) of disease and patterns of transmission or distribution of disease and injury. Such information enables communities to locate points of intervention before people get sick or injured. In this respect epidemiology is the science of prevention.

The methods of epidemiology allow the community health worker to collect, tabulate, analyze, and interpret statistical facts about the occurrence of health problems, risk factors, and deaths in a community. Physicians, nurses, and others trained in clinical sciences sometimes have difficulty standing far away enough from the individual patient to see the larger patterns of disease occurrence in their population of patients, much less in their community. The epidemiological method and perspective on health enables clinical workers and public health officials to specify, describe, and understand such patterns so that they can see the common characteristics of those who have a certain problem in contrast to the characteristics of those who do not have the problem. The comparison may reveal the cause or the source of a disease of unknown origin. Most of the breakthroughs in medicine, especially preventive medicine, that emerged from the laboratory of an immunologist or a physiologist had their first leads from an epidemiologist or other investigator applying epidemiological methods.

Epidemiology's early preoccupation with epidemics gave it its name. The transmission of communicable diseases in populations, when traced systematically, provided clues to the mode of transmission. Some proved to be airborne, some waterborne, some foodborne, and some transmitted by an intermediate **host** or vector such as a rat, mosquito, fly, tick, or bird (Figure 3-9). Such clues enabled community health workers to interrupt the transmission of some diseases through quarantine, pest control, water purification, food protection, immunization, or solid waste disposal.

The methods of epidemiology have turned from communicable diseases to analyzing chronic diseases, degenerative diseases, and even injuries, addictions, and risk factors such as smoking, hypertension, obesity, and other behavioral patterns. These studies, again, have provided the clues and hypotheses on which advice to the public and further research have been based in developing national campaigns against smoking, alcohol and drug misuse, malnutrition, high blood pressure, dental caries, and injuries.

Epidemiological Comparisons

The fundamental tool of epidemiological analysis is comparison. The frequencies and distribution of diseases are compared by measures of incidence and prevalence. **Incidence** refers to the number of new cases or deaths of the disease or conditions that occur during a given time period (week, month, or year). **Prevalence** refers to the number of cases that exist at one point in time. Thus, incidence is influenced entirely by how rapidly a disease is spreading.

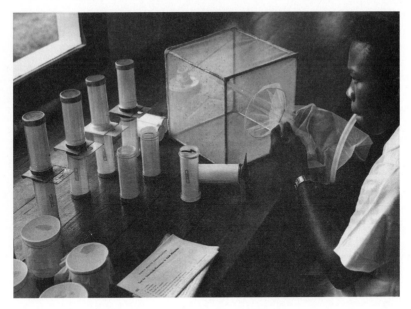

FIGURE 3-9
Studying the behavior of *Anopheles gambiae,* the mosquito that is the main carrier of malaria in Africa, this Liberian entomologist contributes to malaria control efforts.
Photo by P. Almasy, courtesy World Health Organization.

As such, it is the most sensitive measure of an outbreak or epidemic of a communicable or acute infectious or toxic agent disease. Prevalence is influenced both by incidence and by the duration of the disease or condition, hence its wider use in measuring chronic diseases and disabilities. Figure 3-10 illustrates the incidence of deaths from AIDS by year and the prevalence of AIDS cases.

It is difficult to measure the incidence of onset of chronic and degenerative diseases such as AIDS, because they are usually undetected until they reach an acute stage. Incidence rates for morbidity (onset) usually are derived from health department reporting systems that require hospitals, clinics, and even private physicians to report every new case of a communicable or infectious disease they encounter. Prevalence rates usually come from screening and detection programs and special surveys of populations.

To compare the incidence or prevalence of any two groups within a population, or the population of one community with another or with state or national averages, data must be standardized. The all-purpose method of standardization is to construct a **rate** or ratio so that the groups or populations to be compared have a "common denominator." In most comparisons the rate is constructed to make a unit of time, usually a year, the common denominator. Thus, the incidence rate is the number of cases per year. But this basis for comparison is not adequately standardized unless it is known how large the population was in which the incidence rate occurred. An epidemiological rate, then, is calculated as:

Rate = Number of events per population at risk

To make rates even more comparable, they are usually expressed as events per 1000 population, or for

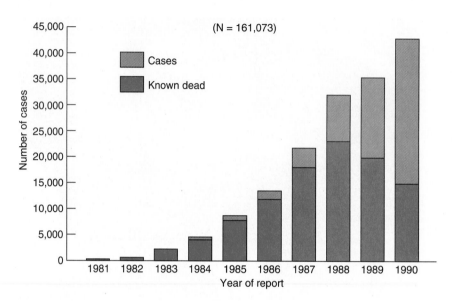

FIGURE 3-10
Acquired immunodeficiency syndrome (AIDS): cases and known deaths, by year of report to CDC, United States, 1981-1990.
Source: Centers for Disease Control and Prevention, 1992.

very rare events, per 10,000 or 100,000 population. Figure 3-11 illustrates the prevalence rates of AIDS cases, per 100,000 population in 1987, which permits a comparison between states or communities.

From demography, we borrow the following formula to calculate **crude death rate:**

$$\text{Crude death rate} = \frac{\text{All deaths during a calendar year}}{\text{Population at midyear}} \times 1000$$

This rate would be expressed as deaths per thousand population.

Age-specific rates. Because mortality varies so much by age, age-specific death rates need to be calculated whenever a comparison is being made between two communities or populations with different age distributions. Finding this **age-specific**

rate is done simply by dividing the number of deaths within each age group (usually 5-year or 10-year groupings) by the midyear population of the corresponding age groups, and multiplying each of these quotients by 1000. This procedure yields a series of rates for comparison, as shown for the city of Baltimore:

Death rates per 1000 population by age and race

	White	*Black*
All ages	15.2	9.8
< 1 year	13.5	22.6
1-4	0.6	1.0
5-17	0.4	0.5
18-44	1.5	3.6
45-64	10.7	18.8
65 and over	59.7	61.1

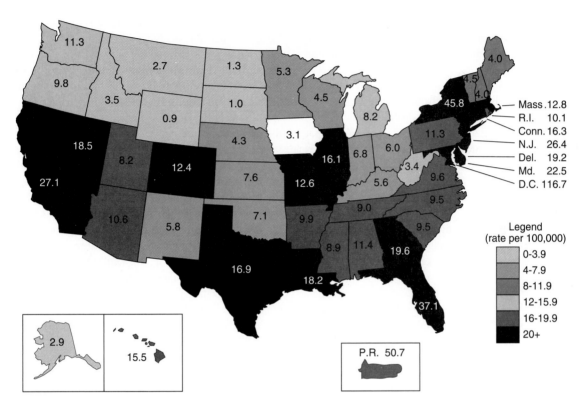

FIGURE 3-11

Annual rates of U.S. AIDS cases per 100,000 population, by state, October 1991 through September 1992.

Source: Centers for Disease Control and Prevention: *HIV/AIDS surveillance,* third quarter edition, Oct. 1992.

Several things about such a tabulation of age-specific and race-specific rates should catch your eye. First, you should be surprised to note that the overall rate for whites is higher than the rate for blacks, especially when you note further that each of the age-specific rates is lower for whites. How can the overall rate for whites be higher than that for blacks if each of the age-specific rates for whites is lower? Herein lies one of the most important lessons of demography and epidemiology. Think about this paradox while we examine a few other features of the tabulation.

Note that the most dramatic differences appear to be between the infant mortality rates and the rates for the 45- to 65-year age group. Infant and childhood mortality will be examined in Chapter 5, adolescent and adult mortality in Chapters 6 and 7, and mortality of the elderly in Chapter 8. For now, it is sufficient to note the high rates at the youngest and oldest age ranges, and the greatest differentials between races at the youngest and middle-adulthood age ranges. Once children of either race survive the vulnerable infancy stage, their death rates go down dramatically, then gradually upward from age 9 onward. This pattern of age-specific death rates is typical of developed countries, where the communicable diseases of childhood are largely under control. In developing countries, the rates for all ages are higher, but most distinctly higher for the childhood ages.

Relative risk. The substantial differences between age-specific and race-specific rates can be translated in terms of risk. This is precisely what insurance companies do in setting the premiums people have to pay for their policies. Rather than using the simple differences between rates, however, relative risk is conventionally expressed in epidemiology as a ratio. The **relative-risk ratio** states the proportionate or multiple risk of death, injury, disease, or disability among those exposed to a risk factor relative to those not exposed.

Relative risk =

$$\frac{\text{Incidence among those exposed}}{\text{Incidence among those not exposed}}$$

Note that the term *incidence* is used. This means that relative risk can apply to any condition for which data are available on the number of cases occurring or discovered over a specified period. With vital statistics such as births and deaths, and with reportable diseases, the period is usually one year. The same rates can be used in relation to pregnancies, automobile crashes, reported symptoms, absenteeism, and other events of community health significance. The risk factor can be a demographic characteristic such as age or race, or it can be a behavioral, environmental, or organizational characteristic.

Cause-specific rates. Data are available from death certificates on the cause of death. Tabulating the causes of death for people in a community, then dividing the total for each cause by the midyear population of the community, yields a series of **cause-specific rates** of mortality. In developed countries the specific mortality rates for heart disease and cancer are much higher than those for communicable

diseases. The opposite is true in developing countries, although this is changing.

Age-adjusted rates. In examining the question of how the total death rate for whites in Baltimore can be higher than that for blacks when each of the age-specific rates for whites is lower, one must consider the relative risks of death between ages. The population of Baltimore, like that of many cities in the eastern United States, consists disproportionately of older whites and younger blacks. If one multiplies the higher rates for older people by the larger proportions of whites in those age groups, one gets high numbers for whites. Then if you add up the products of the multiplications across the entire range, the result will be a higher total for whites than for blacks in the race-specific death rates. This is why comparisons over time, as in Figure 3-12) or between communities or other large, heterogenous groups, are usually age-adjusted. **Age-adjusted rates** are much like the weighted sum of age-specific rates, except that instead of using the proportions in each age group of the population as the weight by which to multiply each age-specific rate, one uses the proportion (between 0 and 1) of some standard population, such as the national proportion in that age group.

Crude death rate versus age-adjusted death rate. Part of the historical trend in declining death rates in developed countries is masked when the comparisons over time are limited to crude death rates, as seen in Figure 3-12. Age-adjusted death rates control for the changing age composition of the population by applying the current age-specific death rates for each age group to a standard population's age distribution. The standard population chosen for the trend analysis shown in Figure 3-12 was the population of the United States in 1940. Thus, the crude death rate and the age-adjusted death rate were equivalent for 1940. Why should the age-adjusted rate be so much lower than the crude death rate today than in earlier years? Why is the

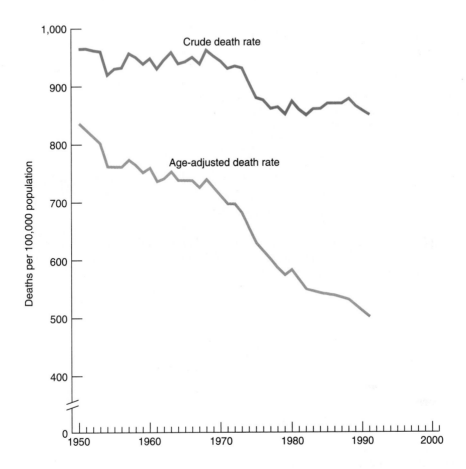

FIGURE 3-12
The decline in the crude death rate has been less dramatic than the decline in the age-adjusted death rate because the crude rate is based on a population containing more elderly people each year, whereas the age-adjusted rate is based on the standard 1940 U.S. population.

Source: National Center for Health Statistics: Annual summary of births, marriages, divorces, and deaths, United States, 1991, *Monthly Vital Statistics Report* 40(13):5, Sept. 30, 1992.

gap between the two rates still growing in the 1980s?

Crude death rate versus age-specific rates. Age-specific death rates are generally higher for older age groups than for younger ones. This means that for any given year the crude death rate, which is weighted by the proportions in each age group that year, will tend to reflect the age-specific rates of the larger age groups more than the rates of the smaller age groups. How might this explain the paradox of the Baltimore data? In the early decades of this century, the younger age groups (under age 25) represented around 50% of the total population of the United States, as seen in Figure 3-13. As their proportion declined in subsequent decades, the propor-

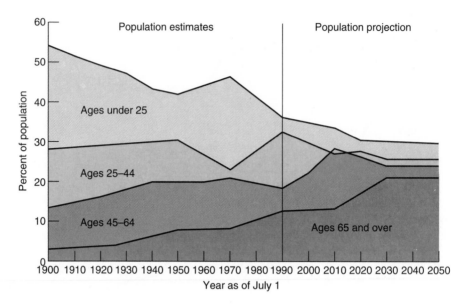

FIGURE 3-13
Younger age groups are becoming smaller as older age groups grow in their proportion of the total population of most countries. The trends here are projected based on assumptions of constant net immigration of 450,000 persons per year and a slow improvement in life expectancy to 84 years for females and 75 years for males by the year 2050.
Courtesy Metropolitan Life Insurance Co.

tion of the older age groups (with higher age-specific death rates) increased. This weighting of the population distribution with older and older ages made the crude death rate look as though there was no decrease in mortality during the postwar decades, as reflected in Figure 3-12.

Birth rates. Even the age-adjusted death rate seems to have stalled in its decline during the 1950s and early 1960s, according to the lower slope in Figure 3-12. Why should the death rate have declined faster during World War II than after the war? This phenomenon can be attributed largely to the "baby boom" of the postwar years. It reflects not so much a slowing of progress in reducing premature death as a rebounding of the proportion of the population

made up of infants and children (see the series of peaks in the middle of Figure 3-13). At the same time, the oldest age groups continued to increase, so that the ratio of the three oldest age groups and the youngest age group (under 1 year) to the total population weighted both the crude death rates and the age-adjusted death rates of the 1950s and 1960s with larger numbers of deaths in the age groups with highest mortality. The dramatic decline in the birth rate in the 1960s allowed the decline in death rates to resume.

These and other rates used by demographers and epidemiologists to compare the fertility, mortality, and health status and trends of populations or communities will be discussed throughout the following chapters.

Host, Agent, and Environment

Concepts underpinning the epidemiological approach to community health include the interaction of disease host (the person in which the disease resides), the disease agent (that which carries or delivers the disease to the person), and the environment. Epidemiology adds the element of **agent** to the ecological concept of human-environment interaction. The development of the germ theory in the late nineteenth century gave rise to the understanding of the role of agents in carrying disease. Water supplies were placed under greater control when it was realized that they harbored agents of disease.

The epidemiological approach to the host has been to build host resistance to disease and to quarantine the host of a disease so that he or she could not transmit it to others. Community health programs apply the principle of host resistance in mass immunization programs, in maternal and child nutrition programs, and in physical fitness programs designed to strengthen the ability of people to ward off infection or disease.

The epidemiological approach to the environment has been directed primarily at controlling water, air, food, and waste products so that agents of communicable disease could not be harbored in those parts of the environment that came into contact with people. In addition, the control of flies, mosquitoes, rats, and rabid animals that transmitted communicable diseases from one part of the environment to another (vector control) was responsible for much of the reduction in yellow fever, malaria, plague, and other pandemic diseases in the last century.

Today, the tools and concepts of epidemiology are being turned to understanding such concerns as the ''host resistance'' of young children to false advertising on television, the automobile and alcohol as ''agents'' of injury and disease, and the social ''environment'' as a context for shaping life-styles harmful to health. These new applications of epidemiological concepts are essential to meet the challenge presented by the dramatic shift (the ''second epidemiological revolution'') from communicable diseases to chronic and degenerative diseases and injury as the leading causes of death.

Epidemics and Pandemics

The term *epidemic* means ''around people'' and denotes a condition from a common cause that has affected a large number of people. The term *pandemic* literally means ''all people'' and is used to denote spread of a disease over a considerable area. Generally the term describes a nationwide, continentwide, or worldwide outbreak. A community or even statewide outbreak of a disease may be regarded as an epidemic. The past has seen devastating pandemics of bubonic plague, yellow fever, cholera, smallpox, typhus fever, and syphilis. The 1918-1919 influenza-pneumonia pandemic caused 400,000 deaths in the United States, 10 million deaths in India, and more than 20 million deaths throughout the world. In some of the underdeveloped nations of the world during the past decade epidemics of acute infectious diseases such as cholera have occurred. These epidemics usually have been confined to a single nation or to a small group of nations. Even in the underdeveloped nations there are not likely to be devastating pandemics of acute infectious diseases such as occurred in the past, but moderately severe outbreaks can be expected for decades to come. In the more developed nations scientific advances in the field of epidemiology make even a moderate pandemic of an acute infectious disease highly unlikely.

The term **endemic** means ''within people'' and denotes a condition that persists within geographical areas. Chronic infections still plague vast segments of the population in many nations of the world. At the present time there are more than 200 million malaria cases in the world, 260 million hookworm cases, 650 million people with ascarids (a roundworm), and 5 million cases of leprosy, of which 3 million are in Asia. Asia has 335 million people who harbor the parasitic ascarid. Each of these Asians will harbor between six and nine adult ascarids. The worms thus carried by these 335 million Asians will consume as much food each day as a population of more than 40,000 people.

Indonesia had 15 million cases of yaws before a staff of Indonesians trained by United Nations technologists and supplied with penicillin from the United Nations proceeded to wipe out the disease. One injection of penicillin usually cures yaws, so that virtually the entire Indonesian population is now free of the disease.

In Australia, Europe, and North America diphtheria, influenza, measles, meningitis, encephalitis, poliomyelitis, and other infectious diseases that conceivably could break out in pandemic form can be controlled effectively. It is possible, however, that a mutant pathogen of humans may arise; such an occurrence will challenge society's ability to control the spread of disease. Our ability to solve disease control problems that might arise will depend on rapid application of our knowledge of infection and its control.

LIFE SPAN VERSUS LIFE EXPECTANCY

Life span and life expectancy are distinct phenomena, one biological and the other epidemiological. Life span is the recognized biological limit of life. Based on present knowledge, biologists tend to set the maximum human life span at 120 years. They do not possess reliable data of human beings living beyond this age. The usual report of people living beyond 120 years emanates from primitive areas where unreliable records or no records at all exist. Biologists suggest that in all probability even the person who lives to age 115 years has shortened his or her life by adverse health practices or circumstances. Scientists recognize that improper dietary practices, infections, excessive fatigue, prolonged exposure, inadequate rest, and other factors may

well have shortened the life of the person who lives to age 115.

Obviously, not all people have a life span of 120 years. Some people likely have a life span considerably below 100 years. This is indicated by failure of any member in some lineages to reach the age of 60 years. Life span is an inherited characteristic that is determined at the time of the fertilization of the ovum by the sperm. The person can do nothing to extend the inherited span but inadvertently or unwisely does many things to prevent the realization of his or her life span.

Life expectancy, on the other hand, is an epidemiological concept that refers to the average duration of time that individuals of a given age can expect to live, based on the longevity experience of the population. These averages are based on the assumption that the longevity experience of the recent past will prevail in the future, even though future developments likely will be favorable to an extension of longevity beyond what past years indicate.

All averages on expectancy apply to the age group's life expectancy at birth. Obviously, individuals within a group will vary, some experiencing an expectancy considerably above the average and some below the average.

Geographic Differences

With all of the United States' medical, hospital, and other health facilities, along with her favorable economic position, it was embarrassing to find that life expectancy in the United States does not compare favorably with that in many other industrialized countries. Of 15 countries with the highest life expectancies for males and for which recent comparable data were available, 9 had higher life expectancies at birth for males than the United States. Japan, Iceland, Sweden, and Norway had the longest life expectancies for males (more than 73 years). For males in the United States life expectancy at birth was 72, for Canada 73 (Table 3-1).

TABLE 3-1

Life expectancy at birth among 15 industrialized nations.

Nation (year)	Total population	Men	Women
Japan (1990)	78.9	75.9	81.8
Iceland (1989-90)	78.0	75.7	80.3
Sweden (1990)	77.6	74.8	80.4
Canada (1991)	77.5	73.0	79.7
Switzerland (1989-90)	77.4	74.0	80.8
Netherlands (1990)	77.0	73.8	80.1
Australia (1990)	77.0	73.9	80.0
Norway (1990)	76.6	73.4	79.8
France (1987)	76.2	72.0	80.3
United States (1991)	75.7	72.0	78.8
Germany, F.R. (1986-88)	75.5	72.2	78.7
Finland (1989)	75.0	70.9	78.9
Denmark (1989-90)	74.9	72.0	77.7
United Kingdom (1985-87)	74.8	71.9	77.6
New Zealand (1987-89)	74.6	71.6	77.6

Source: Metropolitan Life Insurance Co.

The people of seven U.S. midwestern states and the Prairie provinces of Canada consistently have a greater life expectancy than that of the people of most other states and provinces. Iowa, Kansas, Minnesota, Nebraska, North Dakota, Oklahoma, and South Dakota regularly exceed the national life expectancy figures by at least 2 years and occasionally 3 years for both males and females. No acceptable explanation of this phenomenon has been found. The national origin of the population, economic means, climate, vocations, living practices, and other factors have been analyzed, but nothing has been discovered that consistently distinguishes the population of these states from the population of other states.

Two neighboring states, Utah and Nevada, have similar climates and geography but extreme differences of life expectancy, reflecting their differences in life-style (75.8 for Utah; 69.3 for Nevada). Most

of the geographic differences, then, should be traceable to demographic and cultural or social differences that dictate life-style practices and conditions.

Demographic Differences

For females, 9 of the 15 countries with the highest life expectancies had higher life expectancies at birth for females than the United States. Japan, Iceland, Australia, Switzerland, the Netherlands, and Sweden had the longest life expectancies for females (more than 80 years). Life expectancy for females in the United States was 78.8 in 1990 (see Table 3-1).

In every country, life expectancy was greater for females than for males. The increased expectation of life at birth continues the general upward trend with the gradual decline in deaths in younger ages, shown in Figure 3-14. But the increases are slowing and the black male population actually had a decrease in life expectancy in recent years.

Under the mortality conditions prevailing in 1940, an infant born in that year could expect to live an average of 62.9 years. Between 1940 and 1960, 7 years were added to life expectancy. Only 4 additional years were added between 1965 and 1985. Thus the gain in the earlier 20-year period was greater than the gain during the more recent 20 years.

Females have gained more years than males, especially nonwhite females, who now have a longer life expectancy than white males. From 1950 to 1986 white females had a 6.7-year increase, and all other females had a 12.2-year increase. In contrast, white males had only a 5.5-year increase, and all other males had an 8.5 increase during the same period.

Although the difference between life expectancy for males and females has increased, the difference between life expectancy for Caucasians and people of all other races in the United States has been reduced substantially. In 1950 Caucasians could expect to live about 8 years longer than people of all

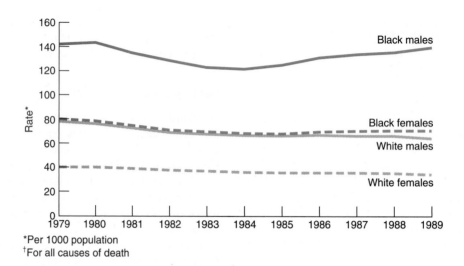

*Per 1000 population
†For all causes of death

FIGURE 3-14
Rates per 1000 population of years of potential life lost before age 65, by sex and race–United States, 1979-1989.

Source: Centers for Disease Control and Prevention, U.S. Department of Health and Human Services, 1993.

other races. By 1986 this differential had decreased to 4 years. Since the mid-1980s, however, the black population in the United States has lost ground. A related measure, **years of potential life lost (YPLL)** before age 65, shows the recent increases for Black males and females on this measure of premature mortality that disregards improvements for the very old (see Figure 3-14).

The greatest gain in life expectancy during the first half of the twentieth century can be attributed to the prevention of deaths in infancy and childhood. In recent years progress has been made in extending the length of life by the postponement of death in the later age brackets, so that in 1985 the life expectancy of a person of 40 was nearly 10 years greater than the life expectancy of a person of 40 in the year 1900.

Risk Factors Determining Life Expectancy

Longevity is a general term that incorporates a vast number of factors significant to individuals who are interested in estimating their own life expectancy. Fortunately, no one knows precisely when he or she will die, but it is possible to establish the approximate probable lifetime by a statistical procedure called health hazard appraisal or health risk appraisal, which weights various characteristics of the individual according to the known correlation of those characteristics with mortality. This allows individuals to identify with some statistical probability how many years they could add to their lives by changing specific health practices, circumstances, or conditions throughout life. Some factors, however, are not changeable.

Race. At the time of birth, the white male has a life expectancy greater than the nonwhite male, and the white female has an expectancy greater than the nonwhite female. After age 74, however, there is a crossover in the white-nonwhite races for both sexes. Whites enjoy lower mortality rates until age 74, when nonwhite mortality becomes lower and remains so. Nonwhites who have surmounted the economic barriers and environmental hazards to health may represent a hardier group of survivors compared with their white counterparts of similar age. This makes the years of potential life lost before age 65 a more sensitive measure for purposes of detecting differences that may be preventable in earlier years (Figure 3-14).

Inheritance. Long-lived parents tend to have long-lived offspring. What actually is transmitted is not the abstraction, long life, but rather the adequate body structure, the efficiently functioning organs and systems, the resistance to diseases, the ability to recover from injury or disease, the capacity to produce necessary body enzymes, and the various other attributes necessary for long life.

Dr. Raymond Pearl, a U.S. biometrist, found that for his subjects 90 years of age or over (longevous group), 46% had two long-lived parents, while in the other subjects (control group), only 12% had two long-lived parents. The significant difference in the two percentages doubtless represents inherited endowment.

In considering the influence of inheritance on the length of life, one should not overlook the fact that living in a long-lived family usually means certain environmental advantages that could be favorable for longevity. Having both parents living to look after his or her welfare should be an aid to an individual in obtaining his or her highest possible potential, both in quality of health and length of life. Certainly gains in the longevity of the general population must be attributed to environmental improvements rather than genetic changes. Inherited longevity still has its advantages in determining one's length of life, but with new knowledge and its applications these advantages are not as great as they were in earlier decades.

Gender. At birth, the U.S. white female has an expectancy greater than that of the male, as seen in Table 3-1 and Figure 3-14. Although the differential between the life expectancy of the female and that of the male declines during the ensuing years, she tends to have an advantage all through life. The female appears to inherit a better set of long-wearing qualities. She has less bulky musculature and more flexible soft tissues. She is less prone to heart disorders and arteriosclerosis. She has lower blood pressure and a higher white cell count, both of which are to her advantage. She engages in less hazardous occupations and less reckless behavior, resulting in injury death rates much lower than those of the male. In the past, she has worked under less daily tension. Even as women increase the intensity of their daily living and the tension that they experience in vocational pursuits, they seem to possess both the means and the social encouragement to give release to their emotions, a practice the male could emulate to his benefit.

With emancipation of the female, however, her advantage in longevity may decrease. Adolescent groups now contain more female cigarette smokers than male smokers, although females smoke fewer cigarettes and inhale less. Unfortunately, they find it more difficult to stop smoking than do males, and recidivism is higher in females. The habit of cigarette smoking is equated with freedom and social advancement in the advertisements directed at females. Another disadvantageous factor is that obesity is more prevalent in females than in males, particularly in the lower socioeconomic groups. As more females seek employment and achieve economic parity with males, the differential in mortality may decline.

Education and occupation. The long-standing recognition of occupation as a factor in longevity (see Table 1-1) incorporates a number of variables, such as the types of individuals who go into various occupations, the hazards and stresses in the occupations, the economic status afforded by different occupations, and the educational background of people in these occupations. Longest lived are clergymen, lawyers, engineers, teachers, doctors, and farmers, essentially in that order. Next longest lived are business executives, white-collar workers, and skilled tradesmen. Shortest lived are the unskilled workers, miners, quarrymen, and granite workers.

Studies indicate that college graduates have a greater life expectancy than that of the general population. Even noncollege graduates, by the application of sound health principles and the use of available medical and health facilities and services, can extend their life expectancy considerably beyond the average.

Income. Favorable living conditions, associated with adequate income, have a definite influence on longevity. Families with a favorable income are able to avail themselves of medical care, proper nutrition, good housing, and other advantages that make a longer life possible. People living in cities with a high average level of income live longer than those living in cities with a low level of income. The advantage conferred by high income is no longer operative, however, in very old age groups, that is, those over 85 years. After this age, genetic endowment is dominant, and socioeconomic status has little influence on further life expectancy.

Marital status. Married men live longer than single men. Many men in poor health remain single, which partially accounts for the shorter life expectancy of single men. The orderly life of the married man apparently operates to his advantage in preserving his life. Among women, the picture of longevity varies. Up to the age of 40, married women have a greater life expectancy than single women, but thereafter married women and unmarried women have the same life expectancy.

Body build. An individual inherits a particular type of body that can be modified very little through nutrition or other means. Although people of certain body builds live longer than those of other body types, no one is doomed to a short life expectancy merely on the basis of his or her body build. People of average height and weight tend to live longest.

As a group, people of very large stature do not live as long as those who are smaller than average in height and weight. Being extremely underweight during young adulthood has an adverse effect on length of life, whereas those who are somewhat underweight in later years tend to have a favorable life expectancy. Obesity, particularly in the later years of life, has an adverse effect on longevity: people more than 25% overweight have a 75% higher death rate than those in the average weight category.

Life-style and habits. Overeating, alcohol and drug misuse and general excessiveness associated with high-tension living tend to shorten life. Cigarette smoking and heavy drinking both reduce life expectancy. Manual labor, even heavy manual labor, before the age of 40 does not appear to affect the length of life, but hard manual labor continued after the age of 40 years does seem to shorten life expectancy. Generally, people of a temperament that leads to a pattern of moderation in living reap benefits in terms of more years added to their lives.

Blood pressure. Low blood pressure, unless extremely low, favors longevity. The higher the blood pressure, the shorter the life, partially as a result of the relationship of blood pressure to heart and kidney disorders and stroke. Individuals with high blood pressure need not assume that they are doomed to a short life and can do nothing to extend their expectancy. Modern medical treatment and behavioral changes in relation to diet, exercise, and stress management can have a significant effect on reducing blood pressure. Blood pressure, tobacco, diet and alcohol together account for more than three-fourths of the premature deaths.

COMMUNITY APPLICATIONS

Both the individual and the community can take effective measures to extend life expectancy, starting with study of the most likely causes of death. More than 76% of all deaths this year in the United States, Canada, Australia, Japan, Singapore, and most European nations, will result from three causes: cardiovascular diseases, cancer, and injuries. Breaking these data down on the basis of age groups allows a community to be more specific in concentrating attention on the most fruitful points of intervention to prevent premature deaths. In addition, if the citizens of a community were informed about what they could do to promote their own quality of health and postpone death, life expectancy could be extended appreciably in that community. Ten of the twelve leading causes of death are subject to reduction, chiefly through informed individual actions, particularly related to tobacco, diet, and alcohol.

A community can contribute to life expectancy through an effective program of health education that gives citizens a knowledge of what they as individuals can do to promote their present health. Individuals should be concerned about the condition of their heart, arteries, kidneys, lungs, and other vital structures. Periodic health-risk appraisals, self-monitoring, and health examinations would give them an assessment of the condition of these structures. Such assessments would also warn them against the development of the various chronic disorders of adulthood. People need to adopt a positive health-oriented mode of behavior, emphasizing proper diet and rest, regular exercise, avoidance of tobacco, and moderate use of alcohol. A life-style of moderation in a community with a value system consistent with health can result in zestful living and longevity. A community program of health promotion should include health education, organizational and environmental changes conducive to healthful living, and periodic tests or examinations with suitable follow-up. Such a program should yield tangible results in reducing disease and disability. Any community with adequate and accessible health services and facilities is contributing to the quality of life of its citizens. The extent to which these services and facilities actually contribute to the postponement of

death and the quality of life will depend on the understanding that citizens have of these services and facilities and the extent to which they avail themselves of health services as well as other, nonmedical resources and opportunities for health promotion in their community.

Research and the diffusion of new knowledge about prevention and control of heart disease, cancer, injury, and other principal causes of death will largely determine the future extension of active and functional life expectancy. A breakthrough in the problem of cancer may have a slight influence on life expectancy. New methods and techniques in heart surgery could increase life expectancy at age 50 by a few months. Reducing automobile-related deaths could have a larger effect on life expectancy.

TABLE 3-2
Health status indicators

Indicators of health status	
Mortality	
All causes	Lung cancer
Infant mortality	Breast cancer
Motor vehicle accidents	Cardiovascular diseases
Work-related injuries	Homicides
Suicides	

Incidence

Acquired immunodeficiency syndrome
Measles
Tuberculosis
Primary and secondary syphillis

Indicators of Risk	

Low birth weight
Births to adolescents
Lack of prenatal care
Children in poverty
Poor air quality

TABLE 3-3

Community objectives for monitoring and surveillance of health

Focus	Objective	Indicator
Community health assessment	1. By _____ the community will conduct community health assessments on a periodic basis.	Availability of community health assessment
Health statistical and epidemiological consultation and capacity	2. By _____ the community will have available health statistical and epidemiological consultation and the capacity to: a. Carry out investigations, special studies, and data analyses b. Institute appropriate measures to control conditions of public health significance in the community c. Evaluate the impact of control measures.	A demonstrable system to provide immediate telephone consultation as well as timely on-site assistance for investigation, control, and evaluation
Quality laboratory services	3. By _____ the community will have access to quality laboratory services necessary for the timely diagnosis/confirmation/ identification of diseases, risk factors, and conditions of public health significance.	A demonstrable system of timely access to quality laboratory services
Identification of underserved populations	4. By _____ the community will be served by an official health agency with capability to conduct surveys in order to identify underserved populations and those demonstrating special needs.	a. Number of surveys conducted b. Availability of survey results
Assessment, monitoring, and evaluation of programs	5. By _____ the health agency will establish a mechanism for the assessment, monitoring, and evaluation of existing programs to measure progress, identify factors that interfere with program effectiveness or efficiency, and determine the need for continuation, refinement, reduction, redirection, or expansion of operations.	Assessment and evaluation mechanisms
Current directory of community programs	6. By _____ the community will have available a current list of community health programs.	List availability
Systematic review of community health services	7. By _____ the community will have a systematic and periodic process to review community health services.	Periodic reports to governing bodies, legislative bodies, elected officials, and the public on current services

TABLE 3-3
Community objectives for monitoring and surveillance of health—cont'd

Focus	Objective	Indicator
	8. By _____ health services agencies will establish and maintain a system to review their programs periodically for their sensitivity to individual, family, and community needs, values, experiences, awareness, understanding, language and cultural differences, rights, and dignity.	1. Existence of system to include: a. Policies that provide for public participation in the agency decision-making process b. Documentation of consumer representation on agency boards, councils, committees, commissions, and task forces c. Written guidelines for and documentation of solicitation of public participation in health care programs d. Existence of consumer education programs e. A stated policy of public access to program information without individual identifiers 2. Agency personnel composition compared to the community it serves in terms of ethnicity, cultural differences, and principal language spoken in a community a. Existence of a written consumer grievance policy and procedures manual

But the primary purpose of community health promotion should be reduced morbidity and improved quality of life.

MEASURING PROGRESS

The United States published *Objectives for the Nation* in disease prevention and health promotion in 1981. Since then several editions of model standards for community attainment of the national objectives have inspired other nations, states, provinces, and communities to formulate their community health plans with quantified objectives and target dates. *Healthy People 2000* is the second decade plan for disease prevention and health promotion in which the United States laid out 300 specific objectives. A national committee of state and local county health officers, together with national organizations, then developed a set of 18 health status indicators that

would be commonly adopted by all states to measure progress toward the objectives for the nation. These are shown in Table 3-2.

The *Healthy Communities 2000: Model Standards* document outlines a series of specific objectives for translating national objectives into achievable community health targets. Each objective or "model standard" provides for the community to set its own reasonable target date for accomplishment of the objective. Each objective also carries one or more indicators of success that can be used to assess progress or attainment of the objective. A set of community model standards or objectives that address the demographic and epidemiological capabilities of the community to assess its health needs and services is shown in Table 3-3.

Future surveillance systems will need to track changes in the public's knowledge of risk factors for particular diseases and conditions, monitor the extent to which people are making changes in their behavior in efforts to reduce their risks, and evaluate their success in maintaining the changes they make. Surveys conducted during the 1970s and 1980s have accumulated a good deal of the necessary baseline data.

SUMMARY

Promoting community health will have no influence on life span and little influence on life expectancy except in the high-risk and poorest sectors of the community. Maternal, infant, and child health programs, adult health programs, prevention of disorders, communicable disease control measures, safety promotion, industrial hygiene programs, reduction of alcoholism, improved sanitation, disaster relief programs, and the extension of community health services directly and indirectly influence the quality of life that all people of the community will enjoy. Because we know the specific leading causes of death and the population distribution of these risk factors, we have specific targets toward which to aim our efforts. Programs can be directed into channels leading to likely dividends. Knowing statistically what the causes of disease, disability, and death are most likely to be, and using population screening, health education, and methods such as health risk appraisal, the community can take advantage of all of the measures, devices, and services available to aid in improving and extending life.

An ecological perspective, supported with demographic and epidemiological methods of analysis, enables the community to understand its health conditions and trends in more comprehensive terms than medical data alone would permit.

QUESTIONS FOR REVIEW

1. What evidence is there that human beings possess an inherent drive to survive?
2. What evidence is there that the advances in health

sciences have had a dysgenic effect on human populations?

3. What is meant by the conservation of human resources?
4. For the past 40 years the Alaskan glaciers have been shrinking rapidly. What interpretation do you make of this, and what is the significance of the phenomenon?
5. What effect would a constantly rising world temperature have on life expectancy, health, the economy, and the general culture of Canada, Russia, the Scandinavian nations, and the Mediterranean nations?
6. In what type of nation does hunger pose the greatest threat?
7. One county with a rate of natural increase of 16 has a neighboring county with a rate of 4. What differences would you expect to find between the two countries?
8. What has been the effect of the development of DDT on the health and culture of the world?
9. What has been the effect of advances in agricultural technology on the health and culture of the world?
10. Why does Sweden have a greater life expectancy than the United States and Canada?
11. What factors probably account for the poor life expectancy of the North American male at age 50?
12. Why do females in the United States and Canada live longer than males?
13. Why can a child born in North America expect to live a greater number of years after his first birthday anniversary than could have been expected after the day on which he was born?
14. How does your community measure up on the objectives in Table 3-3.
15. What is the role of economics in life expectancy?

READINGS

Braithwaite RL, Taylor SE: *Health issues in the black community,* San Francisco, 1992, Jossey-Bass.
Comprehensive review of the health problems facing the black community of the United States.
Healthy communities 2000: model standards, ed 3, Wash-

ington, DC, 1991, American Public Health Association.

The third edition of this widely used community health planning guide articulates with the national objectives for disease prevention and health promotion.

Holland WW, Detels R, Knox G, editors: *Oxford textbook of public health,* ed 2, vol 2: *Methods of public health,* Oxford, 1991, Oxford University Press.

This volume of the *Oxford Textbook of Public Health* covers the demographic and epidemiological methods used in the development and analysis of community health information systems, surveys, and demographic data.

National Center for Health Statistics: *Health, United States, 1991 and prevention profile,* Hyattsville, Md, 1992, Public Health Service.

Each year a statistical report on the health of the nation is presented to the president and to Congress. The 1992 report contains the fifth in a series of prevention profiles documenting progress toward achievement of the 1990 and 2000 objectives in disease prevention and health promotion.

Wunderlich GS, editor: *Toward a national health care survey: a data system for the 21st century,* Washington, DC, 1992, National Academy Press.

Evaluates a plan for national surveys, identifies current and future data needs concerning access, quality, costs, and outcomes of health care. Recommends linking data systems to provide for study of the impact of illnesses over time.

BIBLIOGRAPHY

Aday LA: *At risk in America: the health and health care needs of vulnerable populations in the United States,* San Francisco, 1993, Jossey-Bass.

Centers for Disease Control: Trends in years of potential life lost before age 65 among whites and blacks—United States, 1979-1989, *MMWR* 41:889, 1992.

Chung CS, Tash E, Raymond J et al: Health risk behaviors and ethnicity in Hawaii, *Int J Epidemiol* 19:1011, 1990.

Davis JE: *Contested ground: collective action and the urban neighborhood,* Ithaca, NY, 1991, Cornell University Press.

Fee E, Fox DM: *AIDS: the making of a chronic disease,* Berkeley, 1992, University of California Press.

Frerichs RR: Epidemiologic surveillance in developing countries, *Annu Rev Public Health* 12:257, 1991.

Fries JF, Green LW, Levine S: Health promotion and the compression of morbidity, *Lancet* 1:481, 1989.

Green LW, Simons-Morton D: Education and life-style determinants of health and disease. In Holland WW, Detels R, Knox G, editors: *Oxford textbook of public health,* ed 2, Oxford, 1991, Oxford University Press.

Hardin G: The tragedy of the commons, *Science* 143:1243, 1968.

Homicide among young black males—United States, 1978-1987, *MMWR* 39:869, 1990.

Hopkins K, Kennedy P: *Promoting cultural diversity: strategies for health care professionals,* Newbury Park, Calif, 1992, Sage.

Institute of Medicine: *The second fifty years: promoting health and preventing disability,* Washington, DC, 1990, National Academy Press.

Jacobs DR, McGovern PG, Blackburn H: The U.S. decline in stroke mortality: what does ecological analysis tell us? *Am J Public Health* 82:1596, 1992.

Klein RJ: Health status indicators: definitions and national data. In *Healthy people 2000 statistical notes,* vol 1, no 3, Hyattsville, Md, 1992, National Center for Health Statistics.

Last JM, Wallace RB: *Maxcy-Rosenau-Last public health and preventive medicine,* ed 13, Norwalk, Conn, 1992, Appleton & Lange.

Lederberg J, Shope RE, Oaks SC Jr, editors: *Emerging infections: microbial threats to health in the United States,* Washington, DC, 1992, National Academy Press.

National Center for Health Statistics: Advance report of final mortality statistics, 1990. In *Monthly vital statistics report,* vol 41, no 7, suppl, Hyattsville, Md, 1993, Public Health Service.

Nowjacker R, Gift HC: Contributing factors to maternal and child oral health, *J Pub Health* 50:370, 1990.

Parkerson GR, Broadhead WE, Tse CKJ: The Duke health profile—a 17-item measure of health and dysfunction, *Med Care* 28:1056, 1990.

Stoto MA: Public health assessment in the 1990s, *Annu Rev Public Health* 13:59, 1990.

Strickland GT: *Hunter's tropical medicine,* ed 7, Philadelphia, 1991, Saunders.

Temple NJ, Burkitt DP: Towards a new system of health: the challenge of western disease, *J Community Health* 18:37, 1993.

Torrey BB, Kingkade WW: Population dynamics of the United States and the Soviet Union, *Science* 249:1548, 1990.

Walker D: Linking research activities with policy and program design, *Can J Public Health* 83:181, 1992.

Yeager PC: *The limits of law: the public regulation of private pollution,* Cambridge, 1991, Cambridge University Press.

Yu ESH, Liu WT: U.S. national health data on Asian Americans and Pacific Islanders: a research agenda for the 1990s, *Am J Public Health* 82:1645, 1993.

Yu PA: Population genetics: diversity and stability, Cooper Station, NY, 1990, Harwood.

Chapter 4

Human Behavior and Community Health Education

❖

*Health is the ability to perform certain valued
social roles.*

TALCOTT PARSONS

OBJECTIVES

When you finish this chapter, you should be able to:

- Assess and set behavioral objectives for the factors contributing to a community health or social problem

- Assess and set educational objectives for the factors influencing behavior and life-style in the community or population

- Identify principles of, and resources for, educational intervention in community health problems and community development needs

SCIENCE AND APPLICATION

In addition to biomedical sciences, ecology, demography, and epidemiology considered in the previous three chapters, the behavioral and social sciences constitute a fifth scientific foundation in community health. These foundations are interdependent. The relevance of behavior to community health is chiefly a matter of how human behavior influences biological, ecological, demographic, and epidemiological processes. As was shown in Figure 2-2, the behav-iors of individuals become the life-style norms of populations when practiced by large segments of the community. Norms of fertility and migration behavior show up in demographic trends; norms of health behavior show up in social and epidemiological trends.

In the social history of health, normative behavior becomes organized. Organized behavior of a community has a greater impact than individuals on the environment and therefore on the ecology of health. Community organization can work both to enhance the environment and to offset or control the destructive effects of human behavior on the environment. Finally, the environment, especially the social and economic environment, influences behavior.

These interactions give rise to subspecialties among the foundation disciplines. They include scientific fields such as environmental epidemiology, behavioral ecology, behavioral medicine, health psychology, social medicine, medical geography, and social epidemiology. The application and delivery of the scientific products of these subspecialties fall largely to community health workers, especially through health education. Community **health education** employs a combination of methods designed to facilitate voluntary adaptations of behavior conducive to health. It too has subspecialties in patient education, school health education, population education, environmental education, sex education, nutrition education, and public health education. The broader efforts of community health *promotion,* to be described in subsequent chapters, may go beyond voluntary changes in behavior. They include certain regulatory and environmental control strategies designed to channel, restrain, or support those types of behavior related to the most pressing health or social problems of a community.

HEALTH BEHAVIOR AND LIFE-STYLE

Human behavior relates to health in both direct and indirect ways. Personal or social behavior has a direct effect on health (arrow *a* in Figure 4-1) when it exposes an individual, group, or population to more or less risk of injury, disease, or death. Sometimes the exposure is subtle, as with small but repeated doses of a substance that may become addictive or cumulative in their effect. Drugs and fatty food are examples. Other times behavior may pose an immediate and excessive risk; eating a poisonous or infected food is one example of such behavior. Acute risks to health in food production, distribu-

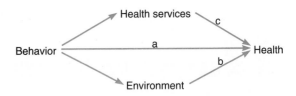

FIGURE 4-1

Health behavior and life-style have both direct (*arrow* **a**) and indirect effects on health through the influence of behavior on environmental exposure or control (*arrow* **b**) and on the development and use of health services (*arrow* **c**).

tion, advertising, and consumption have been minimized in the social history of health by the environmental and regulatory controls administered by public health agencies.

The risks today more often accumulate in smaller doses. For example, chemicals and less lethal or virulent substances (e.g., high-fat food) or actions (e.g., tanning) have cumulative effects that are nearly imperceptible until they reveal themselves in chronic conditions. These may be obesity, elevated blood pressure or serum cholesterol levels, skin wrinkling, reduced lung function or physical conditioning, drug dependency, lead poisoning, or the diseases themselves (heart disease, cancer, emphysema, atherosclerosis, stroke). Sometimes the first notice of a problem that has been developing for years is sudden death, as with a heart attack or stroke.

Direct behavioral risks and benefits to health also have been referred to in previous chapters (Figure 2-2) as part of the natural cycle of health. In this cycle, self-protective behavior is a response to prior adaptive experience and environmental influence. The direct ways that behavior influences health, then, involve preventive behavior, health-enhancing behavior, and self-care behavior, including diet and physical fitness actions.

As part of the social history of health, behavior has additional *indirect* influence on health through social norms, culture, organization, and environment (Figure 2-3). The organizational and environmental routes to health exert additional influences on health, but they, too, are related to behavior. They usually require social action (collective behavior) and planning at a community level.

The relative importance of behavior among the four factors in the health field concept is illustrated in Figure 2-3. In addition to the direct influence of behavior on health, much of what can be accomplished in the environment and in the organization of health services depends on human behavior. Behavior can influence health indirectly through the environment (arrow *b* in Figure 4-1) to the degree that people will plan individual or community actions to bring about changes in the environment. Examples of behavior in community environmental concerns include participating in efforts to control toxic waste disposal, organizing a lead paint removal program in the neighborhood, or voting on referenda or for elected officials in support of community water fluoridation, drunk-driving laws or other automobile safety provisions, food and drug labeling, air and water pollution controls, and regulation of the production, distribution, and advertising of harmful substances.

In addition to the direct effects of behavior on health and the indirect effects of behavior through environmental exposures or control, behavior can influence health indirectly through health services (arrow *c* in Figure 4-1). This can happen in three ways: (1) the public creates and distributes services through individual and community action in the legislative and health planning process, (2) the public uses available services in a timely and appropriate way, and (3) the public follows the medical or preventive regimens prescribed by its health service providers.

COMMUNITY HEALTH EDUCATION

Health education in the community seeks to elicit, facilitate, and maintain positive health practices by assuring that people have the understanding, skills, and support needed for their voluntary adoption of activities conducive to their health. Health education concerns itself not only with current behavior such as preventive actions, appropriate use of health services, health supervision of children from birth to adolescence, and adherence by adults and children to appropriate medical and nutritional regimens, but also with the development in children and youth of a foundation for future health. Within their families and with peers at school, children form predispositions—knowledge, attitudes, and values—that can prevent or promote many of the health problems of later adult life (Figure 4-2). Planning is required to

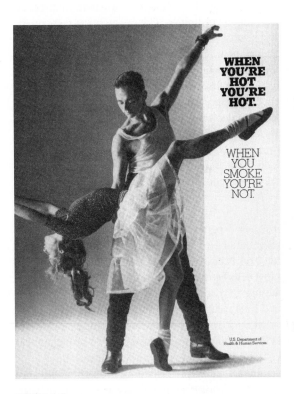

FIGURE 4-2
School health education has become a compulsory element in many primary and secondary schools in the United States. To complement this education, federal agencies have directed mass media messages such as this one to adolescents.
Source: Office on Smoking and Health, Centers for Disease Control and Prevention, U.S. Department of Health and Human Services.

assure that these various channels of influence on health are appropriately combined and designed to support voluntary behavior patterns conducive to health.

Components of Health Education

Health education in the community systematically applies theories and methods from the social and behavioral sciences, epidemiology, ecology, administrative science, and communications. Community health education assumes that beneficial health behavior in both children and adults will result from a combination of planned, consistent, integrated learning opportunities. This assumption rests on direct scientific evidence from the evaluation of health education programs in schools, at worksites, in medical settings, and through the mass media. It also rests on indirect evidence borrowed from experiences outside the fields of health and education. Community development, agricultural extension, social work, marketing and other enterprises in human services and behavior change all have contributed to the understanding of planning for change at the community level.

Planned experiences to influence voluntary changes in behavior, as distinct from incidental learning experiences, link the educational approach to community health. Other change strategies that may be excessively permissive, legal, or coercive must also be distinguished. Behavioral changes resulting from education are by definition voluntary and freely adopted by people, with their knowledge of alternatives and probable consequences. Some behavioral change strategies may have unethical components. Behavior modification techniques, for example, qualify as health education only when the patient or consumer has freely requested or consented to apply the techniques to achieve a specific behavioral result, such as controlling eating or smoking habits, that he or she desires. Principles of community health education planning call for the participation of consumers, patients, or citizens in the planning process.

Use of the mass media qualifies as an educational channel for community health up to the point that the media are controlled exclusively by commercial or political interests whose use of the media is strictly for profit or propaganda. The regulation of advertisers and the media may be necessary as a more coercive, economic, or legal strategy to protect consumers from, for example, deceptive advertising claims concerning the health value of food products. Such was the case when communities took action to restrict the advertising of certain foods and toys on Saturday-morning television programs directed at young children. Several countries restrict the advertising of tobacco and alcohol in the mass media. Third World nations have taken action to restrict the marketing of powdered milk formula for bottle-feeding of babies because it was leading to the use of unsanitary water and bottles in place of breast-feeding, which is safer and more critical to health in those regions.

Whether people truly have the resources or support necessary to make independent decisions and to take voluntary actions depends on some factors beyond their control. Whether or not they were born in a democratic country to affluent and loving parents will set some limits on their ability and will to act independently.

These considerations set some limits on how much health education alone can achieve health objectives without placing undue responsibility for change on people who are relatively powerless to make such change. This overreliance on health education has been referred to as "victim blaming." Combining health education with policy and regulatory actions that empower the relatively powerless and restrain the more powerful who might exploit them, overcomes this risk of blaming the victim.

Even when regulatory or environmental controls on behavior are required, as in the case of drunk driving, seat belts (Figure 4-3), or deceptive adver-

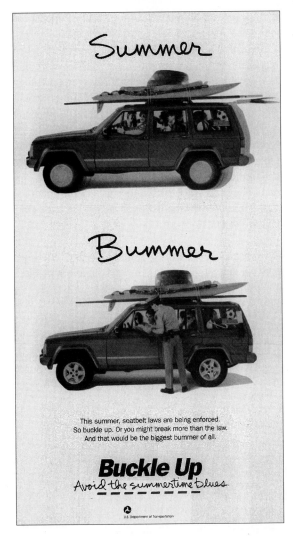

FIGURE 4-3
The alternative to public health education to achieve some
health objectives is legislation and law enforcement. But these
require education of the electorate to pass laws and education
of the public to achieve compliance with the laws.

Source: U.S. Department of Transportation.

tising, health education in a democratic society must
precede such controls to gain the public understanding and support required to pass legislation or to
accept new regulations. Community **health promotion,** then, is the combination of health education
with related organizational, environmental, and economic supports to foster behavior conducive to
health. Health promotion will be the subject of
Chapter 12.

Principles of Health Education

The principle of cumulative learning. Behavior is
the sum of a lifetime of personal and cultural experience; social, economic, and environmental circumstances; and genetic inheritance. Food preferences, driving habits, exercise patterns are all
conditioned since childhood. Therefore to effect behavioral change, health education in any setting requires a planned sequence of experiences and activities over time, tailored as much as resources will
allow to the circumstances and prior experiences of
specific groups and even individuals.

The principle of multiple targets. Health education objectives such as knowledge, attitudes, and behavior are intermediate to the final goals of a community health program. To achieve these ultimate
population health objectives, several causes of
health problems must be addressed by the health
education program. This means that the program
must take into account not only the characteristics
and predispositions of the target population, but also
the social systems that enable its behavior and the
motivation and ability of providers, parents, teachers, employers, and peers to communicate and reinforce the preferred behaviors.

**The principle of aggregating educational tar-
gets.** The difference between developing teaching
programs based on the classroom model and developing health education programs based on the com-

munity model is similar to the difference between the clinical-medical model and the community-epidemiological model. Prescribing for a patient based on the medical history and symptoms of that one person differs from providing the right balance in treating a community or population in which many histories and symptoms vary. A health education program must be flexible and broad enough to accommodate these varied personal histories, because an educational diagnosis cannot be carried out on each patient or consumer. Community health education must be designed to adapt the educational strategies for various subpopulations on the basis of visible or easily identified characteristics, such as age, sex, neighborhood, and ethnic identity because it is seldom possible to analyze each individual's educational needs in community programs.

The principle of participation. The prospects for success of programs requiring citizen, consumer, or patient cooperation are greatly increased when members of the community as well as staff and health service-provider organizations are included early in the program genesis. The *early* involvement of both consumers and providers in identifying problems, assessing their causes, and anticipating barriers to change provides greater assurance that the health education effort will pursue relevant and realistic goals, will employ acceptable methods, and will proceed with the commitment of those involved to the program activities and goals (Figure 4-4).

The principle of situational specificity. Methods used in the accomplishment of educational objec-

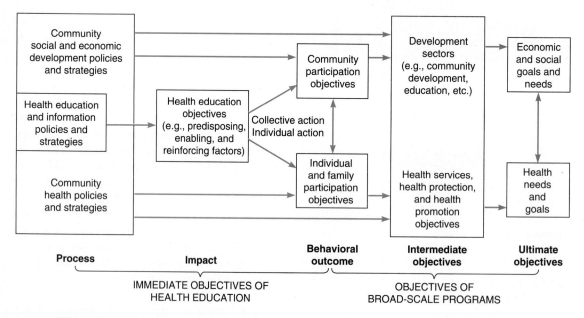

FIGURE 4-4
Health education seen in the context of broader community policies and strategies for social, economic, and health development contributes to individual and collective behavior that supports community development and health goals.

tives range from instructional methods, such as group discussion, individual counseling, behavior modification, educational technology, and staff development, to community methods, such as the use of mass media, political actions, and community organization. There is nothing inherently superior or inferior about any of these methods. The latest technology, such as computer-assisted instruction, is not necessarily appropriate in all circumstances. Appropriate application of methods depends on the situation. For each situation—whether it is a group of mothers discussing infant nutrition, the PTA president advocating an appropriation before the city council, or an in-service training session with outreach workers—theories and principles based on previous research and evaluation should guide the selection of methods and their coordination with the overall educational component of the community program. The selection of methods, then, should be based on an explicit educational diagnosis of the situation.

The principle of intermediate targets. Health education seldom has an immediate, direct impact on behavior. It predisposes behavior primarily through changes in knowledge, attitudes, beliefs, values, and perceptions. It also reinforces behavior by strengthening the social supports of relatives and significant others. It can enable or facilitate behavior through changes in community resources, skill development, and referrals. These represent the full range of variables through which health education should be expected to influence health behavior and which therefore should be considered the intermediate objectives or the immediate targets of health education.

The principle of multiple methods. Because there are multiple targets for health education, no single educational input should be expected to have significant, lasting impact on health behavior unless it is supported by other educational input. Health education strategies must be cumulative and mutually

supportive of the several factors facilitating a behavior conducive to health.

The principle of diversity. The best combination of educational methods, media, and messages for some people is not necessarily the best combination for others or for the same people in other situations. Therefore educational methods within programs should vary according to the audience's characteristics and circumstances. This means that a variety of learning opportunities or experiences must be provided to ensure that different people are exposed to the methods most likely to facilitate their decisions and behavior relating to health.

The principle of health promotion. Health education cannot claim and should not be expected to accomplish more than voluntary behavior change. Unless the additional organizational, economic, and environmental supports for the behavior also change, health education might only frustrate the learner. For example, health education may succeed in changing the dietary knowledge, motivation, and skills of a population of pregnant women, but unless the diet prescribed is economically accessible and culturally compatible in that population, the effectiveness of the health education methods may be limited. The success of a health education component may be impaired by organizational, legal, or economic factors that must be addressed with health promotion interventions beyond health education. These will be addressed in Chapter 12.

The principle of administration. The educational component of community health programs should have (1) the education plan written not separately or independently but within the context of the larger health program plan, (2) the responsibility for coordination of the educational component fixed on a designated person, (3) the responsibility for each educational intervention assigned to specific people, and (4) a budget for personnel, materials, and other costs. The process of health education may then be defined as any combination of learning opportunities designed to facilitate voluntary changes in behavior that are conducive to health. The principles of administration are implied by the terms *combination* and *designed.*

Diagnostic Stage of Educational Planning for Community Health*

A community health plan begins with an analysis of social problems or quality-of-life concerns. It then assesses the incidence, prevalence, and cause of the health problems associated with the social problem in a given population (Figure 4-5). The first step, then, is a social diagnosis of the *ultimate* community concerns or outcomes (Figure 4-5, *bottom*) rather than with immediate input (Figure 4-5, *top*). Step 2 is an epidemiological diagnosis. Step 3 is a behavioral analysis of the priority health problem to determine specific behaviors causing it. For each behavior implicated in the cause of each health problem, a further analysis of the factors influencing the behavior is needed in step 4 before educational methods are selected. Health education based more on favorite techniques than on systematic analysis of behavior and of the learning problems influencing the behavior will tend to be inefficient if not ineffective. Indeed, the selection of appropriate behavioral objectives and adequate methods and materials that make up an educational intervention (step 5) depend to a considerable extent on the accuracy of

---

Epidemiological Diagnosis Example

Consider an example* of health statistics to be reviewed in the epidemiological diagnosis of a community. They include the following rates of maternal and child health in a rural area that is populated mainly by a low-income minority group:

- A community maternal death rate of 65.5 per 100,000 births compared to a rate of 18.4 for the state
- A community infant death rate of 34.5 per 1000 compared to a rate of 21.0 for the state
- A community fetal death ratio of 24.9 despite an overall decline in the state to 14.6

The health problems that might be identified from these statistics are a high incidence of prematurity, low infant birth weights, a pattern of fetal distress and respiratory distress at delivery, and observed failure of infants to thrive. A visiting nurse service also might report data such as the prevalence of anemia and the incidence of gastrointestinal infections and respiratory diseases.

At this stage difficult decisions must be made to place greater priority on some problems than on others. Patients, consumers, parents, and various health service providers within the community may perceive the problems of mothers and children differently than the sponsoring health agency. The two groups may differ also in ranking the priority or urgency of various health problems. How would you reconcile these competing priorities and perspectives?

---

*Adapted from Green LW, Wang VL, Deeds S et al: Guidelines for health education in maternal and child health, *Int J Health Educ Suppl* 21:1, 1978. The maternal and child health examples refer to Chapter 5, but the same approach to health education planning can be applied to the problems described in subsequent chapters. A full application of this community diagnosis and planning framework is illustrated in Chapter 12 in relation to drug misuse.

---

*Based on Green LW: Toward cost-benefit evaluations of health education: some concepts, methods, and examples, *Health Educ Q* 2 (suppl 1):34, 1974. The framework described here is referred to as PRECEDE (predisposing, reinforcing and enabling constructs in educational diagnosis and evaluation). For the latest version of the fuller model combining health education and health promotion, see Green LW, Kreuter MW: *Health promotion planning: an educational and environmental approach,* Mountain View, Calif, 1991, Mayfield.

5 Administrative diagnosis
Interventions are matched with educational and behavioral objectives from steps 3 and 4, budgeted, sequenced, and coordinated.

4 Educational diagnosis
These factors need to be analyzed for each behavior.

3 Behavioral diagnosis
Each behavior defined in terms of timing, frequency, quality, range, duration.

2 Epidemiological diagnosis
Defined by health professionals in terms of morbidity, mortality, fertility, etc.

1 Social diagnosis
Defined by community in terms of unemployment, days lost from work or school, family disruption, and other dimensions of their quality of life.

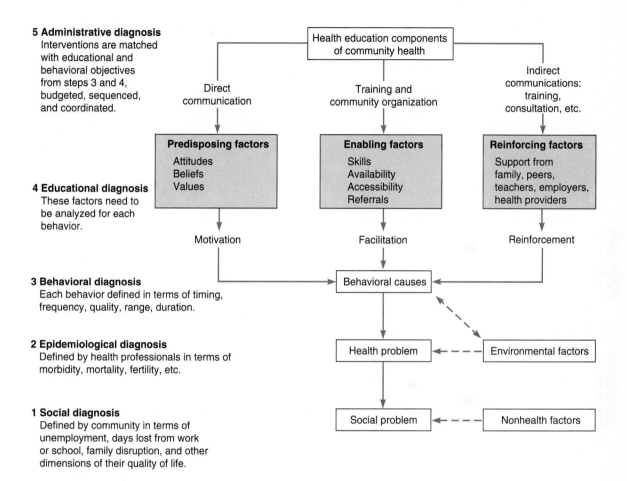

FIGURE 4-5

The PRECEDE model for health education planning begins at the end of the causal chain with the social diagnosis. Subsequent steps correspond to the causal relationships among factors linking health education to ultimate health and social goals.

Source: Adapted from Green LW: Prevention and health education. In Last JM, Wallace RB, editors: *Maxcy-Roseneau-Last public health and preventive medicine,* ed 13, Norwalk, Conn, 1991, Appleton-Century-Crofts.

the preceding steps in problem diagnosis. Political and legislative decisions often determine some of the priorities and direction of community health programs. Local health planners then develop, from the best epidemiological evidence available, a sound and rational basis for setting the broader objectives of health programs before planning the health education components of the program.

Social diagnosis. The starting point should be some assessment of the social concerns of the community to ensure that the health planning is cast in the proper context of the social problems or quality-of-life concerns paramount in the community. This step requires an understanding of the subjective concerns and values of the community, as well as objective data on social indicators such as unemployment, housing problems, teenage pregnancy, violence, and poverty.

Consideration of varying community perceptions should take place early in program development. Health programs are not likely to be successful without community support and participation in the planning process.

Epidemiological diagnosis. The educational components of community health programs are developed within the context of a social concern or quality-of-life issue in the community that has been analyzed and redefined as a health problem. This becomes the ultimate target or an overall program goal. The sponsoring agency should use the most recent available demographic, vital, and sociocultural statistics to define the characteristics of the subpopulations experiencing the health problem. The problem should be further analyzed on the basis of the experience of related agencies and a review of previously published reports. To gain perspective on the experience of the community with the health problem, similar data from other cities, states, or regions should be compared. Particular attention should be paid to the rates in subpopulations (age, sex, race, and income groups) within the community relative to comparable rates in other communities or in national statistics.

Consumer participation in the planning process at this stage helps identify population subgroups within the community, such as adolescent mothers and preschool youth, who may have special problems and needs. Information on these subpopulations should be assembled, information that includes geographical distribution; occupational, economic, and educational status; age and sex composition; ethnicity; health indicators, including age-specific morbidity; and service utilization patterns. Representatives of the consumers or target groups indicated should then be recruited to assist in step 3.

Behavioral diagnosis. The foregoing information and definition of the health problem, the program

goal, and the high-risk subpopulations should lead to the task of specifying behavioral problems or barriers to the community solution of the health problem (Figure 4-6). The following guidelines should be considered in the behavioral diagnosis.

- The behaviors presumably contributing to the health problem should be specified as concretely as possible. An inventory of as many possible behavioral causes as one can imagine should be made.
- The nonbehavioral factors (environmental, human biology, and technological factors) contributing to the problem should be identified so that they may be recognized as determinants for which strategies other than health education must be developed.
- There should be a review of research evidence that the behaviors identified as possible causes are amenable to change through educational interventions and that such change will improve the health problem in question.
- For each health problem, one or more of the following relevant dimensions of health behavior should be identified:

Behavioral dimension	*Example*
Time or promptness of the behavior	Prenatal care begins with the first trimester of pregnancy
Frequency of the behavior	Prenatal visits are every sixth week in the second trimester
Quality of the behavior	Foods with low fat content are selected over those high in fat
Range of health behaviors	Prenatal care is obtained, plus diet control regimen followed, plus smoking stopped
Persistence or follow-through with health behavior	All booster shots are obtained following initial immunization or medical care is continued through prenatal, delivery and postnatal periods

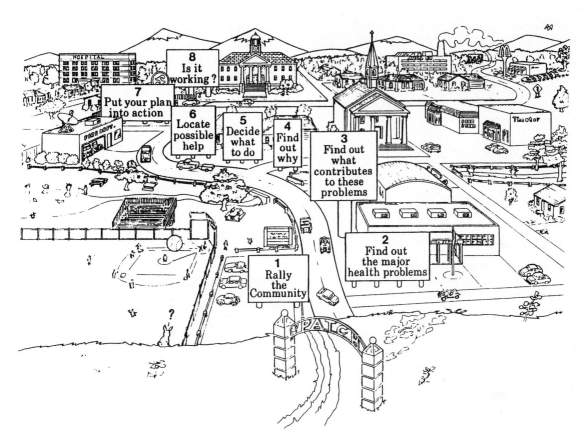

FIGURE 4-6

The U.S. Centers for Disease Control and Prevention provide technical assistance to communities to apply an adaptation of the PRECEDE model for health education planning, called PATCH (Planned Approach to Community Health). PATCH programs have been developed also in Australia and Canada.

Source: Center for Chronic Disease Prevention and Health Promotion, Centers for Disease Control and Prevention, U.S. Department of Health and Human Services.

● An assessment should lead to the selection of specific behaviors that will be the target of the educational interventions. Rarely, if ever, does an agency have the resources necessary to influence all the behaviors contributing to a health problem. An initial selection of some of the behaviors should be made. The selection often must be influenced by policies governing required services of the agency, legal and economic factors affecting the desired behaviors, agency resources and expertise available, political viability of the educational interventions, the possibility of continued funding, and the probability of quick program success. The reasons for selecting specific behaviors as the priority focus of the educational interventions should be justified.

Behavioral Diagnosis Example

The behavioral diagnosis identifies factors influencing the health problem and suggests the actions people can take to reduce the problem.

Examples of nonbehavioral factors influencing the previously defined health problems include the following:

- Genetic factors
- Economic base
- Occupation
- Environmental isolation

Examples of behavioral remedies of the previously defined health problems include the following:

- Consumption of proper nutritional diet
- Acceptance of medical supervision at each stage from prenatal to postnatal year for mother and child
- Postponement of pregnancy to age 18 and avoidance after age 40
- Spacing of pregnancies over 24 to 30 months
- Reduction in total number of pregnancies
- Avoidance of physical and emotional stress during pregnancy
- Avoidance of fetal insult (reduction in smoking and in use of alcohol, aspirin, and other drugs)

The two most important objective criteria for selection of priority behavioral targets for health education are (1) the evidence that the behavioral change will make a difference in the reduction of the health problem, and (2) the evidence that the behavior is amenable to voluntary change.

Educational diagnosis. The behaviors selected should be subjected to further analysis for assessment of their causes. The following sets of factors should be considered as *causes* of each behavior:

Predisposing factors: Knowledge, attitudes, beliefs, and values that motivate people to take appropriate health actions.

Enabling factors: Skills and the accessibility of

resources that make it possible for a motivated person to take action.

Reinforcing factors: The attitudes and climate of support from providers of services, families, and community groups that reinforce the health behavior of an individual who is motivated and able to adopt the behavior but who will discontinue the behavior if it is not rewarded.

Representatives of the various segments within the agency and community who will be affected by the program should be consulted in these analyses.

Failure to assess some of these factors and to develop a community health education program ad-

---

Educational Diagnosis Example

By assessing the predisposing, enabling, and reinforcing factors influencing the health behaviors in the earlier example, you can identify the most useful targets on which to concentrate health education. By consulting with the women themselves, you could adapt the health advice to fit the circumstances of these women more appropriately. Examples of the factors identified in an educational diagnosis of maternal and child health follow:

Predisposing factors: Attitude toward pregnancy as a way of fulfilling needs other than reproduction; belief that pregnancy and childbearing are the only acceptable roles for young women.

Enabling factors: Scarcity and cost of recommended foods; inaccessibility of emergency care; transportation problems in getting to clinics for prenatal and well-child care; clinic hours that preclude attendance by working women.

Reinforcing factors: Husbands do not support contraceptive behavior; loss of income from inability to work in fields may be an incentive for family planning for some, but exemption from work may reward pregnancy for others; crowded clinic and waiting time does not reward clinic attendance.

How would you use this information?

dressed to all three sets would seriously limit the impact of the program. Figure 4-4 summarizes the relationships among the factors that were considered in the foregoing procedures. The methods of health education will be decided last in the administrative diagnosis.

Administrative diagnosis. Selecting the health education methods for a community health program follows almost automatically from a thorough identification and ranking of predisposing, enabling, and reinforcing factors influencing the health behaviors. Administrative diagnosis then includes the assessment of available resources to support needed methods. The coordination and budgeting of these methods into a timetable that corresponds to the community health program is the next step. Both require constructive participation by staff, other organizations, and area residents. In addition to understanding and defining the program's intent, they must also contribute to the setting of priorities; the determination of acceptable approaches, informational content, and phraseology; the suggestion of barriers and facilitators to the achievement of pro-

gram objectives; the identification of indigenous resources; and the review (pretesting) of educational media and materials. By including other organizations and community members in the planning, one obtains their personal commitment to realizing program success. Most importantly, their participation enables program planners to incorporate the interests, perspectives, and values of various stakeholders into the educational activities of the program. The principle of participation applies usually to representatives of related agencies, institutions, and organizations in the community, to the agency staff who will implement the program activities, and to community residents in the target population.

Resources in the community may already be channeling funds and efforts into areas related to the proposed educational program. Other resources may have been active in related areas in previous years. It is important to survey these activities and organizations to avoid overlap and to integrate services.

The program plan is based on survey information obtained from organizations and agencies at national, state or provincial, and local levels (e.g., schools (Figure 4-7), citizens' groups, industry, la-

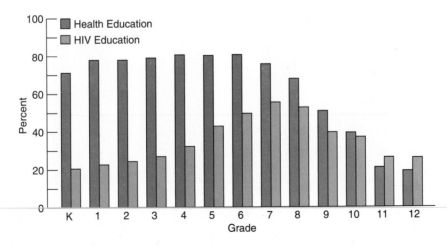

FIGURE 4-7
Percent of U.S. schools requiring HIV and health education units, by grade, in 1991.
Source: Centers for Disease Control: *HIV/AIDS prevention: 1992 HIV fact book,* Atlanta, 1992, Centers for Disease Control.

bor organizations, religious groups, colleges, advertising agencies, drama groups, pharmacies); local facilities (e.g., libraries, health centers, hospitals (Figure 4-8), training centers, town halls, gathering places); personnel (e.g., volunteers, agency staff, social workers) whose functions relate to health education, training, experience, and supervision; community events (e.g., fairs, festivals, conventions, public and private meetings); communications resources (e.g., numbers of telephones and use of radios, billboards, local television and radio stations, newspapers, newsletters, organization bulletins); and funding sources available for the educational program through the health service agency itself and related organizations. This identification and assessment of available resources should lead to the further refinement of objectives, strategies, and methods. Some previously written objectives may be accomplished earlier or more extensively if more resources are obtained. Additional intermediate objectives may be needed for the development of resources that are inadequate.

PLANNING FOR THE DELIVERY OF COMMUNITY HEALTH EDUCATION

The planning steps outlined in this section are not entirely sequential. They begin during the preceding diagnostic stages and continue through the organizational, implementation, and evaluation stages.

Priority Target Populations for Specific Educational Components

The people at risk, or those who are affected by the health problem, are easily identified once the problem has been defined. They are the target for and the beneficiaries of most of the educational interventions, and thus constitute the primary target group that the planners should consult. Education must also be directed toward groups not affected by the health problem but in a direct position to influence those who are. These "gatekeepers" and social reinforcers (parents, spouses, teachers, peers, employers, and "opinion leaders") are often an inter-

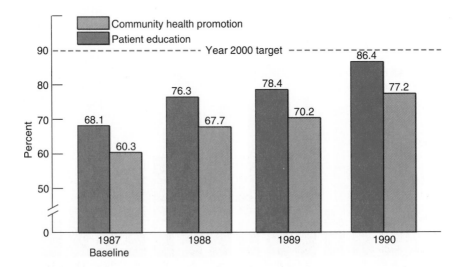

FIGURE 4-8
Increasing percentages of U.S. community hospitals offering patient education and hospital-based community health promotion, 1987-1990.
Source: American Hospital Association Annual Survey of Hospitals, 1987-1990, and Public Health Service, U.S. Department of Health and Human Services.

mediate or additional target population for educational interventions.

As implied in Figure 4-4, the primary target group will receive direct communication designed to influence their predisposition to accept the recommended health practices. One intermediate target group for community organization efforts would be directors of other agencies who control resources that would enable or facilitate the health behavior to be practiced. Another intermediate target group would receive training, consultation, or supervision in reinforcing the recommended health behavior. In relation to the predisposing factors, the primary target population should be described in terms of geographical, occupational, economic, educational, age, sex, and ethnicity distributions. The characteristics that provide the basic analysis for the specification of community health programs are also the basis for the development of educational interventions. Representative persons from the described population and cooperating agencies should be included in the further development of the educational plans. In relation to the enabling and reinforcing factors, intermediate target groups—controllers of needed resources for the health behavior—and those who can reinforce the behavior—transmitters of information—should be contacted and their participation in planning solicited.

Behavioral Objectives

The behavioral objectives stage overlaps with the previous planning stage. It is at this point of specifying behavioral objectives and the consequent educational objectives, however, that the educational component of the community health program should begin to emerge as an entity distinct from other technologies and services.

The objectives derive from the findings of the behavioral and educational diagnoses. The proper statement of the objectives should lend purpose to the program plan and direction to its implementation. The test of objectives is their ability to communicate expected results. Lucidity and precision in their formulation should (1) provide limits to expenditure of time and effort on specific educational interventions, (2) identify criteria for measurement of program achievement, (3) lead to task analyses for selection, training, and supervision of staff, and (4) provide orientation to cooperating agencies and to the general community.

Time spent on the formulation of objectives in educational planning is sometimes more important than in the planning of some administrative and service components because education appears to be more abstract and difficult to define or measure than some of the other activities of community health programs.

Objectives should be expressed as intended outcomes. They may apply to providers and to the organization or system as well as to the consumers. Each objective should answer the question, *Who* is expected to achieve or become *how much* of *what* by *when* and *where?*

Who—target groups or individuals expected to change

How much—the extent of the condition to be obtained

What—the action, change in behavior, or health practice to be obtained

When—the time in which the desired condition is to be obtained

Where—the place in which change will be observed, usually implied within the specification of who

The desired behaviors (what) derived from the behavioral diagnosis should describe what the participants will do or not do as a result of the program that they could not or did not do (as much) before the program. The conditions of the action should be stated in the following way:

Who—some logical portion (percentage) of the target group

How much—or to what extent, an amount of change that will depend on available resources

Where—geographical, political, or institutional boundaries derived in part from the original description of the health problem

When—or how soon, or within what time period, will be determined by the urgency of the health problem in the community and by the rate of change that can be expected from the amount and type of effort devoted to the program

In most community health or population-based programs, "how much" refers to the number of people or percentage of the population, whereas for

---

Example of Setting Objectives

The stated program goal for the earlier example—to raise the survival rate of mothers, infants, and children through raising the quality of prenatal care and promoting the optimum growth and development of children—suggests the following health objectives for the community health program:

- To reduce maternal mortality within counties A and B by 10% within the first 2 years and by an additional 15% the next 3 years, continuing until the state average rate is reached
- To reduce infant mortality to the state average within 10 years

Behavioral objectives then could take the following form:

- In the county 900 women under 40 who are at high risk of problem pregnancy will obtain women's health checkups the first year of the program
- In this group 80% of pregnancies will be detected within the first trimester
- Of the pregnant women 90% will obtain monthly prenatal care for the remainder of their pregnancy

In the first behavioral objective, the following apply

Who—Women in the county who are under 40 and have selected characteristics (e.g., age, socioeconomic status) associated with high-risk pregnancies
How much—900
What—Obtaining women's health checkups
When—During the first year of the program

---

individuals "how much" would refer to the level of accomplishment (e.g., monthly prenatal visits).

Objectives should be so explicated as to lead to assessment criteria. They should be stated in concrete terms with at least an implied if not stated scale of measurement that can be used to evaluate progress and achievement of the objective.

Educational Objectives

Educational objectives become the intermediate or subobjectives to the behavioral objectives (Figure 4-9). These must be accomplished before it is possible to achieve a change or development in behavior. These intermediate changes are defined by an analysis of the predisposing, enabling, and reinforcing factors referred to in the educational diagnosis, along with the assessment of the barriers and facilitators, which are discussed in the following section. To avoid a shotgun approach to communications, the planners should consider the knowledge, attitudes, skills, organization, and training required of people to move toward stated objectives. The various types of educational objectives that flow from these causes of behavior can be described as follows.

Informational objectives. Informational or cognitive objectives relate to the understanding and beliefs necessary on the part of individuals or groups to address or cope with the health problem, services, and activities. In other words, who will comprehend how much of what information?

Attitudinal objectives. Attitudinal or affective objectives relate to the predispositions or feelings people hold toward certain health problems or practices or toward means to be employed in certain health measures (e.g., contraceptives or immunizations). What will sufficiently motivate people to take appropriate health action?

Competency objectives. Persons may have to learn certain skills, such as reading thermometers,

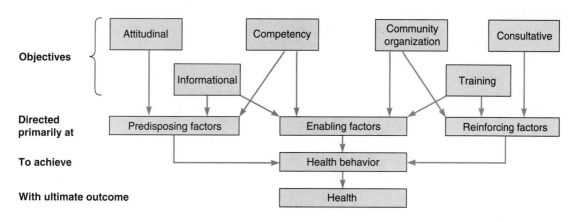

FIGURE 4-9
Types of educational objectives and their relationship to behavioral objectives and health status objectives of community health programs.

recording observations, and judging symptoms, to be able to use services or self-care procedures effectively.

Community organization objectives. Making services accessible through community organization may require the reordering of community priorities or the redistribution of resources.

Training objectives. Training to bring about specified changes in knowledge, behavior, and attitudes of staff, parents, teachers, employers, peers and others who have direct influence over the people whose behavior needs to change can encourage and reinforce desired behavior. Training may take various forms such as consultation, group work, supervision, or continuing education.

Assessment of Barriers and Facilitators to Implementation

Implementing the educational plan requires an assessment of factors that may impede carrying out program activities. At the same time, some characteristics of the community may facilitate program

success. Both the barriers and supports to the program should be assessed.

Barriers to the achievement of educational objectives can assume several forms. Some examples of *social, psychological,* and *cultural* barriers include citizen and staff bias, prejudice, misunderstanding, taboos, unfavorable past experiences, values, norms, social relationships, official disapproval, rumors. *Communication* obstacles include illiteracy and local vernacular. *Economic* and *physical* barriers include low income and inability to pay for prescribed drugs or the means of transportation to medical services, and long distances over difficult terrain to medical facilities. Legal and administrative barriers include residence requirements to be eligible for services, legal requirements that the program operate within defined geographical boundaries, and policies or regulations that restrict program implementation.

Facilitators to the achievement of program objectives go beyond the mere absence of barriers. The predispositions of area residents favorable to the implementation of the program may include past and favorable experience with similar programs, and high credibility of the program sponsoring agency.

Other capabilities facilitating the program might be high education levels of consumers, dynamic and supportive local leaders and organizations, skilled staff with experience, open channels of communication with consumers, and support from other agencies. In addition, some geographical and physical enabling factors may serve as program assets (e.g., population distribution and density, access to facilities).

The introduction of new or unfamiliar schemes for promoting awareness and health behavior has its greatest opportunity for success when integrated into existing systems of knowledge transfer and influence within the community. Schools, local media, clubs, churches, neighborhoods, and ethnic associations are the most effective channels of communication. Also, the identification of barriers should be included in additional objectives that indicate how much and when each of the barriers is to be surmounted in the program.

THE IMPLEMENTATION STAGE

Implementation of the educational components of the community health program follows the development and refinement of the planning operations. At this stage, if involvement of concerned persons has been obtained and planning is detailed and thorough, staff, volunteers, and cooperating agencies will be in agreement over the program's aims and general strategies. They should be committed to assuming their roles in the educational efforts. To initiate the program will require more specific logistical planning and resource identification, equipment and materials assembly, design of procedures, and training and orientation of staff, volunteers, and cooperating agencies.

Priorities for Implementation

Resources always seem scarce in relation to the great needs in community health; and the health ed-

ucation component is often the first to be reduced when budgets are cut. To ensure the most economical use of the resources available, priorities among alternative educational activities must be considered. Related to this pressing need for efficiency is the need for effectiveness. This requires the selection of the most effective combination of educational interventions and activities available. The first step is to determine which procedures are feasible, given limited staff, services, money, and time, and then to combine these resources to achieve the best support of program objectives.

To set priorities, obtain opinions and contributions from community members on priorities for educational services (Figure 4-10). Delineate the areas that will provide the greatest benefits to the most recipients. Phase program activities with a gradual beginning; limiting number and range of activities, with initial emphasis on areas most amenable to quick and early success and activities requiring minimum staff training, can help get a program started. Most of these decisions should be guided by reviewing the most recent scientific literature on the evaluation of health education methods relevant to the local program.

A contingency plan should be developed to aid program survival in the event of future reduction of resources. Beyond these general principles, the selection of educational efforts in strategic patterns or combinations depends on the particular circumstances of each site, the particular objectives, and the expectations for sustaining or institutionalizing the program.

Development of Educational Methods and Media

Having set priorities and selected strategies, the program manager can proceed to develop and schedule the use of educational tools, tactics, and methods. Methods, media, and materials may be classified according to visual, audio, interpersonal, and multimedia attributes. Media can be pretested in the in-

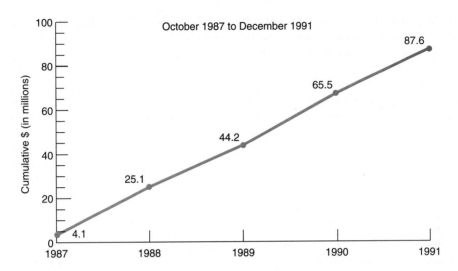

FIGURE 4-10

Cumulative dollar values of donated television and radio time (public service advertising) on HIV/AIDS in support of the CDC campaign, *American Responds to AIDS,* from October 1987 to December 1991. The equivalent of $20 million has been contributed consistently each year by community stations and national networks, which amounted to 72,425 free airings in 1991. This equals an average of 56 exposures or "audience impressions" for every U.S. adult at a cost to CDC of about 1 cent per audience impression.

Source: Centers for Disease Control: *HIV/AIDS prevention: 1992 HIV fact book,* Atlanta, 1992, Centers for Disease Control.

tended audience to determine their acceptability to the particular group and their convenience (time demands, personnel requirements, situational concerns—light, sound). They should also be selected on the basis of their efficiency (fixed costs, continuing costs, space and maintenance requirements, staff and time needs to convey a message), and presumed effectiveness (in communicating messages, arousing attention and interest, promoting interaction, using suitable repetition and message retention techniques, encouraging desired attitudes and adoption of practices).

Interpersonal or two-way communication processes provide the most favorable environment for learning, and it generally has greater long-term behavioral effects. One-way communication, such as use of pamphlets, may be appropriate if the early phases of a program or when other methods with more lasting outcomes are not feasible. A single educational intervention, however, cannot be relied on to have a significant, lasting impact on an individual's health behavior. Only through repeated educational reinforcement by health staff, aides, community leaders, friends, and family, can health education affect human behavior in the context of today's complex community health problems.

Orientation and Training

Some health workers and allied personnel may be uninformed about methods of health education, while others may feel that educational efforts are too slow, complex, and of dubious efficacy. Training can provide people time to discuss their concerns and develop their competence and confidence. Health education training should be differentiated from technical training related to health and medical content. Health education training underscores the attitudinal and behavioral factors essential to long-term health maintenance, the cultural perceptions of the target population, and the necessity of well-planned and properly sustained action. These help achieve the health behavior changes required by the objectives of the community health program.

Staff training may include orientation aimed at sensitizing the staff members to their educational function and to the general objectives of the education program. It may also include preparation in recognizing educational opportunities, communication skills, and reinforcement techniques, training priorities for those staff members in contact with consumers, and continuing education.

Volunteers are not free of cost. Proper use of volunteers requires continuous, careful supervision and training. These should be budgeted in the educational plan. A thorough plan for training volunteers might include a content designed to foster their interest in health education and in the program's need for their insight into the attitudes, reactions, and daily lives of the target population; training in communications skills and teamwork roles; and limits of volunteers' responsibility and authority.

Data Collection and Records

Statistics and financial accounts are used for educational planning and replanning; for continuous monitoring of program impact; for supervision, training, and staff development; and for evaluation of program process and outcome. Information collection requiring additional paperwork must always be weighed against other demands for time. Small additions and checklists may be integrated into existing records with little effort and with staff acceptance. For more intensive narrative reporting and recording, special efforts during limited time periods may be acceptable and provide sufficient data without generating staff resistance and unmanageable

amounts of paperwork. The educational plan should clearly identify the use and purpose of new forms and records.

Scheduling Implementation

Timing is crucial to the success of the educational plan of action. It requires an analysis of when, where, and who is responsible for implementation. This analysis will provide the starting and completion date required for each activity in relation to the total program. Consideration of the training required, production schedules for material, and staff loads guides the development of timetables.

A task analysis and time sequence of activities should integrate the educational implementation with the total program plan. External events should be considered in the scheduling for coordination with community happenings, school openings, holidays, and related community schedules.

The implementing stage is a logical progression from the previous stages of diagnosis, planning, and organizing. Very little can be stated in a program plan about implementation that is not already covered in preceding sections of the plan.

THE EVALUATING STAGES

Good records and documentation, supervisor reports on quality control, and other process evaluation can provide immediate feedback on whether things are working satisfactorily. Peer review among health professionals helps to maintain quality control, but it must be based on standards and documentation of practice. Feedback on patients' or clients' utilization and satisfaction should provide data for program adjustment and replanning. Community surveillance will aid in continuous health education planning and evaluation.

Evaluation is the comparison of an object of interest against a standard of acceptability. It is, at the very least, an assessment of the worth of a program, a method, or some other object of interest. It may provide an estimate of the degree to which spent resources result in specified activity and the degree to which performed activities attain goals. The determination of whether goals have been met is based on criteria indicated by precise statements of objectives along with subjective impressions and reporting. Hard data are sometimes available and can be used to maintain continuous evaluative research efforts. Evaluation can suggest which of several alternative educational strategies is the most efficient and which steps have an effect on the behavior specified. Evaluation provides accountability for time spent. Results usually offer a sense of accomplishment to staff and consumers or sponsors of the program.

Formative and Process Evaluation

Formative evaluation is the earliest phase of **process evaluation.** The terms refer respectively to preliminary and continuous observation and checking to see whether the program activities are taking place with the quality and at the time and rate necessary to achieve the stated objective. Sources of data for formative evaluation usually include pretesting of materials for their readability and acceptability to the target audience. Process evaluation requires ongoing sources of data that often include budget reports on monthly expenditures in specific categories where rate of expenditures would indicate amount of program activity relevant to achievement of objectives.

The standards of acceptability in formative and process evaluation usually are based on professional consensus. Process evaluation also may be based on statistics or observations from daily encounters with consumers, patients, or clients, such as clinic attendance records that are tabulated weekly, monthly, or quarterly for total numbers of new and old patients attending specific clinic sessions. Systematic sam-

ples of the records can be tabulated to obtain more detailed estimates of progress or status on such variables as broken appointment rates, sources of referral for specific clinics or problems, and trimester of first visit for pregnant women. A third type of data available for process evaluation is administrative records. Personnel records on the number of home visits attempted, the number completed, the number of group sessions conducted, and the time allotted for various educational functions can be tabulated periodically.

Feedback mechanisms should be set up so that the information collected can be used by supervisors and peers in reviewing performance. Time should be set aside on the agenda of staff and community meetings for consideration of strengths, weaknesses, and readaptation of ongoing programs. There should be a plan for charting records over time or comparing progress statistics with other programs or standards.

Outcome Evaluation

Outcome evaluation, sometimes referred to as **summative evaluation,** is when the achievement of objectives is assessed by measurement of expected outcomes. The precision with which objectives are stated determines the usefulness of this assessment. Information and data should be determined in advance. Baseline information should be obtained on a period prior to the program's inception for comparison with similarly gathered data from the period of the program or the period following the program. Statistical procedures to assess differences in outcomes should be selected in advance of data collection.

Outcome evaluation asks the following questions: What are the measurable results of program efforts in the promotion of health behavior? Has there been any change in the attitudes of the clients toward recommended actions, or change in their ability to carry out the recommended action, or change in the resources and social support for such actions in the community?

The evaluation of a specific educational component (e.g., a pamphlet or a group discussion) should not depend on the comparison of people who receive only that method with people who receive nothing. The comparison should be made between a group receiving a comprehensive health education program and another group receiving everything *except* the component to be evaluated. Thus there should be overall outcome statistics (knowledge, attitude, and behavioral outcomes) for the entire program and separate statistics on subgroups who were exposed to the entire program except for specific methods or materials of interest. The finding of no significant difference would indicate methods or materials that could be eliminated from the program to reduce costs and increase efficiency.

Reporting on progress or outcomes should occur at any stage in which important or unusual observations or decisions are made. Program developments and results need to be made available to the affiliated organizations, agencies, and institutions participating in the program and to the clients and general public. Their continued participation can be encouraged by noting their contribution to, or influence on, the program. Case histories and reports should be published in professional journals and newsletters for use by other departments, programs, or projects and to contribute to the advancement of professional knowledge and practice.

THE HEALTH EDUCATION SPECIALIST

The person assigned the responsibility for planning and implementing the community health education program ideally has training in public health or community health education and experience in a community health agency or institution. Competencies tested for the Certified Health Education Specialist (CHES) include the following:

1. Planning at the community level including epidemiological and sociological research methods, community organization, and health services administration
2. Assessment and adaptation of communications to attitudinal, cultural, economic, and ethnic determinants of health behaviors
3. Educational evaluation within the context of community health (as distinct from formal curriculum evaluation), including biostatistics, demography, and behavioral research methods

When these skills are not available within the staff of a community health agency, consultation for the planning and preparation stages of health education programs may be obtained from other organizations in the same way that specialized medical, nursing, statistical, engineering, or administrative consulta-

---

U.S. Objectives for the Nation to Enhance Educational and Community-based Programs, by the Year 2000 . . .

Objectives target increasing years of healthy life, increasing the high school graduation rate, achieving access to developmentally appropriate preschool programs, increasing quality school health education, increasing health promotion programs at postsecondary institutions, increasing worksite health promotion activities, increasing worksite health promotion for hourly workers, increasing health promotion programs for older adults, increasing family discussion of health issues, establishing community health promotion programs, increasing health promotion programs for racial and ethnic minority groups, increasing patient education and community health promotion programs, increasing partnerships between television networks and community organizations, and increasing the proportion of people who are served by a local health department that is effectively carrying out the core functions of public health.

tion is used to supplement the expertise of the agency. Continuing education and in-service training are important to maintaining up-to-date knowledge and skills in all community health staff.

SUMMARY

Human behavior accounts for approximately half of the years of an average person's life lost prematurely in Western societies. Behavior is developed and modified through learning processes that can be designed in health education to empower people to take control of their own health and to make voluntary adaptations of behavior conducive to health. In addition, health promotion (see Chapter 12) can build further supports for health behavior through organizational, economic, and environmental adaptations in the community. The planning and implementation steps outlined in this chapter apply to most of the following chapters, which will relate health education to the broader health and social development strategies.

QUESTIONS FOR REVIEW

1. Identify a trend you have noticed in recent years in your community or among your friends in health behavior and health concerns. Can you find objective data to support your observations? If not, how would you go about verifying your subjective view of the trend in health behavior?

2. Identify a national or community health campaign or program spanning a number of years. How do you account for the public concern with different health problems at different times? What were the major features of the health education component of the program? Why have different programs or problems at different times required different health education methods?

3. Among the demographic groups (geographic location, age, sex, etc.) of a population (students, patients,

workers, residents), whose quality of life would you most like to improve? How would you involve the members of the population in identifying their quality-of-life concerns?

4. What health problems are related to the quality-of-life concerns identified in your population?

5. How would you rate (low, medium, high) each health problem according to (a) its relative importance in affecting the quality-of-life concerns and (b) its potential for change?

6. How would you justify your ratings of health problems as having high priority in terms of their prevalence, incidence, cost, virulence, intensity, or other relevant dimensions?

7. What evidence supports your ratings potential for change of health problems in question 5? Refer to the success of other programs or to the availability of medical or other technology to control or reduce the high-priority health problems you have selected.

8. How would you write a program objective for the highest priority health problem, indicating who will show how much of what improvement by when?

9. In relation to the highest priority health problem identified in your program objective in question 8, what specific behaviors in your population might be causally related to the achievement of that objective?

10. How would you rate (low, medium, high) each behavior in your inventory according to its (a) prevalence, (b) epidemiological or causal importance, and (c) changeability?

11. How would you write a behavioral objective for your population (who) showing what percentage (how much) will exhibit the behavior or change the behavior (what) by a given date or amount of time from the beginning of a program (by when)?

12. For one of the high-priority behaviors you selected, what are the predisposing, enabling, and reinforcing factors you can identify?

13. How would you rate each factor believed to cause the health behavior according to each of two criteria: importance and changeability?

14. How would you write educational objectives for the

three highest priority determinants of the health behavior: one objective for a predisposing factor, one for an enabling factor, and one for a reinforcing factor?

15. For the population and health problem you have analyzed, what three educational methods would appear to be most appropriate?

16. How would your program affect and be affected by other programs and units within a health agency or educational institution?

17. What interorganizational coordination would be required to achieve the objectives of your program?

READINGS

Gold R: *Microcomputer applications in health education,* Madison, Wisc, 1991, William C. Brown.

This book reviews the state of the art in applying computer technology and concepts of computer-assisted instruction to health education.

Green LW, Kreuter MW: *Health promotion planning: an educational and environmental approach,* ed 2, Mountain View, Calif, 1991, Mayfield.

This second edition of the text previously titled *Health Education Planning: A Diagnostic Approach* shows the roots of health promotion in health education and how adding environmental targets of change to behavioral targets has broadened the PRECEDE model to include new elements in planning, implementation, and evaluation referred to as PROCEED, an acronym for policy, regulatory, and organizational constructs in educational and environmental development.

Kreuter MW: PATCH: its origin, basic concepts, and links to contemporary public health policy, *J Health Educ* 23:135, 1992.

This lead article in a special issue of the *Journal of Health Education* introduces the Planned Approach to Community Health (PATCH), an application of the PRECEDE model to community health education planning by the U.S. Centers for Disease Control and Prevention.

Prohaska TR, Albrecht G, Levy JA et al: Determinants of self-perceived risk for AIDS, *J Health & Soc Behav* 31:384, 1990.

Five factors influencing people to perceive their level of risk of contracting AIDS are examined: sexual practices, moral evaluations of people with AIDS, emotional response to AIDS, protective actions in response to AIDS, and demographic characteristics.

BIBLIOGRAPHY

Berman SH, Wandersman A: Fear of cancer and knowledge of cancer: a review and proposed relevance to hazardous waste sites, *Social Sci & Med* 31:81, 1990.

Brunk SE, Goeppinger J: Process evaluation: assessing reinvention of community-based interventions, *Eval & Health Professions* 13:186, 1990.

Champion VL: Breast self-examination in women 35 and older: a prospective study, *J Behav Med* 13:523, 1990.

Chavis DM, Wandersman A: Sense of community in the urban environment: a catalyst for participation and community development, *Am J Commun Psychol* 18:55, 1990.

Chung CS, Tash E, Raymond J et al: Health risk behaviors and ethnicity in Hawaii, *Int J Epidemiol* 19:1011, 1990.

Council on Scientific Affairs: A role for physicians and the efficacy of health education efforts, *JAMA* 263:1816, 1990.

Dabbagh L, Green LW: Application of the PRECEDE model in diarrhea prevention in Arab countries, *Int Q Community Health Educ* 12:293, 1991-92.

Dignan MB, Michielutte R, Sharp PC et al: Use of process evaluation to guide health education in Forsyth County project to prevent cervical cancer, *Public H Rep* 106:73, 1991.

Duchin SP, Brown SA: Patients should participate in designing diabetes educational content, *Patient Educ & Couns* 16:255, 1990.

Edet EE: The role of sex education in adolescent pregnancy, *J Royal Soc Health* 111:17, 1991.

Farquhar JW, Fortmann SP, Flora JA et al.: Effects of community-wide education on cardiovascular disease risk factors: the Stanford 5-city project, *JAMA* 264:359, 1990.

Fried JL, Rubinstein L: Attitudes and behaviors of dental hygienists concerning tobacco use, *J Public Health* 50: 172, 1990.

Gottlieb NH, Eriksen MP, Lovato CY et al: The impact of restrictive work site smoking policy on smoking behavior, attitudes and norms, *J Occup Med* 32:16, 1990.

Green LW: Hospitals and health care providers as agents of patient education, *Patient Educ Couns* 15:169, 1990.

Green LW: TV and teens, *J Adol Health Care* 11:91, 1990.

Green LW: The revival of community and the obligation of academic health centers to the public. In Bulger RE, Reiser SJ, editors: *Integrity in health care institutions: humane environments for teaching, inquiry and practice,* Des Moines, 1990, University of Iowa Press.

Green LW: Prevention and health education. In Last JM, Wallace RB, editors: *Maxcy-Roseneau-Last public health and preventive medicine,* ed 13, Norwalk, Conn, 1991, Appleton-Century-Crofts.

Green LW, Gottlieb NH, Parcel GS: Diffusion theory extended and applied. In *Advances in health education and promotion,* vol 3, London, 1991, Jessica Kingsley.

Green LW, Kreuter MW: CDC's planned approach to community health as an application of PRECEDE and an inspiration for PROCEED, *J Health Educ* (special issue on PATCH) 23:140, 1992.

Green LW, Mullen PD, Friedman RB: Epidemiological and community approaches to patient compliance. In Cramer JA, Spilker B, editors: *Patient compliance in medical practice and clinical trials,* New York, 1991, Raven Press.

Green LW, Simons-Morton D: Education and life-style determinants of health and disease. In Holland WW, Detels R, Knox G, editors: *Oxford textbook of public health,* ed 2, Oxford, New York & Toronto, 1991, Oxford University Press.

Harrison JA, Mullen PD, Green LW: A meta-analysis of studies of the Health Belief Model in adults, *Health Educ Res* 7:107, 1992.

Holund U: Effect of a nutrition education program, Learning by Teaching, on adolescents' knowledge and beliefs, *Comm Den Or* 18:61, 1990.

Jang M, Forst M, Moore M et al: AIDS education and prevention programs for intravenous drug users: the California experience, *J Drug Educ* 20:1, 1990.

Kok G, Green LW: Research to support health promotion in practice: a plea for increased co-operation, *Health Promotion Int* 5:303, 1990.

Kottke TE, Solberg LI, Conn S et al: A comparison of 2 methods to recruit physicians to deliver smoking cessation interventions, *Arch Intern Med* 150:1477, 1990.

Kreitler S, Chaitchi S, Kreitler H: The psychological profile of women attending breast-screening tests, *Social Sci Med* 31:1177, 1990.

Kreuter MW: PATCH: its origin, basic concepts, and links to contemporary public health policy, *J Health Educ* 23:135, 1992.

Kumanyik S: Behavioral aspects of intervention strategies to reduce dietary sodium, *Hypertension* 17:1190, 1991.

Lawrence RS: The role of physicians in promoting health, *Health Affairs* 9:122, 1990.

Lovato CY, Green LW: Maintaining employee participation in workplace health promotion programs, *Health Educ Q* 17:73, 1990.

McCoy HV, Dodds SE, Nolan C: AIDS intervention design for program evaluation: the Miami Community Outreach Project, *J Drug Issues* 20:223, 1990.

McCuan R, Green LW: Multivariate analysis in evaluation of health education and health promotion programs. In *Advances in health education and promotion,* vol 3, London, 1991, Jessica Kingsley.

Nutbeam D, Smith C, Catford J: Evaluation in health education: a review of progress, possibilities, and problems, *J Epidemiol Comm Health* 44:83, 1990.

Seffrin JR: The comprehensive school health curriculum: closing the gap between state-of-the-art and state-of-the-practice, *J Sch Health* 60:151, 1990.

Simons-Morton DG, Mullen PD, Main D et al: Characteristics on controlled studies of patient education and counseling for preventive health behaviors, *Patient Educ Couns* 19:175, 1992.

Tabak ER, Mullen PD, Simons-Morton DG et al: Definition and yield of inclusion criteria for a meta-analysis of studies of patient education in clinical preventive services, *Eval Health Professions* 14:388, 1991.

Vickers RR, Conway TL, Hervig LK: Demonstration of replicable dimensions of health behaviors, *Prev Med* 19:377, 1990.

Weiss TW, Slater CH, Green LW et al: The validity of single-item, self-assessment questions as measures of adult physical activity, *J Clin Epidemiol* 43:1123, 1990.

Winett RA, Altman DG, King AC: Conceptual and strategic foundations for effective media campaigns for preventing the spread of HIV infection, *Eval Prog Planning* 13:91, 1990.

PART TWO

· ·

Community Health through the Life Span

Promoting the health of a community means developing and supporting the will and capabilities of people to address their own special health needs. Different health problems or needs will be of primary concern to the various segments within the population. Many health problems are common to expectant mothers, infants, children, adolescents, adults, and the elderly, but each category has special aspects of these common problems, as well as its own unique problems. Whatever the objective epidemiological data may indicate about the health problems of any specific population, these data must be cast in social perspective by consulting with the population itself at the community level.

Community measures to promote the health of the whole population often apply to the needs of all groups. Community attention to the specific needs of a particular segment of the population will serve to protect and promote the health and general well-being of that group. This principle of specificity applies to age groups as well as to ethnic, occupational, residential, and socioeconomic groups, and other divisions of the population. Public health traditionally has given priority to the needs of the highest-risk populations and to the problems that affect the greatest number of people. Community health must address these problems as well as the less dramatic, everyday health concerns of people who are well and at average risk.

The following chapters in Part Two specify high-priority problems for disease prevention and health promotion, based on national and international assessments. From these assessments, objectives for entire nations, states or provinces, and communities can be proposed. This book adapts such objectives for the United States, which represents some 25 developed nations insofar as its vital rates are near the average for other English-speaking and European countries. The objectives for the United States in disease prevention and health promotion are positive expressions of what the nation should be able to achieve by 2000 if it applies the knowledge and technology now available. No assumptions are made about new break-throughs in research, such as new cures for cancer or new immunizations. The objectives for 2000 are based in part on the highest levels of health or the lowest morbidity and mortality rates already achieved in certain other countries or in certain communities.

These objectives are contrasted with the situation in developing countries and with the situation in North America through rates for different ethnic or socioeconomic groups. The intent in formulating the objectives for the nation was to challenge both public- and private-sector organizations at national, state or provincial, and local levels to work toward the elimination of disparities between the haves and the have-nots, between regions or communities, and between races and cultural groups. It is hoped that you might feel challenged to adapt the objectives to populations within the communities in which you live or work.

Chapter 5

Reproductive, Infant, and Child Health

Well begun is half done.
    HORACE

OBJECTIVES

When you finish this chapter, you should be able to:

• Identify the leading health problems, trends, and needs as they relate to reproduction and to the infants and children of a community

• Describe strategies to improve reproductive, infant, and child health

---

From a community health perspective, reproductive health includes the social and biological preparation of men and women for the responsibilities of pregnancy and parenthood. Maternal, infant, and child health (MCH) encompasses community preventive care and education of infants, children, and mothers before and after delivery. It includes education of parents about immunization, dental care, nutrition, family planning, child care and child abuse, substance misuse, physical fitness, and stress. Special attention is given in this chapter to preventive health service and health promotion approaches that should be incorporated in prenatal care, preparation for parenting, and school health, such as proper nutrition and the avoidance of alcohol, drug consumption, and smoking.

REPRODUCTIVE HEALTH

Men and women face critical choices in reproductive health related to preparing for parenthood, maintaining sexual health, family planning, pregnancy, and safe and healthful childbearing. These choices require concern about the health and well-being of all involved.

Family Structure and Health

Family composition is changing. Formally, **family** is defined as a group of two or more people related by birth, marriage, or adoption residing together in a household. This definition, of course, does not include most extended families in Western societies or many of the new forms of cohabitation that have developed in recent decades. The number of two-parent families has steadily declined (see Figure 5-1). In Canada, as of 1991, 1 in 10 couples lived in a common-law union, a 104% increase over the 1981 figure. Single-parent families made up 13% of all Canadian families. Families are important shapers of individual health. It is in families that an individual first learns to make choices that promote physical, emotional, and community health.

Health conditions are likely to be affected by other family circumstances. Nearly one quarter of American children aged 6 years and younger live below the federal poverty level, many of them living with a single parent in female-headed families. Although these families may offer important nurturing, they are more likely to be economically and educationally disadvantaged. In addition, there is evidence that the health of children is affected by the marital status of their parents. Higher infant mortal-

ity, less prenatal care, and a greater risk of developing health problems are found in families with a single parent.

Family Planning

Family planning is the process of establishing the preferred number and spacing of children in one's family and selecting the means by which this objective is achieved. Achievement of family planning goals takes information, motivation, exercise of personal responsibility, community support, and effective means of family planning. Communities, through their multiple institutions, such as government, churches, and voluntary agencies, may influence individual choice in acceptable family planning methods. For example, in the 1980s U.S. federal documents recommending effective means of family planning were listed as ''childbearing, adoption, abstinence from sexual activity outside of

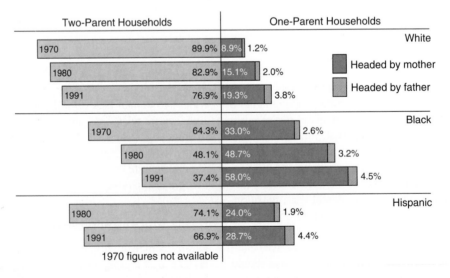

FIGURE 5-1

Increases in single-parent families between 1970 and 1991, United States.

Source: Bureau of the Census, U.S. Department of Commerce.

among women aged 15 to 24 years, 67% of the pregnancies were unintended, with over 86% of the pregnancies of unmarried women unintended. Health education plays a role in family planning by providing men and women with learning experiences that enable them to make choices about reproduction. One objective of these efforts is to increase the number of intended pregnancies. The first objective of the nation (see the box below) is to reduce the number of unintended pregnancies from 56% to 30% by the year 2000. Over 57% of all unintended pregnancies were of women who were not using a contraceptive method.

Birth Control Methods

The most common methods used to decrease the number of unintended pregnancies are shown in Table 5-1. These methods vary in their popularity and their estimated effectiveness, risks, benefits, convenience, availability, and cost. Health education and clinical service programs need to consider these

a monogamous relationship, use of contraceptive methods, natural family planning, and treatment of infertility.'' While these remain viable methods of family planning, their order of priority and program emphasis are likely to change with changes in federal leadership.

Intended and Unintended Pregnancy

In 1988 American women reported that 56% of their pregnancies in the last 5 years had been ''unintended,'' either occurring too soon or when unwanted. The percentage of unintended pregnancies varies with age and socioeconomic status. For example, a 1989 New York State survey found that

TABLE 5-1
Frequency of use, and pros and cons of selected contraceptive methods

	Condom	Diaphragm with spermicide	IUD	Birth control pills	Birth control implant	Vasectomy (male sterilization)	Tubal ligation (female sterilization)
Estimated effectiveness							
	64 to 97%	80 to 98%	95 to 96%	97% (mini) 99% (comb.)	99%	Over 99%	Over 99%
Percent of users							
	6.7%	4.5%	4.0%	15.6%	<1%	25.7%	25.7%
Risks							
	Rarely, irritation and allergic reactions	Rarely, irritation and allergic reactions; bladder infection; constipation; very rarely, toxic shock syndrome	Cramps, bleeding, pelvic inflammatory disease, infertility; rarely, perforation of the uterus	Blood clots, heart attacks and strokes, gallbladder disease, liver tumors, water retention, hypertension, mood changes, dizziness and nausea, not for smokers	Menstrual cycle irregularity; headache, nervousness, depression, nausea, dizziness, change of appetite, breast tenderness, weight gain, enlargement of ovaries and/or fallopian tubes, excessive growth of body and facial hair; may subside after first year	Pain, infection; rarely, possible psychological problems	Surgical complications; some pain or discomfort; possibly higher risk of hysterectomy later in life

Non-contraceptive benefits						
None	None	Less menstrual bleeding contains no estrogen (estrogen used in some birth control pills may be associated with an increased risk of blood clots)	Less menstrual bleeding and cramping, lower risk of fibrocystic breast disease, ovarian cysts, and pelvic inflammatory disease; protects against cancer of the ovaries and lining of the uterus	None	Some protection against sexually transmitted diseases, including herpes and AIDS	Spermicides may give some protection against sexually transmitted diseases
Convenience						
One-time procedure	One-time procedure	Effective 24 hours after implantation for approximately 5 years; can be removed by physician at any time	Pill must be taken on daily schedule, regardless of the frequency of intercourse	After insertion, stays in place until physician removes it	Applied immediately before intercourse	Inserted before intercourse; can be left in place 24 hours, but additional spermicide must be inserted if intercourse is repeated
Availability						
Surgery	Minor surgery	Rx; minor outpatient surgical procedure	Rx	Rx	Nonprescription	Rx

Source: Food and Drug Administration, U.S Dept. of Health and Human Services, Nov. 1991.

factors, as well as the cultural, social, and political acceptability of these methods to selected subpopulations.

Infertility

Infertility affects an estimated 2.4 million married couples and an unknown number of potential parents among unmarried couples and singles. Factors affecting infertility include problems in ovulation, blocked or scarred fallopian tubes, endometriosis, and low sperm count. The estimated 20% of infertility that arises from sexually transmitted diseases is the most preventable. The year 2000 objective for infertility is to reduce the prevalence of infertility from 7.9% to 6.5% of married couples with wives aged 15 to 44 years.

TRENDS IN MATERNAL MORTALITY AND MORBIDITY
Rates

Maternal deaths are those associated with deliveries and complications of pregnancy, childbirth, and **puerperium.** Rates are based on number of mothers dying per 100,000 live births occurring in a given year (see Figure 5-2).

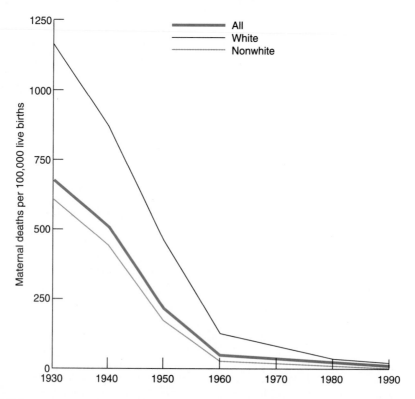

FIGURE 5-2
Maternal mortality by race, United States, 1930-1990, showing the relative rates of decline and the reduced gap between mortality rates for whites and nonwhites.
Source: National Center for Health Statistics, U.S. Department of Health and Human Services.

Causes

The causes of **maternal mortality** have altered, reflecting the relative decline of hemorrhage, infection, and toxemia. Anesthetic misadventures are relatively more common now, since other causes have decreased and since the number of patients receiving anesthesia for childbirth has increased. Paradoxically, advances in medicine have provided challenges in obstetrics: women with congenital heart disease and juvenile diabetes are now able to become pregnant, but their safe delivery demands skill. **Abortion** as a cause of maternal mortality has declined with safe, legalized abortions replacing clandestine, septic abortions.

Widespread availability of effective contraceptive techniques has reduced the number of unintended pregnancies, which in turn has reduced maternal mortality. The radical changes in abortion laws and contraceptive use are the result of societal pressures to which public health, education, and medicine have responded. Teenage pregnancy remains a major problem in the United States, especially in the under-15 age group. This issue will be addressed in the next chapter.

DES. Women were exposed to the drug diethylstilbestrol (DES) when their mothers took the drug before their births from the 1940s into the 1970s for pregnancy complications. These DES daughters are at increased risk of cancer of the vagina and cervix. DES daughters are also more likely to have problems in their pregnancies. The rate of unfavorable birth outcomes for a group of women exposed to DES was nearly twice that of unexposed women, where *unfavorable birth outcome* was defined as a miscarriage, a stillbirth, or an ectopic pregnancy.

Cesarean deliveries. Cesarean delivery rates in the United States increased through the last two decades to a high of 24.4 per 100 deliveries in 1989. In these deliveries the baby is removed surgically through the abdominal wall of the mother, rather than vaginally. In 1970 only about 5.5% of deliveries were

cesarean; in contrast, 1990 was the first year in the two decades since in which the rate dropped to 22.7%. The rate is still considered high, especially since there is no evidence to suggest that such deliveries have improved maternal or child health for their $1.3 billion price tag. Reasons for the high rate include misdiagnosis, widely varying physician practices, convenience to mothers and physicians, increased revenue from deliveries, and physicians' concerns about malpractice suits. The slight decrease in 1990 is attributed to better patient education and organized programs to reduce such deliveries. The objective for the year 2000 is to reduce the cesarean delivery rate to no more than 15 per 100 deliveries.

Ectopic pregnancies. In recent years dramatic increases in the number of women delaying pregnancy until after age 35 and in diseases and procedures affecting the fallopian tubes have increased the rate of ectopic pregnancy. An ectopic or tubal pregnancy occurs when the mass of cells that develops from

Historical and Comparative Perspectives

Consider maternal health conditions at the turn of the century, when the population in the United States was about 76 million. More than 20,000 women died in childbirth each year. Some 90 years later, with a population of more than 230 million—three times the number of people at risk—the yearly number of deaths of women resulting from complications of childbirth has been reduced to fewer than 400. The chances of a woman's surviving childbirth in the United States and in most other developed countries today are about 8999 out of 9000, and the survival rate continues to improve. How do you account for this dramatic reduction in the risks of childbearing in the more developed countries? Why do the maternal mortality rates for the least developed countries remain at levels as high as those in the United States at the turn of the century?

the fertilized egg fails to move through the fallopian tube to attach to the wall of the uterus, where it is supposed to grow; instead, it attaches to the wall of the fallopian tube. In 1980 there was 1 ectopic pregnancy for every 250 normal pregnancies; by 1990 there was 1 for every 70 normal pregnancies, a fourfold increase. Ectopic pregnancies are now the leading cause of maternal mortality in the United States; the relative risk of death from an ectopic pregnancy is 10 times greater than from childbirth and 50 times greater than from a legal abortion.

Pelvic inflammatory disease (PID). PID causes damage to the fallopian tubes. This can lead to infertility and can cause a pregnancy to be ectopic. PID is an infection of the uterus and the fallopian tubes caused by sexually transmitted disease or sometimes by postsurgical infection. If the disease is treated quickly, damage to the reproductive structures can be prevented.

Abortions. Abortion may be spontaneous or artificial. A spontaneous abortion, also called a miscarriage, occurs when a pregnancy ends spontaneously before the beginning of the twentieth week of pregnancy. A miscarriage is due to the separation of the developing fetus and the placenta from the inner wall of the uterus. Usually the cause is unknown.

A pregnancy that ends artificially is also called an abortion, but the medical term is termination of pregnancy. In 1973 the United States Supreme Court ruled in *Roe* v. *Wade* that women have a constitutional right to abortion for any reason during the first 24 weeks of pregnancy and, after that, if the pregnancy endangers the mother's life. In 1969 abortions were legalized in Canada if performed by a doctor in an approved hospital and medically certified that continuation of the pregnancy would likely endanger the life or health of the mother. In 1988 approximately 1½ million abortions were performed in the United States; in 1990 there were approximately 71,000 abortions in Canada.

The states are free to restrict abortion, as long as they do not place an "undue burden" on a woman.

Those restrictions have increased. As of 1992, 16 states have non-enforced laws requiring parents of teenaged pregnant women to be notified before abortion; 20 states have enforced parental-notification laws; 26 states allow minors to bypass parental notification with a court order; 26 states require mandatory counseling about fetal development and abortion alternatives; 13 states have a waiting period; 30 states allow no public funding, except when a mother's life is endangered.

Despite its legal status, abortion remains controversial (Figure 5-3) and is not equally available to all women. With increased restrictions, access to abortion services depends on judges, doctors who may or may not choose to perform them, and lawmakers who decide on public funding for abortion services. Although the medical community over-

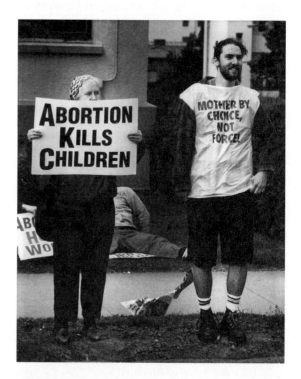

FIGURE 5-3
Anti-abortionists and pro-abortionists have a stand-off near the clinic at Vancouver General Hospital.
Photo courtesy *Vancouver Courier*, Eike Schroter.

whelmingly favors abortion rights, in practice few doctors perform abortions. Eighty-three percent of the counties in the United States have no known abortion provider. A similar disparity exists between countries in Europe and in Latin America. For example, over 4000 women from Ireland cross the Irish Sea each year to have legal abortions in England because they cannot obtain them in Ireland.

Strategies to provide abortion services could include counseling a woman facing an unintended pregnancy to apprise her of her options; starting freestanding clinics in more populous regions; encouraging physicians in hospitals to provide the services; and establishing clinics in county hospitals, with satellite clinics providing services to smaller communities at a distance from the main facility.

Pro-Choice and Pro-Life Controversy

Abortion is a highly controversial meeting ground for legal, political, economic, religious, social, and public health interests. Women find themselves with an unintended pregnancy, and health care workers find their decisions and actions pulled by many interests. A woman exercising her legal right to choose an abortion may face a gauntlet of pro-life supporters who believe that her choice constitutes murder. Health care workers who support a woman's right to choose found themselves ''gagged'' in 1988 by a federal rule that prohibited abortion counseling in federally funded family planning clinics. A physician in the southeastern United States who offered abortion services in several unserved counties was murdered in 1993 by a pro-life supporter who believed that the physician's services constituted murder.

The abortion debate continues at national and local levels in North America. In 1988 the Supreme Court of Canada overturned the 1969 amendment legalizing abortions. The Court's decision left Canada without an abortion law. Shortly after his inauguration; President Clinton approved by executive order new policies that lifted federal abortion limitations imposed by the previous Republican administrations. These included lifting the ''gag rule,'' eliminating a ban on federal fetal tissue research, and forcing a decision on the ban to import RU-486, the ''abortion pill.''

How are political changes in North America likely to affect the pro-choice and pro-life controversy? Why is access to abortion services of concern to public health? What are the options for health care workers who find their personal beliefs at odds with professional requirements? How have abortions affected maternal mortality?

PROMOTING MATERNAL HEALTH

Couples have choices available in planning for children by means of contraception, termination of unintended pregnancies by abortion, prenatal care, continuation of schooling or work during and following maternity leave, and services for safe deliv-

---

U.S. Objectives for Maternal and Prenatal Care

- By 2000 reduce the maternal mortality rate to no more than 3.3 per 100,000 live births. Baseline: in 1989 the overall rate in the United States was 7.9. Despite declines in maternal death rates for both whites and blacks, the rate for black women in 1989 was 18.4, more than three times the rate for white women, 5.6.
- By 2000 increase abstinence from tobacco use by pregnant women to at least 90% and increase abstinence from alcohol, cocaine, and marijuana by pregnant women by at least 20%. Baseline: in 1985 75% of pregnant women abstained from tobacco use.
- Increase to at least 90% the proportion of all pregnant women who receive prenatal care in the first trimester of pregnancy. Baseline: in 1989 76% of all women who had live births met this objective. Baseline rates were lower for blacks—60.4%, American Indian/Alaska Native women—60.5%, and Hispanic women—61.2%.
- By 2000 reduce iron deficiency to less than 3% among women of childbearing age. Baseline: 5% for women aged 20 to 44 years. For black, low-income women in the third trimester the baseline rate is 41%.

ery. The community role lies in assuring access to these services, in making potential users of these options aware of them, and in counseling as to appropriate choice. Early and reliable pregnancy testing and genetic counseling are now available.

Prenatal Care

Prenatal care should be sought early in pregnancy, preferably during the first 3 months. Health education, early detection of abnormalities, and identification of the high-risk mother and infant are the major purposes of prenatal care. At the first visit a complete medical, surgical, obstetric and genetic history is obtained, and a physical examination is performed (Figure 5-4). Routine laboratory data are obtained, including blood type and Rhesus (Rh) factor determination; urinalysis; complete blood count; rubella titer; tests for syphilis, gonorrhea, and abnormalities of hemoglobin synthesis (sickle cell); and cervical smear. A social worker or genetic counselor may interview the woman or the couple and discuss available community resources or potential birth defects.

Early care reduces infant mortality and low birthweight. Although this is widely known among professionals, about one fourth of all infants born in the United States are born to mothers who receive late or no care. Adequate care is defined as care in the first trimester *and* nine or more visits during a full-term pregnancy.

Infants of women who receive no prenatal care have about 10 times the risk of dying in the first months of life. Prenatal care is also a bargain. Every dollar spent on prenatal care for low-income, poorly educated women saves about $3 in intensive care for infants born with birth defects.

Health Education

Community information campaigns about the importance of prenatal care can be directed to the

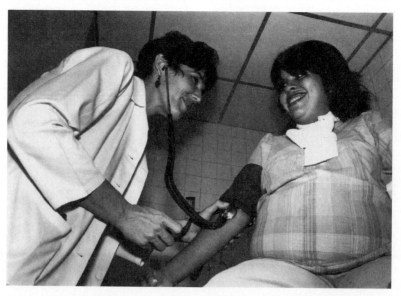

FIGURE 5-4
Prenatal care confers advantages to the fetus and the mother.
Photo by Marsha Burkes, courtesy University of Texas Health Science Center at Houston.

groups least likely to seek care. These include teenagers, especially those who already have children, low-income and uninsured women, women over age 35, recent immigrants, and high-risk minorities. One-shot, short-lived campaigns seldom have much impact on public attitudes or personal health behavior.

The prenatal visits provide an opportunity for counseling and education about health-related behavior, including dental care, avoidance or reduction of alcohol and cigarette smoking, use of seat belts, balanced exercise, and rest. A supportive, nonjudgmental, warm, sympathetic climate is maintained so that communication and cooperation between patient and provider is enhanced and responsibility is shared. For high-risk groups (defined by medical history), exposures to harmful substances or physical abuse might be discussed.

Education for childbirth should start at school in human biology studies. During pregnancy the most effective education is in peer group sessions, when

---

Barriers for Prenatal Care

Important barriers to women seeking prenatal care include costs, available services, and public understanding of the importance of such care. The greatest barrier is financial. More than 14 million American women of reproductive age have no insurance to cover medical care. A growing shortage of obstetric providers, attributed to rising malpractice insurance rates, contributes to service delivery issues for all women. This is a particular problem for poor women who face inadequate facilities or clinical practices, such as long waits and poor interpersonal skills of staff, that make clinic visits difficult or unpleasant.

Although recent congressional mandates have expanded Medicaid, making more women eligible for prenatal and postpartum care, difficulties remain in getting eligible women into care. Lack of understanding about the benefits of prenatal care, along with transportation problems, personal or cultural beliefs, and lack of child care, may deter these women from accessing services.

---

experienced mothers can lead others. Removing fear is a great benefit, and the attendance of fathers is valuable. Visiting the hospital's delivery and newborn suites and meeting the staff can benefit the apprehensive woman. Various professional and lay groups endorse different plans of preparation for and practices during childbirth, but the common thread is open discussion, question and answer, and removal of fear. Couples in such programs enjoy the emotional experience of pregnancy and delivery. Studies have shown reductions in the amount of analgesia and anesthesia used by women who participated in childbirth classes, as well as shortened labor.

Precautions in the early stages of pregnancy include avoidance of three risk factors that can cause congenital defects: infection, exposure to irradiation, and ingestion of alcohol and drugs, including tobacco (Figure 5-5).

Nutrition

A strong relationship exists between pregnancy weight gain of the mother and birth weight of an infant. Since the infant's birth weight is a determinant of potential for survival and future development, recommended weight gain for the mother is important to achieve. In general, women who are normal weight or slightly overweight have better pregnancy outcomes than those who are underweight. Weight gain during pregnancy needs to consider not only caloric intake but also nutritional quality. Other factors influencing weight gain include smoking, strenuous physical work, and chronic illness. The social pressure on women to be thin may make it difficult for some to allow themselves adequate weight gain during pregnancy.

Pregnancy is an ideal time for nutritional counseling for women and their families. It provides an opportunity to educate women not only about their own nutritional needs during pregnancy but also about the future needs of their infants, themselves, and their families. Nutritional counseling needs to consider the recommended balance of food and

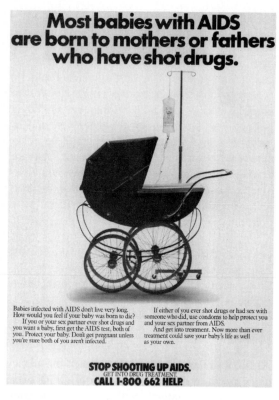

Most babies with AIDS are born to mothers or fathers who have shot drugs.

Babies infected with AIDS don't live very long. How would you feel if your baby was born to die?

If you or your sex partner ever shot drugs and you want a baby, first get the AIDS test, both of you. Protect your baby. Don't get pregnant unless you're sure both of you aren't infected.

If either of you ever shot drugs or had sex with someone who did, use condoms to help protect you and your sex partner from AIDS.

And get into treatment. Now more than ever treatment could save your baby's life as well as your own.

STOP SHOOTING UP AIDS.
GET INTO DRUG TREATMENT.
CALL 1-800 662 HELP.

FIGURE 5-5
Drug abuse invades all aspects of the lives of users and often the lives of others, including the unborn.
Source: National Institute on Drug Abuse, U.S. Department of Health and Human Services.

should be sensitive to the cultural preferences and economic circumstances of the mother. If necessary, women may need referral to appropriate governmental or voluntary agency programs for assistance with their nutritional needs.

Detection of Abnormalities and Risk

High-risk pregnancies should be identified so that these cases can be given special care. Predictors are age, particularly under 15 years or over 35 years; previous obstetric difficulty, such as unexplained

stillbirths, premature deliveries, and spontaneous abortions; women who attend clinics for sexually transmitted diseases, have multiple sex partners, a history of prostitution, or sexual partners who were IV drug users; and women who are under 60 inches tall or those who smoke cigarettes daily or use alcohol or drugs (Figure 5-5).

Many procedures during pregnancy relate more to the health of the fetus and newborn than to the health or safety of the mother, but in the final analysis these considerations are inseparable.

Amniocentesis provides the means to assess many previously undetectable genetic abnormalities in the fetus. A sample of amniotic fluid, drawn from the expectant mother's uterus by means of a hypodermic needle, can be cultured in the laboratory and tested for biochemical and chromosomal defects. Genetic counseling and amniocentesis detect and provide the opportunity to prevent abnormal or defective births. Estimates of the incidence and prevalence of genetic diseases and congenital abnormalities vary. Some 36% of all spontaneous abortions are caused by gross chromosomal defects (amounting to more than 100,000 per year in the United States). At least 40% of all infant mortality results from genetic factors, and genetic defects are present in 5% of all live births.

Many serious genetic disorders can be detected from the fourteenth to the twentieth week of pregnancy, when therapeutic abortion is medically feasible and legally permissible in most states. If the fetus has abnormalities, the prospective parents can choose not to terminate the pregnancy but still gain from the time to prepare for the birth. Increasingly, medical science offers the potential to correct some problems in utero.

Most tests are negative, providing relief from fear and anxiety for prospective parents with any reason to suspect a genetic or congenital abnormality.

One type of screening that has become a standard of care for women is maternal serum alpha-fetoprotein (MSAFP) testing. This test can be used to detect neural tube defect in fetuses, twin pregnancy, central wall defects, Down syndrome, and fetal demise. Because the test is not informative other than in the fifteenth to eighteenth week of pregnancy, early prenatal care is essential.

In the long run, the total cost to the community of caring for the diseases and disabilities of children with genetic and congenital defects far outweighs the cost of prenatal counseling, screening, diagnosis, and abortion. The cost–benefit ratios run as high as $20 saved for every dollar spent on these procedures.

PROMOTING PERINATAL HEALTH

Perinatal mortality is the number of late fetal deaths (stillbirths) from the twenty-eighth week of pregnancy plus the number of deaths in the first week of life per 1000 live births (Figure 5-6). This reproductive index makes up both intrauterine and extrauterine deaths and is a measure of the quality and efficiency of obstetrical and neonatal services. Perinatal mortality is most heavily influenced by low birthweight, formerly called the **prematurity rate,** which is the percentage of all babies born who

> ### U.S. Objectives for Perinatal and Neonatal Health
>
> - By 2000 reduce the fetal death rate to no more than 5 per 1000 live births plus fetal deaths. Baseline: 5.5 per 1000 live births plus fetal deaths in 1989. For blacks and others, the baseline was 11.4 in 1989.
> - By 2000 reduce the incidence of fetal alcohol syndrome to no more than 0.12 per 1000 live births. Baseline: 0.22 per 1000 live births in 1987. American Indians and Alaska Natives are a special population target. Their baseline rate of 4 in 1987 was 33 times higher than whites. The year 2000 target for this population is 2.
> - By 2000 increase to at least 95% the proportion of newborns screened by state-sponsored programs for genetic disorders and other disabling conditions and to 90% the proportion of newborns testing positive for disease who receive appropriate treatment. Baseline: for sickle cell anemia, approximately 33% of live births were screened in 1989.

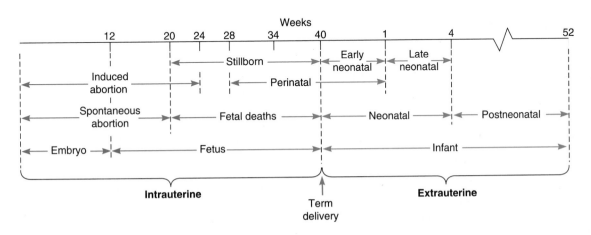

FIGURE 5-6
Reproductive and perinatal mortalities are based on numbers of fetal and infant deaths in each of eight periods, some of which overlap.

weigh 2500 grams (5 pounds, 8 ounces) or less. The rate of survival of such infants is naturally lower than that of term-sized infants, mainly because the respiratory system of premature infants is not sufficiently mature to adapt to extrauterine life. Advances in neonatology, through the use of intensive care nurseries or prematurity centers, have been tremendous, so the survival rate is improving for all birthweight ranges.

Although perinatal mortality is decreasing, its decline is limited by the low-birthweight rate, which has remained constant since 1950 in the United States. It was thought that the low-birthweight rate would fall in response to improved social conditions, but a complex interaction of factors has been operating. A high proportion of births now derive from adolescent mothers and those in lower socioeconomic strata. Mothers aged less than 15 years have a prematurity rate twice that of other mothers, and black babies are twice as likely as white babies to be born prematurely. Low-birthweight infants include newborns who are born too early and those whose intrauterine growth is retarded. Risk factors for low birthweight include (1) previous history of a low-birthweight infant, (2) younger and older maternal age, (3) low socioeconomic status, (4) low educational level, (5) late entry into prenatal care, (6) low pregnancy weight gain or low pregnancy weight, and (7) smoking and substance abuse. These factors are interrelated and are amenable to community influence through nutrition, family planning, health education, and more general socioeconomic support and improvement.

PROMOTING INFANT HEALTH
Infant Mortality

Infant mortality is the number of deaths of children under 1 year of age per 1000 live births. Deaths in the first week of life contribute to rates for both perinatal and infant mortality (Figure 5-7).

At the beginning of this century about 100 of

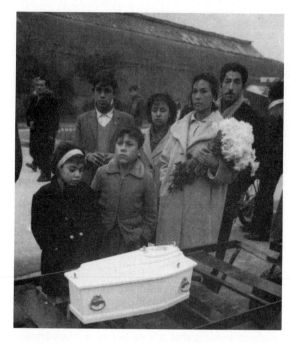

FIGURE 5-7
The baby's coffin and the faces of the mourning family tell the tragic story of infant mortality.
Photo by P. Almasy, courtesy World Health Organization.

every 1000 infants born in the United States died in the first year of life. This figure has progressively declined to 29.0 per 1000 infants in 1950, 20.0 in 1970, and 8.6 in 1992. However, large differences persist in infant death rates among subgroups of the population and between geographical areas. A black child in 1977 was twice as likely as a white infant to die before reaching 1 year of age. Now the difference is three times (Figure 5-8). The rate of infant deaths in Washington, D.C., in 1988 was 19.9 per 1000 live births for whites and 26.0 for blacks; in Minnesota the rate was 7.2 for whites and 19.5 for blacks.

Infant mortality can be divided into two components: (1) **neonatal mortality,** occurring in the first 28 days after birth, which largely reflects prenatal and perinatal circumstances and events, and (2)

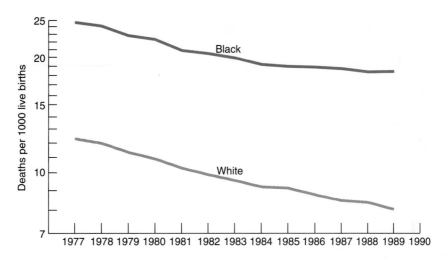

FIGURE 5-8
Infant mortality rates by race, United States, 1977 to 1990.
Source: National Center for Health Statistics, National Vital Statistics System.

postneonatal mortality, occurring between 28 days and 365 days of age, which is dependent on parenting and other aspects of the infant's environment (Figure 5-6). Problems and intervention strategies differ for these two stages.

Neonatal health. Family planning, prenatal care with risk assessment and management, obstetrical technology, breastfeeding, and newborn intensive care represent our major weapons to combat neonatal deaths.

Postneonatal health. Parenting instruction, especially for new mothers, including care and feeding of infants, illness surveillance and care, and use of pediatric services, are techniques to reduce postneonatal infant deaths. Neonatal mortality accounts for more than two thirds of infant deaths, and it is in this category that the largest gains were being made until 1985.

Halted progress. The death rate for babies under 28 days fell dramatically—from 7.6 to 6.5—be-

tween 1982 and 1988; but for infants aged 28 days to 11 months the rate fell only slightly in the same period—from 3.7 to 3.6. The concentration of this effect in black infants can be seen in Figure 5-8.

International rates. Infant mortality in advanced countries is mostly influenced by deaths in the first month of life, which make up 70% of the deaths in the first year. This high proportion results from the reduction in deaths caused by infectious diseases, which earlier in this century contributed to the high infant mortality. Reduction of infant mortality depends now on reducing deaths immediately following birth, which in turn means reducing the low-birthweight rate. Countries that have low infant mortalities—for example, Norway and Sweden—have low-birthweight rates of about 3.0%, whereas the rate is 6.9% in the United States (5.6% for whites, 12.4% for blacks). Weight for weight, babies have a high survival rate in the United States relative to most countries because of advanced neonatology. But the United States must contend with relatively

---

U.S. Objectives for Infant Health

- By 2000 reduce the infant mortality rate to no more than 7 per 1000 live births. Baseline: 10.1 per 1000 live births in 1987. Blacks, American Indians, and Puerto Ricans have infant mortality rates substantially higher than the United States average.

Infant mortality per 1000 live births	1987 Baseline	2000 Target
Blacks	17.9	11
American Indians/Alaska Natives	12.5	8.5
Puerto Ricans	12.9	8

- By 2000 reduce low birthweight to an incidence of no more than 5% of live births and very low birthweight to no more than 1% of live births. Baseline: 6.9% and 1.2%, respectively, in 1987.
- By 2000 reduce the incidence of fetal alcohol syndrome to no more than 0.12 per 1000 live births. Baseline: 0.22 per 1000 live births in 1987. American Indians and Alaska Natives are a special population target. Their baseline rate of 4 in 1987 was 33 times higher than whites. The year 2000 target for this population is 2.

---

more low-birthweight babies, which adversely affects reproductive indexes (see Table 5-2).

Improvements in the survival of infants will also stem from reduction in the needless waste of infant lives caused by injuries and by infectious diseases. Community action is effective here in providing a safe environment and requiring infant car seats by legislation; immunization programs; reduction of burns, alcoholism, and child abuse; and education of mothers to bring their children to a physician early in illness when infectious disease may be successfully treated. Adequate community resources to provide alternate child care facilities for working mothers is imperative.

Breastfeeding

Breast milk alone, without supplements, is the optimal choice for feeding full-term infants for the first 6 months. Mother's milk contains an ideal balance of nutrients, enzymes, immunoglobulin, antiinfective and antiinflammatory substances, hormones, and growth factors that protect the infant and encourage growth. Breast milk changes over time to match the changing needs of the infant. For the mother, breastfeeding facilitates the physiological return to the prepregnant state and offers hygienic and economic benefits over bottlefeeding. For both infant and mother, breastfeeding confers an intense opportunity for bonding and interaction. Breastfeeding is not recommended for women with the AIDS virus, those who abuse drugs or alcohol, and those receiving certain kinds of therapeutic agents, such as chemotherapy.

The percentage of American mothers who breastfeed at birth declined 13% from 1984 to 1989. The percentage of mothers who continue to breastfeed their infants at 6 months fell by a quarter, from 24% to 18%. Again, the average rates mask differences in subpopulations. Breastfeeding rates are highest among women who are older, well-educated, relatively affluent, and who live in the western United States and lowest among low-income, black women under 20 years of age living in the southeastern United States.

Barriers to breastfeeding include the public portrayal of bottlefeeding as the norm, along with lack of information about the advantages and techniques of breastfeeding. As natural an act as breastfeeding is, sometimes mothers need help and support to initiate and sustain it. Voluntary groups such as the La Leche League can provide such assistance free of charge. Other barriers include work policies and facilities that discourage breastfeeding and societal attitudes about women's bodies that lead to the inappropriate perception that breastfeeding in public is a sexual rather than a nurturing act.

TABLE 5-2
Infant mortality

Country	Rate* 1982† Infant deaths per 1,000 live births	1987‡	Average annual percent change	Country	Rate* 1982† Infant deaths per 1,000 live births	1987‡	Average annual percent change
Japan	6.6	5.0	−5.4	Belgium	11.1	9.7	−2.7
Sweden	6.9	5.7	−3.7	Austria	12.8	9.8	−5.2
Finland	6.8	6.2	−1.8	Italy	13.1	9.8	−5.6
Switzerland	7.7	6.9	−2.2	New Zealand	12.0	10.0	−3.6
Canada	**9.1**	**7.3**	**−4.3**	**United States**	**11.5**	**10.1**	**−2.6**
Singapore	10.7	7.3	−7.4	Israel	13.9	10.7	−5.1
Hong Kong	9.9	7.5	−5.4	Greece	15.1	12.6	−3.6
Netherlands	8.3	7.6	−1.7	Czechoslovakia	16.2	12.8	−4.6
France	9.5	7.8	−3.9	Cuba	17.3	13.3	−5.1
Ireland	10.5	7.9	−5.5	Puerto Rico	17.1	14.2	−3.6
Federal Republic of Germany	10.9	8.2	−5.5	Portugal	19.8	14.2	−6.4
Denmark	8.2	8.3	0.2	Bulgaria	18.2	14.8	−4.1
Norway	8.1	8.4	0.7	Kuwait	22.8	15.7	−8.9
Scotland	11.4	8.5	−5.7	Hungary	20.0	17.3	−2.9
Australia	10.3	8.7	−3.3	Costa Rica	19.4	17.4	−2.2
Northern Ireland	13.7	8.7	−8.7	Poland	20.2	17.5	−2.8
German Democratic Republic	11.4	8.8	−5.0	Chile	23.6	18.5	−4.8
Spain	11.3	9.0	−7.3	Romania	28.0	22.5	−4.3
England and Wales	10.8	9.2	−3.2	U.S.S.R.§	25.1	25.4	0.3

*Number of deaths of infants under 1 year per 1000 live births.
†Data for the U.S.S.R. are for 1983.
‡Data for Kuwait are for 1986; and data for Spain are for 1985.
§U.S.S.R. now divided into several countries.

COMMUNITY HEALTH PROGRAMS FOR CHILDREN

Basic health services for the prevention of disease and the early identification of illness or disability should be available to all children. Well-child clinics providing assessment of growth and development, nutrition information, nurturing and anticipatory guidance, and immunization for all children should be available. Well-child care should be at regular intervals and may be performed by allied health personnel other than physicians. Competent pediatric nurse practitioners, experienced public health nurses, and all physician's assistants working in tandem with psychologists and educators can assess the progress of a child, interpreting the steps already taken and the next steps to be expected for the person caring for the child.

Parent-infant bonding and anticipatory counseling to prevent problems will enable the child to grow up in a healthful and well-structured atmosphere. Early recognition of social and psychological problems will permit early and simple correction of adverse circumstances. School health is an essential component of community health.

Status of Child Health

Children are healthier today than ever before, certainly as measured by the usual morbidity and mortality indicators. Today, however, there are different threats to the health of children and youth, often characterized as the "new morbidity," for which environmental (social, physical, familial, and economic) and behavioral factors have been identified as causative or contributive. Some special childhood problems of concern to those who will work with these age groups are learning disorders, inadequate school functioning, behavioral problems, speech and vision difficulties, mental retardation, child abuse and neglect, and injuries.

The family has profound effects on the health and educational status of its members. The national goals to improve the health of children and youth and to prevent consequences of the "new morbidity" are highly dependent on the family environment. But the family is no longer seen as the sole agent of children's socialization; the emerging understanding is that both the child and the family are affected by every institution of society. The focus now on children in the context of living in a complex world of family interactions, mass media, and other societal forces. The attention to the impact of families and school on children's health will make children targets to an increasing degree for delivery of health, educational, and other community programs.

Immunization Programs and Procedures

Many infectious diseases stimulate the production of protective antibodies that usually confer long-lasting, even lifelong, protection against reinfection. Vaccines and toxoids stimulate production of these antibodies without causing disease. At present there are eight diseases for which routine vaccination is widely recommended: seven (diphtheria, measles, mumps, pertussis, polio, rubella, and tetanus) through vaccination of all children in the first years of life (annual birth cohort in the United States, approximately 3 million), and one (influenza) through routine annual vaccination of individuals at high risk of complications or death from influenza infection (approximately 40 million in the United States, most over 65 years of age).

Decisions to recommend routine use of immunizing agents are typically based on the risk of acquiring the disease, the severity of the disease or its consequences, the efficacy of the vaccine, the safety of the vaccine, and the number of doses required for initial immunization or boosters.

Progress. From the 1950s through the mid-1970s remarkable progress was made in the reduction of

---

U.S. Objectives for Childhood Health

- By 2000 90% of children under 2 years of age will have the basic immunization series. Baseline: 70% to 80% estimated in 1989.
- By 2000 increase to at least 90% the proportion of all children entering school programs for the first time who have received oral health screening, referral, and follow-up for necessary diagnostic, preventive, and treatment services.
- By 2000 reduce iron deficiency to less than 3% among children aged 1 through 4 years. Baseline: 9% for children aged 1 through 2 years. For low-income children aged 1 to 2 years the baseline is 21%.

vaccine-preventable diseases throughout the world. Immunization programs historically have focused primarily on the protection of children against the childhood diseases, which only 30 years ago produced extensive mortality and residual disability in even the most advanced countries. In the United States the 1955 Poliomyelitis Vaccine Assistance Act, later expanded by the Vaccine Assistance Act of 1962, supported extensive growth in state-level programs to provide all children with immunizations against the major childhood vaccine-preventable diseases. As more vaccines were developed, the list of diseases to be combated was expanded, and the number of reported cases fell as the vaccines came into wide use. As the incidence of disease fell, however, efforts to immunize all children did not receive priority, and levels of immunity to many of these diseases crested and, in some places, declined.

Strategy. Nationwide immunization campaigns in the United States periodically must raise the percentage of children fully protected against these diseases back up to 90%. Although an effective national assessment of the preschool population has not been developed, the immunization level is believed to be approximately 70% to 80% with certain pockets of the population having levels lower than 50%. Special efforts need to be made to reach black and Hispanic populations who have substantially lower immunization levels than the general population. Particular attention must be paid to the gap between immunization levels in affluent communities and those in low-income areas and to the differences in levels between school-age and preschool children.

Canada has less of a problem in maintaining high immunization levels because its universal health care system provides access for all income groups to child-care services, including immunizations. Canada also has maintained controls on the pricing of drugs, including vaccines. President Bill Clinton tackled the U.S. drug industry's pricing of vaccines

in his first week in office. The components of the increase in private-sector costs of vaccines recommended for a 2-year-old child between 1982 and 1992 are shown below.

Component of cost	1982	1992
DPT (diphtheria, tetanus, whooping cough)	$1.48	$21.64
+ federal tax		18.24
OPV (oral polio vaccine, 3 doses)	8.25	28.86
+ federal tax		0.87
MMR (measles, mumps, rubella)	10.44	20.85
+ federal tax		4.44
HIB (bacterial meningitis, 4 doses)	—	61.16
Hep. B (hepatitis B, 3 doses)	—	32.13
Totals	**$20.17**	**$188.19**

The federal taxes were levied by Congress in 1986 to create the Vaccine Injury Compensation Fund, providing no-fault compensation to children suffering severe side effects from vaccines. The liability of drug companies to pay such compensation before 1986 had driven several drug companies out of the business of manufacturing vaccines. Liability suits have also had the effect of causing some parents to fear the vaccines, but the actual risks of side effects remain lower than the risks of disease complications. Another factor in the price increase has been research financed largely by the drug companies. This research has resulted in the two new vaccines for bacterial meningitis and hepatitis B since 1982.

The same set of vaccines cost the public sector only $89.78 because the state and federal governments buy in bulk at a discount of over 50%. Government programs alone, however, have not been adequate to achieve the immunization targets. Many public health clinics require a physician's referral or a complete physical examination before they will administer a vaccination. In the 11 states that purchase all vaccines for free administration to all children, regardless of income, the increase in immunization rates over the national average of 58% is only to 61%. The problem then is not just price. Community coordination such as that achieved during the 1960s with the ''Oral Polio Sundays'' is needed with support from a variety of national and community organizations.

Coordination. Such organized professional groups as the American Academy of Pediatrics, the American Academy of Family Practice, the National Medical Association, the National League of Nursing, and the American Hospital Association all make substantial contributions to these periodic national immunization efforts. Local chapters of such voluntary groups as the National Council of Negro Women, the General Federation of Women's Clubs, the Parent-Teacher Association, and the American Red Cross participate extensively at the local chapter level. Organized sports provide publicity, with the National Basketball Association, the National Football League, and major league baseball donating time for immunization messages during broadcasts of games.

Many states have stepped up enforcement of school entry immunization laws and have expanded the requirements to include more diseases. Today all 50 states and 10 Canadian provinces have school immunization statutes that will help ensure that North American children are protected against vaccine-preventable childhood diseases.

Schedule of vaccines. The generally recommended age to begin routine immunizations is 2 months. The first vaccines given are diphtheria and tetanus toxoids combined with pertussis vaccine, or **DPT,** and oral poliovirus vaccine, OPV. Measles vaccine for rubeola is most effective when given after 1 year of age. However, in some populations where natural measles occurs frequently in the first year of life, it is preferable to administer the rubeola vaccine as early as 6 months of age. If this is necessary in a community, a repeat dose of measles vaccine needs to be given after the age of 1 year to immunize any infants whose earlier vaccine response had been blocked by passive immunity.

Selected Screening Programs

Screening for tuberculosis should be performed routinely prior to rubeola vaccination. In addition, a hematocrit for anemia should be done on all children during the first 6 months of life. This is particularly important in the low-birthweight infant who has grown quickly.

Other diseases screened will depend on the community and the population at risk. Thus screening for sickle cell anemia, Tay-Sachs disease, thalassemia, and other genetic diseases should be done if the population is of the corresponding ethnic group at risk.

Screening for illness should be carefully performed prior to placement in day-care centers. It should be repeated for the preschool or school physical examination, and hearing, speech, and eye examinations should be performed. These routine screenings can be performed by trained paramedical personnel. Dental evaluation and fluoride therapy for the prevention of caries are also necessary.

Health Services for Chronic Diseases

Special health services for children with chronic diseases and disorders such as cerebral palsy, epilepsy, and congenital malformations require careful planning within the community. Various health professionals need to be involved. Continuity and comprehensiveness of care are essential to afford the child the best quality of life possible. Much of the care may be given by nonmedical providers, particularly in the school setting and in other areas in the community. Unfortunately, because of the large number of U.S. programs that provide services for problems, attempts to obtain care may reveal a fragmented and frustrating maze. Many programs provide only part of the full care needs for each child, and each program may have different eligibility rules as well as a separate point of entry that is often difficult to locate. The comprehensiveness of Canada's health care system overcomes many of these difficulties.

In the case of complicated congenital deformities, such as meningomyelocele, children frequently require the services of more than one program or need a service that is not provided within the community in which they live. There is no greater deterrent to the effective and efficient care of children with chronic diseases than the fragmentation of services as a result of the isolation of categorical programs. For example, habilitation programs for children with orthopedic deformities may not be available for children damaged by trauma. Confusing eligibility and elimination rules may result in children slipping through the cracks between programs that are narrowly defined and poorly coordinated. Health education can help families by providing information not only on community resources, options, and requirements but also on strategies for negotiating among them. Such strategies may include clarifying needs, identifying questions to get answered, training in child care (Figure 5-9) and identifying key decision makers.

Organization

Many programs have been developed by the federal governments and by the states and provinces of the U.S. and Canada to provide health services for children. These programs have had a major role in improving the health of the nations' children, but for a number of reasons some of them are now less effective. The U.S. federal Maternal and Child Health (MCH) and Crippled Children's Services (CCS) programs of Title V of the Social Security Act, for example, were created in 1935 to provide national leadership in the field of maternal and child health and to direct the state Maternal and Child Health and state Crippled Children's programs. Thus the state Maternal and Child Health programs remain the major providers of basic health services for

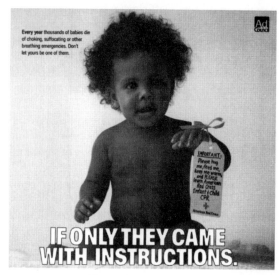

FIGURE 5-9
Child   includes looking after the safety and well-being of children. The American Red Cross advertises its cardiorespiratory resuscitation program.
Courtesy Ad Council.

mothers and children, and the state Crippled Children's programs remain the major public system for providing the special health services required for children with chronic diseases and disorders. The legislation that created these programs did not link them to community health programs and services.

Other categorical programs created by Congress have independent organizational structures at the federal, state, and community levels; these include Title I programs, the Developmental Disabilities program, the Early and Periodic Screening, Diagnosis, and Treatment (EPSDT) program, and the Supplemental Food Program for Women, Infants, and Children (WIC). Some of these function at the national, state, and community levels parallel to, or even in open competition with, each other and with the MCH and CCS programs. The result is a duplication of services, inefficiencies in administration, and increased costs. More important, the fragmentation of service results in some children receiving suboptimum care or not receiving needed services. Table 5-3 suggest ways that these programs could overcome their problems of coordination and fragmentation.

Some states and different communities have established special units in their mental retardation programs for the identification and care of such children. Mental health programs for children frequently dovetail with the adult services, and some function through the schools. Psychological services may be obtained through mental health programs or the school system.

Each community must determine the organization of its own community child health services. The purposes of such services should be strongly influenced by national and state or provincial goals, and adapted by the community after careful study of that community's needs. The organization of local child health service should be the responsibility of the community itself. Thus the number and type of health services provided will vary a great deal. Certain services and programs—for example, those concerned with teenage pregnancy and abortion counseling, sexually transmitted disease, and child abuse—should be available for all children who need them.

INTERNATIONAL CHILD SURVIVAL

In the next hour, 1700 children will die of illness and malnutrition. Television has brought many of these starving faces into our homes on the nightly

TABLE 5-3
Shifting the focus of child health services

Current system	Proposed system
Deficit/treatment model	Health promotion model/promotes health and well-being
Often responsive at point of irreversible damage	Supports families in identifying risks and resolving problems early
Focus on individual problem	Focus on family and individual strengths
Multiple agencies: multiple sites and service agents	Single points of entry, care coordination, and service teams
Services located in bureaucratic settings	Services available at natural "touchpoints" (e.g., hospitals, schools, child care agencies)
Inflexible, restrictive funding	Flexible and integrated funding across agencies
Focus on process data (e.g., number of clients served)	Added focus on outcome data (e.g., reduction in teen pregnancy)
Separate services, separate goals, and service plans	Integrated services, integrated service plans.
Tendency to enforce client compliance and client dependency	Focus on consumer independence and self-determination
Many services delivered by state	Most services delivered by community
Many funds managed at state level	Most funds managed at local level
Inflexible choices for servicing children and families	More options for serving children and families
• Child left in home with minimal services from house or community	• Tailor services to meet strengths and needs of child, family
• Primary out-of-home, restrictive, or out-of-community placements	• Family support and community services balanced with secure and intensive treatment placements
• Limited family involvement in service decisions	• More family involvement in service decisions

Source: Adapted from Oregon Legislative Committee on A Positive Future for Children and Families, 1993.

news. Most of the children live in developing countries. That number of deaths amounts to 40,000 a day, 15 million a year. Many millions more will live out their lives with mental and physical handicaps. Yet much of this is preventable. Less than 100 years ago, when the United States was a developing country, children were ravaged by the same diseases that now prevail in the Third World, and its infant mortality rate was as high.

Education and socioeconomic development, improved sanitation and other public health measures in Europe, North America, and a growing number of countries in the Western Pacific, have enabled over 95% of their children to survive through the preschool years. In developing countries as many as 25% of all children die before their fifth birthday. The techniques to save at least half of these children are available, even without immediate improvements in socioeconomic development (Figure 5-10). The international Campaign for Child Survival refers to these techniques as GOBI and FFF, which stand for growth monitoring, oral rehydration therapy, breastfeeding, and immunization, plus female education, food supplements, and family planning.

Growth Monitoring

Recording a child's weight gain once each month, and using a chart that costs only 10 cents can indi-

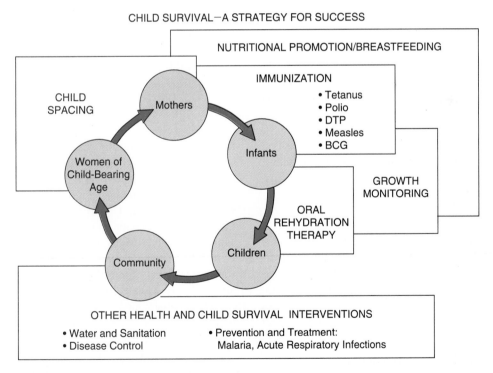

CHILD SURVIVAL–A STRATEGY FOR SUCCESS

FIGURE 5-10

The U.S. Agency for International Development is promoting a Child Survival Program with component strategies related to the life cycle, which links reproductive, infant, and child health to the community.

Source: USAID Health Information System.

cate malnutrition before it causes serious damage to a child's health. At this early stage, a community health worker can educate a family on ways to improve a child's nutritional health, even when food and money are scarce.

Oral Rehydration Therapy

Of the annual toll of 15 million, five million children die of dehydration from diarrhea. It is the single biggest killer of young children. Preparation of a simple mixture of sugar, salt, and water from a 10-cent packet can enable a child to absorb 25 times more fluid and salts than before. However, only 15% of families in the world know of this ORT method so far, although ORT is saving half a million children each year.

Breastfeeding

Infant formulas marketed in developing countries are often mixed with contaminated water. The baby has not yet developed immunities against the organisms found in the water. Therefore, infants receiving these formulas have as much as three times greater risk of dying in infancy than babies who are breastfed. Breast milk provides the best possible nutrition. It also provides natural immunities against childhood diseases during the first 6 months of feeding.

Immunization

Six diseases—measles, whooping cough, tetanus, polio, tuberculosis, and diphtheria—account for over 3.5 million preventable childhood deaths yearly. Only 10% of children in the developing world receive immunizations against these diseases. The cost of the full set of immunizations is only $5.

Education, Food Supplements, and Family Planning

Health education can make these techniques readily available to families with little dependence on im-

proved access to medical facilities or personnel. More general education for women can also make them more willing and able to take advantage of new innovations. The level of a mother's education is the single most influential factor in the health of her children.

Food supplements of only a few hundred calories a day for chronically malnourished women who are pregnant can reduce low-birthweight deaths by 50%. A 2-cent megadose of vitamin A every 6 months or a daily handful of leafy green vegetables can prevent the deficiency that causes vision impairment in 10 million young children and blindness in up to one half million children each year.

Spacing of births allows couples to provide more care and family resources to each infant, thereby assuring its survival with greater certainty. Spacing also gives the mother more time to regain her strength and to resume her education or career before the next pregnancy. Education for family planning remains a high priority for public health in the Third World.

CHILD DAY CARE PROGRAMS

As more women enter the work force, the need for accessible, affordable, quality day care for children has risen. Approximately 67% of married women who have children under 18 years of age work outside the home in the United States; nearly 70% of Canadian women with children under 16 years of age do the same. Many European countries have passed laws that guarantee working mothers and sometimes fathers time off and wage replacement after delivery to care for their infants. In Canada women are guaranteed 15 weeks off work with 60% replacement of their salaries. No such policies currently exist in the United States. Children of working families are cared for in a variety of ways (Figure 5-11). Parents themselves provide care for 28% of working mothers, other relatives 19%, commercial day care 28%, and neighborhood day care 20%. Studies show that poor child care practices, whether

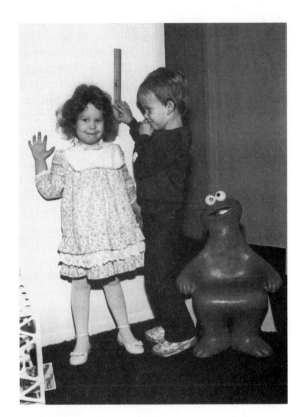

FIGURE 5-11
Child care provides for the development of social skills, but also brings greater risks of communicable disease transfer.
Photo by Marsha Burkes, courtesy University of Texas Health Science Center at Houston.

by parents or others, are linked to violence, crime, illness, depression, and immature moral development. Child care centers are targeted with special objectives for the nation's health with regard to immunization levels, food service, and infectious diarrhea. Health education strategies directed at families can clarify child care options and identify criteria for selecting among options. Health education strategies directed at child care workers need to focus on year 2000 objectives.

Head Start programs in the United States have been found in long-term studies to have saved $4.75 in reduced costs of special education, public assis-

tance, and crime for every dollar invested in quality preschool education. Fewer than half of the disadvantaged 4-year-old children eligible for Head Start participated in the program in 1990. This was increased to 55% in 1991. The year 2000 target is 100 percent.

SCHOOL HEALTH PROGRAMS

Comprehensive school health programs that educate children about parenthood, sexuality, personal hygiene, substance abuse, and nutrition should be instituted on a community-wide basis. These programs should be supported by health services and environmental protection within the school setting and in the community. Community health should seek the cooperation of the schools. Children are a captive audience during their school hours. Attendance of parents at school functions enables an extension of health education to the family.

More than 40 million U.S. children and youths spend most of the day in school. Teachers provide instruction that can help young people make decisions that promote health and prevent disease. Parents enhance the opportunities for good health for their children by fostering healthful personal habits and by ensuring availability and use of appropriate childhood health services.

The dramatic shift in child and youth health priorities suggests the need for the reassessment of health strategies—services and policies organized for the enhancement of health and the prevention of disease. The challenge to schools to participate in future programs in child health has been eloquently stated in the U.S. Objectives for the Nation. Four objectives focus on the school setting. Objective 8.2 addresses increasing high school graduation rates and is identical to one of the National Education Goals. The 1990 baseline for people ages 19 to 20 years who had earned regular or alternative credentials was established at 83% for all races; the year 2000 target is 90%. In 1990 the high school graduation rate was 78% for blacks, 60% for Hispanics,

---

U.S. Objectives for Child Care Centers

- By 2000 95% of children in licensed child care facilities and kindergarten will have the basic immunization series. Baseline: 94% for children in licensed child care and 97% for children entering school.
- By 2000 reduce infectious diarrhea by at least 25% among children in licensed child care centers. Children in licensed child care centers have three to four times as much diarrheal disease as do those not in child care.
- By 2000 increase to at least 90% the proportion of child care food services with menus that are consistent with the nutrition principles in the *Dietary Guidelines for Americans* (or the *Canadian Food Guide*).

---

and 87% for whites. Objective 8.3 targets ensuring access to developmentally appropriate preschool programs for disadvantaged children and children with disabilities. This objective is discussed in the preceding section on child day care. Two other objectives are shown in the box on p. 145. More will be covered on school health in later chapters.

Public health people too often view the school as a convenient repository or channel of information transfer rather than as an active partner in community health. Community health agencies, frustrated in their own attempts to reach young people, often find the school a convenient scapegoat for community problems such as drug abuse, teenage pregnancies, and highway injuries and deaths among youth.

Schools have been criticized and blamed for many things pertaining to the generation gap, including the decline of reading and writing skills, couch-potato television viewing, and the decline of physical fitness in youth. A recent survey found a 42% increase (from 24% in 1984 to 34% in 1991) in the number of children aged 3 through 17 years considered overweight.

Recognizing their accountability for the decline

of reading and writing skills, schools are resistant to accepting any new responsibilities for the education of children and youth with respect to health and safety, sexuality, and substance abuse. Where they have accepted educational responsibility for these, they often have drawn the line excluding their accountability for behavior.

Part of the debate has centered on the question of responsibility. The health sector has had limited opportunity—given its current structure—to reach well children. Health professionals have assumed that it was the school's responsibility to provide most of the health and safety education as well as to provide many health services and health protection needs. The schools in turn have seen most of these needs as outside their purview and have abrogated the responsibility to parents, and parents can avoid paying much attention to the health and safety needs of their children so long as the children are well. When their children suffer illnesses, injury, or dysfunction, they look to the health sector for help or relief, thus completing the circle of transferred responsibility.

The way out of this cycle is to share and coordinate the responsibility among schools, parents, and health agencies, while developing the knowledge and skills of children, so that they can assume a greater role in protecting themselves and promoting their own health.

There must be a larger role, however, for the public health sector than merely facilitating the sharing of responsibility between schools and parents. What about the adequate labeling of foods so that even children could use the labels? What about advocating the availability of healthful food choices in restaurants frequented by children and possibly the restriction of permissible fat content in standard servings such as in triple cheeseburgers, which contain 15 teaspoons of fat?

Even school gaps need to be closed and responsibilities shared among school health teachers, school lunch personnel, physical educators, and school health services personnel. Similarly, school

Objectives for School Health

By 2000 at least 50% of schools should provide comprehensive school health education at elementary and secondary levels. Figure 5-12 shows the states requiring school health education, with course content determined by grade level. By 2000 the number of schools that provide nutrition education from preschool through twelfth grade will increase to at least 75%, preferably as part of quality school health education. Baseline: only 12 states mandate nutrition as a core content area.

counseling personnel and administrators should share responsibility for the early identification and treatment of physical and emotional health problems and in the building of a physical and social environment that is conducive to healthy growth and development.

The strategies required to accomplish these intersectoral and multidisciplinary collaborations must include coalitions and team building at the community level. Coalitions provide shared responsibility and resources and the development and strengthening of broader power bases. A broader community power base can provide political advo-

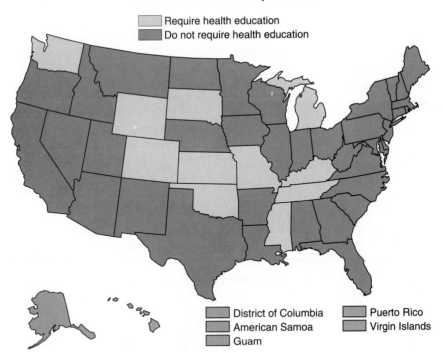

1990 Health Education Requirements

Require health education
Do not require health education

District of Columbia
American Samoa
Guam

Puerto Rico
Virgin Islands

FIGURE 5-12
States and territories requiring school health education as of 1990, with content varying by grade level.
Sources: National Association of State Boards of Education, Council of Chief State School Officers. *AIDS, HIV, and school health education: state policies and programs 1990,* Alexandria, Va, 1991, National Association of State Boards of Education.

cacy for the health of children and youth, who cannot vote for themselves.

SUMMARY

Mortality of mothers, infants, and children does not tell the entire story of reproductive, infant, and child health, but a knowledge of what causes deaths at the various fetal, infancy, and childhood stages should be of benefit in any community health program. Specific death rates point out where specific emphasis must be placed if we are to save the lives of mothers, infants, and children. Comparisons between countries (see Table 5-2) indicate the potential for improvement.

To propose that all of these deaths could be prevented is unrealistic, but to say that at least half of them could be prevented with our present knowledge and means is a reasonable objective for the United States. Certainly injury deaths, which loom so prominently in the statistics of childhood, can be reduced. Deaths from infectious diseases can be controlled better than is indicated in the statistics. The health of mothers and children in all countries can be further improved.

Reproductive, infant, and child health care programs are the foundation of community health promotion because they are the basis for health education, immunization, early diagnosis and treatment, and the development of health habits that sustain later health habits. In the spirit of disease prevention and health promotion, reproductive health is essential to successful infant health outcomes, which in turn provide the foundation for successful community health programs directed at children, youth, adults, and eventually the elderly.

QUESTIONS FOR REVIEW

1. Why is it desirable for a couple to have a premarital medical examination and genetic counseling to determine their capacity for childbearing?

2. What is the reciprocal obligation of the expectant mother and society?

3. Why is the U.S. maternal mortality rate higher than New Zealand's even though obstetrics is just as far advanced in the United States as it is in New Zealand?

4. To what extent is legislation of benefit in maternal health promotion?

5. What economic factors in your community are significant in maternal health?

6. What is one of the leading causes of infant deaths, and what are some measures for reducing the number of infant deaths from this cause?

7. Where in the field of infant health could time and funds for research be best invested?

8. What were the causes of infant deaths in your community during the past 5 years?

9. What are the contributions of voluntary agencies to the infant health program in your community?

10. How would you educate parents about the advisability of taking apparently healthy children to their family physician, pediatrician, or child health clinic for a checkup at regular intervals?

11. What are some of the special social and mental health problems associated with disability in childhood, and what is a community's responsibility in dealing with these problems?

12. Does the school assume the role of the parent when it concerns itself with the pupil's health?

13. What official and voluntary agencies are available in your community for helping a family with a child needing orthopedic services?

READINGS

Bush PJ, Iannotti RJ: Alcohol, cigarette, and marijuana use among fourth-grade urban schoolchildren in 1988/89 and 1990/91, *Am J Public Health* 83:111, 1993.
Self-reported alcohol use, use without parental knowledge, and smoking more than a puff of cigarettes declined in Washington, D.C. Marijuana use and cigarette experimentation did not. Perceived peer pressure to use declined.

Chen LC, Amor JS, Segal SJ, editors: *AIDS and women's reproductive health,* New York, 1991, Plenum.

This compilation provides an examination of AIDS and women's reproductive health epidemiology, policy, roles of sexually transmitted diseases, contraception, and sexual behavior in facilitating or interrupting HIV transmission, issues of mother-to-child transmission, and program strategies.

Oregon Legislative Assembly: *A positive future for Oregon's children and families. A report of the Children's Care Team,* Portland, 1993, Oregon Legislative Assembly.

Summarizes the recommendations for a reconfiguration of the state social and health service systems to improve the services to children and their families. Emphasis on prevention and a "wellness" model breaks from traditions of focus on more intensive problems with children.

Wallace HM, Patrick K, Parcel GS, Igoe JB, editors: *Principles and practices of student health,* Oakland, Calif., 1992, Third Party.

This three-volume reference covers health status indicators for school-age children, nutrition priorities in student health services, historical and organizational perspectives on school health, worksite health promotion for school personnel, and other topics.

Went S, editor.: *A healthy start,* Victoria, Australia, 1991, Monash University.

Reviews the experience of the Health in Primary Schools project, based on the premise that school–community cooperation requires broad community support and involvement.

BIBLIOGRAPHY

Alexander MA, Sherman JB, Clark L: Obesity in Mexican-American preschool children: a population group at risk, *Public Health Nurs* 8:53, 1991.

American Public Health Association and American Academy of Pediatrics: *Caring for our children: national health and safety performance standards for out-of-home child care programs,* Washington, DC, 1992, American Public Health Association.

Bush PJ, Zuckerman AE, Taggart VS et al: Cardiovascular risk factor prevention in black school children: the "Know Your Body" evaluation project, *Health Educ Q* 16:215, 1989.

Frazier PJ, Horowitz AM: Oral health education and promotion in maternal and child health: a position paper, *J Public Health Dent* 50:390, 1990.

Germain A, Holmes KK, Piot P et al. *Reproductive tract infections,* New York, 1992, Plenum.

Greenberg LW: Pediatric patient education: the unanswered challenge to medical education, *Patient Educ Couns* 17:3, 1991.

Hawks SR: Fetal alcohol syndrome: implications for health education, *J Health Educ* 24:22, 1993.

Hayes CD, Palmer JL, Zaslow MJ: *Who cares for America's children?* Washington, DC, 1990, National Academy Press.

Healthy communities 2000: Model standards, ed 3, Washington, DC, 1991, American Public Health Association.

Heatherington SE: A controlled study of the effect of prepared childbirth classes on obstetric outcomes, *Birth* 17:86, 1990.

Hogue CJR, Hargraves MA: Class, race, and infant mortality in the United States, *Am J Public Health* 83:9, 1993.

Institute of Medicine Subcommittee for a Clinical Applications Guide: *Nutrition during pregnancy and lactation: an implementation guide,* Washington, DC, 1992, National Academy Press.

Klerman LV: Alive and well? *A research and policy review of health programs for poor young children,* New York, 1991, National Center for Children in Poverty, Columbia University School of Public Health.

Kotch JB, Blakely CH, Brown SS et al. *A pound of prevention: the case for universal maternity care in the U.S.,* Washington, DC, 1992, American Public Health Association.

Lindstrom B: Children and divorce in the light of salutogenesis—promoting child health in the face of family breakdown, *Health Prom Int* 7:289, 1992.

Lochhead YJ: Failure to immunize children under 5 years—a literature review, *J Adv Nurs* 16:130, 1991.

Malloy MH, Hoffman HJ, Peterson DR: Sudden infant death syndrome and maternal smoking, *Am J Public Health* 82:1380, 1992.

McMurry MP, Hopkins PN, Gould R et al: Family-oriented nutrition intervention for a lipid clinic population, *J Am Diet Assoc* 91:57, 1991.

Mesters I, Meertens R, Crebolder H, et al. Development of a health education program for parents of preschool children with asthma, *Health Educ Res* 8:53, 1993.

Michaels ML, Roosa MW, Gensheimer LK: Family characteristics of children who self-select into a prevention program for children of alcoholics, *Am J Community Psychol* 20:663, 1992.

Minkler M, Roe KM: *Grandmothers as caregivers: raising children of the crack cocaine epidemic,* Newbury Park, Calif, 1993, Sage.

Mitchell A, Cooperstein E, Larner M: *Child care choices, consumer education, and low-income families,* New York, 1992, National Center for Children in Poverty, Columbia University School of Public Health.

Mitford J: *The American way of birth,* New York, 1992, Dutton.

Nordstrom M-L, Cattingius S, Haglund B: Social differences in Swedish infant mortality by cause of death, 1983 to 1986, *Am J Public Health* 83:26, 1993.

Porter CP: Social reasons for skin tone preferences of black school-age children, *Am J Orthopsychiatry* 61: 149, 1991.

Redman S: Women and reproduction. In Saltman D, editor: *Women and health,* Sydney, 1991, Harcourt Brace Jovanovich.

Rifkin SB: *Community participation in maternal and child health/family planning programmes: an analysis based on case study materials,* Geneva, 1990, World Health Organization.

Rosen M: Health maintenance strategies for women of different ages: an overview, *Ob Gyn Clin* 17:673, 1990.

Sciarillo WG, Alexander G, Farrell KP: Lead exposure and child behavior, *Am J Public Health* 82:1356, 1992.

Siskind V, Del Mar C, Schofield F: Infant feeding in Queensland, Australia: long-term trends, *Am J Public Health* 83:103, 1993.

Slutsker L, Smith R, Higginson G, et al. Recognizing illicit drug use by pregnant women: reports from Oregon birth attendants, *Am J Public Health* 83:61, 1993.

Stewart DD: Child passenger safety: current technical issues for advocates and professionals, *Fam Community Health* 15:12, 1993.

Taggart VS, Zuckerman AE, Sly RM et al: You can control asthma—evaluation of an asthma education program for hospitalized inner-city children. *Patient Educ Couns* 17:35, 1991.

Chapter 6

Adolescent Health

❖

*We abandon the young people at adolescence at
the time when the negative peer group cultures
are beginning to pull in ways that can be very
troublesome. During that time, young people do
tell us to go away, but they do not mean too far.*
JAMES P. COMER

OBJECTIVES

When you finish this chapter, you should be able to:

- Assess the special health problems and needs of the adolescent population of a community

- Identify programs appropriate to health promotion and disease prevention in these populations

---

Among American and Canadian adolescents 20% suffer at least one serious health problem, and 25% are believed to be at high risk for school failure, delinquency, early unprotected sexual intercourse, or substance abuse. Yet teenagers in both countries see physicians less often than do other age groups. In the United States, they are more likely than any other age group to be underinsured or uninsured. Increasing numbers of adolescents are poorly housed, poorly fed, and poorly educated. Parental guidance and nurturing have been made less accessible to adolescents by the changing family structure described at the beginning of the preceding chapter. The community must fill these voids if it is to de-

pend on this generation to become the adults who must take responsibility for the community's health and well-being in the years ahead.

In the absence of community supports for adolescent development and a positive, preventative approach, the community is left to pick up the pieces of neglected needs and missed opportunities. Indeed the consequences of neglected needs in early prenatal care and early childhood development described in Chapter 5 accumulate into adolescence. The cost to the community of waiting too long to intervene on these problems is that they get worse and increasingly hard to change. They sometimes lead, if uncorrected, to behavior and health problems

149

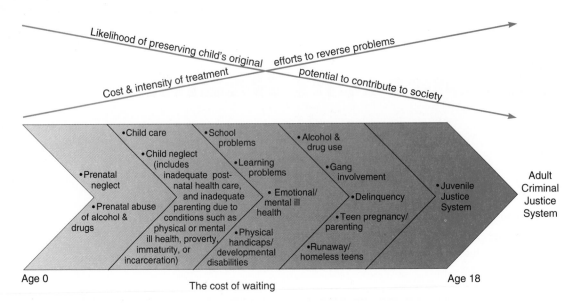

Likelihood of preserving child's original efforts to reverse problems

Cost & intensity of treatment   potential to contribute to society

•Child care   •School
                    problems
        •Child neglect   •Alcohol &
         (includes   drug use
•Prenatal inadequate post-   •Learning
  neglect   natal health care, problems   •Gang
            and inadequate   involvement
•Prenatal abuse parenting due to • Emotional/   •Juvenile   Adult
of alcohol &   conditions such as mental ill •Delinquency Justice Criminal
drugs   physical or mental health   System   Justice
               ill health, poverty, •Teen pregnancy/   System
               immaturity, or •Physical parenting
               incarceration) handicaps/
                            developmental •Runaway/
                            disabilities homeless teens

Age 0   Age 18
              The cost of waiting

FIGURE 6-1
The potential of a child or adolescent to contribute to the community declines with the failure to intervene
early, and the cost of treating or reversing problems increases with neglect.
Source: Oregon Legislative Committee on a Positive Future for Children and Families, 1993.

that spill over into the community's well-being in the form, of school disruption, delinquency, and crime, as shown in Figure 6-1.

EARLY ADOLESCENCE AND TRANSITION

At the threshold between childhood and young adulthood, usually between ages 10 and 14, teen-agers become adolescents by virtue of **puberty.** This is a time when new hormones are racing through the body, creating some confusion of feel-ings, mood swings, and sexual awakening. Matu-ration to adult roles and characteristics brings with it a search for greater independence, new relation-ships, new freedoms. This places the young adoles-cent at particular risk of making decisions and be-havioral choices at times of vulnerability to unaccustomed feelings, often without the needed adult guidance and understanding. Some of the be-

havioral decisions, such as smoking or alcohol use, can lead to addictions; some can permanently injure the mind or body. Some place friends, family, or community at risk of injury or damage. These tur-bulent years set the stage for later adolescence, when still greater independence will take a greater toll if the earlier developmental process has led to self-destructive, self-indulgent, or self-demeaning be-havior patterns.

Adolescents 12 to 14 are quite different from those in the ages 15 to 19. The transitions from el-ementary to middle or junior high school and from there to high school are momentous changes in the lives of young people. The transition from high school to work or college is also stressful and some-times fraught with new threats to health if not to life. The mortality risks for the broad age groups tell only part of the story of life-span variations in health. The problems of coping and adaptation to life-span transitions have additional health consequences that are more pervasive than mortality risks at that age.

Transitions in the life span. Anticipating the potential health problems of individuals or populations so that they can be educationally prepared for them requires prediction based on past experience with other people who have been exposed to the same agents under similar circumstances. The best predictor of potential health problems in populations is age. Transitions from one age range to another could be the most propitious times to intervene for purposes of primary prevention of problems anticipated in the next developmental stage in the life span.

As suggested in Table 6-1, each transition in the life span has one or more major tasks of coping and adaptation associated with it. The life-span transitions are demarcated by important events affecting

most people as they age. The tasks of coping and adaptation associated with those events or transitions lead to positive health consequences if they are carried out successfully and to negative consequences if the individual fails to cope or adapt effectively.

Other transitions. The adolescent and adult years bring an increasing number of challenges to coping and adaptation in addition to life-span transitions. Transitions from one status, role, or circumstance to another also require adaptations of lifestyle (Figure 6-2). They present problems of stress and coping similar to those of the life span. For example, the high degree of mobility in American life poses to communities the problems of uprooting, discontinuity of social support, isolation, confusion, stress, and economic insecurity. Unemployment clearly

TABLE 6-1

Examples of issues for health promotion related to life-span transitions

Developmental transitions	Major tasks of coping and adaptation	Health consequences
Infant→child	Avoidance of hazards	Safety and injury control
Preschool→school	Selection of foods	Dental caries, obesity, nutritional deficiencies
Elem.→jr. high (early adolescence)	Resistance to peer pressure; changing bodily functions	Smoking, alcohol, drugs, pregnancy
Jr. High→high school (middle adolescence)	Development of autonomous identity and confidence	Substance abuse, pregnancy, auto accidents, sexually transmitted diseases
High school→work or higher education	Development of autonomous function and role; coping skills; uprooting	Suicide, homicide, alcoholism, addictions
Single→married and/or pregnancy and parenthood	Curtailed freedom and increased responsibility for life-style; uprooting	Congenital defects, infant mortality, low birth weight, obesity
Young adult→middle age ("midlife" transition) Parent→"empty nest"	Reduced parenting roles, changing bodily function, reduced activity	Hypertension, digestive disease, atrophy, obesity, alcoholism
Working adult→retired adult or widowed	Reduced social roles; sedentary living; bereavement	Loneliness, reduced self-esteem, atrophy, loss of reasons for living and the will to live, or zest for living

Reproduced with permission from Green LW: Modifying and developing health behavior, *Annu Rev Public Health*, vol 5, © 1984 by Annual Reviews, Inc.

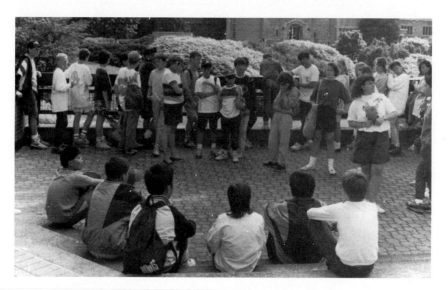

FIGURE 6-2
Early adolescence creates challenges of transition from elementary or middle school to high school and new peer relations.
Photo courtesy University of British Columbia.

represents a challenge to coping and adaptation with known health consequences. These transitions, then, account for some of the typical or prevalent health problems and causes of death found in the adolescent and adult populations of most communities. The question for community health is whether strategies can be designed to intervene effectively and preventively in relation to these transitions.

A MODEL OF COMMUNITY INTERVENTION

The suggestion was made in the foregoing paragraphs that communities should be able to organize a social history of intervention that anticipates critical transitions and prepares individuals for them.

Transition-Based Programs

The advantage of the life-span perspective is that it allows community health professionals to identify whole populations at risk, according to readily available demographic markers such as age, graduation, application for driver's license or marriage licenses, birth certificates, and applications for unemployment compensation. Other populations at risk of maladaptation to critical transitions can be identified from vital records such as divorce and death certificates and social agency records on newcomers to the community, disaster victims, school dropouts, and applicants for welfare or medical assistance. Clusters of transitions for an individual or for populations signal potential problems of coping with loss, bereavement, uprooting from social ties, and adaptation to new circumstances.

The advantage of being able to use such demographic markers to identify high-risk populations within the community is that it is unnecessary for health agencies to wait for the problems to surface in the form of patients, clients, or victims before taking some action. This precept is fundamental to any preventative approach at the community level.

In the prevention of vaccine-immunizable diseases, it was possible to obtain nearly 100% coverage with the requirement that all children had to be immunized before entering school. Efforts toward the prevention of adolescent health problems resulting from life-style (see Table 6-1) cannot be quite so coercive or regulatory.

Justification for Intervention

Communities could justify legal coercion in the prevention and control of communicable diseases on the grounds that they were protecting the population at large from the negligence or carelessness of individuals. With most of the life-style diseases and disabilities today, the individual often is harming only his or her own health, so that coercive measures are difficult to justify in a democratic society. One can advance the argument that the harm people do to themselves usually spills over into the lives of others, especially family and friends. That case can be persuasive to the point of justifying coercive legislation prohibiting such individual behavior as drunk driving, child abuse, and other violent behavior. It can even carry over to more subtle infringements of individual life-style on the well-being of others, as we have seen in recent years with the passage of "clean air" acts prohibiting smoking in crowded workplaces and restaurants in some cities and states. Legislation raising the age of driver's licensing and of alcohol purchasing also have successfully reduced overall automobile injury rates and especially alcohol-related injuries in the 15 to 19 age group.

For most of the individual life-styles influencing health, however, the justification for intervention must be based on a more generalized or collective sense of the well-being of the community, including notions of social and economic health, quality of life, and responsibility. Such value-laden notions require that interventions remain largely noncoercive in their offering and voluntary in their selection. Restated from a different perspective, the individual retains the freedom to engage in the potentially harmful practice, but the community must find ways to minimize the damage done by rampant or widespread practices that place a burden on the health and social resources of the community and ultimately on its quality of life and economic survival.

The major advantage of the life-transitions approach to health promotion is that it is not limited to any particular disease. Each application anticipates a great number of potential problems known to compromise host resistance and resources and to produce risk factors for most of the leading causes of death and disability. It is a model, in short, that applies broadly to the range of behaviors posing threats to health, including smoking, alcohol and drug misuse, overeating, inactivity, reckless or violent behavior, and other dysfunctional ways of coping with stress.

DEMOGRAPHY AND EPIDEMIOLOGY OF ADOLESCENT HEALTH

The lines between childhood and adolescent status and between adolescence and young adult status are blurred by differences between psychosocial maturation and biological maturation. Psychosocial maturation is concerned with mental, emotional, moral, and social development. The ability of an adolescent to move through the life tasks associated with these ages signals psychosocial maturation (see Table 6-1). Biological maturation for this age group centers on physical growth and development such as height and weight, and on a set of sexual characteristics such as menstruation for females and voice change for males.

Psychosocial and biological maturation may occur at different rates, making it difficult to characterize the adolescent population by the usual developmental or chronological criteria. For example, biologically mature youth may lack the emotional maturity their physical size suggests; biologically immature youth may be asked to work or engage in social roles their physical size does not support. For these and other reasons, common age groupings for health analysis for adolescents and young adults vary between 10 and 24 years.

Demographic Trends

The proportion of adolescents in most Western countries relative to the general population is on the decline, having reached a peak in the mid-1960s, when the post–World War II babies, the "baby boomers," reached their teens. In 1980, 10- to 19-year-olds made up 17% of the U.S. population; by 1990, their percentage decreased to 14%. With an increase in the percentage of children under 5 years of age, resulting from the 1980s "baby boomlet," the percentage of younger adolescents is expected to rise again in the 1990s.

The adolescent population of North America mirrors the increasing cultural diversity of Canada and the United States. Although whites comprise the largest proportion of adolescents, their overall percentage in the North American population fell relative to Hispanics, blacks, Native Americans, Eskimos, Asians, and other races during the 1980s. The number of Asian and Pacific Islander youth more than doubled between 1980 and 1990 in both the United States and Canada. The percentage of adolescents living in poor or near-poor families also varies with race and ethnicity. The overall U.S. dropout rate for high school is 12.6%. This varies from 12.4% for whites, to 13.8% for blacks, and 33% for Hispanics. These demographic changes have implications for school health curriculum, community health activities, and community health services.

Today's adolescents, those born in the early 1980s in the United States, have an overall life ex-

Objective for High School Graduation Rates

• By 2000 increase the high school graduation rate to at least 90%.

pectancy of 73.7 years. Life expectancy is affected by many factors; gender and race are two important ones. For adolescents born in 1980, white females have a life expectancy of 78.1, black females 72.5, white males 70.7, and black males 63.8. On the average, whites live longer than blacks, women live longer than men. These statistics reveal the importance of considering the characteristics of subpopulations in planning community services. Needs vary.

Epidemiological Trends

The overall U.S. death rates for those 15 to 24 years of age have decreased dramatically since the beginning of the century when there were nearly 600 deaths per 100,000 population. Communicable diseases were then among the leading causes of death. In 1983 the long-term decline in the death rates for children 1 to 14 years of age continued, exceeding the 1990 objective for the nation by 1985 (Figure 6-3, *A*), but for 15- to 24-year-olds, the death rates reversed (Figure 6-3, *B*). This age group experienced increases for much of the remainder of the decade. Differences among races continued, and the leading causes of death changed. This is the only age group that has sustained a reversal in its death rates in recent decades.

In 1990 there was another 4% increase in the death rate for the 15 to 24 age group. Declines in death rates for cancer and heart disease (6% and 1%, respectively) were offset by increases for injuries and homicides (up 4% and 25%, respectively). Motor vehicle crashes are the leading cause of death for white youth in this age group. They account for 78% of the injury deaths in 1990; over one half are associated with alcohol. Homicide is the leading killer of black adolescents and young adults. The homicide rate increased from over 13% in 1980 to 20% in 1990. These deaths, too, are associated with alcohol and other drugs. Most suicides, the third leading cause of death, are among white males, although females attempt suicide approximately three times more often.

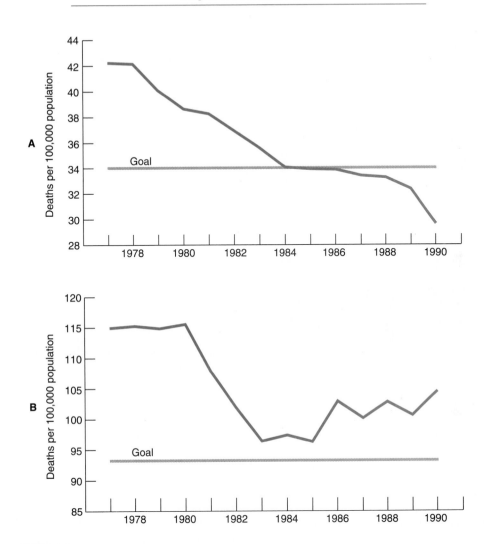

FIGURE 6-3
A, Death rates for children 1 to 14 years of age, United States, 1977-90, and 1990 goal. **B**, Death rates for adolescents and young adults 15 to 24 years of age, United States, 1977-90, and 1990 goal. NOTE: 1990 data are provisional.

Source: National Center for Health Statistics, National Vital Statistics System.

The corresponding comparisons for black and white U.S. adolescents ages 10 to 14 and 15 to 19 are shown in Figure 6-4 for each of the leading causes of death. The three leading causes of death in these age groups—injuries, homicide, and suicide—are amenable to health-promotion strategies. The increases in these types of deaths will be shown in later sections to be caused in turn by another set of social, behavioral, and health problems, including alcohol and drug misuse, stress, and family disruption. For now, it will suffice to say that the inequities in life chances for survival and health

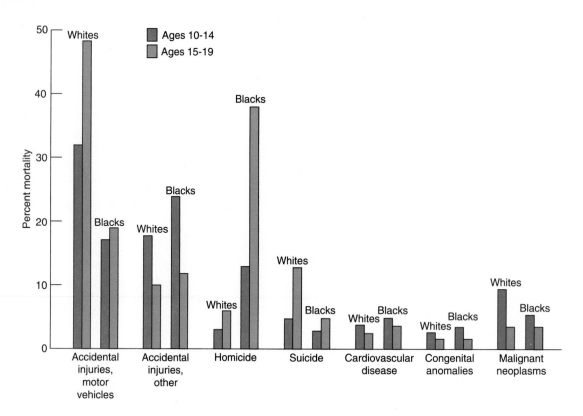

FIGURE 6-4
Percent mortality attributable to seven leading causes of death for black and white U.S. adolescents ages 10 to 14 and 15 to 19, 1987.
Source: Office of Technology Assessment, 1991.

take dramatic shape with the homicide experience of blacks compared to whites in the teenage years.

ADOLESCENT HEALTH CARE

A broad definition of adolescent health includes aspects of more traditional definitions, such as presence or absence of physical disease and disability. In addition, it includes consideration of developmental changes, social competence, health-enhancing or compromising behaviors, perceived quality of life, and social and physical environments. Most important, a definition of adolescent health needs to go beyond a view of adolescence *solely* as a transitional period between childhood and adulthood. Adolescence is to be lived, not lived through.

Recommendations for Preventive Services

The U.S. Preventive Services Task Force (1989), building on the work of the Canadian Task Force on the Periodic Health Examination, recommends a specific set of screening, counseling, and selected other clinical procedures for adolescents. Table 6-2 shows the specific clinical services recommended for ages 13 to 18. Within the table are 15 "high-risk categories" associated with some procedures. These

TABLE 6-2

Recommendations, U.S. Preventive Services Task Force for clinical prevention procedures for adolescents

---

Screening

History	*Physical exam*	*Laboratory/diagnostic procedures*
Dietary intake	Height and weight	**HIGH-RISK GROUPS**
Physical activity	Blood pressure	Rubella antibodies (HR3)
Tobacco/alcohol/drug use	**HIGH-RISK GROUPS** (see Table 6-3)	VDRL/RPR (HR4)
Sexual practices	Complete skin exam (HR1)	Chlamydial testing (HR5)
	Clinical testicular exam (HR2)	Gonorrhea culture (HR6)
		Counseling and testing for HIV (HR7)
		Tuberculin skin test (PPD) (HR8)
		Hearing (HR9)
		Papanicolaou smear (HR10)[4]

Counseling

Diet and exercise	*Sexual practices*	*Dental health*
Fat (especially saturated fat), cholesterol, sodium, iron,[2] calcium[2]	Sexual development and behavior[3]	Regular tooth brushing, flossing, dental visits
Caloric balance	Sexually transmitted diseases: partner selection, condoms	*Other primary preventive measures*
Selection of exercise program	Unintended pregnancy and contraceptive options	**HIGH-RISK GROUPS**
Substance use	*Injury prevention*	Discussion of hemoglobin testing (HR13)
Tobacco: cessation/primary prevention	Safety belts	Skin protection from ultraviolet light (HR14)
Alcohol and other drugs: cessation/ primary prevention	Safety helmets	
Driving/other dangerous activities while under the influence	Violent behavior[5]	
Treatment for abuse	Firearms[5]	
HIGH-RISK GROUPS	Smoke detector	
Sharing/using unsterilized needles and syringes (HR12)		

Immunizations & chemoprophylaxis

Tetanus-diphtheria (Td) booster[1]	**HIGH-RISK GROUPS** Fluoride supplements (HR15)	

Remain alert for:

Depressive symptoms Suicide risk factors (HR11)	Abnormal bereavement Tooth decay, malalignment, gingivitis	Signs of child abuse and neglect

---

This list of preventive services is not exhaustive. It reflects only those topics reviewed by the U.S. Preventive Services Task Force. Clinicians may wish to add other preventive services on a routine basis, and after considering the patient's medical history and other individual circumstances. Examples of target conditions not specifically examined by the Task Force include: Developmental disorders; Scoliosis; Behavioral and learning disorders; Parent/family dysfunction.

1. Once between ages 14 and 15. 2. For females. 3. Often best performed early in adolescence and with the involvement of parents. 4. Every 1-3 years. 5. Especially for males.

are identified as HR1 through HR15 in Table 6-2 and defined in Table 6-3. Screening and counseling for all adolescents are recommended to include history and current status of health behaviors and measures of physical growth and blood pressure. Additional laboratory tests and counseling are recommended for selected high-risk groups such as intravenous (IV) drug users and those with multiple sex partners. Getting accurate information on such sensitive topics is important to planning health-promotion strategies, but it may be perceived as intrusive and, therefore, the information may be difficult to obtain.

Access to Health Care

Despite recommendations for preventive screening and counseling, 22% of American 16- to 24-year-olds were not covered by private or government health insurance in 1990. These 7 million adolescents and young adults have limited or no access to health services. Although this age group makes proportionally fewer visits to healthcare providers, health status indicators do not suggest that adolescents and young adults have the least need for medical care. In fact, this age group has substantial rates of both acute and chronic medical conditions and socially related health problems.

ADOLESCENT HEALTH BEHAVIOR

Adolescent behavior is often of greater concern to the community than adolescent health. The health-related behavior of greatest emotional and political concern, although it does not show up directly in the mortality statistics, is the increase in sexual activity among teenagers. The associated consequences of

TABLE 6-3
Ages 13-18 high-risk categories for clinical prevention services in Table 6-2

HR1 Persons with increased recreational or occupational exposure to sunlight, a family or personal history of skin cancer, or clinical evidence of precursor lesions

HR2 Males with a history of testicular atrophy

HR3 Females of childbearing age lacking evidence of immunity

HR4 Persons who engage in sex with multiple partners in areas in which syphilis is prevalent, prostitutes, or contacts of persons with active syphilis

HR5 Persons who attend clinics for sexually transmitted diseases; attend other high-risk health care facilities (e.g., adolescent and family planning clinics); or have other risk factors for chlamydial infection (e.g., multiple sexual partners or a sexual partner with multiple sexual contacts)

HR6 Persons with multiple sexual partners or a sexual partner with multiple contacts, sexual contacts of persons with culture-proven gonorrhea, or persons with a history of repeated episodes of gonorrhea

HR7 Persons seeking treatment for sexually transmitted diseases; homosexual and bisexual men; past or present intravenous (IV) drug users; persons with a history of prostitution or multiple sexual partners; women whose past or present sexual partners were HIV-infected, bisexual, or IV

drug users; persons with long-term residence or birth in an area with high prevalence of HIV infection; or persons with a history of transfusion between 1978 and 1985

HR8 Household members of persons with tuberculosis or others at risk for close contact with the disease; recent immigrants or refugees from countries in which tuberculosis is common (e.g., Asia, Africa, Central and South America, Pacific Islands); migrant workers; residents of correctional institutions or homeless shelters; or persons with certain underlying medical disorders

HR9 Persons exposed regularly to excessive noise in recreational or other settings

HR10 Females who are sexually active or (if the sexual history is thought to be unreliable) aged 18 or older

HR11 Recent divorce, separation, unemployment, depression, alcohol or other drug abuse, serious medical illnesses, living alone, or recent bereavement

HR12 Intravenous drug users

HR13 Persons of Caribbean, Latin American, Asian, Mediterranean, or African descent

HR14 Persons with increased exposure to sunlight

HR15 Persons living in areas with inadequate water fluoridation (less than 0.7 parts per million)

Source: U.S. Preventive Services Task Force.

adolescent pregnancy and sexually transmitted diseases, including AIDS, produce high emotional and social costs not accounted for in most vital statistics (Figure 6-5).

Teenage Sex and Contraceptive Use

Since the 1970s sexually transmitted diseases, unintended pregnancies, and other problems that result from sexual activity have increased among adolescents in Canada and the United States. Among American students in grades 9 to 12 in 1990, 54% reported having had sexual intercourse. Male students were significantly more likely than female students to have had sexual intercourse, 61% and 48%, respectively. Black students were significantly more likely than white or Hispanic students to have had sexual intercourse, 72%, 52%, and 53%, respectively. In Canada the rates are reported by age, with one third of 15-year-old girls, more than one half of the 17-year-olds, and nearly three fourths of the Canadian 19-year-olds reporting they had engaged in sex.

Among currently sexually active American students in 1990, approximately 77% used contraception. The methods reportedly used by adolescents, such as birth control pills, condoms, and withdrawal, vary in effectiveness (see Chapter 5, Table 5-2). White female students were significantly more likely to use contraception than black or Hispanic female students.

National objectives related to adolescent sexuality, developed during the late 1980s, include abstinence, combined method contraception, and parent involvement. At the local level, nearly all school-based clinics provide counseling to students about choices related to sexual activity and birth control methods. Many clinics do not prescribe contraceptives, however, because of community resistance.

FIGURE 6-5
This magazine ad for condom use was sponsored by the National AIDS Network, the American Foundation for AIDS Research, and the Advertising Council.

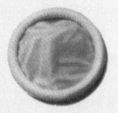

USING IT WON'T KILL YOU. NOT USING IT MIGHT.

Maybe you don't like using condoms. But if you're going to have sex, a latex condom with a spermicide is your best protection against the AIDS virus.

Use them every time, from start to finish, according to the manufacturers' directions. Because no one has ever been cured of AIDS. More than 40,000 Americans have already died from it.

And even if you don't like condoms, using them is definitely better than that.

HELP STOP AIDS. USE A CONDOM.

Many school-based clinics operate in areas servicing low-income, minority adolescents who have limited access to other sources of health care. In addition to family planning, these clinics provide services such as physical examinations, immunizations, and nutrition counseling.

Teenage Pregnancy and Birth

Adolescent childbearing is a major concern for its social and economic consequences as much as for its health effects. The birth rates for females aged 15 to 17 years showed a steady decrease between 1970 and the mid-1980s. Between 1986 and 1989,

---

Objective for Adolescent Pregnancy Rates

• By 2000 reduce pregnancies among girls aged 17 and younger to no more than 50 per 1000 adolescents. Baseline: 71.1 pregnancies per 1000 girls aged 15 to 17 in 1985.

---

however, the birth rate for black teenagers increased by 18% as did the birth rate for white teenagers (Figure 6-6).

Some 31% of all births to unmarried women in 1989 were to those between 15 and 19 years of age. Of the 1.1 million girls in this age group who become pregnant each year, an estimated 84% did not intend to get pregnant. About one half of these adolescents obtain abortions, and about one half of them give birth (Figure 6-7). In 1989 black girls aged 15 to 17 years were almost five times as likely to have a second baby and seven times as likely to have a third baby as were white girls in the same age group.

The costs of adolescent pregnancy are high to young women and to society. There are higher risks of infant mortality and low birthweight, especially for infants born to very young mothers. These mothers face probable discontinuance of their education at an early age, which, in turn, diminishes employment prospects and increases the probability of welfare dependence. The Center for Population Options estimates that U.S. taxpayers spent $25 billion in

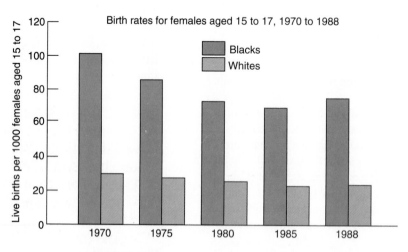

FIGURE 6-6
Birth rates for females aged 15 to 17, United States, 1970-1988.
Source: National Center for Health Statistics.

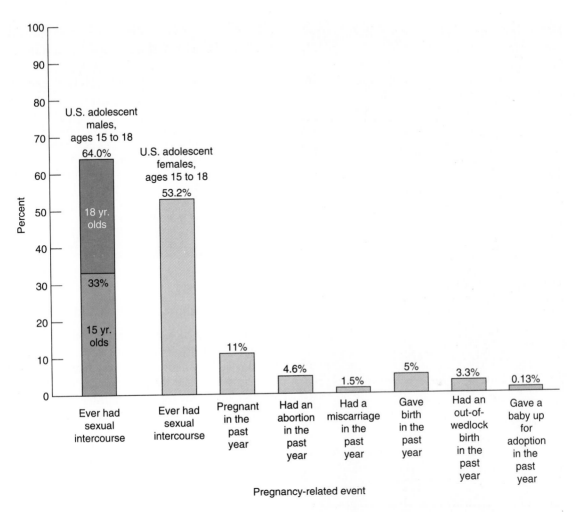

FIGURE 6-7
Disposition of sexual unions among U.S. adolescent males and females, estimated from various sources.
From U.S. Congress, 1991.

federal dollars to assist families begun by a birth to a teenager. From 1989, through Aid to Families with Dependent Children (AFDC) and Food Stamps, support for these families increased by 16% to $3.5 billion in 1990. Finally, the growing threat of heterosexual transmission of HIV infection and AIDS has multiplied the risks of pregnancy for adolescent women and their babies (Figure 6-8).

The causes of adolescent pregnancy are complex. Caution needs to be taken against simple stereotypes in characterizing them. The debate too often begins and ends with the need for abstinence or to provide more accessible contraceptive services. Greater efforts are needed to consider adolescent attitudes, beliefs, and values in counseling about choices about sexuality (Figure 6-9).

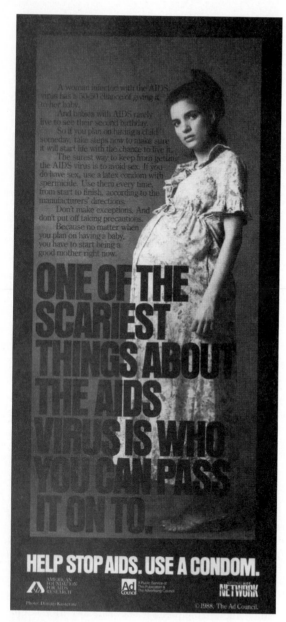

ONE OF THE SCARIEST THINGS ABOUT THE AIDS VIRUS IS WHO YOU CAN PASS IT ON TO.

HELP STOP AIDS. USE A CONDOM.

FIGURE 6-8
Another ad on AIDS and current or future pregnancy, by the same sponsors as Figure 6-5.

Objectives for Adolescent Family Planning

- By 2000 reduce the proportion of adolescents who have engaged in sexual intercourse to no more than 15% by age 15 and 40% by age 17.
- By 2000 increase to at least 90% the proportion of sexually active, unmarried people aged 19 and younger who use contraception, especially combined-method contraception, that both effectively prevents pregnancy and provides barrier protection against disease.
- By 2000 increase to 85% the proportion of people aged 10 through 18 who have discussed human sexuality with their parents and/or have received instruction from them.

Sexually Transmitted Diseases and AIDS

Sexually active adolescents are not only at risk for pregnancy but also for problems associated with involvement in unprotected sexual intercourse, including AIDS and sexually transmitted diseases (STDs), infections spread by transfer of organisms from person to person during sexual contact. By age 21 approximately one out of every five young Americans has required treatment for an STD. Because only some teenagers are sexually active, this amounts to a rate of at least 25% among all adolescents who are sexually active and over 40% in the older teens.

Between 1960 and 1988 gonorrhoea increased four times among 10- to 14-year-olds. Data from the Centers for Disease Control suggest that in 1989 30% of newly reported gonorrhea cases and 10% of newly reported syphilis cases in the United States occurred among 10- to 19-year-olds. These and other STDs can cause serious complications, including pelvic inflammatory disease, sterility, ectopic pregnancy, and blindness.

Acquired immunodeficiency syndrome (AIDS), the sixth leading cause of death for 15- to 24-year-olds, can also be transmitted through sexual activity.

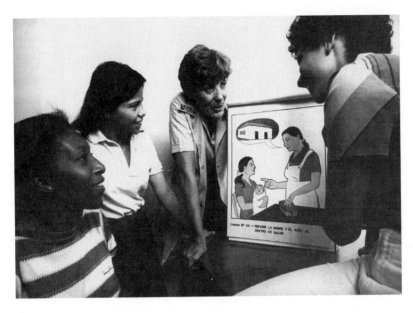

FIGURE 6-9
Nurses provide much of the counseling to young mothers and teenagers of migrant families, requiring language skills and sensitivity to cultural perspectives.
Photo courtesy National Council for International Health.

Although AIDS has gained considerable attention, the control of other STDs has benefited from the professional and public efforts to control the spread of AIDS. Provisional data for 1990 suggest a decline in the death rate from AIDS.

More than one half of the 15- to 19-year-olds in 1988 reported having sexual intercourse in the past 3 months, but only 25% reported they always used condoms. Condoms are the only known protection against AIDS for those engaged in sexual intercourse. The National Adolescent Student Health Survey in 1989, however, found that many adolescents do not know how to avoid getting STDs, nor can they identify common early signs. Misinformation among adolescents was clear. Some 12% of surveyed students thought birth control pills provided protection against the HIV virus, and 23% believed it possible to tell by looking at a potential partner whether he or she had AIDS.

Objectives for Sexually Transmitted Diseases

- By 2000 increase to at least 60% the proportion of sexually active, unmarried 15- to 19-year-old women who used a condom at last sexual intercourse. Baseline: 25% used a condom at last sexual intercourse in 1988.
- By 2000 include instruction in sexually transmitted disease transmission prevention in the curricula of all middle and secondary schools. Baseline: 95% of schools in 1988.

Alcohol, Tobacco, and Illicit Drug Use

The use of alcohol, marijuana, and cocaine by high school seniors decreased throughout the 1980s. The use of tobacco, however, remained relatively constant. By age 18 over 90% of adolescents have tried alcohol, over 40% have tried marijuana, and over

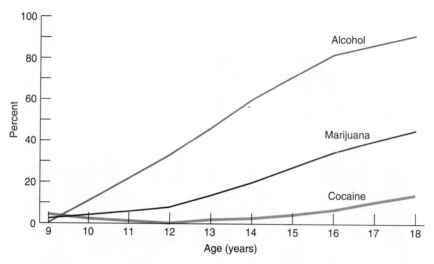

*Unweighted sample size = 11,631 students.

FIGURE 6-10
Uptake of first use of selected drugs by age, United States, 1990.
Source: Centers for Disease Control and National Institute on Drug Abuse.

10% have tried cocaine (Figure 6-10). Use of these substances in adolescent years has the potential to set patterns for future behaviors that have an impact on health beyond the adolescent years.

Alcohol use. In 1980 nearly three quarters of high school seniors had tried alcohol in the past month; by 1990 that percentage had dropped to 57%. Alcohol, however, remains the major drug of choice for adolescents. Of the nearly 21 million U.S. students in grades 7 to 12, 8 million drink alcohol monthly, and 454,000 have five or more consecutive drinks at least once a week. Of those who engage in such binge drinking, 59% are male and 41% are female (Figure 6-11).

Drinking is more prevalent among those aged 18 to 24 than in any other age group. Alcohol use by adolescents that impairs judgment has serious consequences for injuries and homicides. One half of all motor vehicle accidents for 15- to 24-year-olds

> **Objectives for Adolescent Alcohol Use**
>
> • By 2000 reduce deaths among people aged 15 through 24 caused by alcohol-related motor vehicle crashes to no more than 18 per 100,000. Baseline: 21.5 per 100,000 in 1987.
> • By 2000 reduce the percentage of 12 to 17 year old youth who have used alcohol in the past month to 12.6 percent. Baseline: 25.2 percent in 1988.

involve alcohol. Laws that make it illegal to sell alcohol to minors discourage but do not prevent adolescents from obtaining alcohol. Educational intervention intended to reduce alcohol use by adolescents needs to be aimed not only at youth, but at those who give or sell alcohol to them.

Tobacco use. The Youth Risk Behavior Survey by the Centers for Disease Control in 1991 showed that

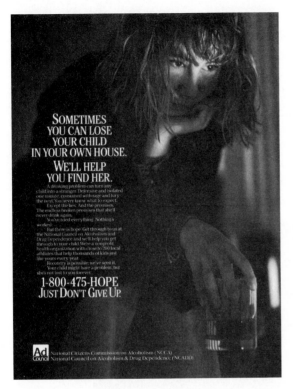

FIGURE 6-11
A partnership of a voluntary association and a federal agency, together with the Ad Council, sponsored this public service ad on teenage alcoholism.

70% of all students in grades 9 to 12 had tried cigarette smoking. The prevalence of frequent cigarette use was significantly greater among white students (15%) than among Hispanic (7%) or black (31%) students. The percentage of students who tried cigarette smoking increases significantly between grades 9 and 12.

The percentage of high school seniors who had used cigarettes in the previous month hovered near the 30% level during the 1980s. Although the rate for females dropped during the 1980s, the rates for males increased. By 1990 smoking rates for male and female seniors in high school were 29%.

Objectives for Teenage Smoking Reduction

By 2000 reduce the initiation of smoking by youth to no more than 15% as measured by the prevalence of smoking among people ages 20 through 24. (Baseline: 29.5% in 1987.)

What needs to be done in communities to support the continuing reductions?

Objectives for Tobacco Use Reduction by Adolescents

- By 2000 reduce the initiation of cigarette smoking by children and youths so that no more than 15% have become regular cigarette smokers by age 20. Baseline: 30% of youths had become regular cigarette smokers by ages 20 to 24 in 1987.
- By 2000 reduce smokeless tobacco use by males aged 12 to 24 to a prevalence of no more than 4%. Baseline: 6.6% among males aged 12 to 17 in 1988.

Health education efforts in the 1980s were directed at female adolescents whose smoking rates had surpassed that of their male counterparts in the mid-1970s.

Smokeless tobacco use was reported by over 10% of all students in the 1991 Youth Risk Behavior Survey. This rate is higher in rural areas. Significantly more males than females are likely to use this form of tobacco. Although cigarettes are associated with damage to the respiratory system and lungs, smokeless tobacco causes damage to the mouth, lips, and tongue. Both forms of tobacco are associated with increased cancer rates.

Illicit drug use. The use of illicit drugs such as marijuana, cocaine, inhalants, hallucinogens, heroin, or nonprescription use of psychotherapeutic drugs (sedatives or stimulants) appears to be far less common among adolescents living at home than the use of alcohol or tobacco (Figure 6-12). The percentages of high school seniors who had tried marijuana or cocaine in the previous month were more than halved during the 1980s to 14% and 2%, respectively, by 1990. White students are three times more likely than black students to have used either drug in the previous month. Black youth who may daily see the crime and horror of drug use in their communities have compelling reasons for turning

Objectives for Illicit Drug Use Reduction
• By 2000 reduce the percentage of 12- to 17-year-olds who used marijuana in the last month to 3.2%. Baseline: 6.4% in 1988.
• By 2000 reduce the percentage of 12- to 17-year-olds who used cocaine in the last month to 0.6%. Baseline: 1.1% in 1988.

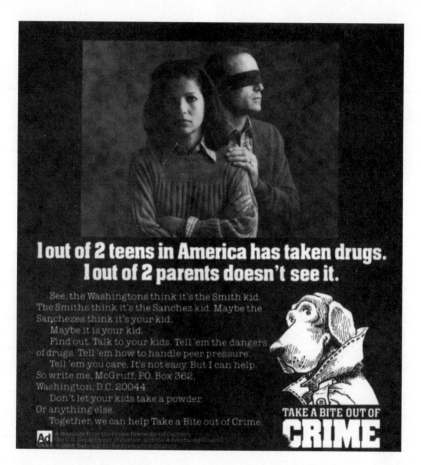

FIGURE 6-12
The Community's concern about teenage drug abuse grows as the problem is seen to affect middle-class kids (not just the poor) and to relate to crime and delinquency.

away from illegal drug use, but their economic circumstances may make drug dealing seem the only viable alternative for financial success.

Between 1991 and 1992, after a decade of decline, the rate of illicit drug use went up slightly among 13- and 14-year-olds.

Diet and Physical Fitness for Adolescents

Dietary patterns. Dietary patterns established during youth may extend into adulthood and increase the risk for cancer and other chronic diseases. Diets that are high in fat and low in fruit, vegetables, and grain are of particular concern to future health. In 1991 13% of American youth in grades 9 to 12 reported consuming five or more servings of fruit and vegetables during the day preceding the survey. Males were more likely than females and whites more likely than blacks or Hispanics to eat more fruit. Of all students, 65% reported eating no more than two serving of foods typically high in fat content during the day preceding the survey. Only 64% of teenagers regularly eat breakfast.

Weight and physical activity. Data for adolescents on fitness and nutrition are limited. Physical activity and dietary patterns of adolescents contribute to problems of obesity. Close to 55% of American youth between 5 and 17 years were of average weight in proportion to their height. Another 38% were overweight, and the remaining 8% were underweight. There is almost a linear relationship between family income and the probability of being overweight. Poor children were almost three times as likely as children in families with higher incomes to be overweight. Black children, regardless of sociodemographic characteristics, were the most likely to be overweight and the least likely to be underweight. More than twice the proportion of black children were reported as overweight compared with Hispanic children and white children.

Steroids. The use of steroids among adolescent athletes and body builders is considered a growing problem. An estimated 1 million Americans, one half of them adolescents, use black-market steroids. Countless others are choosing from among more than 100 other substances, legal and illegal, to enhance physical size and performance. The problem received worldwide attention during the 1988 Olympics when Canadian runner Ben Johnson was forced to forfeit his gold medal because of steroid use. The risks of steroid use are considerable, including damage to muscles, sex organs, and the nervous system. In addition to its physical dangers, steroid use can lead to aggression, violence, and a vicious cycle of dependency. The encouragement to use steroids comes from a personal competitive de-

---

Objective for Weight Control for Adolescents

- By 2000 reduce overweight to a prevalence of no more that 15% among adolescents aged 12 to 19.

Objective for Steroid Use Reduction

- By 2000 reduce to no more than 3% the proportion of male high school seniors who use anabolic steroids. Baseline: 4.7% in 1989.

Objective for Physical Activity for Adolescents

- By 2000 increase to at least 75% the proportion of children and adolescents aged 6 to 17 who engage in vigorous physical activity that promotes the development and maintenance of cardiorespiratory fitness 3 or more days per week for 20 minutes or more per occasion. Baseline: 6% for youth aged 10 to 17 in 1984.

sire, peers, some coaches, and even parents. Over one half of the teens who use steroids start before age 16, sometimes with the encouragement of their parents.

Mental Health of Adolescents

Abuse and neglect. The U.S. Child Abuse Prevention and Treatment Act clarifies child abuse and neglect as the physical or mental injury, sexual abuse or exploitation, negligent treatment, or maltreatment of a person under the age of 18 by a person responsible for the child's welfare. The most recent national incidence study estimates that nearly 1 million American children nationwide experienced demonstrable harm as a result of maltreatment in 1986 and that 1.5 million experienced abuse or neglect. Abuse can be physical, emotional, or sexual, the latter remaining the least frequent type of abuse. Neglect includes physical, educational, and emotional failure to provide for a child or adolescent's basic needs. In 1986 1100 children died as a result of abuse or neglect, a 51% increase from 1980. A 1992 study in Canada reported that teenagers and children comprised a larger proportion of victims of sexual assault than adults. Four out of every 10 sexual assault victims were under 12 years old, 4 between 12 and 19 years old, and 2, 20 years old or over.

The reasons for abuse and neglect are multiple and include individual characteristics of parents or children, family interactions, and environmental conditions. An adolescent's race, ethnicity, or geographic location has no significant impact on the incidence of maltreatment, but small family size de-

creases and large families increase the possibility. Females experience more abuse than males.

The maltreatment of children and adolescents is a community problem; no single agency, individual, or discipline has the necessary knowledge, skills, resources, or societal mandate to provide the assistance needed by those who are abused or neglected.

Suicide. Rates for suicide among adolescents 15 to 19 years of age have quadrupled from nearly 3 per 100,000 in 1950 to over 11 in 1988. Suicide is the third leading cause of death among adolescents. Attempted suicide is a potentially lethal health event, a risk factor for future completed suicide, and a potential indicator of other health problems such as substance abuse, depression, or adjustment and stress reactions. The Youth Risk Behavior Survey done in 1990 by the Centers for Disease Control found that in the preceding 12 months 27% of all American students in grades 9 to 12 reported they had thought seriously about attempting suicide.

Female students were significantly more likely than male students to report they had thought seriously about suicide and made an attempt that required medical attention. Black students reported lower levels of suicidal thought than white or Hispanic students.

Delinquency and homelessness. In recent years the number of U.S. adolescents confined to public and private juvenile facilities for delinquent acts has been increasing. Most of the increase has apparently been due to an increase in the number of adolescents confined for minor offenses. In 1988 there were 1.6 million arrests of adolescents (Figure 6-13).

Objective for Adolescent Abuse and Neglect Reduction

• By 2000 reduce rape and attempted rape of women aged 12 to 34 to no more than 225 per 100,000. Baseline: 250 per 100,000 in 1986.

Objective for Adolescent Suicide Rates

• By 2000 reduce suicides among youths aged 15 to 19 to no more than 8.2 per 100,000. Baseline: 11.3 per 100,000 in 1988.

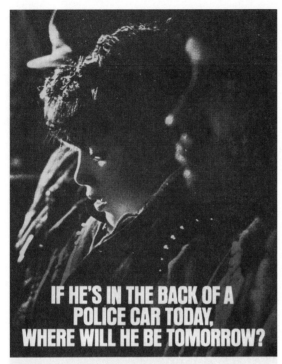

IF HE'S IN THE BACK OF A POLICE CAR TODAY, WHERE WILL HE BE TOMORROW?

He's not a bad kid, really. But one night, while spraying graffiti on a brick wall, this 12 year-old had his first brush with the law.

Where do you go before things get out of hand?

He got help at a local Youth Center. They got help from the United Way. All because the United Way got help from you.

Your single contribution helps provide therapy for a child with a learning disability, rehabilitation for a cocaine abuser, and a program that sends a volunteer to do the shopping for a 79 year-old woman.

Or, in this case, a place where a kid can toss a basketball around after school. A place where a basically good kid can stay that way.

United Way

It brings out the best in all of us.

FIGURE 6-13
The United Way, a voluntary association, and the Ad Council, sponsored this public service ad on teenage problem prevention.

Adolescents may be homeless either on their own or with their families. In 1984 the United States estimated that there are as many as 1 million homeless and runaway adolescents each year (Figure 6-14).

Anorexia nervosa and bulimia. Anorexia and bulimia are compulsive eating disorders with consequences similar to those of malnutrition. Both disorders involve the depletion of nutrients and both are considered epidemic in adolescent and young women in North America. Societal pressures on women to be thin, especially media images, contribute to the problem for adolescents. The fixation on slimness causes the anorexic to starve herself, the bulimic to "binge and purge"—eating compulsively, then regurgitating. The bulimic person, male or female, also suffers from upper intestinal and oral tissue damage from the frequent exposure of the throat and mouth to stomach acids. Dentists are of-

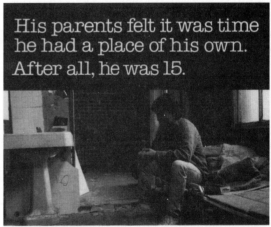

His parents felt it was time he had a place of his own. After all, he was 15.

Every year hundreds of thousands of kids are thrown away. Put out onto the streets. With no job, no money and nowhere to go. But now there is a number for kids to call. The Covenant House Nineline helps kids with food, clothing, a place to sleep and, most of all, someone to talk to.

To get help in your hometown call our Nineline 1-800-999-9999. It's free. **Nineline 1-800-999-9999 Anytime. Anywhere.**

FIGURE 6-14
Teenage homelessness affects all classes of runaway and shutout adolescents, not just the poor. It relates to problems of crime, prostitution, and substance abuse.

Objectives for Violence among Adolescents
• By 2000 reduce by 20% the incidence of physical fighting among adolescents aged 14 to 17. Baseline: not currently available. • By 2000 reduce by 20% the incidence of weapon carrying by adolescents aged 14 to 17. Baseline: not currently available.

ten the first to detect the bulimic, recognizing their pattern of tooth erosion.

Adolescent Health Education and Services

As a complement to school health education and school health services, a major responsibility of community health education and ambulatory care services in the community is to recognize the special needs of adolescents beyond the classroom and the school. Teenagers are confused by peer pressure, parental disapproval, their individual values, and their decision-making ability. This confusion may preclude their seeking help before they begin using alcohol or become sexually active, especially with pregnancy or automobile accidents already a possibility.

It is the responsibility of the personnel of ambulatory (walk-in) clinics and programs to be aware that teens who are seeking services will have different levels of information, education, and experience. Because adolescents vary in their knowledge levels, attitudes, cultural background, and behavior, no single program activity can meet all of their needs. Teens may or may not be living with their parents or attending school, and regardless of the family's income they may be unable to pay for medical services. Health services staff members must be prepared to deal with these variations in developmental levels, social situations, the teenagers' degree of communication with the parents, their ability to plan, and their willingness to recognize the risks of alcohol, drugs, or sexual activity and to take pre-

Historical Perspective on Teenage Sex
At the turn of the century, girls had their first period at an average age of 15. Today, the average age at which menstruation begins is 12. In 1900, menstruation began at the age when most girls were about to complete their education, marry, and begin their families. Society's norms were more closely coordinated with nature's biological clock. Today, because of improved nutrition, the biological clock ticks faster, offering sexual and reproductive maturity at a younger age. But social organization has delayed the other rights and responsibilities of maturity. With improved educational and employment opportunities, marriage and childbearing are delayed, leaving an ever-increasing gap between the age at which sexual maturity occurs and the age of first intended pregnancy. How does this historical perspective bear on the teenage pregnancy and abortion rates?

ventive measures against pregnancy or drunk driving.

The guidelines that follow were developed for adolescent health services and community projects.

• Adolescents often have vague and sometimes incorrect knowledge of drugs and sex. There is a need for open discussion of their ideas and beliefs about sex and reproduction; both sexes should be involved when possible. Teenagers need to be clearly informed about the possible results of alcohol or drug misuse and of sexual intercourse. Group discussions may be an effective way for adolescents to gain necessary information but should not replace individual counseling. Adolescents should be told through media and outreach programs that they are welcome at the ambulatory care clinic, that their privacy is protected, that their records are confidential, and that education and counseling are free.

• Teenagers must be given sufficient knowledge at their level of understanding to make a responsible decision about engaging in sexual activity that may lead to pregnancy, to make an informed choice of a method of birth control, to be aware of possible side effects and contraindications of use of the various contraceptive methods, and to become thoroughly aware of the physical, emotional, and social consequences of sexual activity for both participants, their families, and their communities.

- Risk taking with alcohol, drugs, or sex is often associated with other teenage problems. Health care providers can assist by referring teenagers to employment agencies, alternative school programs, and drug or alcohol misuse agencies. Counseling services must be available to a teenager in urgent need of discussing problems. Delay in getting to ''talk to somebody'' can cause the person to change his or her mind about asking for help.

- A project should identify the resources of the community and other resources available under state or province and federal programs that are potential sources of assistance and cooperation. Projects can also use the materials and experience of national groups (e.g., March of Dimes, National Organization for Women, Salvation Army) that are also dealing with the problem of teenage pregnancy. Local chapters of those organizations should be involved with the project's activity (Figure 6-15).

- Effective ways must be found to reach the teenage population. Techniques and means of contact need to be selected uniquely for the population; these might include teen-oriented radio stations, television, bulletin-board notices at teen hangouts, school group activities, and youth groups. Organizations such as the Parent-Teacher-Student Association, local school boards, churches, and Big Brother and Big Sister organizations have an interest in helping teenagers. Work with them can help to develop a broad base of support in the community. Work with the schools can promote educational programs to alert teenagers about health issues related to smoking, drugs, drinking, and adolescent sexual activity.

Develop community awareness. Projects should develop a plan for community education to increase awareness of adolescent pregnancy and health problems. This can be done by:

1. Publicizing the scope and implications to the community of teenage sexual or substance misuse activity (e.g., number of school dropouts due to pregnancy, number of teens with out-of-wedlock births, number of teen abortions, venereal disease rates, number of births to teenage girls, number of automobile injuries and deaths involving alcohol). National media and data can be used (Figure 6-16).

2. Identifying community leaders and groups who can help to make contact with teens and remove barriers to their receiving services and continuing their education. These people could be school board members, social service workers, or youth workers. Parent groups can be highly effective in the review of materials and in initiating public action and may not have the same constraints as school administrators and teachers.

3. Developing programs to educate parents about the extent of teenage sexual or drinking activity, the knowledge and guidance teens may need, and where they can get information and help.

4. Providing a central source of information, resource material, and personnel. This could also mean helping libraries and bookstores acquire accurate and acceptable references, arranging displays for fairs and exhibitions, providing speakers for community groups, and notifying newspapers and radio and television stations of the availability of these resources.

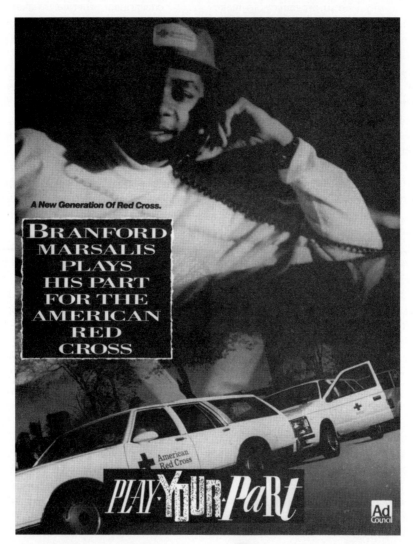

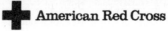
FIGURE 6-15
Voluntary associations seek greater participation of teenagers, as suggested by this appeal
from the Red Cross.

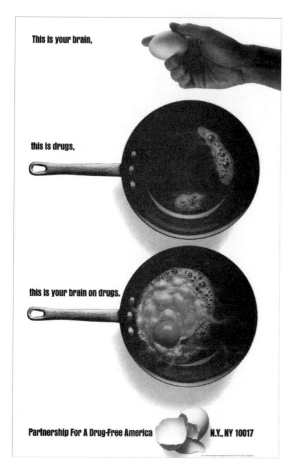

This is your brain,

this is drugs,

this is your brain on drugs.

Partnership For A Drug-Free America   N.Y., NY 10017

FIGURE 6-16
The most widely recognized public service advertisement among teenagers in 1991 was this ad by a business coalition on drug abuse prevention.

Develop adolescent awareness. Teenagers today are faced with adapting to the mores of a rapidly changing society and, although lacking sufficient life experience in their developmental years, are forced to make decisions that can greatly affect their adult lives. It is the responsibility of health services staff members to be aware of the varying levels of knowledge and education of the adolescents who come to them for services, so that the individual can be given appropriate information about human re-

production, contraception, alcohol, drugs, or other topics of concern. Sexually active teens need information about the specific services available to them. Efforts must be made to reach teenagers, whether in the community or in family planning clinics. The following activities have been found to be effective.

1. Identify all access points of contact with adolescents (e.g., schools, homes, recreation centers, shopping malls, employment agencies, local hangouts, teen-youth programs, and radio and television).

2. Devise strategies to reach teenagers at their locations (e.g., put up posters at public places such as sports arenas, educate adults working with teens about availability of counseling and referral, furnish spot announcements regarding family planning clinics for use by radio and television stations, send flyers to other health and social service agencies, and form discussion panels for church groups or youth clubs).

3. Use audiovisual materials suitable to adolescents of different ages and different environments. Project developers should also be aware that many materials already are available from sources such as the National Clearinghouse for Family Planning Information, the National Health Information Clearinghouse, the National Clearinghouse for Smoking and Health, Health Canada, and national clearinghouses for alcohol information. Materials developed locally should be age-appropriate and easily understood, with the information directed to assist teenagers' decision making: whether to have sexual intercourse, how to choose a contraceptive, where and when to get tests for venereal disease or pregnancy. Teenagers can help with the preparation of some materials and can act as valuable "reviewers."

4. Make special efforts to reach teens who are not in school. One approach is to identify

hangouts such as bowling alleys, video parlors, hamburger stands, and beaches and swimming pools and then establish rapport with the informal leaders.

5. Publicize the availability of services in terms that are meaningful to teenagers; teens may not know that family planning clinics, community health centers, or other ambulatory care projects are relevant to their needs. Teens need to know that family planning services are not only for adults or married couples.

Counseling. Counselors and educators should have thorough training in adolescent growth, development, and behavior patterns and should be screened for their ability to relate to teenagers. The two major concerns of the counseling process are (1) to impart sufficient knowledge to help the individual make a responsible and intelligent choice about smoking, alcohol, and sexual intercourse and, if indicated, about a birth control method and (2) to instill the necessary motivation and skill to enable the individual to follow through with the decision to use birth control or not to smoke or use alcohol.

Crisis counseling should be available to teenagers in urgent need of discussing their problems. Teens need more counseling than is usually provided for adults; many who come to the clinics are uncertain or worried about the risks they are taking. Teens should be encouraged to include their sex partners or friends in the counseling sessions. Males should be encouraged to come to the clinic for educational counseling services. If they will not participate, educational materials should be sent to them through the teenage girls being counseled.

Complete and thorough discussions about sexual development, human sexuality, reproduction, and the choices of contraceptive care must be given. Contraceptive methods discussed should include abstinence, natural family planning, barrier methods (diaphragms, condoms, and foam), and oral contraceptives and intrauterine devices (IUDs).

Services. An ambulatory care clinic should examine its service-delivery system to evaluate its usefulness and attractiveness to adolescents. Many teenagers coming to the facility lack knowledge about many things: confidentiality of services, medical procedures, cost of services, and necessary follow-up of a positive pregnancy or sexually transmitted disease test. Teenagers are entitled to the full range of medical and other services offered by an ambulatory care clinic. To be encouraged to accept the project services, teenagers need special assurance that confidentiality will be honored. They are concerned with privacy, so services should permit anonymity, either with clinics made available through multipurpose health centers or with separate entrances or hours established for teen use. Appointments should be available on short notice; drop-ins should be seen, if the project has sufficient personnel. Teens should receive pregnancy testing or treatment for sexually transmitted infections as quickly as possible.

It must be made plain to teenagers that project services are free or low-cost, and if there is a charge, they should be allowed to make deferred payments. The inability to pay for services, regardless of family income, is a serious deterrent to their seeking help. Many will pay for services if they can do so in installments and without being billed at home.

Pregnancy testing services are highly attractive to teenagers. Studies have shown that a pregnancy scare is often a prime motivation for a teenager to attend a family planning clinic. Providers wishing to attract teenagers should provide easily accessible pregnancy testing services and should not turn away or refer a teenager who requests only a pregnancy test and declines birth control assistance.

Staff members working with teenagers should be sympathetic and sensitive to various teen-specific needs. They must avoid ambiguous language. For example, they should not assume that sexual activity is understood by a teen to mean sexual intercourse. Teenagers need to know what will happen at the clinic and should be told what to expect during the physical examination.

Training. Family planning and health professionals who provide care to teenagers should have training that is specific to teenage needs. This training should cover adolescent growth and development, human sexuality, responsibilities of a sexual relationship, decision making about the use of contraceptives (for different relationships, ages, motivations, and developmental levels), health risks and problems specific to young females, responsibility of males, and alcohol and drug use and effects. Staff members may need special training in counseling or may need to supplement their skills by working with counselors who are alert and sensitive to the concerns of teenagers.

People outside the medical service disciplines who have contact and good rapport with adolescents should be enlisted to counsel and to help disseminate information about family planning services. Some experienced providers suggest that the training of people who are not medical professionals and who can communicate well with young people is an excellent way of increasing teen use of available services (Figure 6-17). Training for counseling should be thorough in all phases, with emphasis on the ability to communicate at the teenager's level of comprehension. It may be advantageous to have counseling given by a young person or one who appears young, for many adolescents will not express themselves or listen to an individual who is not regarded as a contemporary. The training of volunteer peer counselors (other teens) is a technique that recognizes adolescent communication patterns. Teen counselors can be an important resource in the community.

Special efforts should also be made to develop education and discussion sessions for parents on a communitywide basis. Although much teen learning comes from peers, parents are key to the development of their children's values, attitudes, and sense of responsibility. Frequently parents are overlooked

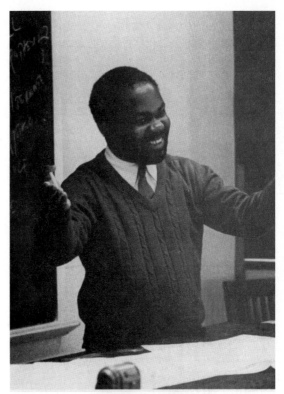

REACH FOR THE POWER. TEACH.

No other profession has this power. The power to wake up young minds. The power to wake up the world. Teachers have that power. Reach for it. Teach. For information call:

1-800-45-TEACH.

Recruiting New Teachers, Inc.

FIGURE 6-17
Teachers are sometimes the best channel for communicating effectively with teens.

as important members of the team. Teenagers can also play a role in supporting their parents in managing adult health problems; they will soon encounter such problems themselves. This brings us to adult health.

SUMMARY

Adolescence is a tumultuous period. Challenges to health from the adaptation to growing independence from adult authority are compounded by social trends making adult support and guidance more problematic. Communities must help fill this gap through the organization of services, programs, and projects in schools, clubs, and recreational environments.

QUESTIONS FOR REVIEW

1. Why is it important to consider adolescent health to be on a life-long health continuum rather than a separate, discrete stage?
2. In what ways might prevention efforts for adolescents be the same as those for children and adults? In what ways might they be different?
3. How do biological and psychosocial maturation affect health differently? The same?
4. What factors account for adolescents as the only age group that has sustained a reversal in death rates in recent decades?
5. Review Table 6-1. How can health education programs use the major tasks of coping and adaptation for adolescents to address health consequences faced by this age group?
6. What implications do demographic changes among adolescents have for school health curriculum, community health activities, and community health services?
7. In which leading causes of adolescent ill health is alcohol use involved? How would alcohol use by adolescents be addressed differently through health promotion, health protection, and health service efforts?

8. What are the costs of adolescent pregnancy to the infant, the teenage mother, significant others, and society at large?
9. What are the pros and cons of arguments about placing condoms in schools for easier access by adolescents?
10. How did health education contribute to the decline in adolescent female smoking in the 1980s?
11. What are the multiple factors that converge to make suicide the third leading cause of death for adolescents?
12. What existing services and facilities in your community meet the needs of adolescent health? What additional services are needed?

READINGS

Allen KF, Moss AJ, Giovino GA et al: Teenage tobacco use: data estimates from the Teenage Attitudes and Practices Survey, United States, 1989. In *Advance data from vital and health statistics,* no 224, Hyattsville, Md, 1992, National Center for Health Statistics. For many adolescents, the benefits of smoking were perceived to outweigh the risks. The smokers overestimated their ability to quit smoking. Quit attempts often met with failure. Detailed breakdown of data on smokers, former smokers, and never smokers.

Cornelius LJ: Health habits of school-age children, *J Health Care Poor Underserved* 2:374, 1991.
Analyzes data on disadvantaged children and youth aged 5 to 17 from the National Medical Expenditure Survey. Income and education of the highest wage earner in the family were significantly related to the number of good health habits.

Hendee WR, editor: *The health of adolescents: understanding and facilitating biological, behavioral, and social development,* San Francisco, 1991, Jossey-Bass. For clinical and community professionals, this book offers suggestions for promoting the health of adolescents in 22 chapters covering normal adolescent growth and development, precursors of adolescent health problems, access to health care, and improving the health of adolescents.

Kann L, Anderson JE, Holtzman D et al: HIV-related knowledge, beliefs, and behaviors among high school students in the United States: results from a national survey, *J Sch Health* 61:397, 1991.

Estimates of the prevalence of sexual intercourse and illegal drug injection from a national sample of U.S. high school students indicate that nearly all knew the major modes of transmission of HIV infection; 3% reported injecting illegal drugs, 1% shared needles; 59% reported having sexual intercourse, and 40% of those reported having four or more sexual partners.

Kobokovich LJ, Bonovich LK: Adolescent pregnancy prevention strategies used by school nurses, *J Sch Health* 62:11, 1992.

A survey of school nurses in the mid-Atlantic region found that the structure of school nursing services often does not permit adequate time or opportunity to engage in adolescent pregnancy prevention efforts.

BIBLIOGRAPHY

Alteneder RR, Price JH, Telljohann SK et al: Using the PRECEDE model to determine junior high school students' knowledge, attitudes, and beliefs about AIDS, *J Sch Health* 62:464, 1992.

Altman DG, Rasenick-Douss L, Foster V et al: Sustained effects of an education program to reduce sales of cigarettes to minors, *Am J Public Health* 81:891, 1991.

American Medical Association: *Healthy youth 2000: national health promotion and disease prevention objectives for adolescents,* Chicago, 1991, Department of Adolescent Health, The Association.

BC Youth: *Youth talks: your views, your ideas, your future; final report,* Victoria, 1992, *BC* Youth Council.

Berg CL, Swanson DJ, Juhl N: Total blood cholesterol and contributory risk factors in an adolescent population, *J Sch Health* 62:64, 1992.

Brown LK, Nassau JH, Levy V: "What upsets me most about AIDS is . . ." A survey of children and adolescents, *AIDS Educ Prev* 2:296, 1990.

Carnegie Council on Adolescent Development: *Turning points: preparing American youth for the 21st century,* New York, 1989, Carnegie Corporation of New York.

Centers for Disease Control: Tobacco use among high school students—United States, 1990, *MMWR* 40:712, 1990.

Centers for Disease Control: Attempted suicide among high school students—United States, 1990, *MMWR* 40:633, 1991.

Centers for Disease Control: Accessibility of cigarettes to youths aged 12-17 years—United States, 1989, *MMWR* 41:485, 1992a.

Centers for Disease Control: Sexual behavior among high school students—United States, 1990, *MMWR* 40:885, 1992b.

Centers for Disease Control: Selected tobacco-use behaviors and dietary patterns among high school students—United States, 1991, *MMWR* 41:417, 1992c.

Cockburn J, Hennrikus D, Scott R et al: Adolescent use of sun-protection measures, *Med J Austr* 151:136, 1989.

Contento IR, Kell DG, Keiley MK et al: A formative evaluation of the American Cancer Society *Changing the Course* nutrition education curriculum, *J Sch Health* 62:411, 1992.

DePanfilis D, Salus MK: *A coordinated response to child abuse and neglect: a basic manual,* Washington, DC, 1992, National Center on Child Abuse and Neglect, U.S. Department of Health and Human Services.

DiFranza JR, Richards JW, Paulman PM et al: RJR Nabisco's cartoon camel promotes Camel cigarettes to children, *JAMA* 266:3149, 1991.

Dijkstra M, deVries H, Parcel GS: The linkage approach applied to a school-based smoking prevention program in the Netherlands, *J Sch Health* 63:339, 1993.

Dougherty D, Eden J, Kemp KB et al: Adolescent health: a report to the U.S. Congress, *J Sch Health* 62:167, 1992.

Duval B, LaVoie M: Sélection des comportements devant faire l'objet d'une intervention en éducation pour la santé: application à la prévention des MTS chez les adolescents [How to select target behaviors in health education—a model applied to the prevention of STD in teenagers], *Revue Canadienne de Santé Publique* 81:363, 1990.

Dwyer KM, Richardson JL, Danley KL et al: Characteristics of eighth-grade students who initiate self-care in elementary and junior high school, *Pediatrics* 86:448, 1990.

Edet EE: The role of sex education in adolescent pregnancy, *J R Soc Health* 111:17, 1991.

Farrell AD, Danish SJ, Howard CW: Risk factors for drug use in urban adolescents: identification and cross-validation, *Am J Community Psychol* 20:263, 1992.

Feighery E, Altman DG, Shaffer G: The effects of combining education and enforcement to reduce tobacco sales to minors, *JAMA* 266:3168, 1991.

Gerstein DR, Green LW, editors: *Preventing drug abuse: what do we know?* Washington, DC, 1993, National Academy Press.

Hamburg DA: *Today's children: creating a future for a generation in crisis,* New York, 1992, Times Books.

Hardy JB, Zabin LS: *Adolescent pregnancy in an urban environment.* Baltimore, 1990, Urban & Schwarzenberg.

Health and Welfare Canada: The *health of Canada's youth: views and behaviours of 11-, 13- and 15-year-olds from 11 countries,* Ottawa, 1993, Health and Welfare Canada.

Hechinger FM: *Fateful choices: healthy youth for the 21st century,* New York, 1992, Hill & Wang.

Holund U: Effect of a nutrition education program, Learning by Teaching, on adolescents' knowledge and beliefs, *Community Dent Oral Epidemiol* 18:61, 1990.

Jemmott JB III, Jemmott LS, Fong GT: Reductions in HIV risk-associated sexual behaviors among black male adolescents: effects of an AIDS prevention intervention, *Am J Public Health* 82:372, 1992.

Jessor R, Donovan JE, Costa FM: *Beyond adolescence: problem behavior and young adult development,* New York, 1992, Cambridge University Press.

Klein JD, Slap GB, Elster AB et al: Access to health care for adolescents: a position paper of the Society for Adolescent Medicine, *J Adolesc Health* 13:162, 1992.

Lemberg R, editor: Controlling eating disorders with facts, advice, and resources, Phoenix, Ariz, 1992, Oryx.

Liburd LC, Bowie JV: Intentional teenage pregnancy: a community diagnosis and action plan, *Health Educ* 20:33, 1989.

Olsen TL, Anderson RL, Dearwater SR et al: The epidemiology of low back pain in an adolescent population, *Am J Public Health* 82:606, 1992.

Price JH, Telljohann SK: School counselors' perceptions of adolescent homosexuals, *J Sch Health* 61:433, 1991.

Sarason IG, Mankowski ES, Peterson AV Jr et al: Adolescents' reasons for smoking, *J Sch Health* 62:185, 1992.

Schinke MA, Orlandi M, Schilling RF et al.: Feasibility of interactive videodisc technology to teach minority youth about preventing HIV infection, *Public Health Rep* 107:323, 1992.

Simons-Morton BG, Brink SG, Parcel GS et al: *Preventing alcohol-related health problems among adolescents and young adults: a CDC community intervention handbook,* Atlanta, Ga, 1989, Centers for Disease Control.

Tower CC: The role of educators in the protection and treatment of child abuse and neglect, Washington, DC, 1992, National Center on Child Abuse and Neglect, U.S. Department of Health and Human Services, DHHS Pub No (ACF) 92-30172.

U.S. Congress, Office of Technology Assessment: Adolescent health, vol 1, summary and policy options, Washington, DC, 1991, U.S. Government Printing Office.

U.S. Preventive Services Task Force: *Guide to clinical preventive services: an assessment of the effectiveness of 169 interventions,* Baltimore, 1989, Williams & Wilkins.

Vincent M, Clearie AF, Schluchter MD: Reducing adolescent pregnancy through school and community-based education, *JAMA* 257:3382, 1987.

Williams DP, Going SB, Lohman TG et al: Body fatness and risk for elevated blood pressure, total cholesterol, and serum lipoprotein ratios in children and adolescents, *Am J Public Health* 82:358, 1992.

Chapter 7

Adult Health

❖

*John Wolf died of lung cancer in New York at a
relatively young age. He had been a careful,
conscientious, attentive, even elegant man—most
of his life—but his deep restlessness and
unrelieved pessimism could only be numbed and
disguised by smoking 3 packs of unfiltered
cigarettes per day from the time he was 18. Like
many busy men who maintain an otherwise calm
and managed air about themselves, John Wolf
smoked himself to death.*

JOHN IRVING *The World According to Garp*

OBJECTIVES

When you finish this chapter, you should be able to:

- Assess the special health problems and needs of the adult populations of a community
- Identify programs appropriate to health promotion and disease prevention in these populations

This chapter focuses on the chronic diseases that are among the leading causes of death for adults: cancer, heart disease, liver disease, chronic lung disease, and diabetes (Figure 7-1). In addition, we discuss arthritis, the most common chronic disease in adults. Other leading causes of death among adults—injuries, homicide, HIV infection, and suicide—are discussed respectively in chapters on injury control, communicable disease, and mental health. The three leading causes of death—cancer, heart disease, and injuries—account for approximately 62% of all deaths in this age group. More importantly from a community perspective, many of the leading causes of death in this age group are related to life-style practices that are amenable to community programs.

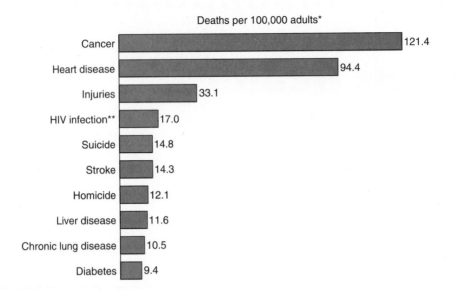

Deaths per 100,000 adults*

Cancer	121.4
Heart disease	94.4
Injuries	33.1
HIV infection**	17.0
Suicide	14.8
Stroke	14.3
Homicide	12.1
Liver disease	11.6
Chronic lung disease	10.5
Diabetes	9.4

*Provisional 1990 data
**HIV infection includes ages 25 and over

FIGURE 7-1
Leading causes of death for adults aged 25 to 64, United States, 1990.
Source: National Center for Health Statistics, Centers for Disease Control and Prevention, U.S. Department of Health and Human Services.

SHIFTING PERSPECTIVES ON HEALTH

More than once the preceding chapters have adjusted the lens through which you have been asked to view community health. The complexity of community health requires you to wear mental bifocals, trifocals, and even quadrifocals to shift back and forth from one perspective to another. At the very least you will encounter the perspectives of various disciplines, each of which views the field of community health from one of the four spheres previously reviewed in Figure 1-1 that overlaps with it. These disciplines bring their own traditions, nomenclature, skills, and philosophies to the analysis or solution of community health problems. The beginning of this chapter will review some of the dominant perspectives as an introduction to the subject of adult health. Keep in mind that these perspectives

apply to each of the age groups and to each of the health promotion, health protection, and health services chapters to follow.

The Historical Perspective

At the beginning of this century, when community health professionals concentrated their efforts on the prevention and control of communicable diseases, their emphasis was on the school-age child. It soon became apparent, however, that proper control measures required going back to the preschool child. Eventually attention shifted to infant health. Because a truly preventive approach to infant health required increasing attention to prenatal factors, intensified efforts in maternal health resulted. This legitimized some shift in resources from infant and child health to adolescent and adult health, at least for females.

With the advances in communicable disease control and the prevention of death in the early years of life, greater proportions of the population survived through **adolescence** to **adulthood** and into old age. The chronic and degenerative diseases, usually most prevalent in adulthood, became the leading causes of death and disability (Figure 7-2). These changes led the health professions to expand their approach to the health of the adult population. Among the noncommunicable diseases now in the list of the leading causes of death in the United States are "accidents" (fourth in age-adjusted death rates, behind cancer and vascular diseases), suicide (eighth), and homicide (eleventh). These three causes show up most dramatically in the adolescent and early adult years.

Demographic and Epidemiological Perspectives

The overall shift in the configuration of causes of death from the first half of the century is reflected in Figure 7-2. The specific causes of death for all ages in 1900 and 1990 are detailed in Figure 7-3. Heart diseases in 1990 account for more than three times as many deaths as injuries and cerebrovascular disease (stroke).

The death rates for these most common causes of death have been decreasing at least since the late 1960s. This outweighs by a large margin the increases in cause-specific death rates for the less frequent causes lower on the chart, including AIDS. The substantial decrease in the overall death rate can be traced largely to the reductions in mortality from heart disease, stroke, and injuries.

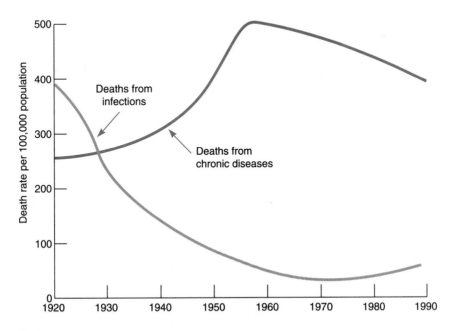

FIGURE 7-2
The "diseases of civilization" have virtually reversed their position relative to the infectious diseases as causes of death since 1920 in the more industrialized countries. AIDS and HIV infections have brought a slight increase in the deaths due to communicable diseases relative to chronic diseases since 1981.

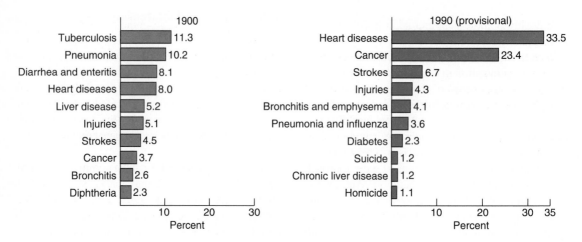

FIGURE 7-3

Changes in 10 leading causes of death for all ages, as a percent of all deaths, United States, 1900 and 1990.

Source: National Center for Health Statistics, Centers for Disease Control and Prevention, U.S. Department of Health and Human Services.

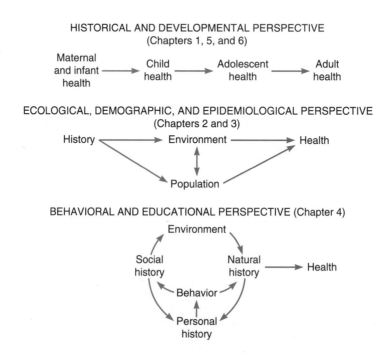

FIGURE 7-4

The main features of the several perspectives from previous chapters are summarized.

Behavioral and Educational Perspectives

From the behavioral and educational perspectives, adult health develops out of the cumulative historical, demographic, and epidemiological forces just described, combined with the attitudes, values, beliefs, and behavior of individuals, as described in Chapter 4. These individual, cultural, and sociopsychological factors make up the personal history that each person brings to bear on the natural history of health, the social history of health, and the environment, as reflected in Figure 7-4.

The Life Span Perspective

One approach to the analysis of adult health relative to that of other age groups, combining the developmental, epidemiological, and behavioral perspectives, is to use transitions in the life span. Recall the epidemiological concepts of host, agent, and environment discussed in Chapter 3.

Host resistance. The ideal intervention in community health is one that anticipates potential problems or requirements for the health of populations and prepares the ''host'' population to resist the problem or to provide for the need. If the environment can be structured to preclude the need for any action on the part of the host, so much the better. If the agent can be isolated and neutralized, better yet.

Unfortunately, the agents of the new leading causes of morbidity and death are pervasive and are tightly woven parts of the fabric of modern living, such as rich foods, alcohol, drugs, sedentary work and leisure, stress, guns, and automobiles and other machinery. Few societies or communities have been willing to turn back the clock on such agents. Although some can be controlled through environmental regulation of their distribution, pricing, taxation, and public use, most of these agents are used privately. There is little choice, then, but to supplement organizational, economic, and environmental strategies with educational interventions that build host resistance.

Life span risks. No variable relates more consistently to mortality and morbidity than age. Age is such a powerful correlate of mortality and morbidity that crude death rates and cause-specific incidence and prevalence rates are difficult to use for comparative purposes without adjustment for age, as we have seen in Chapter 3. Because age is so consistently associated with morbidity and mortality, it serves as a convenient marker for program planning. A community can set its priorities for intervention on the problems of specific subpopulations defined by age. The four leading causes of death, for example, can be seen in Table 7-1 as quite distinct for each of six major age groups.

TABLE 7-1
The four leading causes of death are notably different for each of the six age groups used in the federal disease prevention and health promotion initiative in the United States.

Rank	Infants	1-14	15-24	25-44	45-64	65+
1	Prematurity	Unintentional injuries	Unintentional injuries	Unintentional injuries	Cancer	Heart disease
2	Birth-related	Cancer	Homicide	Cancer	Heart disease	Cancer
3	Congenital defects	Congenital anomalies	Suicide	HIV infection	Stroke	Stroke
4	Sudden infant death	Homicide	Cancer	Heart disease	Injuries	Chronic obstructive pulmonary disease

PRINCIPAL CAUSES OF ADULT DEATHS

The leading causes of death for adults age 25 to 64, shown in Figure 7-1, reflect the long-term decline in this age group's death rate, which continued through the past decade. Between 1980 and 1990 a 20% decline achieved the 1990 goal of 400 deaths per 100,000 population. The three leading causes of death—cancer, heart disease, and injuries—account for about 62% of all deaths in this age group. While rates for leading causes of death continued to decline in 1990, deaths from HIV infection, homicide, and diabetes increased. Over 90% of all HIV deaths occurred in this age group.

The current list of leading causes of death contrasts with the causes of death prevailing in 1900, when tuberculosis ranked first, followed by pneumonia and gastroenteritis. The leading cause of death in all age groups in 1900 does not even appear on the 1990 list (see Figure 7-3). Today many of the leading causes of death in this age group are associated with risk factors related to life-style. It is estimated that 30% of all cancers are associated with smoking and that 35% may be linked to poor eating habits.

As significant as the decline in the general death rate for adults has been, of more immediate interest and value to community health is to consider the trends in principal causes of death projected from the present time into the future. Such an analysis will help identify the particular health problems to be anticipated in the adult age groups where special emphasis must be placed today if some of these problems are to be prevented.

CANCER

Etiology

Cancer is the leading cause of death in adults aged 25 to 64 years. Cancer is a group of diseases characterized by uncontrolled and disordered growth of abnormal cells. Cancer cells displace or destroy normal cells and, if not stopped, spread to other parts

Objective for Adult Health
• Reduce the death rate for adults by 20% to no more than 340 per 100,000 people aged 25 to 64. Baseline: 423 per 100,000 in 1987.

of the body. Thus cancer has two hallmarks: reproduction and invasion. The reproduction of cells is, of course, a normal biological function in growth and repair of tissues. Cancer cells, however, have a higher rate of cell growth than the normal tissues from which they are derived.

Cancer cells invade by three main mechanisms. The first is by direct spread or extension, growing into surrounding tissues and failing to respect the boundaries from which they are derived. Cancer cells may also invade lymph channels and be carried to distant parts of the body. The lymph channels meet at points where there are lymph nodes; there the cancer cells may enlarge and grow.

The cancer cells may also be carried directly into the bloodstream, which enables them to reach distant parts of the body where they grow, attempting to reproduce the tissue of their origin. This new or secondary tumor is called a **metastasis.** The original tumor may be silent—that is, without symptoms such as pain or bleeding—early in its life, and it may spread quickly. These factors make some cancers difficult to treat successfully and thus emphasize the necessity of early diagnosis, which is the objective of most community cancer control programs.

Risk factors. Risk factors for cancer include a familial tendency for the development of cancer, especially of breast, stomach, and large intestine. It is not known to what extent this is truly a genetic factor or to what extent it is caused by environmental factors such as diet, life-style, or occupation that may remain similar from one generation to the next.

Repeated infections, particularly viral, are associated with cancer of the cervix. Radiation stemming from industrial and medical uses of x-rays and radioactive devices may also cause cancer. Older radiologists have been shown to have an excessive mortality from leukemia. Uranium mine workers have been found to develop lung cancer at higher rates than does the general population. The atomic bomb survivors in Japan have experienced an excessive mortality from leukemia.

The risk factor most clearly related to development of cancer is cigarette smoking. Smokers have higher rates of cancer for all the tissues that are exposed to the **carcinogens** in tobacco smoke. These tissues include the larynx, oral cavity, esophagus, lung, and urinary bladder. The impact of cigarette smoking is very large, both because of the prevalence of the habit (about 29% of adults in Canada and 25% in the United States are smokers) and because of the high relative risk of lung cancer that accompanies cigarette smoking.

Specific occupational hazards, such as exposure to asbestos, result in higher cancer rates. The contribution of air pollution is difficult to evaluate because of the long latent period for many cancers (20 to 40 years) between exposure and diagnosis of the cancer, combined with the confounding effect of cigarette smoking.

Social and Epidemiological Diagnosis

Cancer is found in all races and ages of human beings and in all other animal species. Cancer is predominantly a disease of middle and old age; it is not common in children and young adults. Persons age 70 and over account for a higher number of cases than any other age group. The risk of developing cancer increases with age. The death rate for males exceeds that for females; the rate for blacks exceeds that for whites. At present the chance of a person who is less than 20 years old developing cancer sometime during his or her lifetime is about one in four for males and slightly higher for females.

The most common sites for cancer vary by sex. For females the most common sites in 1993 are breast (32%), colon and rectum (13%), and lung (12%). For males, the most common sites are prostate (28%), lung (17%), and colon and rectum (13%). The death rates for different sites vary slightly from incidence rates for most sites, but are significantly higher for lung cancer as a proportion of all cancer deaths.

Trends

In 1990 cancer accounted for 23.4% of all deaths, varying with gender, age, and race. This is an increase from 1970, when cancer accounted for 17.2% of all deaths. Overall, cancer mortality rates have not changed much since 1950, although some changes have occurred in rates of certain cancers. Some of the most prevalent forms of cancer can either be prevented or diagnosed early enough to prevent their spread.

Since 1930 cancer incidence has increased most rapidly for lung cancer for both sexes (Figure 7-5). Both males and females have had decreases in the incidence of cancer of the stomach. Between 1930 and 1989 there has been no change in breast cancer deaths rates for females. The incidence of breast cancer, however, has increased. Between 1980 and 1987 there was a 32.5% increase in the incidence of breast cancer. The increase is attributed in large part to the increase in use of screening mammography, which detects breast cancer at an earlier stage than it would ordinarily be detected (Figure 7-6). It is thought that once the increase in mammography use stabilizes the incidence rate will stabilize and then decline. This appears to be happening.

Deaths from prostate cancer for men have increased from 1930 through the early 1990s. It is estimated that 25 million men over the age of 50 have histologic evidence of prostate cancer. The majority of these men will never develop symptomatic disease. This means that more men will die *with* prostate cancer than *from* prostate cancer.

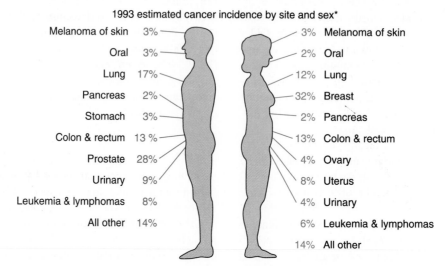

1993 estimated cancer incidence by site and sex*

Melanoma of skin	3%		3%	Melanoma of skin
Oral	3%		2%	Oral
Lung	17%		12%	Lung
Pancreas	2%		32%	Breast
Stomach	3%		2%	Pancreas
Colon & rectum	13 %		13%	Colon & rectum
Prostate	28%		4%	Ovary
Urinary	9%		8%	Uterus
Leukemia & lymphomas	8%		4%	Urinary
All other	14%		6%	Leukemia & lymphomas
			14%	All other

*Excluding basal and squamous cell skin cancers and carcinoma in situ.

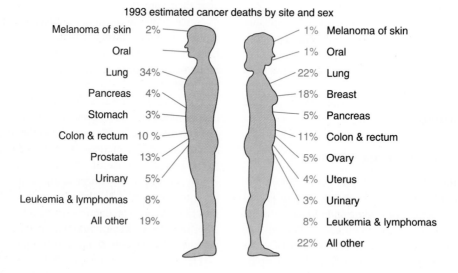

1993 estimated cancer deaths by site and sex

Melanoma of skin	2%		1%	Melanoma of skin
Oral			1%	Oral
Lung	34%		22%	Lung
Pancreas	4%		18%	Breast
Stomach	3%		5%	Pancreas
Colon & rectum	10 %		11%	Colon & rectum
Prostate	13%		5%	Ovary
Urinary	5%		4%	Uterus
Leukemia & lymphomas	8%		3%	Urinary
All other	19%		8%	Leukemia & lymphomas
			22%	All other

FIGURE 7-5
Relative incidence of cancer and proportion of all cancer deaths attributable to each site of cancer for men and women, United States, 1993.

Source: National Cancer Institute and American Cancer Society. From *CA Cancer J Clin* 43:9, 1993.

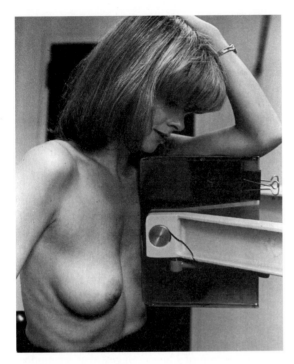

FIGURE 7-6
The mammogram compresses one breast at a time for better radiographic resolution of small lumps that would not be detected by physical breast examination (palpation).
Photo courtesy American Cancer Society.

Objective for Lung Cancer

- By 2000 slow the rise in lung cancer deaths to achieve a rate of no more than 42 per 100,000 people. Age-adjusted baseline: 37.9 per 100,000 in 1987.

Lung cancer rates in most countries have increased dramatically in both sexes. In 1930 the lung cancer death rate for females was approximately 3 per 100,000; by 1989 it rose to 31. For males in 1930 lung cancer deaths were approximately 5 per 100,000; by 1989 the rate soared to 73! In the late 1980s the lung cancer death rate for men was be-

ginning to decline, but the rate for females continues on an upward curve. Even though current smoking rates have dropped, lung cancer death rates reflect higher smoking rates in previous decades. Much of the debt for increased smoking among females since World War II is yet to be paid. Men who were smoking more than women earlier in this century have already paid the heavy price.

Early Detection of Cancer

The most promising method of early detection is screening people who have no symptoms but who, by reason of their age, sex, occupation, ethnicity, or life-style, may be in a high-risk group. The validity of screening methods varies.

Cervical cancer. The Papanicolaou (Pap) smear is an effective screening for cancer of the cervix, the entrance to the female uterus. This exam is both sensitive and specific in detecting precancerous changes in the cervix. The test is reliable and painless and as a result has achieved wide use among health providers and patients. The 5-year survival rate for the earliest, precancerous stage of cervical cancer is 100%. Virtually all women can be saved if the diagnosis is made at this early stage. The community problem is that certain groups of women, including the old, less educated, and low-income, do not seek out the screening test. Community efforts need to

---

Objectives for Pap Smear Screening

- By the year 2000 increase to at least 95% the proportion of women age 18 and older who have ever received a Pap test. Baseline: 88% had the test in 1987.
- By the year 2000 increase to at least 85% the proportion of women age 18 and older who received a Pap test within the preceding 1 to 3 years. Baseline: 75% ''within the preceding 3 years'' in 1987.

be directed toward identifying these women and encouraging them to avail themselves of this preventive procedure.

Breast cancer. Methods of detecting breast cancer include breast self-examination, screening at physicals, and mammography. Monthly breast self-examination should be encouraged in all women. The method is simple to learn and can be taught by demonstrations, films, television programs, and printed material. Fear of finding a "lump" and lack of experience with the technique are barriers to self-examination that health education can address. For some women, partner examinations may be preferable, if the partner is properly trained in the technique. Breast examinations are routinely done by many physicians during clinic visits for Pap smears.

Mammography is an x-ray examination of the soft tissues of the breast to detect cancer in its early stages (Figure 7-6). This test holds great promise of identifying early tumors that are too small or inaccessible to palpate. The recommended frequency of mammography screening varies with risk factors, which include age, previous other cancer, close relative with breast cancer, first menstrual period at age 10 or earlier, no pregnancies, first live birth at age 30 or older, and previous benign breast disease. The U.S. Preventive Services Task Force recommends that women have mammography every 1 to 2 years beginning at age 50, or for women at increased risk beginning at age 35.

Prostate cancer. With the incidence of prostate cancer now exceeding lung cancer for men, new recommendations have been made for screening. In 1992 the American Cancer Society approved inclusion of early detection procedures for prostate cancer in its "Guidelines for Cancer-Related Checkup." The recommended test measures prostate-specific antigen (PSA). When found and treated early, prostate cancer can be cured. Health education

efforts can make men at risk aware of this screening and its importance.

Lung cancer. The gloomy outlook in lung cancer is slowly improving. Although we can identify persons of high-risk—namely, men and women over 45 years of age who smoke more than one pack of cigarettes daily—it is still difficult to detect lung cancer early. This is because changes detectable by x-ray film occur late, and lung cancer cells are difficult to produce and interpret microscopically. Not all tumors exfoliate cells that may be coughed up and recognized as cancer cells under the microscope.

Colorectal cancer. Colon and rectal cancers may be detected by the presence of blood in the stools. Sigmoidoscopy (an exam that allows direct vision of the lower bowel) and x-ray examination of the lower bowel are indicated if blood is present. The American Cancer Society Recommendations for the Early Detection of Cancer suggest that sigmoidoscopy be done every 3 to 5 years in males or females over 50 on the advice of their physician (Figure 7-7). Stool sample tests are recommended annually for this group. Digital rectal examinations are recommended annually for males and females over 40 years of age.

Treatment and Survival of Cancer Patients

Cancer may be treated by surgery, irradiation, and drugs. Surgery may range from simple local excision of the tumor, the surrounding tissues, and the lymph nodes, so that the whole tumor area is removed. This may require diversion of the urinary or alimentary tract. Irradiation may precede or follow surgery and may be applied by different emitters. Drug therapy may involve altering hormonal status if the tumor is hormone-dependent; other chemotherapy involves use of cytotoxic and antimetabolite drugs. The type of treatment used depends on many

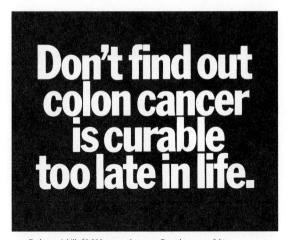

Don't find out colon cancer is curable too late in life.

Each year it kills 60,000 men and women. But what most of them really die of is procrastination. Because colon cancer is 90% curable if caught in its earliest stages.

If you're over 40, you're at risk. See your doctor and request a colorectal cancer checkup. Do it now.

We know it's not the first thing on your mind. We just don't want it to be the last.

Learn more. Call the American Cancer Society at 1-800-ACS-2345.

 AMERICAN CANCER SOCIETY®

FIGURE 7-7
Colon cancer, like most other cancers, is much more curable if detected and treated early. Hence national and community organizations devote considerable health education resources to informing the public about the need for screening.

Source: Courtesy American Cancer Society and Advertising Council.

factors, such as the organ of origin of the tumor, the extent of invasion, the microscopic appearance, and the age and general health of the patient. Often a combination of two or more cancer treatment methods is used, and a second or third course of treatment is often applied.

The dominant factor in the prognosis for cancer patients is the stage at which treatment is first begun. The outlook is markedly improved if the cancer is treated when it is still localized, rather than spread to the neighboring lymph glands or to distant organs of the body.

The 5-year survival rate is an important measure of the success of cancer treatment. The rate varies with the type of cancer, sex, and race. The overall 5-year survival rate between 1983 and 1989 for white women is 57%, for white men it is 48%, for black women 44%, and for black men 33%. Cancers with the highest 5-year survival rate for men are urinary bladder and prostate cancers; for women, melanoma of the skin and uterine cancer. The cancer with the lowest survival rate for both sexes is pancreatic cancer.

Cancer Research

Cancer research has the following three thrusts: (1) to discover the causes of the cancer so that preventive measures may be taken, (2) to pioneer new screening and education programs for early detection and for reducing exposure to cigarettes and other risk factors, and (3) to improve results of treatment for persons with cancer. The public should not be persuaded to believe that if sufficient money is spent, the threat of cancer will be removed. The unfortunate fact is that, in cancers in which the cause has been discovered, the number of cases has actually increased. Lung cancer is the classic example. The cause is clearly identified as cigarette smoking, but prevention involves altering behavior, which is difficult to achieve. Many cancers may be prevented by the modification of life-style to avoid known hazardous customs and by the use of early detection methods already available. The community effort must be directed toward making people aware of this, rather than making them dependent on research results or cures at some future date.

CARDIOVASCULAR DISEASE
Etiology

Multiple terms are used to refer to disorders of the heart and circulatory system. **Cardiovascular disease** (''cardio'' means heart, ''vascular'' means blood vessels) is a broad term that includes heart disease, hypertension or high blood pressure, atherosclerosis, stroke, rheumatic heart disease, and other disorders.

A normal heart is a strong, muscular pump that beats on the average 100,000 times each day and pumps close to 2000 gallons of blood. The normal function of the heart muscle depends on an adequate blood supply. Heart disease is a general, vague term that covers all ailments of the heart, from heart attacks to congenital defects. **Coronary artery disease** refers to the conditions that cause narrowing of the coronary arteries so that blood supply to the heart is reduced. This narrowing occurs when fatty substances, cholesterol, cellular waste products, calcium, and fibrin are deposited on the inner lining of the artery. This build-up is known as plaque. **Atherosclerosis** is a type of thickening or hardening of arteries (''athero'' means gruel or paste, ''sclerosis'' means hardening), in which the blood vessels supplying the heart are less elastic and narrower. As a result of this condition the heart receives an insufficient amount of blood to carry out its function. Damage to the heart muscle caused by insufficient blood supply from obstructed coronary arteries is called **coronary heart disease.** Permanent damage to, or death of, the heart muscle is called a **heart attack** or myocardial infarction. When there is an insufficient supply of blood to the brain, a **stroke** can result.

Trends

Cardiovascular disease—in particular, coronary heart disease and stroke—is the main cause of death for all age groups in industrialized countries and is rising at an alarming rate in much of the developing world. For 25- to 64-year-olds, heart disease is the second leading cause of death. Approximately 7 million Americans are affected by coronary heart disease, 500,000 die annually, and costs to the nation are approximately $43 billion per year in direct and indirect costs. Between 400,000 and 500,000 Americans suffer nonfatal strokes each year. Although deaths from strokes have decreased by 57% since 1972 (Figure 7-8), it remains the sixth

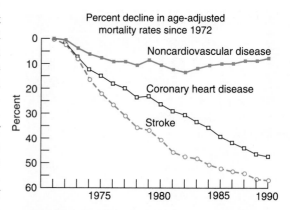

FIGURE 7-8

Reductions in U.S. cardiovascular diseases since 1972 have been five to six times greater than in noncardiovascular diseases. This has been attributed variously to less animal fat in the American diet, better health habits, better control of blood pressure, and better emergency response to heart attacks.

Source: National Center for Health Statistics, Centers for Disease Control and Prevention, U.S. Department of Health and Human Services.

leading cause of death among 25- to 64-year-olds.

Dramatic reductions in mortality from cardiovascular disease have been achieved in recent decades. For example, in the United States coronary heart disease now claims 47% fewer lives than in 1972, stroke 57% fewer lives, and all cardiovascular diseases 35% fewer lives. Similar reductions occurred in Canada and Australia. Trends in cardiovascular disease are reversed in some industrialized countries and in much of the less industrialized world. In some Central and Eastern European countries there have been sharp increases (30% to 80%) over the last 20 years.

Despite the overall decline, deaths from coronary heart disease are higher among men than among women, and are higher among blacks than among whites. Black Americans have nearly twice as many strokes, 10 to 18 times more kidney failure, and 3 to 5 times more heart failure related to high blood pressure.

Social and Epidemiological Diagnosis

Changes in life-style and risk factor reduction were major contributors in the North American declines. Community action in reducing deaths from heart disease and stroke has a long history, during which the role of prevention has continually increased in emphasis compared with that of treatment. Major epidemiological studies conducted in the 1950s and 1960s provided the evidence for defining the risk factors associated with heart disease and stroke and for developing intervention strategies to reduce morbidity.

A **risk factor** is a habit, trait, or condition in a person that is associated with an increased chance (or risk) of developing a disease. Risk factors for cardiovascular diseases can be divided into two types: nonmodifiable and modifiable. Nonmodifiable factors are those that cannot be changed through prevention measures, including age, sex, family history, and personality type. Modifiable factors are those that are amenable to prevention measures and include high blood pressure, high blood cholesterol, overweight, cigarette smoking, and physical inactivity.

The government has addressed these risk factors with various programs in recent decades. The smoking risk factor is one example. In 1964 the U.S. Surgeon General's report on smoking and health was a bold step to address this major contributor to both heart disease and cancer. Efforts by communities to reduce smoking and the risks from smoking continue to expand and have produced positive results. Diet and obesity represent another risk area in which governments continue to promote research and education. Risks due to high blood pressure have received considerable attention and are addressed later in this chapter. Through promoting the positive effects of physical fitness government programs have addressed the problems of inactivity. These efforts have had some impact. A recent national survey, for example, indicated that one third of adult Americans exercised regularly, and that the percentage of persons who do not smoke has increased from 57% in 1974 to 75% in 1991.

Coronary Heart Disease

Over half of cardiovascular deaths are attributed to coronary heart disease. This disease causes reduced blood flow to the heart and results in damage to the heart muscle. A heart attack occurs when the damage to the heart muscle is permanent and may result in death. Nearly a quarter of all heart attacks result in sudden death (within 2 hours). Two thirds of all heart attack victims survive their first attack, but most of the fatalities occur before the patient can reach the hospital. This proportion is declining as communities train more people in cardiopulmonary resuscitation (CPR) and improve their emergency procedures. More than 15 million people in the United States have been trained in CPR procedures. Research, testing, and evaluation of CPR indicates that if performed properly and early enough, as many as 120,000 lives can be saved each year.

The progress in reducing coronary heart disease has been greatest in some of the countries that had (and still have) relatively high rates, with the exception of Japan. Japan has both a low rate (the lowest of any developed country) and a declining rate (third fastest improvement after the United States and Australia). Figure 7-9 compares selected countries on ischemic heart disease (the major component of coronary heart disease) deaths and stroke deaths for males and females.

Nonmodifiable risk factors. Nonmodifiable risk factors for coronary heart disease include age, sex, family history, and personality type.

1. Age. The incidence rates for heart attacks rise steeply from age 35 to 55 years and then fall as those susceptible to the disease are eliminated.
2. Sex. Males below 50 years of age are afflicted by coronary heart deaths in a ratio of 4:1 com-

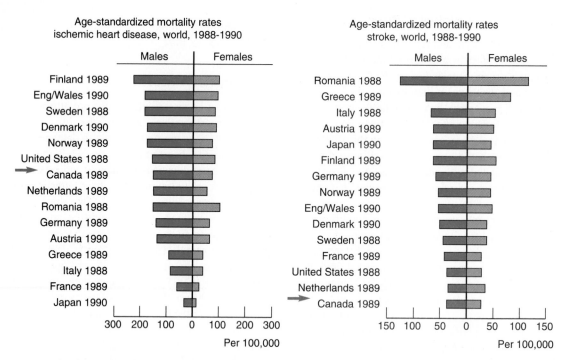

FIGURE 7-9
Comparisons of major components of cardiovascular death rates among selected countries. Note the reversed positions of Japan, the United States, and Canada.
Source: Canadian Centre for Health Information, Statistics Canada.

pared to females. After 50 years of age, the preponderance of male victims is markedly reduced but still persists. This suggests some hormonal factor in the cause.

3. Family history. There is a strong familial tendency toward coronary heart disease, particularly on the male side. Families share many habits and customs of exercise, diet, and lifestyle; thus this familial predisposition reflects a combination of genetic and environmental causes.

4. Personality type. This is included as a nonmodifiable risk factor, for it has not been proved that it can be changed. People with a striving, time-conscious behavior pattern are identified as having a type A personality.

They are involved in a chronic struggle against time or other people. There is no limit to the number of events these persons squeeze into a day. They have an intrinsic drive toward some goal, and the achievement of this goal is opposed by time, persons, and things. Consequently, persons with type A personality often suffer frustration, are constantly in a hurry, and have free-floating hostility. Type A personalities with hostility suffer higher rates of heart attack than those persons with the converse, type B, or type A without hostility.

Modifiable risk factors. The four main modifiable risk factors for coronary heart disease are high blood cholesterol high blood pressure, cigarette smoking, and physical inactivity. Any one of these risk factors increases an individual's chance of developing heart disease, and all four together may greatly increase heart disease risk, perhaps by ten times or more. Obesity and diabetes are other risk factors. High blood cholesterol and high blood pressure are discussed here. Other factors are discussed in more depth later in this chapter, or in subsequent chapters.

High blood cholesterol. It has been estimated that a 1% drop in a population's cholesterol level will result in a 2% to 3% drop in heart disease.

Pure cholesterol is an odorless, white, waxy, powdery substance. You cannot taste it or see it in the foods you eat. It is found in all foods of animal origin. To carry cholesterol through the blood, the body wraps it in protein packages. This combination is called a "lipoprotein." Cholesterol is found in all the major lipoproteins, including the low-density lipoproteins (LDLs)—the "bad" cholesterol—and the high-density lipoproteins (HDLs)—the "good" cholesterol. High LDL levels promote the deposit of cholesterol on artery walls; HDL is thought to carry cholesterol away from the arteries to the liver for excretion.

The cholesterol level is determined by a blood test. In adults a total blood cholesterol level of about 240 mg/dl warrants medical attention. Levels above 200 mg/dl also increase the risk of heart disease and may require further evaluation. It is recommended that all adults age 20 and over have their blood cholesterol measured at least once every 5 years. Community screening programs have contributed to an increased number of adults being aware of their cholesterol level (Figure 7-10).

Individuals who exercise regularly, don't smoke, and maintain a desirable weight are more likely to have higher HDL levels. Nations whose citizens have high serum cholesterol levels, chiefly the westernized countries, have heart attack rates much higher than countries such as Japan that are also highly developed but whose people have low cholesterol levels. Cholesterol levels are closely related

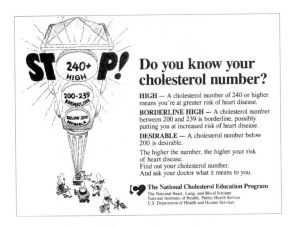

Do you know your cholesterol number?

HIGH — A cholesterol number of 240 or higher means you're at greater risk of heart disease.

BORDERLINE HIGH — A cholesterol number between 200 and 239 is borderline, possibly putting you at increased risk of heart disease.

DESIRABLE — A cholesterol number below 200 is desirable.

The higher the number, the higher your risk of heart disease.
Find out your cholesterol number.
And ask your doctor what it means to you.

The National Cholesterol Education Program
The National Heart, Lung, and Blood Institute
National Institutes of Health, Public Health Service
U.S. Department of Health and Human Services

FIGURE 7-10
Community campaigns to control serum cholesterol levels have emphasized screening to make people aware of their readings.
Source: National Heart, Lung, and Blood Institute, National Institutes of Health, Public Health Service, U.S. Department of Health and Human Services.

to the percentage of saturated animal fats in the diet. Alteration of the national diet is the most promising avenue to reduction of coronary mortality, as well as other chronic diseases (Figure 7-11).

Hypertension. Blood pressure is the force exerted by the blood against artery walls. The heart creates this pressure as it pumps blood. The higher the resistance by the arteries to the pumping, as occurs with atherosclerosis, the greater the pressure required from the heart to pump the blood. Elevated pressure means the heart is working harder than normal and the arteries are under greater strain. This may contribute to heart attacks, strokes, kidney disease, and atherosclerosis.

Chronic high blood pressure or **hypertension** is widely prevalent in the United States. More than 60 million Americans have blood pressure readings of 140/90 mm Hg or higher. Black Americans have almost a 33% greater chance of having high blood pressure than whites. It has been estimated that hypertension costs the nation more than $8 billion per year in medical care costs, lost productivity, and lost wages. Furthermore, hypertension has been found

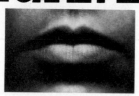

COLON CANCER, BREAST CANCER AND HEART DISEASE CAN ALL START IN THE SAME PLACE.

Too many people get into trouble because they open their mouths without thinking. Unfortunately, the diet that most Americans eat may contain enough fat to increase the risk of certain cancers as well as heart disease.

But you can help reduce your risk by eating a low-fat diet containing lots of fruits, vegetables, whole grain foods, lean meats, fish, poultry and low-fat dairy products. For a free booklet on low-fat eating, call 1-800-EAT-LEAN.

Remember, your brain is only a few inches from your mouth. When you eat, we suggest you use it.

1-800-EAT-LEAN

 A public service message from The Henry J. Kaiser Family Foundation

FIGURE 7-11
Diet, especially the consumption of fat, accounts for the largest part of the deaths from both cancer and heart disease, the two leading causes of death in more industrialized countries. Community campaigns directed at this one risk factor can cut across several diseases.

Source: Henry J. Kaiser Family Foundation and Advertising Council.

to be highly correlated with reduced life expectancy: the higher the blood pressure, the shorter the life (Figure 7-12).

The natural course of hypertension spans some 15 to 20 years, starting on the average around age 35 often ending in premature death around age 50. High blood pressure is often called the "silent killer" because 75% of those who have the condition are without symptoms. When symptoms do occur they are manifested by damage to the heart, brain, kidney, and eye. Hypertension is the single

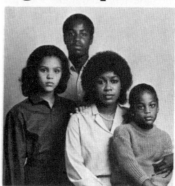

My husband took good care of us. If only he'd taken care of his high blood pressure.

Looking back at it all, it just doesn't make any sense. We have everything we need except a husband and a father.

If you have high blood pressure, take your pills, watch your weight and the salt. And if you think that is too much trouble... well...you just don't know about the trouble you could be leaving behind.

HIGH BLOOD PRESSURE
Treat it for life.

The National High Blood Pressure Education Program
The National Heart, Lung, and Blood Institute, National Institutes of Health
Public Health Service, U.S. Department of Health and Human Services

FIGURE 7-12
Community high blood pressure control programs use public service materials from the National High Blood Pressure Education Program or similar national programs in other countries. Success of this program is credited with part of the remarkable reduction of strokes and other cardiovascular diseases in the United States.

Source: National Heart, Lung and Blood Institute, National Institutes of Health, Public Health Service, U.S. Department of Health and Human Services.

most important risk factor for strokes and heart disease.

The cause of hypertension is unknown in 90% of cases. There is often a family history of hypertension, and relatives of hypertensive persons have been shown to be more likely to be hypertensive (especially children of two hypertensive parents). Obesity and salt consumption are correlated with hypertension, and both of these factors are modifiable. The use of oral contraceptives may increase blood pressure also. Smoking and high blood cholesterol are not associated with development of hypertension, but contribute to a poor prognosis for those who have hypertension. A great advance has been made in the treatment of hypertension with the introduction of effective drug therapy and advances in diet, relaxation, and exercise therapy.

Example of a national program. Federally funded studies in the United States in the late 1960s and early 1970s clearly demonstrated that high blood pressure could be controlled and that reduced disease and death for middle-aged males would result. However, the national health examination surveys indicated that for about 85% of hypertensive individuals, the high blood pressure was either undetected, untreated, or uncontrolled. A national high blood pressure education program and a large-scale study were recommended to provide experience and data on the effectiveness of antihypertensive therapy for both sexes, all races, and both young and middle-aged adults. The results of this campaign and the large-scale study clearly indicated that systematic, effective management of high blood pressure, especially when combined with effective public and patient education, can reduce the death rate for both those with severe and those with mild hypertension.

The National High Blood Pressure Education Program, in participation with government agencies, private industry, voluntary health associations, and professional groups, was effective in decreasing the proportion of undetected cases of high blood pressure. Further, the proportion of those under treatment whose blood pressure is controlled has also increased. The reductions in deaths from heart disease and stroke can at least partially be attributed to the success of the effort to control high blood pressure.

Medical evidence refutes the reliability of self-perceived symptoms for high blood pressure, but many persons continue to believe that they can de-

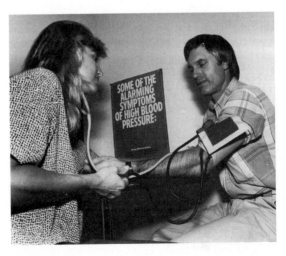

FIGURE 7-13
Blood pressure measures are essential in part because the person cannot rely on any other symptom of high blood pressure, as the poster in the background of this clinical scene implies with the blank space following the colon.
Source: Photo by Marsha Burkes, courtesy University of Texas Health Science Center at Houston.

tect their own symptoms of hypertension (Figure 7-13).

Hypertension lends itself well to community control, because community surveys can be performed to identify people who have high blood pressure and do not know it. People can visit centers in their community and have their blood pressure recorded, after which they can be referred for treatment if needed. (There are some 2000 locally organized hypertension programs in the United States.) Once the cases are identified, the problem then lies in patient education to effect compliance in taking the drugs to maintain normal levels of pressure. The increase in the number of hypertensive persons who have been brought under control because of efficient drug therapy has resulted in reduced mortality and morbidity. This reduction is reflected in a decrease in the number of heart attacks in which hypertension was a factor and also, more importantly, in a decrease in the number of cerebrovascular accidents, or strokes.

Interaction of risk factors. Risk factors for coronary heart disease, including high blood pressure and high blood cholesterol, interact with each other. Stress has been named as another possible risk factor. Stress is difficult to measure either as a source or as a result of emotional tension. Nevertheless, a period of severe stress or excessive fatigue is identified as having preceded a heart attack in many cases. In those who practice regular exercise the outcome of a heart attack is more favorable than in those who do not. The benefits of regular exercise are many and may include reductions in other risk factors such as high blood pressure, cholesterol, and stress, as well as more direct effects on reduced rate of heart attack. Obesity is associated with increased frequency of heart attacks, particularly in the markedly obese. The difficulty is that such patients are frequently hypertensive, of sedentary habit, or diabetic, and it is difficult to identify which risk factor is operative.

In summary, coronary heart disease is multifactoral in origin and is highly preventable. Atherosclerosis and elevated cholesterol levels are usually present, sometimes accompanied by other risk factors.

STROKE

The sixth leading cause of death in the 25- to 64-year-old age group is stroke. A stroke occurs when the blood supply to the brain is interrupted, either gradually or abruptly. An artery of the brain may rupture, usually one with preexisting damage, as the result of atherosclerosis. This is particularly likely if the patient has high blood pressure; the weakened vessel is inadequate to withstand the higher pressure. Such *hemorrhagic* strokes have a high fatality rate and are usually found among older people. Disruption of the blood supply may also result when a blood clot forms in the artery either from atheroma or from a clot formed elsewhere, such as in a damaged valve in the heart itself. The clot blocks the cerebral artery and deprives the brain tissue of oxygen. This type of stroke, termed *embolic,* occurs in younger patients and has a lower fatality rate. Many people recover from the initial stroke, but they are often left with some residual disability. Despite the devoted efforts of therapists and the perseverance of patients, complete recovery after stroke is uncommon. Particularly in older people stroke is a major source of disability. The hope lies in prevention, chiefly by controlling hypertension and preventing atherosclerosis.

LIVER DISEASE

The eighth leading cause of death for 25- to 64-year-olds is liver disease, the most common of which is cirrhosis of the liver. Cirrhosis is a chronic disease that results in slow deterioration of the liver so that it is progressively less able to carry out its functions. The most common cause of this disease in North America is alcohol abuse. Death from cirrhosis declined during the Prohibition Era when alcohol was illegal. Following Prohibition death rates from cirrhosis increased until 1973, when they again began to decline steadily with reductions in alcohol consumption. Community programs to reduce cirrhosis need to focus on efforts to reduce heavy drinking patterns, especially in high-risk subpopulations. Current death rates for nonwhites remain almost 70% higher than rates for whites; the rates for Native American men are triple those of white men. These disparities may represent differential access to health care, differential drinking patterns, or some combination of these and other factors.

CHRONIC LUNG DISEASE

Chronic obstructive pulmonary disease (COPD), which is characterized by permanent airflow obstruction to the lungs, is the ninth leading cause of death for 25- to 64-year-olds. Nearly 80,000 people die each year from this condition. Cigarette smoking accounts for 82% of those deaths. The death rate

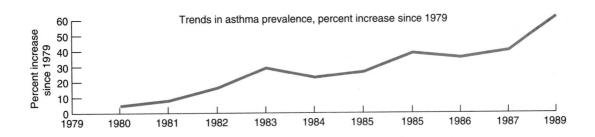

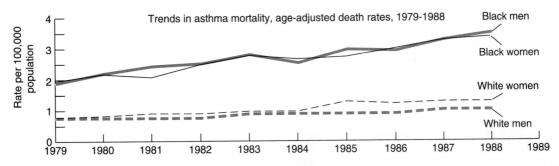

Source: National Health Interview Survey, National Center for Health Statistics

FIGURE 7-14

One of the few chronic diseases that has steadily increased in prevalence and in death rates for the adult population since 1979 is asthma. The 1992 provisional rate indicates a continuing rise to 1.9 deaths per 100,000 for the U.S. population (black and white combined).

Source: National Health Interview Survey, National Center for Health Statistics, Centers for Disease Control and Prevention, U.S. Department of Health and Human Services.

from this disease parallels that of lung cancer. Death from this disease often comes after an extended period of disability and many of those disabled by lung disease die from other causes. Community programs to reduce smoking rates will benefit reduction of this disease. With cessation of smoking, the rate of functional loss declines, but lost lung function cannot be regained. Timely smoking cessation can prevent the development of symptomatic disease.

Asthma is one chronic lung disease that has increased in prevalence and in mortality rates in recent years, especially in the black population in the United States (Figure 7-14). The cause of this increase is unknown, but poor living conditions and air pollution are suspected.

DIABETES

Diabetes is a vascular disease as well as a metabolic disorder. It is characterized by high blood glucose levels caused by a deficiency in insulin production, an impairment of insulin action, or both. Approximately 7 million people in the United States have been diagnosed with diabetes, and an additional 5 million may unknowingly have the disease. In 1990 diabetes was the tenth leading cause of death for 25- to 64-year-olds. A conservative estimate of direct medical costs and lost productivity costs for diabetes is over $20 billion annually.

The morbidity of diabetes is caused by its vascular complications. Coronary heart disease rates are increased by diabetes. Specific preventable complications of diabetes include renal disease; diabetic retinopathy and blindness if the retinal arteries are involved (Figure 7-15); amputations necessitated when blood supply to the limbs is decreased, usually in the foot and calf, with resulting gangrene; and perinatal morbidity and mortality due to diabetes in birth mothers. Because of the role health education can play in these complications, one U.S. objective for the nation is to increase to 75% by the year 2000 the number and percentage of people with diabetes who have received formal patient education about their disease, and resources to assist in the management of it.

High-risk populations for diabetes include blacks, Hispanics, Native Americans, obese people, people with a family history of diabetes, and women

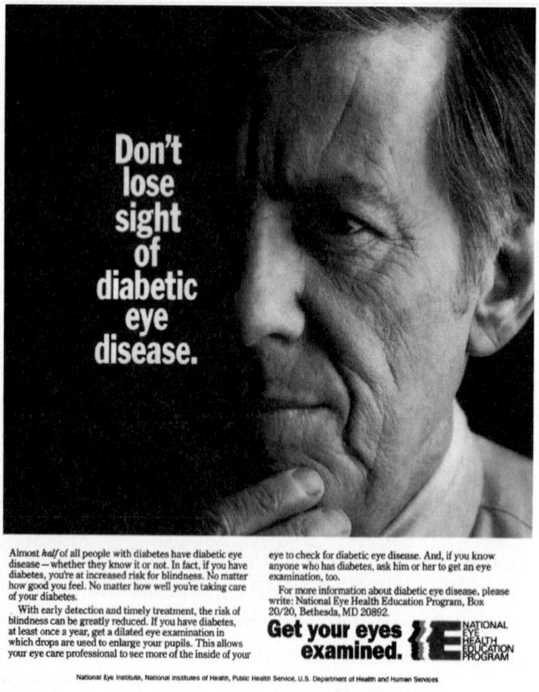

Don't lose sight of diabetic eye disease.

Almost *half* of all people with diabetes have diabetic eye disease—whether they know it or not. In fact, if you have diabetes, you're at increased risk for blindness. No matter how good you feel. No matter how well you're taking care of your diabetes.

With early detection and timely treatment, the risk of blindness can be greatly reduced. If you have diabetes, at least once a year, get a dilated eye examination in which drops are used to enlarge your pupils. This allows your eye care professional to see more of the inside of your

eye to check for diabetic eye disease. And, if you know anyone who has diabetes, ask him or her to get an eye examination, too.

For more information about diabetic eye disease, please write: National Eye Health Education Program, Box 20/20, Bethesda, MD 20892.

Get your eyes examined.

NATIONAL EYE HEALTH EDUCATION PROGRAM

National Eye Institute, National Institutes of Health, Public Health Service, U.S. Department of Health and Human Services

FIGURE 7-15
Among the complications of diabetes, retinopathy is the most common. Blindness can be prevented by adequate control of the blood sugar level and self-management of the disease.
Source: National Eye Institute, National Institutes of Health, Public Health Service, U.S. Department of Health and Human Services.

with previous gestational diabetes. The prevalence of diabetes in the U.S. black population is about 50% higher than in non-Hispanic whites, and the occurrence in Hispanics is about double that of non-Hispanic whites.

Half of all diabetic persons may be treated by diet alone—one that is low in calories and fat. The remainder require insulin or oral hypoglycemic drugs. Community efforts are needed, for the prognosis in diabetes is related to the resources of the patients, their families, and the communities in which they live. Diabetics who are old, poor, or live alone tend to do poorly. The duties of the community toward persons with diabetes are similar to those toward persons with hypertension. Screening programs to uncover the disease early, before it is symptomatic, are of prime importance. After those with diabetes are identified, education is needed to ensure adherence to diet and drug regimens and other life-style modifications.

ARTHRITIS

Arthritis and rheumatic diseases are the most common cause of lost work days annually in most developed countries, although the respiratory diseases account for the greatest number of episodes of sickness. It is difficult to determine the prevalence of types of arthritis because of the range of symptoms and the variability of diagnostic standards. If major mobility limitations are used as the determining factor, the prevalence of some arthritic symptoms is 3%. Rheumatoid arthritis is a systemic inflammatory disease with local joint manifestations, in which the small joints of the hands are often affected early. The disease pursues a chronic course marked by relapses and remissions. The sex ratio shows an excess of females, 2.5 to 1.0. Risk factors include lower socioeconomic status, infections, trauma, winter season, and social stress. The age of onset is young, between 20 and 45 years, commonly 30 to 40 years. In contrast, osteoarthritis affects older persons exclusively and occurs in larger, weight-bearing joints such as the hips and knees. Trauma and obesity are antecedent factors. The community role includes employers providing work for those arthritic persons who are able to work, which is a surprisingly high proportion. Transportation services from home to treatment facilities, home visits, and meals on wheels services are all vital to these people.

As with each of the major chronic diseases (heart, cancer, diabetes, and lung diseases), the U.S. Congress has called for the establishment of regional comprehensive arthritis centers with two distinct purposes: (1) to develop and foster new methods for the prompt and effective application of available knowledge and (2) to develop new knowledge to combat arthritis. In response to this mandate the National Institute of Arthritis, Metabolism, and Digestive Diseases has developed a program of multipurpose arthritis centers, each of which engages in research, education, and community demonstration projects.

The Multipurpose Arthritis Centers have a national distribution ranging from Boston to Hawaii. Many of the projects underway in these centers could not have been started without the interaction of individuals brought together under their aegis. Examples of major efforts of the centers include research into the genetic basis of arthritis; new advances in health services research, such as cost effectiveness studies and analysis of disability; comprehensive education of allied health professionals; and research into the best methods of delivering arthritis health care and education to those least able to obtain it, such as the homebound individual and residents of the inner city.

SUMMARY

Besides periodic health assessments and examinations, individual citizens can contribute to their own health through physical activity adapted to their capacity, relaxation, rest, proper nutrition, avoiding tobacco and limiting exposure to other harmful substances, prevention of disease, early treatment of

disease and disability, promotion of life interests, and attainment of emotional stability are all important in the promotion of a high level of health, the extension of the prime of life, and a greater life expectancy. Time, money, and effort must be devoted to health promotion and must be invested by communities and employers as well as by adult individuals for themselves and their families.

The adult health program must concentrate on specific health problems and at the same time must promote general health education and coping skills. It must deal with the present but must project itself into programs anticipating future needs and emerging patterns of risk factors and risk conditions.

QUESTIONS FOR REVIEW

1. How would the conquest of infection affect the incidence of the degenerative diseases?
2. What is meant by a "disease of civilization?"
3. Why is it important that effort be extended toward research in the treatment as well as in the prevention of the degenerative diseases?
4. What indications exist that adults are taking a more objective attitude toward diseases of the circulatory system?
5. Why is the death rate from vascular lesions affecting the central nervous system higher among females than among males, although males have a higher incidence of hypertension?
6. Why does the United States invest more money in cancer research than in research related to circulation?
7. In the United States in 1900, nephritis ranked sixth as a cause of death with a specific rate of 88.6 per 100,000. Now, more than 90 years later, the rate is less than 5.0 per 100,000. To what do you attribute the decline in this cause-specific death rate?
8. How would you design a program for your community to decrease the incidence of cancer of the respiratory tract?
9. Why is it preferable to teach a respect for cancer rather than a fear of cancer?
10. Using only local funds and resources, how would you design a community program for early discovery of

cancer through the regular medical examination of virtually all adults?

11. What additional services and facilities are needed by your community for an adequate cancer control program?

12. How would you design a program intended to discover all cases of diabetes mellitus in your community?

13. What are the services and facilities available in your community for the diagnosis and treatment of arthritis?

14. What additional services and facilities are needed by your community for an adequate adult health program?

READINGS

Goldbloom RB, Lawrence RS, editors: *Preventing disease: beyond the rhetoric*, New York, 1990, Springer-Verlag.

Based on the work of the Canadian Task Force on the Periodic Health Examination and the U.S. Preventive Services Task Force, this book examines how the recommendations of these two groups can be put into practice by the health care systems of the two countries.

Green LW, Kreuter MW: CDC's planned approach to community health as an application of PRECEDE and an inspiration for PROCEED, *J Health Educ* 23:140, 1992.

Describes how the PRECEDE model, introduced in Chapter 3 of this book, was used in the community chronic disease prevention programs sponsored by the U.S. Centers for Disease Control.

Lauzon R: Heart disease prevention. In Health and Welfare Canada, Stephens T, Fowler GD, editors: *Canada's health promotion survey 1990: technical report*, Ottawa, 1993, Minister of Supply and Services Canada.

Reports on the 1990 national survey of Canadians ages 15 and over, their knowledge and perceptions of the causes of heart disease, and health behaviors people had taken to detect or control blood pressure or cholesterol, quit smoking, exercise, modify diet, or maintain weight.

Tomatis L: *Cancer: causes, occurrence and control*, Oxford, 1990, Oxford University Press.

Is cancer preventable? This book presents the available evidence on the subject by describing the occurrence of, and variations in, the different forms of cancer.

BIBLIOGRAPHY

Airhihenbuwa CO: A conceptual model for culturally appropriate health education programs in developing countries, *Int Q Comm Health Educ* 11:53, 1990-91.

Allegrante JP, Kovar PT, MacKenzie CR et al: A walking education program for patients with osteoarthritis of the knee: theory and intervention strategies, *Health Educ Q* 20:63, 1993.

American Heart Association: Statement on exercise—benefits and recommendations for physical activity programs for all Americans, *Circulation* 86:340, 1992.

Battista RN, Williams JL, MacFarlane LA: Determinants of preventive practices in fee-for-service primary care, *Am J Prev Med* 6:6, 1990.

Bertera RL: Planning and implementing health promotion in the workplace: a case study of the Du Pont Company experience, *Health Educ Q* 17:307, 1990.

Bertera RL, Oehl LK, Telepchak JM: Self-help versus group approaches to smoking cessation in the workplace: eighteen-month follow-up and cost analysis, *Am J Health Prom* 4:187, 1990.

Biglan A, Glasgow RE: The social unit: an important facet in the design of cancer control research, *Prev Med* 20:292, 1991.

Braddy BA, Orenstein D, Brownstein JN et al: PATCH: an example of community empowerment for health, *J Health Educ* 23:179, 1992.

Brunk SE, Goeppinger J: Process evaluation: assessing reinvention of community-based interventions, *Eval Health Professions* 13:186, 1990.

Byles JE, Redman S, Hennrikus D et al: Delay in consulting a medical practitioner about rectal bleeding, *J Epidemiol Community Health* 46:241, 1991.

Byrd T: Project Verdad: a community development approach to health, *Hygie: Int J Health Educ* 11:15, 1992.

Canadian Heart Health Survey Research Group: Canadian heart health surveys: a profile of cardiovascular risk, *Can Med Assoc J Suppl*:1969, 1992.

Canadian Task Force on the Periodic Health Examination: Periodic health examination, 1991 update: secondary prevention of prostate cancer, *Can Med Assoc J* 145: 15, 1991.

Costanza ME: Physician compliance with mammography guidelines: barriers and enhancers, *J Am Board Fam Pract* 5:1, 1992.

Dignan MB, Michielutte R, Sharp PC et al: Use of process evaluation to guide health education in Forsyth County project to prevent cervical cancer, *Pub Health Rep* 106:73, 1991.

Farquhar J: Bridging the gap: science and policy in action, Declaration of the Advisory Board, Victoria, 1992, International Heart Health Conference.

Farquhar JW, Fortmann SP, Flora JA et al. Effects of community-wide education on cardiovascular disease risk factors—the Stanford 5-city Project, *JAMA* 264:359, 1990.

Farr LJ, Fisher LJ: ''Bring your body back to life'': the 1990 Western Australian quit campaign, *Health Prom J Austr* 1:6, 1991.

Gottlieb NH, Eriksen MP, Lovato CY et al: Impact of a restrictive work site smoking policy on smoking behavior, attitudes, and norms, *J Occup Med* 32:20, 1990.

Klag MJ, Whelton PK, Coresh J et al: The association of skin color with blood pressure in United States blacks with low socioeconomic status, *JAMA* 265:599, 1991.

Kumanyik S: Behavioral aspects of intervention strategies to reduce dietary sodium, *Hypertension* 17:1190, 1991.

Lawrence RS: The role of physicians in promoting health, *Health Affairs* 9:122, 1990.

Leppik IE: How to get patients with epilepsy to take their medication: the problem of noncompliance, *Postgrad Med* 88:253, 1990.

Love RR, Davis JE: Screening mammography in clinical practice: a complex activity, *Arch Intern Med* 151:19, 1991.

McCoy CB, Nielsen BB, Chitwood DD et al: Increasing the cancer screening of the medically underserved in South Florida, *Cancer* 67:1808, 1991.

McCoy HV, Dodds SE, Nolan C: AIDS intervention design for program evaluation: the Miami Community Outreach Project, *J Drug Issues* 20:223, 1990.

Nutbeam D, Smith C, Catford J: Evaluation in health education: A review of progress, possibilities, and problems, *J Epidemiol Comm Health* 44:83, 1990.

O'Conner A: Women's cancer prevention practices. In Health and Welfare Canada, Stephens T, and Fowler Graham D, editors: *Canada's health promotion survey 1990: technical report,* Ottawa, 1993, Minister of Supply and Services Canada.

Rakowski W, Assaf AR, Lefebvre RC et al: Information-seeking about health in a community sample of adults: correlates and associations with other health-related practices, *Health Educ Q* 17:379, 1990.

Reynolds KD, West SG, Aiken LS: Increasing the use of mammography: a pilot program, *Health Educ Q* 17: 429, 1990.

Simons-Morton DG, Parcel GS, Brink SG et al: Smoking control among women: needs assessment and intervention strategies. In Ward WB, Lewis FM, editors: *Advances in health education and promotion,* vol 3, London, 1991, Jessica Kingsley.

Singer J, Lindsey EA, Wilson DMC: Promoting physical activity in primary care: overcoming the barriers, *Can Fam Phys* 37:2167, 1991.

Walsh JME, McPhee S: A systems model of clinical preventive care: an analysis of factors influencing patient and physician, *Health Educ Q* 19:157, 1992.

Worden JK, Solomon LJ, Flynn BS et al: A community-wide program in breast self-examination training and maintenance, *Prev Med* 19:254, 1990.

Zapka JG, Hosmer D, Costanza ME et al: Changes in mammography use: economic, need, and service factors, *Am J Public Health* 82:1345, 1992.

Chapter 8

Aging and Health of the Elderly

❖

Our objective should be to die as young as possible—as late as possible.

<small>ANONYMOUS</small>

OBJECTIVES

When you finish this chapter, you should be able to:

- Assess the special health needs of a community's elderly population
- Identify community health programs and services appropriate to the needs of the elderly
- Anticipate future health needs of the elderly

Gerontology and **geriatrics** both study the aging process, including biological, psychological, and social change. Gerontology concerns itself with the natural aging process and with pathological aging. Geriatrics deals with the care of the aged and concerns itself primarily with enabling older people with illness or disability to live productively and enjoyably. The applied field of community health deals more with geriatrics than with gerontology; hence this chapter will be concerned with health as an aspect of geriatrics. Health cannot be isolated from the total life of the community. Circumstances of living that are indirectly related to health must also be considered, hence the use of *social* geriatrics in community health.

Healthy People 2000, the U.S. objectives for health promotion and disease prevention, suggests steps to be taken to maximize well-being at each stage of life. This chapter will review these from the perspective of the elderly. Resist, however, the tendency to accept a narrow age orientation to health and behavior, because many of the problems of old age—such as heart disease, stroke, and cancer—are rooted in circumstances and behavior found earlier in life. Health promotion and disease prevention are lifelong concerns that can produce benefits at any stage of the life cycle, but their benefits for the elderly are cumulative.

This chapter concentrates on the three points of intervention represented by the models of the health field and community health promotion developed in previous chapters. First, the natural history of health behavior among the aging population will be examined. The chapter will then examine the social history of changes in the life circumstances of aging persons that may precipitate, facilitate, or reinforce the processes of change or adaptation represented in Figures 2-2 and 2-4 and in Tables 6-1 and 7-1. You should review these figures and tables now. Discussion will concentrate specifically on three circumstances or transitions of the kind implied by Table 6-1: relocation, retirement, and **bereavement.** Finally, this chapter will suggest a number of health-promoting programs focused on these and other transitions, and targeted to those elderly people most at risk in a community. How you might be able to help mobilize community resources and the elderly themselves in support of such programs will be discussed.

THE NATURAL HISTORY AND DEMOGRAPHY OF AGING

Aging could be thought of as a process that begins with conception, but in practice, aging is regarded as that phase in life when body functioning begins to decline. Technically, then, one could describe everyone over the age of 30 as aging. The problem here is with the particular health factors that are of special importance to a given age. Because the age of eligibility for retirement benefits has been widely accepted as 65, it is customary to think of anyone beyond this age as being in the classification of ''aged.'' Yet a person of chronological age 55 could be older socially or physiologically than another individual of age 75. The arbitrary age of 65 is accepted in health circles as marking off a segment of the population that has health needs different from those of other segments. This grouping is accepted even though it is acknowledged that many of the health problems of the retired population could have

been prevented or at least anticipated constructively with **preretirement counseling.**

The Relativity of Health

Although health is a primary concern of the elderly, illness and age are not synonymous. Data from national surveys indicate that the majority of the elderly in the United States see themselves as well, not sick. Over half of those over the age of 80 who are living in the community (not in nursing homes) report that their health is good. In assessing their health status, the elderly compare themselves not with all people, but with their age cohorts, including those who are institutionalized and those who have died. A high correlation exists between the negative evaluation of health status and the degree to which an elderly person feels economically stressed, lonely, alienated, or useless.

The elderly person who reports that he or she has good to excellent health also more often reports having a positive psychological attitude, feeling financially secure, having a high sense of the worth of things, feeling useful, and feeling personally secure and not being bothered by feelings of anger, tension, restlessness, or confusion.

Natural History

Aging is a natural process involving a number of physiological changes, many of them merely a decline in the rate of functioning. A reduction in the metabolic rate of about 7% occurs every 10 years after the age of 30. There is a retardation of the rate of cell division, cell growth, and cell repair. Tissues, including their cells, tend to dry out. A fatty infiltration usually occurs with cellular atrophy, and a decrease in the speed of muscular response and a decline in muscular strength result. With a reduction in the efficiency of circulation, endurance is adversely affected. Connective tissues suffer a decrease in elasticity, bones become more brittle as the amount of organic material becomes reduced, teeth lose their structural integrity, and functioning of the digestive system declines so that digestion proceeds at a much slower rate. Many people over age 60 produce no hydrochloric acid in their stomach. Some of the nutritional deficiencies of older people can be attributed to poor digestion and inadequate absorption rather than to a poor diet. There is also a general decline in the functioning of the nervous system and special sense organs. Because of the body's delayed response to infection or any other disorder, illness tends to be extended in the older person. The net effect is a notable increase in the proportion of people experiencing limitation of activity in the later ages (Figure 8-1, *A*). But these limitations of activity are also heavily influenced by economic circumstances, as shown in Figure 8-1, *B*.

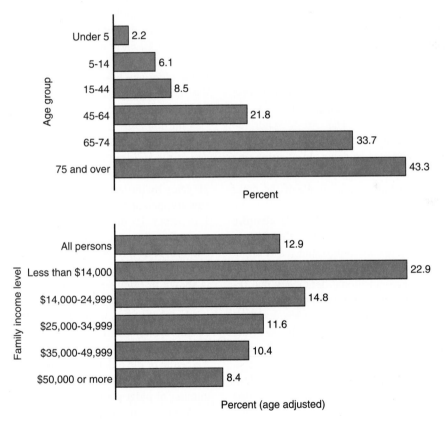

FIGURE 8-1

Percentage of people experiencing limitations of activity by age (**A**) and by income (**B**), 1990. Besides income, educational level also contributes to the decline in functioning with age. Activity limitations are four times as common among people with 8 years of education than among those with 16 years or more.

Source: National Center for Health Statistics, Centers for Disease Control and Prevention, U.S. Department of Health and Human Services.

Factors in Aging Faster

The principal concern of health science, however, is with pathological aging, which means a hastening of the aging process by adverse factors affecting body functioning. Repeated insults to the body leave their mark. The prime of life, as we know it, could be extended and thus the disabling effect of aging could be delayed if all factors that produce pathological aging could be prevented or dealt with summarily.

Low-grade infection, particularly of a chronic nature, takes its toll on the body. Toxins from the environment also hasten the aging process. Extended critical illness from which an individual recovers nevertheless hastens aging. Degenerative diseases such as hypertension, arthritis, and rheumatism tend to produce premature aging. Chronic tension, worry, and fatigue, associated with an inability to relax, can hasten the aging process. The stress syndrome masks a disturbance of biochemical functioning that can contribute to premature aging. In addition, the use of multiple drugs commonly results in overdosages and toxicities that complicate all of the other factors.

Inactivity can be a factor in producing **atrophy** and pathological aging. The level of effectiveness that the circulatory system attains and the strength of the muscular and skeletal systems depend on regular activity. Marked nutritional deficiency that results in emaciation over an extended period of time, such as one observes in some of the underdeveloped nations of the world, has a recognized adverse effect on the retention of the prime of life. Inadequacy of vitamins, proteins, and minerals in the diet can also hasten premature aging. Cigarettes, excessive alcohol, and cholesterol are the most clearly isolated agents today that contribute to early degeneration.

Demographic Trends

That the age distributions of populations (see Figures 3-7 and 3-13) are shifting toward the older groups is general knowledge. The number of people 65 years and older in the United States has increased from 3 million in 1900 to ten times this number in 1990 (31.7 million), while the number of people under 60 years old has increased at only one fourth this rate. Current projections for both developing and developed countries indicate that the older age groups will continue to grow at a faster pace than the rest of the population into the twenty-first century. The growth rate for the elderly population will be somewhat slower in this decade when people born during the depression of the 1930s, constituting a relatively small cohort, reach the age of 60. As persons born during the ''baby boom'' years reach the age of 60 early in the next century, most of the growth in the Western populations will again occur in the older age brackets. Between 1990 and 2030, the oldest age group (85 years and over) of the United States is projected to more than triple in size to 9 million.

With these demographic changes, the average age of the U.S. population has risen from 23 years to 33 years since 1900, and is projected to climb to 38 years by the year 2035. At the beginning of this century, persons 60 years old and over represented 1 of every 16 persons. They now represent 1 of every 7, and by the year 2035 will represent about one fourth of the total population. The distribution of elderly age groups in the 20 largest populations is shown in Figure 8-2. When today's college students are in their 70s, they will represent over one third of the adult population over 25 years old.

The elderly merit an organized community program for the promotion of their health. Concern for the health of the older age segment of the population has been intensified by the rapid increase in the number of older people.

A 65-year-old man can now expect, on the average, to live to 80; a woman of 65, to 85. By the year 2000, life expectancies for 65-year-olds may increase by another 1 or 2 years. The gain in life expectancy during the twentieth century represents an outstanding achievement, but it brings with it substantial changes in society as a whole and enor-

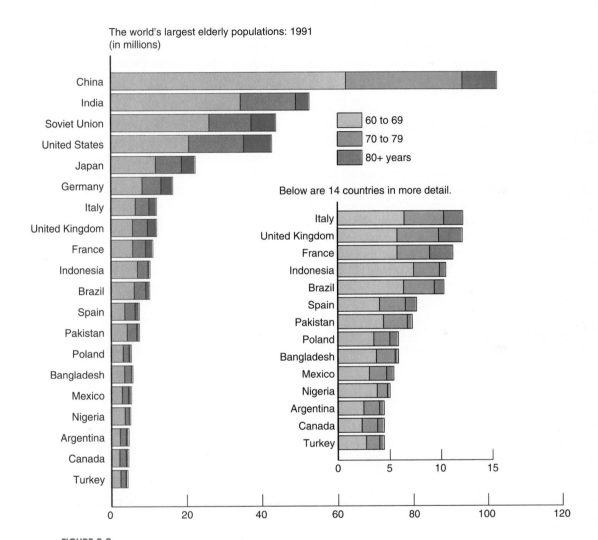

FIGURE 8-2

Twenty largest populations of elderly people in their 60s, 70s, and 80 or more years, in millions, 1991. The Soviet Union is now made up of several separate countries.

Source: Bureau of the Census: *Global aging: comparative indicators and future trends.* Washington, DC, 1991, Economic and Statistics Administration, U.S. Department of Commerce.

mous challenges for communities. The increasing numbers of the ''young-old''—persons in their late 50s, 60s, and early 70s who are retired, are relatively healthy and vigorous, and seek meaningful ways to use their time, either in self-fulfillment or in community participation—challenge the community to use their talents both to enrich their own lives and to improve society at large.

A second set of community issues stems from the even more striking increases in the numbers of the ''old-old''—persons in their mid-70s, 80s, and 90s (Figure 8-2). An increasing minority of the old-old remain vigorous and active, but the majority need a range of supportive and restorative health and social services. The old-old of the 1990s represent a disproportionately disadvantaged group. The reasons are several, including the fact that this group includes many immigrants who were poorly educated and who have spent their working years at low-paying jobs. Many have been unable to accumulate savings or to build up sufficient equity in the Social Security system to sustain them adequately through their years of retirement.

Future populations of young-old and old-old persons will have different characteristics. They will have been better educated and will have received better medical care and nutrition throughout their lives. Because their life experiences as a cohort will have been markedly different from those of the present population of older people, their expectations of life, including their expectations of old age, will be different. As a result, programs suited to the young-old and old-old persons of today will need continuous revisions if they are to be suited to future populations.

THE SOCIAL HISTORY AND EPIDEMIOLOGY OF AGING

Social norms and conditions produce for many older people the following characteristics and circumstances: (1) loss of income and status, and an increased uncertainty about personal worth, (2) insecurity associated with a feeling of inability to meet the demands of life, (3) apprehension about health, (4) difficulty in adjusting from a work routine to one of retirement, (5) inability to find avenues of service that will provide personal gratification, (6) difficulty in handling stresses created by social change, and (7) limited incentive for social participation. These changes are summarized in Figure 8-3.

Just as many of the health problems of the poor are related to problems of racism and class, and just as some problems of women are related to sexism, so too are major problems of the aged related to **ageism.** A community approach to the health of the elderly therefore must concern itself with public and professional attitudes toward aging and stereotypes about the aged. Institutional prejudice also exists to the extent that our community services and institutions discriminate against the aged in ways that threaten their access to health care and other resources. Community health programs should attempt to adjust resources, communications, and organizational arrangements to meet the special needs of older people.

Each day the community sees its elderly people and may assume that they are living more enjoyably and effectively or more unhappily than they really are. Rather than relying on assumptions, the community needs to make a critical appraisal of the status of its elderly citizens.

Compression of Morbidity and Active Life Expectancy

We have witnessed a lengthening of longevity, or mean life expectancy at birth, not because we have lengthened the life span, but because we delayed the premature deaths that were occurring within that biologically set life span. We have, in a word, compressed the *mortality* experience of the population into later and later stages of the life span, as shown in Scenario 3 of Figure 8-4.

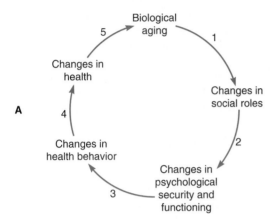

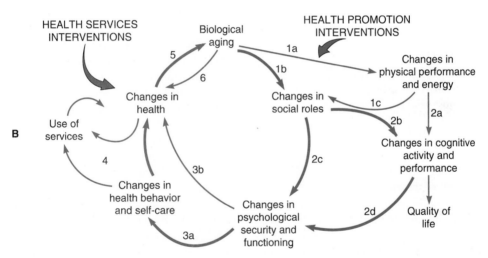

FIGURE 8-3

The cycle of life-style transitions and aging. **A**, Simplified. **B**, elaborated. The cycle shows the natural history of change and points of intervention to modify: (1) the impact of biological aging on social roles and status; (2) the impact of changing social roles and status on psychological security or functioning; (3) the impact of psychological changes on human behavior; (4) the impact of behavior changes on health; and (5) the effects of changing health status on delining biological functioning.

Sources: **A**, Levkoff S, Green LW, Hansel N: Changes in the cycle of lifestyle and aging: implications for health promotion, *Spec Care in Dent* 4:130, 1984; **B**, Green LW: Some challenges to health services research on children and the elderly, *Health Serv Res* 19:793, 1984.

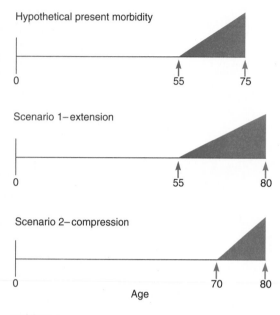

FIGURE 8-4

Rather than merely extending the period of illness and disability by prolonging life, as in Scenario 2, health promotion for the elderly seeks to compress the onset of illness and disability into the latest possible years, as in Scenario 3.

Source: Fries JF, Green LW, Levine S: Health promotion and the compression of morbidity, *Lancet* 1:105, 1989.

As we compress mortality tighter and tighter against the wall of the biological limit, there is less remaining gain to be sought in prolonging life or reducing mortality, but there is much to be gained in delaying the onset of *morbidity,* as shown in Scenario 2 of Figure 8-4. This is the task of health promotion.

The morbidity in question at these older ages is the manifestation of chronic and degenerative conditions that afflict us all. Most adults have some degree of atherosclerosis, some degree of hypertension or hypotension, some degree of osteoporosis and decreased lung function, and some loss of agility, sensory acuity, memory, suppleness, muscle endurance, and circulatory and metabolic efficiency. They are

not diseases to be prevented; they are conditions to be slowed in their progression, limited in their impact, and adapted to as they relate to life-style, functioning, and the quality of life—which brings us to the second concept.

As we seek to compress morbidity against the far wall of our biologically determined maximum life span, we also seek to maintain active functioning in the years of waning biological functions. We might have to slow down in old age, but we should not have to live too many years in pain, social embarrassment, inability to function independently, or incapacity to enjoy life. The concept of **active life expectancy** refers to the quality of the remaining years of *functional* well-being.

Historically, we have compressed mortality mainly by controlling infections and communicable diseases, and more recently by reducing the death rate from cardiovascular diseases in middle-aged men. The former we accomplished largely through environmental interventions, the latter largely through life-style changes. At least in the earlier case, the real gains in longevity came with the suppression of death rates at younger ages, not in the over 65 age groups, but that was partly because the population was concentrated in those ages and more of the deferrable mortality occurred at those ages. The historical and demographic circumstances have changed.

In the decades ahead, the opportunity to compress morbidity and the opportunity to increase active life expectancy appear likely to increase during the older ages. The opportunity can be deceptive, however, for we have little evidence that intervening late in the degenerative processes can make a significant difference in health.

Health and the Three Functions of Age

Figure 8-5 illustrates the biological, social, and behavioral paths through which age influences health status. It indicates the complexity of the social and

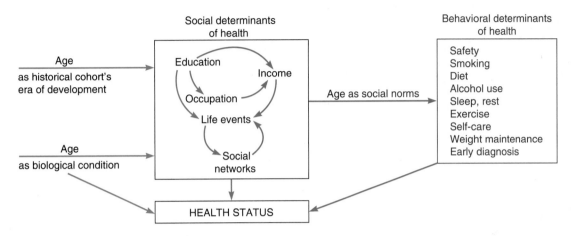

FIGURE 8-5
Health and the three ways age operates to influence health status outcomes.
Source: Green LW, Gottlieb NH: Health promotion for the aging population: approaches to extending active life expectancy. In Andreopoulos S, Hogness JR, editors: *Health care for an aging society,* New York, 1989, Churchill Livingstone.

behavioral determinants of health status that may be addressed in health promotion for the elderly.

When considering the influence of age on health status, it is important to consider three meanings of age: (1) age as maturation or biological condition, (2) age as cohort or historical location, and (3) age as life course or a set of age-related social roles through which each individual passes. These three functions of age are not independent of each other. One's cohort location (for example, those born and raised in the 1920s compared with those born and raised in the 1940s) influences the social norms or expectations held by society for behavior at different ages. It may also influence one's maturation or biological state. Improved nutrition and living conditions in succeeding generations have influenced biological aspects of aging.

So far we have discussed the concept of health promotion in light of current theories concerning the compression of morbidity and active life expectancy. Behavioral patterns and social transitions also produce key elements in improving the quality of life and self-reported health status of older adults.

For each of these entities we suggest intervention strategies for health promotion programs directed to the elderly.

Life-Style Health Practices as a Point of Intervention

Healthful life-style behavior forms a cornerstone of disease prevention and health promotion. As a function of age, the health status of elderly persons is related to their earlier personal health practices. Never smoking, moderate alcohol consumption or abstinence, regular physical activity, and weight maintenance have been associated with lower mortality rates for all causes, as well as from specific diseases for which certain of the practices carry a high relative risk. Although it is not clear (except for smoking among women) that life-style practices among the elderly are associated (independent of age, health status, and income) with mortality, it is well established that these behaviors contribute to overall quality of life and alter the course of various diseases and conditions among older adults. For ex-

TABLE 8-1

Comparisons of 65+ populations of North America with all adults (age 18+ in U.S., 15+ in Canada) on selected health promoting behavior and conditions, 1990 in Canada, 1991 in U.S.

	Percentages	
Parameter	*65+ years*	*All ages*
Physical activity		
U.S.: Exercise strenuously 3 or more times per week	26	37
Canada: Vigorous physical activity	48	48
Usually 30 minutes or more		
Men	43	55
Women	29	42
Three or more times/week		
Men	61	52
Women	49	49
Stress		
U.S.: Experience high levels of stress at least several days a week	21	32
Canada: Perceive their lives as somewhat or very stressful		
Men	31	61
Women	33	60
Smoking		
U.S.: Do not smoke	83	75
Canada: Do not smoke	84	37
Men	82	69
Women	86	72
Alcohol		
U.S.: Do not drink alcohol	60	39
Canada: Lifetime abstainers and former drinkers	38	19
Men	34	15
Women	42	23
Seat belt use		
U.S.: Wear seat belt all the time in front seat of car	71	69
Canada: Always wear seat belt in car	86	79
Men	81	72
Women	90	86

Sources: *Prevention Index 1992: a report card on the nation's health,* Emmaus, Pa, 1993, Rodale; Santé et Bien-être social Canada, Stephens T, Fowler Graham D: Enquête Promotion de la santé Canada 1990: rapport technique, Ottawa, 1993, Ministre des Approvisionnements et Services Canada.

ample, stopping smoking after a myocardial infarction has been shown to reduce the mortality rate, and exercise among elderly persons increases the physical capacity to withstand illness and injury, increases flexibility, and improves cardiovascular functioning.

Data from national health interview surveys compare the prevalence of selected life-style health practices among the elderly and the total population (Table 8-1). Such data are based on self-report. When examining patterns of behavior using such survey data, it is important to remember that we cannot separate the three functions of age as they influence health-related practices. For example, older persons may be less likely to engage in aerobic exercise because they are physically unable to do so, or because the primary socialization of their cohort was in an era when exercise was not popular, or because age-graded norms for exercise stereotype them as fragile, slow, and clumsy, and they are expected not to engage in ''child's play.''

ACTIVE LIFE EXPECTANCY APPROACH TO HEALTH PROMOTION FOR THE ELDERLY

Taking the task for health promotion for the elderly to be the compression of morbidity would lead a community to intervene primarily in smoking, alcohol and drug misuse, exercise, and nutrition in the young and middle-aged populations. These precursors to morbidity have their genesis in early ages, and they are cumulative in their impact on morbidity. Taking the task also to be the extension of active life expectancy would lead the community to emphasize these same interventions plus some others, but more with the older age groups. We need to step back from the problems of a particular age group and ask what preceded that age that might have precipitated the problem. It is perhaps inherent in the concept of health promotion that intervention must precede the problem. In order to intervene before a problem manifests, we must anticipate

the problem, and in health we can only do that probabilistically.

The probabilities used for most health planning are vital statistics and incidence rates. Prevalence rates serve to inform health planning for purposes of allocating facilities and resources for the care of existing problems, but age-specific incidence rates are needed to anticipate and to plan for interventions designed to prevent the emergence of future problems. Unfortunately, incidence rates for the morbidities of old age are the least developed of all health statistics. They simply do not exist for most of the chronic and degenerative diseases because the onset of such conditions is undefined and, as noted earlier, most adults have some of these conditions to some extent.

Community-Wide Approach

How then can we recognize and target health promotion interventions strategically and efficiently? One answer to this question is the community-wide approach to life-style modification. This approach is based on two theories, one epidemiological and the other sociological. The epidemiological theory is that by moving the mean risk factor levels a small amount in an entire community, a statistically greater impact can be achieved on mortality than can be obtained by moving the mean risk factor levels of high-risk groups a large amount. The sociological theory is that by intervening in the community at large, behavioral and environmental changes can be mobilized on a more pervasive scale. This would produce a social influence or normative effect and set into motion a more permanent diffusion process. Both theories and the argument they support for community-wide interventions have merit, but with some limitations for the elderly.

Community-wide approaches are appropriate for reducing the risk of later morbidity and mortality in young and middle-aged populations. For programs directed at older age groups, however, these approaches are less applicable. The elderly represent a distinct community in only a few places, such as retirement villages, mobile home parks, and arguably nursing homes. Community organization and community-wide health education or screening methods are ideally suited to these situations, but they miss most elderly people. Community-wide programs intended for the elderly but applied to the community at large are costly and inefficient in reaching the elderly.

This situation, then, is the dilemma of health promotion for the elderly. Traditional medical approaches are often too late for purposes of prevention and active life expectancy. The traditional public health method of identifying high-risk groups on the basis of incidence rates fails to apply because the new morbidities have undefined onsets and therefore few meaningful incidence rates available. The promising new community-wide strategies for chronic disease prevention do not fit for this demographic group because the elderly seldom make up a geographic community of their own.

Research has demonstrated that it is possible to build a sense of community and self-reliance among even the low-income elderly residing in single-room occupancy hotels in an inner city area. It requires, however, a highly targeted, labor-intensive outreach strategy that engages and organizes unaffiliated elderly people in identifying and solving their own mutual problems. It is not the same as the media-oriented, community-wide interventions used in the general population. The solutions for health promotion for the elderly seem to lie more with an open-ended strategy of involving the elderly in identifying their own needs than with the community-wide, categorical, disease-specific strategy suitable with other population groups (Figure 8-6).

Transitions in Aging

Most older individuals do encounter situational changes associated with aging. The most pervasive of these in their effects on life-style and health are relocation, retirement, and widowhood. The

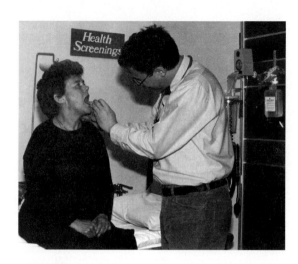

FIGURE 8-6
Periodic health screening examinations detect the onset of chronic or infectious conditions at an early stage when they can be most effectively treated and controlled through life-style management and self-care rather than extensive medical or surgical treatment.

changes produced by these transitions may be accompanied by stress or bereavement. These in turn can make the individual susceptible to both physical and psychological illness.

Many older adults experience transitions without developing any subsequent pathological conditions. Others experience adverse outcomes as measured by health status indicators (nursing home admissions, hospitalizations, operations, acute illness) and psychosocial indicators (depression, psychosomatic illness, low morale, lowered life satisfaction). Factors that appear to influence adaptation or resistance include experiential, environmental, and social aspects of the individual and of the change. For each of the three types of transitions, stressors and protective factors that influence the adaptation process can be identified in the community.

Relocation. Relocation takes the form of various types of moves—from one home to another within the community, from one community to another, from home to institution, from one institution to another, or even within an institution. Studies of the effects of relocation on the elderly have detected changes in mortality rates, physical health status indicators, and social, economic, and psychological outcomes. The effects of relocation depend on the way the move is handled, including the degree of support provided and the degree of preparation for the move, and the degree of environmental change involved. The effects also depend on the relocation's duration, its predictability, whether the move was voluntary or involuntary, and the degree of control felt by the elderly person.

Two factors seem most consistently to act as buffers for an individual's response to relocation stress: the degree of control over the event and the degree of predictability of the new environment. When the elderly person perceives a move as voluntary and feels a sense of control or choice about the relocation process, less stress is experienced and fewer negative physical or psychosocial consequences result. Similarly, the more radical the environmental change, the less predictable the new environment, and the more negative the effect of relocation.

Individual response to relocation stress is influenced by the person's characteristics prior to the move, attitudes about the move, degree of preparation for the move, and degree of physical disability at the time of the move. Individual characteristics consistently associated with the adverse consequences of relocation include advanced age, poor physical health, psychiatric disturbances, and cognitive malfunctioning. Adverse consequences of relocation are also greater in males, those living alone, those having few social contacts with friends and kin, those in poor financial circumstances, those lacking access to various social services, and those who lived in the same place a long time.

Finally, the degree and type of preparation for the move influence relocation outcomes. Uncertainty, and thus stress, may be decreased as predictability of the new environment is increased through anticipatory counseling or preparatory education programs. The increased attention the residents receive as a result of participation in preparatory programs might cause a decline in negative outcomes immediately following the relocation. A protective effect associated with increased social support and attention prior to and immediately following relocation probably results in a delayed and possibly reduced peak in mortality rates among those relocated.

Retirement. In the future a greater percentage of citizens over age 65 will receive Social Security and survivors' insurance benefits. Socioeconomic factors may even produce a retirement age of 60 for the general population. The earlier retirement age and the shrinking resources available from Social Security funds will pose additional problems unless better programs are promoted to prepare people for retirement.

At least half the people over age 65 are potential members of the labor force, and many of them prefer to work. Frequently it is necessary for them to learn a new type of work. Some find that their skills and trades have become obsolete, and for this reason have to find new types of employment. Many of these individuals have an adequate physical capacity as well as an adequate learning capacity to take up new jobs, but industries are reluctant to employ elderly workers because they believe them to be slower and to have higher rates of injury and absenteeism. The older worker, however, is generally meticulous, produces work of a high quality, and is extremely reliable. There is a need to lower work barriers for the elderly who are physically and mentally capable. Employment opportunities need to be increased for those elderly citizens capable of contributing to the community's economy (Figures 8-7 and 8-8). Part-time jobs have their merit, particularly when the elderly person supplements work with other community services and activities. Childcare roles for the elderly seem especially suited to their needs and those of today's communities with growing numbers of working women.

Preparation for successful old age should begin at about age 40, with the development of a wide

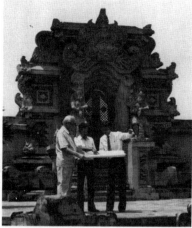

Turn your lifetime of experience into the experience of a lifetime.

IESC Volunteer Gordon Swaney, a retired U.S. manager, on project site in Indonesia.

We're looking for executives who know their way around the trenches as well as the front offices. Because if you're recently retired, there's a whole world out there desperately waiting to be taught what you spent a lifetime learning.

Through the International Executive Service Corps—the not-for-profit organization that sends U.S. managers to help businesses in developing nations—you can volunteer for short-term assignments in foreign countries where you're truly needed. Although you will not be paid, you and your spouse will receive all expenses, plus the personal satisfaction of teaching others while you discover more about yourself.

Think of it. Your experience can make a difference in a land much different from your own. Instead of ending your career, you could be starting the experience of a lifetime.

Send for more information today.

International Executive Service Corps

Ad Council
A Public Service of This Publication

YES, I'd like to share my lifetime of experience with others. I recently retired from my position as a hands-on manager with a U.S. company. I also understand that volunteers and their spouses receive expenses, but no salary. Please send me more information now.

Name_____

Address_____

City_____State_____Zip_____

Write to: IESC, 8 Stamford Forum, P.O. Box 10005, Stamford, CT 06904-2005. Or, for faster response, call this number: (203) 967-6000.

E2

FIGURE 8-7
Volunteer work puts lifetime skills to useful applications and helps the retired person maintain a sense of self-worth and social value.
Source: Advertising Council.

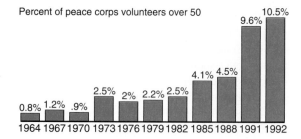

Percent of peace corps volunteers over 50

FIGURE 8-8
In the first year of the Peace Corps only 83 of the 10,078 volunteers, less than 1%, were people 50 or over. In 1992, out of a total of 5300 Peace Corps volunteers, 556 were 50 or older. The biggest increases were between 1988 and 1991, with more than a doubling of the proportion who were older volunteers.
Source: U.S. Peace Corps.

range of interests and channels of community service. Elderly persons must be encouraged to accept change, cultivate a range of interests, maintain a willingness to learn, and participate actively in community affairs.

Some retire freely. Others experience compulsory retirement; but even among those who face compulsory retirement, some willingly retire, while others reluctantly give up the work role. Still others retire for health reasons, while some persons may face retirement after job loss. Given these varied conditions, retired people experience very different physical and mental health outcomes as they pass from working to nonworking life-styles.

Some possible phases in the natural history of the adaptation process might be the honeymoon phase, the disenchantment phase, the reorientation phase, and the stability phase. Such phases are left understandably undocumented, given the difficult task of measuring and verifying their manifestation, duration, and sequence. The notion of retirement adaptation as a transition process is important to health promotion insofar as interventions could be targeted to phases, and different retirement outcomes might be predicted at specific time intervals for different groups of retirees (see Table 6-1).

Widowhood and bereavement. A third common life transition of old age is widowhood. Like retirement, where stress produced by loss of the work role affects and is affected by other variables, widowhood is a complex phenomenon that produces losses and changes beyond the loss of a spouse. For some it may mean the loss of dependable financial resources and a concomitant decline in economic status, while for others it may mean a decline in social interaction and a concomitant decline in social status. Many widowed people suffer from stigma and deprivation, the stigma leading to altered self-concept and isolation and the deprivation to loneliness and depression.

Poor adaptation to the stresses produced by widowhood has been found to be associated with inadequate income, poor physical health, lack of a supportive reference group, and lack of alternative roles to substitute for the lost role of spouse, such as employment or extended family involvement. These studies suggest that the association between widowhood and lower morale or depression may be attributed to factors other than the loss of a spouse per se. These other factors are the concomitant life changes that widowhood may bring. As with relocation and retirement, situational factors that occur along with widowhood rather than widowhood itself may be the causal agents of stress, adaptation, and lower morale among the widowed.

Community Interventions in the Transitions

Considering each major transition separately and applying the model in Table 6-1, what might be appropriate health-promoting interventions?

Relocation. Less negative consequences of relocation are associated with a predictable postrelocation environment, and change that is perceived as voluntary and in one's control. While one may not be able to change the nature of a move, prerelocation preparation might help the relocated person better manage the new environment. In the case of an in-stitutional setting, providing information as to what to expect in terms of new routines, new staff, and new time schedules might make the new environment more predictable and thus more manageable, even with a radical move.

The actual control a resident has over an administrative move within an institution or even a move from the home setting into the institutional one may be limited. Education can at least provide understanding and can actively engage the resident in the relocation process. In this way, the resident perceives that he or she has some control over the relocation process. People of any age who believe that they have control over outcomes can better manage change and are more likely to adopt positive adaptive behavior, leading to a sense of competence and control that may motivate further adaptive behavior. (Figure 8-9).

Providing preparation for the move thus appears to be an important factor in mediating the stress experienced by relocated persons. Group programs can provide the helpful social support needed in times of uncertainty and change. Such support can serve as a protective mechanism against any stresses caused by the change. The group can offer support

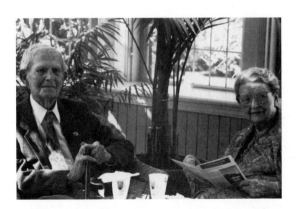

FIGURE 8-9
People who have control over their own selection of housing and social relationships enjoy greater emotional and physical health.

Source: Photo by Judy McLarty, courtesy University of British Columbia.

by mobilizing psychological resources to master emotional burdens, by sharing tasks, and by providing the skills and guidance to improve handling of the situation.

Retirement. For many, the process of retirement is a normal, expected life event that in itself does not constitute a stressful transition, but rather calls forth changes in self-concept, self-identity, and social roles. While these changes do call for new adaptations, they are not necessarily traumatic. Successful adaptation to nonworking status seems to depend on a retiree's health and on the psychological, social, and financial resources he or she brings to retirement. While many resources are fixed, such as finances, others are more amenable to change. Retirees' adjustment to their new roles depends in part on their ability to support consistent, coherent self-images despite major changes in their social system, as well as on the degree of support provided in their social environment. Interventions aimed at helping the individual retiree find meaningful ways of maintaining a positive self-image may be oriented toward anticipatory socialization. This might involve identifying a variety of role options open to the retiree, and then preparing the retiree for the role chosen.

Bereavement. The treatment of widowhood as a unitary phenomenon with similar outcomes for all is equally unsuitable. Interventions should be targeted toward building the knowledge and skills needed to cope with whatever unique sources of difficulty the widow or widower will experience. While some sources of stress may not be amenable to change, interventions might at least enable the bereaved to cope better with certain problems—for example, financial worries. Other situational factors of widowhood are more amenable to direct manipulation and change. If a widowed person is found to lack sufficient family interactions, efforts can be made to increase activity—if not with family members, then with other peers. If difficulties result from lack of work involvement, efforts can be directed at

securing employment. In other words, interventions should be tailored to meet individual needs. A number of programs have been established to ameliorate the loneliness and isolation experienced by the recently widowed. These "widow-to-widow" programs train widowed persons to serve as outreach workers for those more recently bereaved.

Although major life events do not necessarily precipitate crisis reactions in the majority of the aged, many elderly people experiencing these events are at high risk of mental and physical illness. Yet even for those who are adversely affected, it seems that the set of mostly controllable circumstances surrounding the event, not the event itself, constitutes the source of difficulty. Community programs can be directed at these situational factors. Such interventions can be regarded as health promotion insofar as they represent a primary prevention approach to the cycle of deteriorating life-style and health. By anticipating the potential adaptations required in transitions to come, health education can be combined with organizational, economic, and environmental supports for coping strategies and behavior conducive to health in the aging population.

SPECIFIC HEALTH PRIORITIES OF AGING
Physical Health

Many of the disorders of the later years, such as diseases of the heart, arteriosclerosis, and other degenerative diseases, require far more medical care than those of earlier years. Government must bear a larger proportion of the bill for the aged. Primary prevention is still in order for certain infectious diseases, such as influenza and pneumonia, and for injury control. Early detection and treatment (secondary prevention) of malignant neoplasms (cancer) and hypertension could give these older citizens several additional years of active life. Even individuals over age 65 who appear to be in excellent health should have a medical examination every year (Table 8-2). Of course, those who are at high risk should

TABLE 8-2
Periodic screening and health services recommendations of the U.S. Preventive Services Task Force for people 65 and over. (Leading Causes of Death: heart disease; cerebrovascular disease; obstructive lung disease; pneumonia/influenza; lung cancer; and colorectal cancer)

Screening

History	Physical exam	Laboratory/diagnostic procedures
Prior symptoms of transient ischemic attack	Height and weight	Nonfasting total blood cholesterol
Dietary intake	Blood pressure	Dipstick urinalysis
Physical activity	Visual acuity	Mammogram[2]
Tobacco/alcohol/drug use	Hearing and hearing aids	Thyroid function tests[3]
Functional status at home	Clinical breast exam[1]	*HIGH-RISK GROUPS*
	HIGH-RISK GROUPS	Fasting plasma glucose (HR5)
	Auscultation for carotid bruits (HR1)	Tuberculin skin test (PPD) (HR6)
	Complete skin exam (HR2)	Electrocardiogram (HR7)
	Complete oral cavity exam (HR3)	Papanicolaou smear[4] (HR8)
	Palpation of thyroid nodules (HR4)	Fecal occult blood/Sigmoidoscopy (HR9)
		Fecal occult blood/Colonoscopy (HR10)

Counseling

Diet and exercise	Injury prevention	Dental health
Fat (especially saturated fat), cholesterol, complex carbohydrates, fiber, sodium, calcium[3]	Prevention of falls	Regular dental visits, tooth brushing, flossing
Caloric balance	Safety belts	*Other primary preventive measures*
Selection of exercise program	Smoke detector	
	Smoking near bedding or upholstery	Glaucoma testing by eye specialist
Substance use	Hot water heater temperature	*HIGH-RISK GROUPS*
Tobacco cessation	Safety helmets	Discussion of estrogen replacement therapy (HR13)
Alcohol and other drugs:	*HIGH-RISK GROUPS*	Discussion of aspirin therapy (HR14)
Limiting alcohol consumption	Prevention of childhood injuries (HR12)	Skin protection from ultraviolet light (HR15)
Driving/other dangerous activities while under the influence		
Treatment for abuse		

Immunizations

Tetanus-diphtheria (Td) booster[5]	Pneumococcal vaccine	*HIGH-RISK GROUPS*
Influenza vaccine[1]		Hepatitis B vaccine (HR16)

Remain alert for:

Depression symptoms	Changes in cognitive function	Malignant skin lesions
Suicide risk factors (HR11)	Medications that increase risk of falls	Peripheral arterial disease
Abnormal bereavement	Signs of physical abuse or neglect	Tooth decay, gingivitis, loose teeth

This list of preventive services is not exhaustive. It reflects only those topics reviewed by the U.S. Preventive Services Task Force. Clinicians may wish to add other preventive services on a routine basis, and after considering the patient's medical history and other individual circumstances. Examples of target conditions not specifically examined by the Task Force include: chronic obstructive pulmonary disease; hepatobiliary disease; bladder cancer; endometrial disease; travel-related illness; prescription drug abuse; and occupational illness and injuries.

*The recommended schedule applies only to the periodic visit itself. The frequency of the individual preventive services listed in this table is left to clinical discretion, except as indicated in other footnotes. See definitions of high-risk (HR) groups in Table 8-3.

1. Annually. 2. Every 1-2 years for women until age 75, unless pathology detected. 3. For women. 4. Every 1-3 years. 5. Every 10 years.

have periodic checkups more frequently (Table 8-3).

Arthritis and rheumatism, though not commonly a cause of death, are two of the principal causes of disability in the aged. They can usually be treated to relieve patients of much of their pain and enable them to extend their activities. Self-care education has been shown to improve many of the problems of arthritis.

Disorders of vision are common among the elderly (Figure 8-10). Some degree of correction is usually possible even though the individual's vision

with glasses may still not be normal. When the loss of vision has progressed to a state where the individual can no longer read, recordings are available that enable the blind or near-blind to enjoy hearing the literature or feature articles of the day that they would normally read.

Loss of hearing in the later years of life is also common. Hearing aids have been developed to the point where a much higher percentage of the hard-of-hearing are aided to hear adequately for customary needs. Deafness produces a feeling of loneliness. It leads to social isolation and a consequent decline

TABLE 8-3

Ages 65 and over high-risk categories for preventive services or counseling (see Table 8-2).

HR1 Persons with risk factors for cerebrovascular or cardiovascular disease (e.g., hypertension, smoking, CAD,* atrial fibrillation, diabetes) or those with neurologic symptoms (e.g., transient ischemic attacks) or a history of cerebrovascular disease.

HR2 Persons with a family or personal history of skin cancer, or clinical evidence of precursor lesions (e.g., dysplastic nevi, certain congenital nevi), or those with increased occupational or recreational exposure to sunlight.

HR3 Persons with exposure to tobacco or excessive amounts of alcohol, or those with suspicious symptoms or lesions detected through self-examination.

HR4 Persons with a history of upper-body irradiation.

HR5 The markedly obese, persons with a family history of diabetes, or women with a history of gestational diabetes.

HR6 Household members of persons with tuberculosis or others at risk for close contact with the disease (e.g., staff of tuberculosis clinics, shelters for the homeless, nursing homes, substance abuse treatment facilities, dialysis units, correctional institutions); recent immigrants or refugees from countries in which tuberculosis is common (e.g., Asia, Africa, Central and South America, Pacific Islands); migrant workers; residents of nursing homes, correctional institutions, or homeless shelters; or persons with certain underlying medical disorders (e.g., HIV infection).

HR7 Men with two or more cardiac risk factors (high blood cholesterol, hypertension, cigarette smoking, diabetes mellitus, family history of CAD); men who would endanger public safety were they to experience sudden cardiac events

(e.g., commercial airline pilots); or sedentary or high-risk males planning to begin a vigorous exercise program.

HR8 Women who have not had previous documented screening in which smears have been consistently negative.

HR9 Persons who have first-degree relatives with colorectal cancer; a personal history of endometrial, ovarian, or breast cancer; or a previous diagnosis of inflammatory bowel disease, adenomatous polyps, or colorectal cancer.

HR10 Persons with a family history of familial polyposis coli or cancer family syndrome.

HR11 Recent divorce, separation, unemployment, depression, alcohol or other drug abuse, serious medical illnesses, living alone, or recent bereavement.

HR12 Persons with children in the home or automobile.

HR13 Women at increased risk for osteoporosis (e.g., Caucasian, low bone mineral content, bilateral oophorectomy before menopause or early menopause, slender build) and who are without known contraindications (e.g., history of undiagnosed vaginal bleeding, active liver disease, thromboembolic disorders, hormone-dependent cancer).

HR14 Men who have risk factors for myocardial infarction (e.g., high blood cholesterol, smoking, diabetes mellitus, family history of early-onset CAD) and who lack a history of gastrointestinal or other bleeding problems, or other risk factors for bleeding or cerebral hemorrhage.

HR15 Persons with increased exposure to sunlight.

HR16 Homosexually active men, intravenous drug users, recipients of some blood products, or persons in health-related jobs with frequent exposure to blood or blood products.

*Coronary artery disease.
Source: U.S. Preventive Services Task Force.

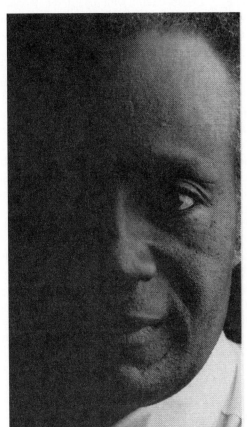

You could be going blind and not even know it.

Glaucoma is an eye disease that can steal your sight. Especially if you're over 60, or Black and over 40. But glaucoma can usually be controlled if it's detected and treated early.

So, get a dilated eye examination in which drops are used to enlarge your pupils.

For more information, write: National Eye Health Education Program, Box 20/20, Bethesda, MD 20892.

Don't lose sight of glaucoma.

NATIONAL EYE HEALTH EDUCATION PROGRAM

National Eye Institute, National Institutes of Health, Public Health Service, U.S. Department of Health and Human Services

FIGURE 8-10

Public service advertisements encourage the elderly as well as black men over 40 to seek screening examinations for glaucoma, the leading cause of blindness in adults over 60.

Source: National Eye Institute, National Institutes of Health, Public Health Service, U.S. Department of Health and Human Services.

in social functioning. This emphasizes the need to develop programs to provide whatever level of hearing can be attained. Indeed, when asked to rank the importance of priorities for disease prevention and health promotion, the elderly gave highest priority to sensory deprivation control.

Mental Health and Mental Disorders

Definitions of health and disease change not only with biomedical advances, but also with social and historical factors—for instance, with changes in social attitudes toward deviant behavior. These changes apply especially to attempts to distinguish mental health and mental disorder, as the next chapter will show. But for older people they pose growing social problems. It is estimated that some 15% of persons over 65 suffer from mental disorders, 5% from severe disorders. Alcoholism and drug misuse appear to be increasing among older persons. One striking fact is that, while this age group constitutes only 10% of the total population, it accounts for over 30% of all suicides. Criminal behavior, on the other hand, drops dramatically with age.

Physical health is a very important element in mental health, but so are social factors. Such social issues as ethnicity, socioeconomic status, marital status, and rural or urban residence may contribute to the incidence, prevalence, cause, diagnosis, and treatment of mental disorders. For instance, industrialization and urbanization are often said to be producing greater social stresses and greater social isolation for older persons, and therefore more mental disorders. But the nature of social stress is not well understood, and studies indicate that social isolation is as often an outcome as a cause of mental illness in older people.

Education and income are highly related to the type of mental illness suffered and also to the type of treatment offered by mental health professionals. There is a relationship also between education and the extent to which people seek help, either professional or nonprofessional. Western society in general has experienced a broadening range of problems for which people seek assistance and a rising level of expectation with regard to outcomes. As new cohorts of the old are increasingly well educated, their needs and expectations of the mental health system are likely to change.

The majority of functional psychiatric disturbances in old age (hypochondriacal states, paranoid reactions, and particularly depression) are responsive to appropriate treatment. Estimates of the prevalence of **Alzheimer's disease** in the over 65 population range from under 5% to over 11%. For the over 85 population, estimates average between 15% and 20% but range as high as 47%. Some 10% to 15% of organic brain syndromes are reversible (those due to coexisting physical illness or to drug intoxication, for instance). No cure has yet been found for Alzheimer's disease.

From the perspective of the mental health system as a whole, there have been striking changes in patterns of use of psychiatric facilities for different age groups. As mental health ideologies have changed, the mental health system has served a smaller proportion of older persons, with a great shift occurring after World War II from the use of mental hospitals to the use of nursing homes. These issues will be discussed further in the next chapter.

COMMUNITY ORGANIZATION AND THE ELDERLY

Community provisions for the allocation of resources and social roles to the aged make a large difference in the quality of life and consequently in the health of the elderly.

Social Networks

To prevent feelings of isolation, older persons need continued involvement in various social networks (such as family, friendship, work, leisure, church and organizational contexts). Dyadic or paired relationships (for example, a confidant) maintained over time seem to be of particular importance, but dyadic bonds have seldom been organized, except for the husband-wife relationship.

Advancing age brings a decline in number of social roles, amount of interaction, and variety of social contacts. Less active persons, however, are likely to be older, in poorer health, and in more deprived circumstances, so it is not clear to what extent the decline is a cause or a consequence of the aging process. It is probably both, creating an isolation-aging cycle. There is evidence that older people living alone more often become institutionalized, and that people with strong social networks survive and remain healthy more than those without social interaction.

Communities cannot ignore the impact on the aged of declining involvement in various social networks. Activity and morale are influenced by the extent to which social networks encourage or discourage continued participation. Therefore a distinction must be made between voluntary and involuntary withdrawal. Furthermore, it is probably the quality of interaction, rather than the frequency, that is important.

Family Networks

Among social networks, the family remains paramount. Although social norms may stress nuclear family independence, older people remain linked to kinship networks. Most older people have close relatives within easy visiting distance, contacts are frequent, and it is children, particularly daughters, to whom older people turn for help.

The family has remained a strong and supportive institution for older people. Most older persons want to be as independent of their families as possible, but when they can no longer manage for themselves, they reasonably expect their children to come to their aid. Not only do such expectations exist, they are usually met. Patterns vary among social classes and ethnic groups, but most older persons see their

children regularly, and a complex pattern of exchange of goods and services exists across generations, with ties of affection and obligation remaining strong. Furthermore, elderly parents appear to have attitudes and values remarkably similar to those of their children and grandchildren.

A trend toward separate households for older persons has developed (*family* is not synonymous with *household*). Yet the latest national data show that the older the individual, and the sicker, the more likely the person is to be found living with a child (the "sandwich generation")—more than twice as likely as to be living in an institution. The trend toward separate households will be affected by economic factors, housing policies, and the increasing number of families in which old-old persons have children who are themselves old. If more effective networks of supportive social and home health services (Figure 8-11) are built, more intergenerational households in which both generations are old may emerge.

The structure of the family has changed in the past few decades, with a larger proportion of older men and women married and living with their spouses, and with accompanying decreases in the proportions of those widowed, divorced, or never married. At the same time, the absolute number of widows is increasing as the difference in **longevity** between the sexes grows greater. Whether these trends will continue will depend on a host of social and economic factors. Changing attitudes toward divorce and remarriage and toward nontraditional forms of family life, such as communal living for people in their later years, will influence these patterns.

Friendship and Membership Ties

Friendship and membership ties complement kinship ties by relieving some of the burden of care from the family. The more characteristics neighbors have in common (such as socioeconomic status, marital status, and value orientations), the more in-

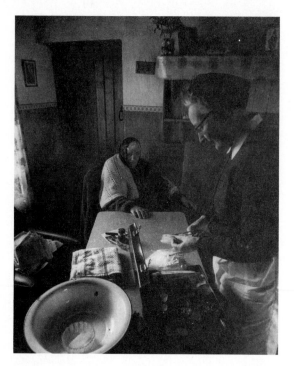

FIGURE 8-11
Home health services provided by health departments or visiting nursing services enable frail elderly people to remain in their own homes. Here a home visiting nurse in Ireland administers medications to an elderly woman.
Source: Photo courtesy World Health Organization.

Church attendance drops off among the very old, but it is not clear how much this relates to such factors as health, residential location, or socioeconomic status. Nor is it clear how age-related factors relate to historical factors in affecting patterns of church attendance or private devotions. In what ways does church attendance among older people reflect broader social trends? To what extent do private devotions replace church attendance? Related questions concern the church as a social institution in the lives of older persons. To what extent and for what subgroup does the church perform a supportive social and psychological function?

tegrated the friendship network. Voluntary membership in associations and participation in various organizations, including old-age clubs and senior citizen centers, depend to a considerable extent on styles established earlier in life.

In recent years more women have been assuming dual roles in the home and workplace. Women have increased the time spent in paid work and have somewhat decreased the time spent in family roles, although not enough to compensate for the increase in paid work time. The allocation of men's time to work and family roles, on the other hand, has remained relatively constant. It appears that as women's participation in the labor force increases, there

is a net transfer of labor away from men and toward women. Many women are under considerable stress resulting from these dual roles, but their opportunities for social ties that will carry over into retirement have been multiplied.

Civic Participation

Elderly people are less connected to the fabric of society because of their displacement from their earlier roles, especially work and family, and thus are correspondingly more alienated from their community. Civic participation is a means of reestablishing this connection.

Within populations with a similar level of education, social class, and ethnic background, the political behavior, community organizational involvement, and volunteer activities of older people are not noticeably different from those of younger people. Voting behavior remains remarkably consistent far into old age; older people do vote, and they tend to vote for the party for which they have always voted. There is no evidence of a voting bloc composed of the elderly. There has, however, been an enormous growth of lobby groups among the elderly. Participation in political activity other than voting is infrequent among older people.

The elderly who participate in community organizations appear to be a very select sample (who may represent their individual needs more than any constituency). The community organization often selects as representatives of the older population those elderly people who can be expected to go along with the organization's practices rather than those who might be critical.

Age-based Organizations

An age-based organization is one that depends on the existence of older persons for its activities. The elderly are its members, its direct or indirect consumers, or its subjects of special concern. Such organizations exist in industrialized nations throughout the world. A few are active in U.S. politics, such as the National Council of Senior Citizens, the Gray Panthers, and the American Association of Retired Persons. Such organizations can play a role in shaping the issues of public policy debate: they gain access to legislators, administrative officials, and political party organizations. They often seek to organize elderly voters as a bloc at the local or national level.

Aging as a Concern of Political Systems

The aged first became a major concern of governments in the late nineteenth century. The birth of the modern welfare state, with economic relief for older persons as a major feature, began with Bismarck in Germany in the 1880s, then spread to other industrialized countries. Relatively late, the United States enacted the Social Security program in 1935 (Figure 8-12).

Income-maintenance policies have undergone innumerable expansions in the intervening decades. The range of efforts for helping older persons has

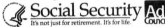

Just who is eligible for Social Security?

More people than you think. Because Social Security isn't just for retirement.

If a serious illness or injury prevents you from working, it can provide disability payments. If your life is cut short, it will pay survivors benefits.

Now you can find out what your benefits might be. Write to Dept. 74, Pueblo, Colorado 81009, to apply for your own Personal Earnings and Benefit Estimate Statement.

Social Security Ad Council
It's not just for retirement. It's for life.

FIGURE 8-12

Social security, enacted in the United States in 1935 as a major source of income security for elderly people, also provides survivors' benefits for dependents and disability payments for injured workers.

Source: Social Security Administration.

broadened. It now includes attempts to meet both personal needs, such as shelter, medical care, and employment training, and group needs, such as better transportation and other community improvements. The evolution of governmental policies toward the aged can be traced to factors ranging from the efforts of individual reformers to various societal changes brought about by long-term economic, demographic, and ideological trends. Organizations such as political parties, labor unions, and professional and commercial organizations have found reason either to advocate or oppose governmental action toward the aging. As they grow in number and in proportion to the total voting-age population, the political power of the aging grows. The costs of health and pension support for the elderly will grow concomitantly (Figure 8-13).

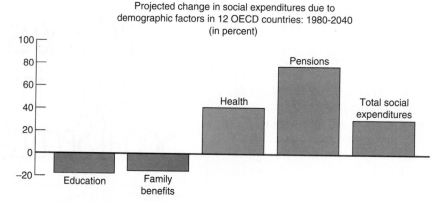

Projected change in social expenditures due to
demographic factors in 12 OECD countries: 1980-2040
(in percent)

Note: The 12 countries are Australia, Belgium, Canada, Denmark, France, Germany, Italy,
Japan, the Netherlands, Sweden, the United Kingdom, and the United States.

FIGURE 8-13

The reductions in educational and family benefit costs will be more than offset by the growing numbers of elderly people requiring health and pension support in the 12 countries of the Organization for Economic Cooperation and Development, including Canada and the United States.

Source: Bureau of the Census: *Global aging: comparative indicators and future trends,* Washington, DC, 1991, Economics and Statistics Administration, U.S. Department of Commerce.

COMMUNITY HEALTH PROMOTION PROGRAMS

Functional programs can best be formulated on the community level. At more distant bureaucratic levels, planned programs often fail to touch individual elderly citizens and their families. Of necessity, the national, state, or provincial program will be removed from the individual and will be less sensitive to local variations in needs and perceptions.

A community program for the elderly has three goals: (1) public education in the field of adult health, (2) integration of all resources and forces in the community that have a service to offer elderly persons, and (3) the acquisition and provision of necessary services that the community does not now have available. A community health agency must be designated to determine health promotion needs and the approaches that should be used. If the official community health center does not provide medical service, it may serve as a center for information, coordination, and health promotion.

The community program must include public health education. The public needs to understand the nature of aging and the phenomena associated with it. The public should understand what can be done to prevent some of the premature deterioration of aging and should have an understanding of measures for the prevention of diseases and disabilities of the advancing years. The public needs to be informed of the importance of self-care and medical supervision and of the contribution that various individuals, agencies, and self-help groups have to make to the elderly citizens of the community. Perhaps most important, the public needs to adjust its perceptions of aging and of the elderly.

To promote the health of elderly people, a community program must provide for the diagnosis, treatment, hospitalization, and rehabilitation of those elderly people who have some disability. It must provide for activities that elderly people can enjoy through participation. The program should also provide some means through which elderly people who are unable to pay for professional services may receive the services required.

Most elderly people in a community are self-sufficient or have members of their immediate family who can provide advice or assistance, but some have no such source of aid. These individuals would greatly benefit from an effective community health program for the elderly.

Nutrition Programs for the Elderly

Community nutrition policies and programs promote better health among older people through health education, counseling, and the limited delivery of food services. Nutrition programs help reduce the isolation of older persons by offering them an opportunity to participate in community activities and to combine food and friendship.

Reasons some elderly people do not eat adequately include: (1) insufficient income; (2) insufficient skills to select and prepare nourishing and well-balanced meals; (3) dental problems; (4) limited mobility; and (5) feelings of rejection and isolation that obliterate the incentive necessary to prepare and eat a meal alone. Such physiological, psychological, and social and economic changes can cause malnutrition and further physical, mental, and sensory deterioration.

Community provision of meals in group settings include schools, churches, community centers, senior citizen centers, public housing, and other public and nonprofit facilities where additional supportive services may be available. Outreach programs identify those older persons most in need. Escort and transportation services bring participants to nutrition program sites.

The nutrition program may provide home-delivered meals to participants who from time to time are unable to attend the meal service site. The program recognizes the need for a network of supportive services, including health services, information and referral, escort services, health and welfare counseling, and consumer education. Nutrition projects act as centers of activity, attracting older persons to a place where, in addition to getting a nourishing meal, they have the opportunity to receive these other services, as well as advice on such important matters as legal rights, housing, shopping assistance, income maintenance, and crime prevention. Older persons also have the opportunity for socialization and recreation and for volunteer service to others. Under the terms of the Older Americans Act, states are encouraged to make nutrition program projects part of the system of services for the elderly.

Health and nutrition education can make older persons, project staff members, and volunteers aware of the relative values of food and its contribution to health and well-being, and can thereby influence selection, purchase, and preparation. Increased public and professional awareness can also lead to advocacy for policy changes at the local level and organization for advocacy at the state or provincial and national levels.

Community programs must give highest priority to low-income persons 60 years of age and over and their spouses, and others who are determined to be in great need. These may include minorities, native populations, and persons who speak little English. Meal sites need to be located in urban and rural areas that have high proportions of older persons in these categories.

Participants should be given an opportunity to contribute to all or part of the cost of the meal. The nutrition program advisory council, which should contain a participant majority, establishes either a contribution schedule based on resources or a single flat sum as a guide to the size of contribution. Each participant determines what he or she is able to contribute. Contributions are received in such a manner that the amount given is known only to the contributor.

While the quantity of food required by the person in the later years of life is not as great as in the earlier years, the qualitative needs are just as important. Diversity of proteins and adequate vitamins and minerals should be included in each day's diet. Food should be attractive because the sense of taste becomes dulled with age. In the later years of life the output of digestive enzymes is reduced and the rate of digestion is much slower. For this reason, many elderly people prefer eating smaller but more frequent meals.

Other Health Promotion Programs

The immediate benefits of smoking cessation (Figure 8-14) and of increasing physical activity are more dramatic for the elderly than for other age groups. A national objective for the year 2000 states that the proportion of adults 65 years and older who regularly participate in vigorous activities that promote the development and maintenance of cardiorespiratory fitness, for 3 or more times per week, 20 or more minutes per occasion should increase from

7.5% to 20%. Vigorous is defined as 60% or greater of maximal cardiorespiratory capacity.

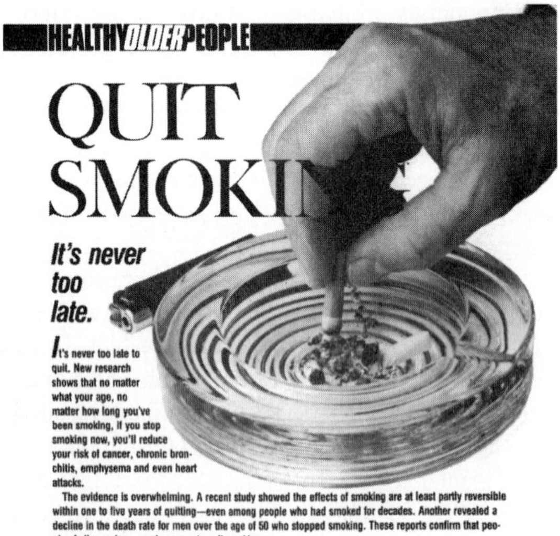

Communities need to support programs that will promote physical activity for older citizens. Efforts might include developing focal points, such as senior centers, to coordinate physical activity services to older citizens. Health care institutions such as hospitals and nursing homes should provide encouragement, equipment, and facilities to enhance the physical activity of their staff and clients. Designs for all multifamily housing should incorporate facilities such as exercise rooms or open spaces and gardens to provide physical activity options.

Moderate activity is highly desirable for the normal elderly person. It can be beneficial in producing a near-maximum level of functioning for the individual. Activity can be purposeful and productive, such as tending a garden. Moderately paced exertion can be rewarding physically, emotionally, and socially.

Intervals of rest during the day should be coordinated with the tasks or activities requiring physical exertion. Midmorning, noon, and midafternoon rest periods will be adequate for some, but others may need more frequent rest. Some elderly individuals do very well without any particular rest periods; this is true of the somewhat restless individual who prefers to be occupied with some task.

Elderly people often go to bed earlier and rise earlier than is the custom of the general adult population. Some seem to require less sleep than they did in earlier years.

FIGURE 8-14
The benefits of quitting cigarettes are notable even in old age. This public service advertisement was issued by a national coalition on Healthy Older People.
Source: Office of Disease Prevention and Health Promotion, Public Health Service, U.S. Department of Health and Human Services.

Injury Prevention Programs

Physical injury and accidental death rates increase in the old-age groups. Slowed reaction time, poor vision, and the inability to adjust readily to changing situations make the old person more injury-prone than younger individuals. Conditions in the home should be made as safe as possible. Living on one floor is an effective safety measure, because falls on stairs constitute a frequent cause of death for old people. Well-lighted rooms and hallways, and even the use of continuous dim light through the night, can be effective safety measures. Old people also have a high fatality rate in motor vehicle-pedestrian accidents. Loss of sensitivity in the skin can result in scalds and **hypothermia.**

Examples of injury prevention programs for the elderly and other high-risk groups will be presented in Chapter 13.

MEDICAL AND LONG-TERM CARE SERVICES

Older people require proportionately more medical services than the general population. Most communities can provide the variety of medical skills necessary for the more complex problems of the aged by calling on the services of the various specialists available in the area. Interest in the health aspects of geriatrics has been rising, as evidenced by increasing numbers of physicians and other professionals who are members of the American Geriatrics Society or the Gerontological Society. Unfortunately, medical and nursing students have shown resistance to working with geriatric patients.

Special geriatrics clinics have been established. Their goal has been to offer coordinated medical and social services to the population of independent, working elderly to aid them in retaining their independence. In addition to providing important diagnostic services to the elderly, the geriatrics clinic is able to formulate a continuing program of health supervision for its clients. These efforts and special projects are most laudable, but as yet most communities rely on the general hospital and medical services that are already available.

Nursing Homes

Although it may be saddening to note that more than 1 million elderly people in the United States are in nursing homes, it is at the same time encouraging to note that over 19 million are not. Most of the geriatric concern has been with the 5% who are institutionalized. This has tended to bias popular and professional perceptions of what old age is like.

Public health departments have been lax in licensing nursing homes in the United States. All 50 states have licensing laws, but their requirements are generally below the minimum standards recommended by national organizations (see Table 8-4). The present situation still calls for legal action for providing desirable conditions through licensing of nursing homes.

Nursing homes should be affiliated with and should cooperate with general hospitals. In such an arrangement, physicians will have elderly patients moved from the general hospital to the less expensive nursing home, where they know the chronically ill can receive the necessary nursing care. Such an arrangement also means a greater likelihood that the majority of the patients in the nursing home will be under medical supervision.

Home Care

Physicians, nurses, occupational therapists, and social workers agree that the aging who are ill should be cared for in their own homes as long as possible. Obviously, certain situations make this impossible or undesirable. But when home conditions are acceptable, some chronically ill patients can be as well taken care of in the home as in the nursing home or the hospital. Visiting nursing services can be used to good advantage, especially when only part-time nursing service is necessary.

Home health care services can include part-time nursing care, physical therapy, home-delivered meals, transportation and escort services, and other programs of assistance and care. Families and professionals are well advised to explore home health care services available in the community before contracting with a nursing or custodial home (Figure 8-15).

TABLE 8-4

Nursing Home Visits Checklist

This checklist for assessing nursing homes can be used by families seeking the best arrangement they can afford, or by professionals who make referrals to nursing homes.

Home A: _____

Home B: _____

Home C: _____

	Home A	Home B	Home C
Location			
1. Is the home close to family and friends?	( )	( )	( )
Layout			
1. Do residents have places to put personal possessions?	( )	( )	( )
2. Is there adequate privacy in bathrooms and around the beds?	( )	( )	( )
3. Are there places for private conversations with visitors?	( )	( )	( )
4. Are there handrails and grab bars in the halls and bathrooms?	( )	( )	( )
5. Are there sufficient smoke detectors and fire extinguishers?	( )	( )	( )
6. Are exits clearly marked and unobstructed?	( )	( )	( )
7. Are there call buttons for each bed and in the bathrooms?	( )	( )	( )
8. Is there additional heat available in the bathrooms?	( )	( )	( )
9. Does the home have a lounge for the residents?	( )	( )	( )
10. Is there an outdoor area that residents use?	( )	( )	( )
11. Is there a public telephone available for residents' use?	( )	( )	( )
Cleanliness			
1. Is the home generally clean and orderly?	( )	( )	( )
2. Are employees clean and well-groomed?	( )	( )	( )
3. Is the home reasonably free of unpleasant odors?	( )	( )	( )
4. Are the bathrooms sanitary?	( )	( )	( )
5. Is the kitchen clean?	( )	( )	( )

	Home A	Home B	Home C
Food			
1. Are weekly menus posted?	( )	( )	( )
2. Is the menu varied, but with balanced, nutritious meals?	( )	( )	( )
3. Are special diets provided for residents who need them?	( )	( )	( )
4. Are adequate between-meal and bedtime snacks provided?	( )	( )	( )
5. Does the food taste good?	( )	( )	( )
6. Are serving sizes ample?	( )	( )	( )
7. Are seconds available?	( )	( )	( )
Atmosphere			
1. Is the general atmosphere of the home warm and cheerful?	( )	( )	( )
2. Are the residents treated with the dignity accorded a guest?	( )	( )	( )
3. Are the staff and administrators courteous, cheerful and enthusiastic?	( )	( )	( )
4. Do residents speak favorably of the home?	( )	( )	( )
5. Is there a varied program of recreational, cultural, and intellectual activities?	( )	( )	( )
6. Are there opportunities to attend religious services both in and out of the home?	( )	( )	( )
Administration			
General			
1. Is the home certified for Medicare?	( )	( )	( )
2. Is the home certified for Medicaid?	( )	( )	( )
3. Does the home have a current state license?	( )	( )	( )
4. Does the administrator have a current state license?	( )	( )	( )
5. Are all costs clearly specified in terms of amount *and* in terms of coverage?	( )	( )	( )

TABLE 8-4
Nursing Home Visits Checklist—cont'd.

	Home A	Home B	Home C	NOTES:
6. Are refunds available for unused services?	( )	( )	( )	
7. Are there written procedures for handling residents' personal funds and valuables?	( )	( )	( )	
8. Was a written statement of residents' rights provided?	( )	( )	( )	
Medical				
1. Is a physician available at all times in case of emergency?	( )	( )	( )	
2. Does the home have an agreement with a nearby hospital in case of emergency?	( )	( )	( )	
3. Are there established procedures for reporting unusual incidents involving the resident to the resident's family?	( )	( )	( )	
4. What is the health care staff-to-resident ratio on the wing?	( )	( )	( )	

Source: Texas Attorney General's Office: *Selecting a nursing home,* Austin, 1992, Attorney General of Texas.

Elderly day care programs have become more common. Many of them include health services such as medication administration, podiatric services, rehabilitation therapies, dietary counseling, and mental and recreational services and programs.

Consumer Issues in Health Care for the Elderly

Nursing homes. The Health Care Financing Administration, which is the U.S. agency with responsibility for Medicare and Medicaid, issued a 75-volume report in December 1988 evaluating the 15,000 American nursing homes then caring for the more than 1.5 million Medicare and Medicaid patients. For each home the report bluntly stated "not met" for criteria similar to those in Table 8-4 if the nursing home was deficient on that standard. More than 40% mishandled food; 29 percent of them improperly dispensed medicines; 25% fell short on isolation techniques to prevent the spread of infection. About 2400 of the 15,000 met all of the 32 health, safety, and care standards. This "consumer guide" to nursing homes was helpful to communities seeking to improve their services and to people looking for a nursing home.

Health insurance. The elderly as health care consumers also face an array of confusing and difficult choices with health insurance. A federal health insurance program was added to Medicare in 1989 to cover "catastrophic" illnesses, costing some elderly people an additional $800 per year as a federal income-tax surcharge. Many viewed this as a discrim-

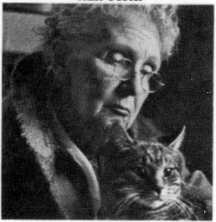

LIKE MOST PEOPLE HER AGE, SHE BELONGS IN A HOME. HER OWN.

For 30 years, it's been her home. But now, she could end up in a nursing home. Simply because she could use a hand shopping for groceries.

Who do you turn to when you're all alone?

She got help through a volunteer shopping program for the elderly. They got help from the United Way. All because the United Way got help from you.

You helped support a program that provides a volunteer to do the shopping for a 79-year-old woman. A woman who wants nothing more than to live out her life in the home she loves.

United Way

It brings out the best in all of us.

FIGURE 8-15

The United Way in most communities seeks to support independent living for elders. Home health care expenditures rose by 30% between 1991 and 1992, compared with an 11.5% increase in overall national health care expenditures.

Source: United Way and Advertising Council.

inatory tax on the elderly. Organizations in the following year succeeded in repealing the law.

Out-of-pocket health costs. The elderly spend approximately 18% of their income—an average of $2,566 in 1990—on health costs. The costs not covered by Medicare, Medicaid, private health insurance, or government amount to 13% of the total. Elderly health care payments went up 12% per year between 1980 and 1990, while their income went up 7.1% per year.

Rehabilitation

Ill or disabled elderly people need more than custodial care. Chronic disease hospitals are not the answer, because they tend to create the conception of lifelong disability. The general hospital can usually provide all of the services necessary for the care and treatment of the elderly patient, without creating the impression of cold-storage institutionalization. Hospital patients should have a combination of medical care and rehabilitation to prepare them for their mode of living after they are discharged from the hospital. Both nursing and social services are necessary before patients are transferred home. The elderly person may need some supervision to make a reasonable adjustment to a normal living routine. Even when the elderly person lives with other members of the family, social work services can be of value in aiding all concerned to understand how to meet the elderly person's needs.

COMMUNICATING WITH THE ELDERLY

Like all members of society, old people must be able to read and grasp the meaning of a great deal of printed and optically projected material if they are to maintain a self-sufficient life-style. But it is not generally recognized that older persons' lack of comprehension, when it occurs, may result from a sensory rather than intellectual failure.

Print Media

One aspect of this sensory failure is that type style, type size, and layout of printed materials affect an older person's reading speed, ease of reading, and interest in written materials. Older persons both prefer and can read faster when shown roman rather than other styles of type. Roman type may be found in newspapers and many textbooks. Increasing the type size beyond a certain point does not facilitate reading for older people.

We know very little about specific benefits or costs of the communications media used to provide information about social services. Isolation from communication flows sometimes accompanies physical isolation. Communication by print—fliers, pamphlets, notices, newspapers, and the like—is the least effective substitute for face-to-face contact between older people and those responsible for interpreting laws, regulations, eligibility, and entitlements.

Electronic Media

Communications other than face-to-face communication are not necessarily inferior. Modern communications media, including the telephone, allow telecommunications in place of transportation, sharing of valuable human resources among underserved populations, and other benefits. These media provide solutions ready and waiting to alleviate problems.

Over half the services provided to clients by public social service agencies are information exchanges of one sort or another and hence are directly amenable to enhancement by telecommunications. Older adults watch television, on the average, 3 hours per day—slightly less than the average for the total population. On the other hand, adult television viewing increases with age. A majority of old people consider television viewing as an important recreational activity; in fact, television viewing ranks first among all activities of the elderly, according to some surveys. It has been reported that old people prefer personal, nonfiction programs in which people like themselves play important roles, either as members of the studio audience or as contestants.

Radio and television have brought religious services into the home for elderly shut-ins, and this has been supplemented by the churches' providing additional, more personal, services to the shut-ins. These personalized services need not be of a strictly religious nature. Church people are in a strategic position to give the type of personal service that will help the older shut-in to attain and maintain the frame of mind and general well-being so essential to physical and mental health.

Telephone Contact

Telephone reassurance provided by daily telephone contact with an older person who might otherwise have no outside contact for long periods of time can be an important service. Persons receiving telephone reassurance may be called at a predetermined time each day. If the person does not answer, help is immediately sent to his or her home; usually a neighbor, relative, or nearby police or fire station is asked to make a personal check. Such details are worked out when a person begins receiving this service. Telephone reassurance has been credited with saving many lives by the quick dispatching of medical help. In one case, an alert caller noticed a slight slurring of speech in a client she talked with regularly. Although the client reported no difficulties, the caller reported the slurred speech to her supervisor,

---

Out of Sight, Out of Mind?

The older woman is far more likely than the older man to live alone. This isolation impairs communication, making both the diagnosis and the treatment of physical and mental illness more difficult in older women. Many women may be diagnosed as suffering from senile dementia or Alzheimer's disease when in fact they are lonely, isolated, and depressed. How do loss of vision or hearing, which are common health problems of the aged, lead to misunderstandings and misdiagnoses?

who sent someone to check the situation. The client had suffered a heart spasm and was rushed to the hospital in time. Telephone reassurance generally costs little and can be provided by callers of any age, from teenagers to older people themselves. It is sponsored by a variety of organizations and agencies in the United States ranging from women's clubs to police departments. For example, in one community, residents of a home for the aged make calls to the elderly living alone. In another, older persons who cannot leave their homes are called daily by senior center members. In a third, a hospital auxiliary and the Business and Professional Women's Club make daily calls.

TRANSPORTATION

The elderly require access to the services, facilities, resources, and opportunities necessary for existence. Transportation, whether for visiting and traveling, taking the individual to a health service or facility, or bringing a service provider to the individual, influences the effectiveness of other services for the elderly. Basic priorities and accompanying funding for transportation will remain inadequate, forcing communities to choose between improvements for the elderly or improvements for all travelers.

Mass Transit

Mass transportation systems have become increasingly important with the growing problems of the automobile as the primary mode of transportation. Automobile ownership declines with age. This decline is mostly a result of the lower incomes of the elderly, but it is also influenced by their decreasing physical or psychological ability to drive. Studies indicate a greater dependence on walking among the aged, but walking is limited by the inadequacy of pedestrian accommodations and security. Studies also indicate that public transportation is least adequate for those most in need of it: the physically

frail, individuals with no friends or relatives to drive them, minority group members, and the poor.

Many communities and civic organizations either now offer or are experimenting with various forms of assistance to help meet the transportation needs of the older population. In European countries, public transportation systems are far better suited to the needs of the elderly than those of North America.

U.S. Federal and State Support

The National Mass Transportation Act of 1974 included a number of provisions that aided older riders. The act required that any public transit system receiving capital assistance funds from the Urban Mass Transportation Administration of the U.S. Department of Transportation charge half fare or less for the elderly. Other programs administered by the Urban Mass Transportation Administration include research and development grants to test innovative approaches to transportation problems and funding for capital assistance and the acquisition of vehicles and other needed equipment.

Several other avenues of assistance can be used to provide transportation services for the elderly. Under Title III of the Older Americans Comprehensive Services Amendments, which authorizes support for state and community programs, the U.S. Administration on Aging awards grants to the designated state agencies on aging to assist state and local agencies in the development of comprehensive and coordinated services to the elderly. The designated state agency can identify potential sources of funding for transportation, provide advice on how best to plan for and implement a project, and coordinate efforts with other agencies and organizations that might be involved in planning and supporting transportation projects.

Community Programs

Many communities operate transportation projects. Some are relatively inexpensive, using volunteer drivers in small towns and rural areas. Others use sophisticated demand-responsive or regularly scheduled transit vehicles, often designed to meet the special needs of the elderly.

Free or reduced fares on public transportation vehicles are enabling the elderly in many parts of North America and Europe to travel during midday, night, and weekend hours. Many areas that permit older people to ride free during off-peak transit hours also offer reduced fares during rush hours.

One community mobilized service to the elderly and handicapped where little or none existed before. Eligible riders have access to specially equipped minibuses that offer door-to-door service, nominal fares, and transportation by advance reservation, weekly subscription, or telephone request, as well as charter service.

participation in social activities and associations cannot be offered as a substitute for health care.

Zest for living is extremely important in the health of the elderly. On a large-group basis, concerts, lectures, dancing, parties, excursions, and outings can be highly important in the lives of the elderly and can contribute measurably to their outlook. Checkers, chess, cards, and shuffleboard are popular games that can be organized and promoted among the elderly. Social action groups such as the Gray Panthers provide a vehicle for productive civic participation. Communities without such organizations should provide avenues for the development and promotion of a zest for living. This aids older people in their feeling of security, which is a primary need of every person, but it also brings returns to the community in the continuing participation of the aging in community life.

LEISURE-TIME ACTIVITIES

The value of recreational and social participation is generally acknowledged, but for no group are these of greater health value than for the aging (see Chapter 10). With a great deal of newly found time on their hands, the elderly need activities that will occupy them profitably and enjoyably. Some have business interests, trade skills, voluntary association memberships, or a garden to occupy their attention and time, but many are in need of help in developing satisfying leisure-time activities. Most of the elderly seek and enjoy the companionship of others. A community can provide for individual instruction for recreation purposes, but provision for instruction and supervision on a group basis is usually more practical.

Small groups of elderly people can take up arts and crafts, music, dramatics, poetry, and creative writing. The mutual encouragement, the sociability, and the general elation that come from such participation can do more for many of these people than can the physician or the hospital. On the other hand,

SUMMARY

Community responsibility for the health of the aging population encompasses concern for the citizen's total living. A community health program for the elderly should include or take into account medical services, hospital facilities, nursing home services, housing conditions, health education, health counseling, recreation programs, and individual and group participation in productive and enjoyable activities. The community health department alone cannot carry the whole program, but it can be the agency that integrates all community resources having a contribution for the elderly. Social service, education, communication, and transportation agencies can complement the health department and initiate action necessary for the promotion of the well-being of the elderly.

The compression of morbidity thesis and the goal of extending active life expectancy lead us to seek points of intervention for health promotion that will head off the downward, cumulative spiral characterizing the degenerative process. The most effective prevention, as usual, would be early prevention, but it is difficult to mount programs, capture resources, and sustain the attention and motivation of people who have yet no symptoms and for whom the benefits of the recommended actions are years away. Conventional public health strategies do not fit the needs of the elderly because the early onset of most conditions cannot be identified, incidence data are largely unavailable, and community-wide interventions are too costly and inefficient in reaching the dispersed elderly population.

Health promotion programs designed and evaluated to date have been directed primarily at more affluent people, leaving the search alive for approaches that use the development of community ties, and those that use early warning signs or life events as points of intervention. Clearly identified transition points such as retirement, relocation, and widowhood enable professionals to intervene in anticipation of the adaptations people and communities need to make in their lifestyles in order to adjust. Successful adjustment reduces the development of dysfunctional coping and the harm to health that usually follows. This anticipatory approach to transitions serves both the primary prevention purposes of health promotion and the health enhancement purposes, strengthening the coping abilities of older people.

4. To what extent do changes in the economy affect thepopulation age distribution of a county or a state?
5. What factors are essential if an individual is to be relatively "young" at age 75?
6. What is the general social status of the elderly people of your community and what is the significance of their social status in terms of their health?
7. To what extent is the community health program for aging people primarily a program of curing illness rather than of promoting health?
8. What does your state or provincial health department have in the way of an agency and a program for the promotion of the health of the elderly?
9. What special activities in the interest of better health for the elderly are carried on by your official community health department?
10. What are the voluntary health agencies of your community doing on behalf of the health of elderly citizens?
11. What are the contributions of other institutions in your community, such as churches, to the health and general well-being of the senior citizen?
12. How interested in and how well informed about matters relating to the health of elderly people is the general public in your community?
13. What would be a good routine of daily living for a man or woman of age 70 without impairments?
14. Why are sensory losses so important to the elderly?

QUESTIONS FOR REVIEW

1. What are some signs of "ageism" in your community?
2. Why must gerontology concern itself with social and psychological aging as well as with physiological aging?
3. List 10 persons of your acquaintance who are over 65 years of age. What percentage have good health, what percentage have fair health, what percentage are ill but up and around, and what percentage are disabled? What percentage have health impairments that could be corrected or at least reduced?

READINGS

Chatman EA: *The information world of retired women,* Westport, Conn, 1992, Greenwood.

Highlights the information needs of older women, identifying their help-seeking behaviors and the role professionals can play in supporting them.

Institute of Medicine: *The second 50 years: promoting health and preventing disability,* Washington, DC, 1990, National Academy Press.

This report proposes specific strategies and priorities to do more to promote health and prevent disability in the elderly.

Nordin R, Hamid AM, Adnan WAW: Preparing the young to look after the old, *World Health Forum* 13: 300, 1992.

The number of Malaysian people aged 60 or more has increased steadily. This article describes an innovative introduction of geriatrics to the medical curriculum in that country.

Schaie KW, Blazer D, House JS, editors: *Aging, health behaviors, and health outcomes,* Hillsdale, NJ, 1992, Erlbaum.

This collection includes analyses of social stratification, social structure, and behavior as these affect aging and health status in the general population and in minorities.

BIBLIOGRAPHY

Andreopoulos S, Hogness JR, editors: *Health care for an aging society,* New York, 1989, Churchill Livingstone.

Bellin C: Relocating adult day care: its impact on persons with dementia, *J Gerontol Nurs* 16:11, 1990.

Betancourt RL: *Retirement and men's physical and mental health,* New York and London, 1991, Garland.

Bureau of the Census: *Global aging: comparative indicators and future trends,* Washington, DC, 1991, Economics and Statistics Administration, U.S. Department of Commerce.

Canada pension plan, old age security act, and pension benefits standards act, with regulations, ed 9, Don Mills, Ontario, 1992, CCH Canadian Limited.

Chappell NL, Segall A, Lewis DG: Gender and helping networks among day hospital and senior centre participants, *Can J Aging* 9:220, 1990.

Committee on a National Research Agenda on Aging, Division of Health Promotion and Disease Prevention, Institute of Medicine: *Extending life, enhancing life: a national research agenda on aging,* Washington, DC, 1991, National Academy Press.

Denke MA, Grundy SlM: Hypercholesterolemia in elderly persons: resolving the treatment dilemma, *Ann Int Med* 112:780, 1990.

Ebrahim S, Williams J: Assessing the effects of a health promotion programme for elderly people, *J Public Health Med* 14:199, 1992.

Erben R, Franzkowiak P, Wenzel E: Assessment of the outcomes of health intervention, *Soc Sci Med* 35:359, 1992.

Fiatarone MA, Marks EC, Ryan ND et al: High-intensity strength training in nonagenarians: effects on skeletal muscle, *JAMA* 263:3029, 1990.

Fries JF, Green LW, Levine S: Health promotion and the compression of morbidity, *Lancet* 1:105, 1989.

Fulmer TT: The debate over dependency as a relevant predisposing factor in elder abuse and neglect, *J Elder Abuse Neglect* 2:51, 1990.

Glickstein JK, Neustadt GK: *Reimbursable geriatric service delivery: a functional maintenance therapy system,* Frederick, Md, 1992, Aspen.

Gordon RM, Tomita SK: The reporting of elder abuse and neglect: mandatory or voluntary, *Canada's Mental Health* 38:1, 1990.

Green LW: Some challenges to health services research on children and the elderly, *Health Serv Res* 19:793, 1984.

Green LW, Gottlieb NH: Health promotion for the aging population: approaches to extending active life expectancy. In Andreopoulos S, Hogness JR, editors: *Health care for an aging society,* New York, 1989, Churchill Livingstone.

Kapp MB: *Ethical aspects of health care for the elderly,* Westport, Conn, 1992, Greenwood Press.

Kohn M, Donley C, Wear D, editors: *Literature and aging: an anthology,* Kent, Oh, 1992, Kent State University Press.

Leutz WN, Capitman JA, MacAdam M et al: *Care for frail elders: developing community solutions.* Westport, Conn, 1992, Greenwood Press.

Levkoff S, Green LW, Hansel N: Changes in the cycle of lifestyle and aging: implications for health promotion. *Spec Care Dent* 4:130, 1984.

McDonald PL: *Elder abuse and neglect in Canada,* Toronto, 1991, Butterworths.

Minkler M, Estes CL, editors: *Critical perspectives on aging: the political and moral economy of growing old,* New York, 1990, Baywood.

Minkler M, Robertson A: The ideology of ''age/race wars'': deconstructing a social problem, *Ageing and Society* 11:1, 1991.

Moschis GP: *Marketing to older consumers,* Westport, Conn, 1992, Quorum.

Parkerson G, Broadhead WE, Tse CKJ: The Duke Health Profile: a 17-item measure of health and dysfunction, *Med Care* 28:1056, 1990.

Patla AE, Frank JS, Winter DA: Balance control in the elderly: implications for clinical assessment and rehabilitation, *Can J Public Health Suppl* 2:29, 1992.

Pillemer K, Bachman-Prehn R: Helping and hurting: predictors of maltreatment of patients in nursing homes, *Research on Aging* 13:74, 1991.

Robertson A: The politics of Alzheimer's disease: a case study in apocalyptic demography, *Int J Health Services* 20:429, 1990.

Sandler IN, West SG, Baca L et al: Linking empirically based theory and evaluation: the family bereavement program, *Am J Community Psychol* 20:491, 1992.

Savishinsky JS: *The ends of time: life and work in a nursing home,* Westport, Conn, 1991, Bergin & Garvey.

Wagner EH, LaCroix AZ, Buchner DM et al: Effects of physical activity on health status in older adults I: observational studies, *Ann Rev Pub Health* 13:451, 1992.

Wahl JA: Elder abuse: the hidden crime, Toronto, 1991, Advocacy Centre for the Elderly and Community Legal Education Ontario.

PART THREE

· ·

Promoting Community Health

In this part, the strategies for health promotion in the community are outlined, beginning with community mental and social health, stress, and suicide prevention. Community recreation and fitness and the development and support of healthful life-styles and policies round out this presentation of health promotion.

Health promotion goes beyond health education in its emphasis on social and environmental supports for individual, organizational, and community action. It seeks to make the community conducive to health by altering the forces making it difficult for individuals to maintain their own health.

Chapter 9

Community Mental and Social Health

❖

Health is a state of complete physical, mental and social well-being and not merely the absence of disease or infirmity.
WORLD HEALTH ORGANIZATION

OBJECTIVES

When you finish this chapter, you should be able to:

- Analyze and assess the mental health concerns and needs of a community
- Identify strategies appropriate to address those needs
- Identify resources in the community to support a comprehensive mental and social health program

---

Communities have learned to deal with less fear and superstition with mental health and mental disorders. The prejudices once associated with ''madness'' have given way to more enlightened and tolerant perspectives on the full range of stresses in daily living, problems of coping, emotional setbacks during times of critical transitions and events, and minor neuroses and compulsions that afflict everyone at some time. The gradient from these common states of mind to peak performance and happiness at one extreme and the depths of psychotic disorientation and antisocial violence at the other reflects the distribution of mental health and mental illness in a community.

Research on the brain, the nervous system, and emotions can be applied to organize a highly effective community mental health program. Such a program first assesses the social problems or quality-of-life concerns of a community, considering what the people perceive to be their own priorities for improving the quality of their lives. Applying knowledge from the sciences of mental health and public health to the subjective concerns of a community is the essence of community mental and social health.

In this chapter we will discuss the concept of mental health; the epidemiology of mental distress, illness, and disorder; issues in promoting mental health; the social pathology of divorce, suicide, and violence; resources for community action in mental health; and provisions for the rehabilitation of those who have been mentally ill. The control of stress and violence in the community, now considered a priority objective of many health agencies, will be included. Community actions to control violence and the abuse of alcohol and drugs will be considered in Chapters 12 and 13.

CONCEPTS OF MENTAL AND SOCIAL HEALTH

The term **mental health** refers to the emotional and social well-being as well as the psychological resources of the individual. Emotions are feelings with physiological as well as psychological components. Anger, for example, is more than a mental state; it evokes physiological responses, some of which are beneficial in preparing the individual to cope with circumstances. Over time, however, any chronic emotional state or stress becomes a strain on the body's organs and physiological systems. Thus, physiology both contributes to mental health and is affected by it. Stress also underlies many of the other behavioral and immunological problems that account for much of the chronic disease and infectious disease in the community. Stress and **coping** (the ability to adjust to stress) influence smoking, drinking, compulsive eating, resistance to infections, reckless driving, and various forms of violence. Interventions to reduce stress and to help people manage stress might represent a powerful program of primary prevention in relation to most of the leading causes of death and disability in modern society.

Modern Definition of Community Mental Health

The Canadian Ministry of Health and Welfare defines mental health as "the capacity of the individ-

---

> ### Spiritual Dimensions of Health
>
> Spirituality may enhance health by providing:
>
> - A personal system of belief or faith that both includes and extends beyond the physical self, giving one a sense of belonging
> - A locus of power and empowerment that provides opportunities for self-realization and community
> - A system of unconditional meaningfulness and purpose that provides the self with a sense of positive direction and the possibility of fulfillment
> - Peace and calm in the face of stressful life circumstances.

ual, the group and the environment to interact with one another in ways that promote subjective well-being, the optimal development and use of mental abilities (cognitive, affective and relational), the achievement of individual and collective goals consistent with justice and the attainment and preservation of conditions of fundamental equality." This interactive definition moves mental health from an individual psychological perspective to a community social-psychological perspective.

The Canadian definition also minimizes the view of mental health as a static trait of the individual but, rather, recognizes it as a dynamic combination of energy, strengths, and abilities of the individual interacting effectively with those of the group, the family, and the community. It places mental health on a continuum from optimal to minimal, with the two ends of the continuum defined by the harmony and integration of individual, group, and environmental factors.

Social Health

Social health must be assessed by community criteria of productivity and quality of life. The goal of "Health for All by the Year 2000" has been declared by the World Health Organization (WHO) and the United Nations Children's Fund (UNICEF) to be a level of health such that all people are capable of working productively and participating actively in the social life of their community.

The breakdown of social health is signaled by problems of family breakdown through divorce or separation, the alienation of young people from community norms, racial and ethnic conflict, crime, high unemployment, homelessness, and growing or persistent poverty accompanied by conspicuous consumption and opulence in the same community. These reflect social pathologies that undermine the foundations for physical and mental health.

No one lives perfectly efficiently, nor does any person experience continuous happiness. The best that most people can do is attain happiness occasionally, and then only for short periods. It would not be fair to label an occasional lapse of "socially considerate behavior" a mental disorder. Imperfect people in an imperfect world means that even the highest level of mental health is not perfect health. Varying degrees of mental health are distributed broadly in the community in accordance with the normal curve characterizing the distribution of most natural phenomena. The goal of community mental health is to shift the average for the population toward more positive levels and to prevent, control, and alleviate suffering at the negative end of the curve.

EPIDEMIOLOGY OF MENTAL HEALTH AND ILLNESS

No two individuals are alike; each person is unique. Yet most of us, in terms of mental health, fit within the overall pattern or range accepted as the usual. This allows for the wide span of individual differences to be found among persons whose conduct is regarded as quaint, faddish, eccentric, or avant-garde, but within accepted patterns. Within this range of mental health we find various points on a continuum.

Distribution of Characteristics

At the extreme positive end, some individuals function efficiently on a high level and derive unusual enjoyment in their living. They encounter frustration, disappointment, and failure, but with a minimum of friction. They freely and effectively use their abilities in harmony with life's demands and gain a maximum of personal satisfaction in their accomplishments.

Another group of individuals, still a standard deviation or more from the population average, adjusts to frustration, disappointment, and failure and experiences only a moderate amount of disturbance from the friction they encounter in life. This is a desirable quality of mental health and perhaps should be rated as good mental health. Doubtless, many of the individuals in this group could attain an even higher level of mental health with better understanding and organized community efforts.

A third group constitutes a majority of people in some populations. These individuals are not mentally disordered, although they do experience occasional or even more frequent emotional upsets. Their distinguishing characteristic is that they seldom seem to reach a dynamic level of adjustment in which they attain considerable accomplishment with an accompanying great amount of enjoyment. They tend to operate in second gear and live rather uninteresting, uninspired, and passive lives. They drag through life, getting a half-measure of what life really has to offer. These individuals possess a fair level of mental health. Many of them, through understanding and community support, could enjoy life more.

At the negative end of the continuum, one or more functional disorders dominate the lives of some people. Some of these disorders, such as depression, strike most people at some times, but for the chronically mentally distressed they persist and make it difficult if not impossible for the individual to carry out the functions of daily living. Functional incapacity strikes most notably in relation to those functions involving interaction with other people.

These mental disorders affect nearly one third of Americans with one or more acute mental disorders over the life span. During any given month, over 15% of Americans will experience some mental disorder (Figure 9-1).

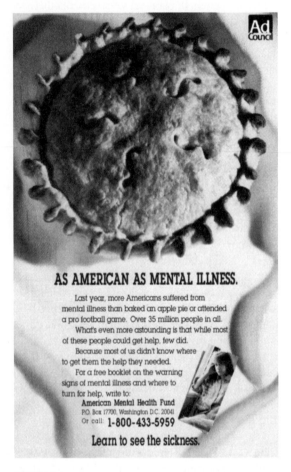

AS AMERICAN AS MENTAL ILLNESS.

Last year, more Americans suffered from mental illness than baked an apple pie or attended a pro football game. Over 35 million people in all.
What's even more astounding is that while most of these people could get help, few did.
Because most of us didn't know where to get them the help they needed.
For a free booklet on the warning signs of mental illness and where to turn for help, write to:
American Mental Health Fund
P.O. Box 17700, Washington D.C. 20041
Or call 1-800-433-5959

Learn to see the sickness.

FIGURE 9-1
Mental illness is more common than most people assume. One out of three Americans will experience some mental disorder during their lifetime. This public service newspaper ad encourages help-seeking behavior. As with most conditions that can become chronic, early diagnosis and treatment or counseling can usually head off the worst outcomes.
Source: Courtesy, American Mental Health Fund.

Long-term community care for the mentally ill has grown to a point where state hospitals now play a minor role. Most states have proprietary hospitals that specialize in the care of the mentally ill, but these facilities are used by a small and declining percentage of mentally ill patients. The severely mentally ill need special medical and hospital services, and this is the province of the psychiatrist or the medical practitioner. **Psychiatry** is that medical specialty that concerns itself with the diagnosis, treatment, and cure of mental disorder.

The present psychosomatic approach to mental illness indicates that the physical and the psychological are interrelated and that mental disorders can have their genesis in a physiological disturbance. Mental illness, which was once regarded as primarily a problem of custodial care, is now regarded as a problem of medical care. This change has come about because of the development of specific medication in the treatment of mental disorder and the concept that a mental hospital is a place where one can go for a short time for treatment. Cold-storage institutionalization has become obsolete, and today mental illness is regarded as truly remediable. Advances in the 1980s indicate that a major breakthrough in the treatment and care of mental disorder has occurred and that the problem is yielding to the united efforts of the many disciplines attacking it. The general public is not yet aware that the success of **chemotherapy** in dealing with the symptoms of mental illness represents a landmark in the progress of the public's health.

Epidemiology of Mental Illness

Epidemiology uses population-based rates to identify the incidence and prevalence of a specific condition, its distribution, and changes in the occurrence of phenomena; from all these factors it infers the likely causes of the condition and suggests points of intervention in the natural history of its spread in the population. Currently, one in five adults suffers from a diagnosable mental disorder, including severe mental illness such as schizophrenia, affective disorders, and substance abuse.

Whether mental disorder is on the increase in the United States is difficult to assess. People today are more inclined to use professional services and facilities. Chemotherapy has not reduced hospital admissions significantly but has shortened the length of stay and increased the use of outpatient services.

Symptoms of Mental Illness

Sometimes inappropriate or extreme behavior can be a warning sign of mental illness. Some of the common warning signs people can learn to recognize:

- Marked personality change over time
- Confused thinking; strange or grandiose ideas
- Excessive anxieties, fears, or suspiciousness; blaming others
- Withdrawal from society, lack of friendliness; abnormal self-centeredness
- Denial of obvious problems; strong resistance to help
- Thinking or talking about suicide
- Numerous, unexplained physical ailments; marked changes in eating and sleeping patterns
- Anger or hostility out of proportion to the situation
- Abuse of alcohol or drugs
- Growing inability to cope with problems and daily activities such as school, job, or personal needs

Today, in America, over 35 million people suffer from some form of mental illness. It is indiscriminate. It strikes people from all walks of life. It affects one in four families. In fact, mental illness is the most prevalent disease in America, more prevalent than cancer, heart, and lung disease combined.

Mental illness is not one disease but a broad classification of many. More than 13 million Americans suffer from anxiety disorders, over 9 million from depression, and over 2½ million from schizophrenic disorders. Twelve million children suffer from au-

tism, depression, hyperkinetic disorders, and other diseases. Drug and alcohol abuse, suicidal tendencies, obsessive-compulsive disorder, Alzheimer's disease, anorexia nervosa, and bulimia can all be classified as mental illness.

Many mental disorders have a biological origin. Schizophrenia and depression, for example, may result from chemical imbalances, deficiencies, or structural abnormalities that can create a malfunction in the brain's signaling system. This awareness has led to new research and progress in the treatment of mental illness.

Using advanced technologies, many chemical imbalances can be corrected, thus controlling the manifestations of many forms of mental illness. These advances have set the stage for new techniques in psychotherapy. With proper treatment, two out of three victims of mental illness can expect to get better and lead productive lives.

Despite these statistics, only one in five people with mental illness seeks professional help, because they do not understand the symptoms and the wide variety of treatments available to them.

Types of Mental Illness

The four most common mental disorders in lifetime incidence and prevalence rates are substance abuse, anxiety disorders, severe cognitive disorders, and affective disorders. These categories have been revised in the 1992 International Classification of Mental and Behavioral Disorders, as shown in Table 9-1. Future statistical tabulations will increasingly classify mental and behavioral disorders as they appear in this table. Within each broader category is contained at least one subcategory associated with biological etiology and one subcategory associated more with environmental or developmental conditions.

Substance abuse. Substance abuse disorders are diagnosed in 16% of all adults over 18 at some time during their lives. Alcohol abuse accounts by far for

TABLE 9-1
Structure of ICD-10 classification of mental and behavioral disorders

Organic mental disorders	
1. Organic and symptomatic disorders	**F0** Organic, including symptomatic mental disorders
2. Alcohol and drug disorders	**F1** Mental and behavioral disorders due to psychoactive and other substance use

Psychotic mental disorders	
1. Schizophrenia and related disorders	**F2** Schizophrenia, schizotypal, and delusional disorders
2. Affective disorders	**F3** Mood (affective) disorders

Neurotic, stress and personality disorders	
1. Neurotic and stress disorders	**F4** Neurotic, stress-related and somatoform disorders
2. Adult personality and behavior disorders	**F5** Behavioral syndromes and mental disorders associated with physiological dysfunction
	F6 Disorders of adult personality and behavior

Disorders of childhood, adolescence, and development	
1. Mental retardation	**F7** Mental retardation
2. Disorders of childhood, adolescence, and development	**F8** Disorders of psychological development
	F9 Behavioral and emotional disorders with onset usually occurring in childhood or adolescence

Source: World Health Organization: *The ICD-10 classification of mental and behavioral disorders,* Geneva, 1992, World Health Organization.

the majority of these disorders, with 13% of Americans likely to have an alcohol problem during their lives. This is more common than abuse of all other drugs combined, for which 6% of Americans will have problems in their lifetime (Figure 9-2). These rates add to more than 16% because some people abuse both alcohol and other drugs. Chapter 11 will address the substance abuse disorders and community strategies to prevent them.

Anxiety disorders. After substance abuse, anxiety disorders make up the second most common lifetime mental illness, but they are even more common at any given point in time. These include phobias, panic disorders, and obsessive-compulsive disorders such as anorexia nervosa. These affect 15% of Americans during the course of their lives and 7% in any given month.

Severe cognitive disorders. Severe impairment of intellect is quite uncommon below the age of 65, except in those with injuries to the head or congenital anomalies. It increases in incidence rapidly after age 65 as a result of strokes and dementia. For example, Alzheimer's disease results in loss of mental functioning as well as previous relationships.

Affective disorders. Chronic depression can be expected to affect 8% of Americans during their lives and 5% at any given time. At least one episode of

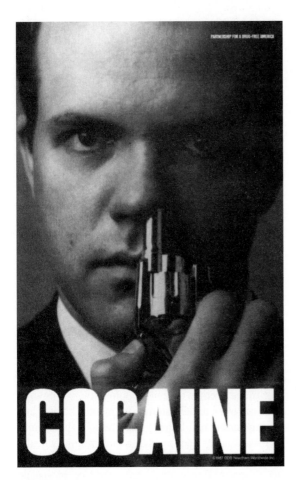

FIGURE 9-2
Partnership for a Drug-Free America, a coalition of public and private organizations, sponsored a public service advertising campaign that obtained $1 million per day worth of donated television air time and print media space during its peak in the early 1990s. This was during a period, however, when cocaine use was declining and alcohol abuse remained a more serious threat to health than all the illegal drugs.
Source: Partnership for a Drug-Free America.

disabling depression will strike an estimated 15% to 25% of the population during their lives. An estimated 20,000 suicides a year are attributable to depression.

Major mental illness affects more than 35 million Americans and costs more than $40 billion in direct care. Another $50 billion will accrue in the indirect costs of mental illness, such as lost work time and wages. More than 9.5 million children under 18 suffer from mental-emotional disorders

Etiology of Mental Illness

Potential risk factors and situations contributing to mental illness include genetic heritage, family history, poverty, chronic illness, disruption of family stability, abuse and neglect, social isolation, substance abuse, or sudden stressful events such as divorce, bereavement, or unemployment. Continuing epidemiological research will help link these risk factors and situations more specifically to the symptoms and diagnoses of mental illness. George Albee, an early leader in prevention for mental health, proposed the following formula for the ratio of difficult life circumstances to available strengths and resources accounting for the incidence of psychopathology:

$$\text{Incidence of psychopathology} = \frac{\text{Organic factors} + \text{Stress} + \text{Exploitation}}{\text{Coping skills} + \text{Self-esteem} + \text{Social support}}$$

A broad range of studies on psychopathology during the past decade promoted the theory that most of the major psychoses stem from a combination of biogenetic and environmental factors. In other words, a genetic susceptibility to schizophrenia and manic-depressive psychosis induces vulnerability within the nervous system. This, together with multiple environmental factors (physical and social), triggers one of these two disorders, each of which affects 1% of the population.

Organic factors. Biological integrity can be compromised by genetic or congenital conditions before birth and by illness, trauma, malnutrition, lead poisoning, and abuse or neglect in childhood. Injury to the head and substance abuse at any point in life can cause permanent damage to mental capacities or neurological functioning. Strokes, sensory decline, and dementia later in life account for most of the adult deterioration in mental capabilities. Studies of adopted offspring and identical twins have strongly suggested genetic factors influencing both schizophrenia and depressive disorders.

Stress. Probably the most pervasive determinant of stress is the confrontation of situations over which the person has, or perceives to have, no control. The same situation will produce more or less stress for different people depending on how much control they have or feel they have over it. Thus a poor person or a person with a disability will encounter more circumstances over which they have little control than will a person with more resources at his or her disposal. When the sources of such stress persist on a daily basis, the individual employs conscious and unconscious defense mechanisms. Chronic and habitual use of some defense mechanisms such as denial, repression, anger, or substance abuse, can lead to dysfunctional coping styles that spill over into all areas of living and interacting with other people.

Social conditions. Stress derives from a combination of stressors and the absence of controls or buffers. Two people confronting the same source of stress (stressor) can have quite different reactions, because one feels alone in dealing with the stress whereas the other feels the support of others. Social support can come immediately from coworkers or classmates in a supportive work or classroom situation or secondarily from a solid family and friendship network to fall back on. Self-help groups have been organized in many communities to provide social support for those who have common problems or needs. These have been especially beneficial for single people living long distances from family and long-standing friends. The average American moves 12 times in a lifetime, according to the Census Bureau. This makes for a nation of uprooted strangers, having few of the natural social supports traditionally provided by extended family and friendship networks. This, in turn, has made the work setting an increasingly important source of social support.

People need to understand why they do certain things, what gives rise to certain emotions, what they must do to adjust to their emotional responses, and what personality qualities they need to fortify or develop. This is the area in which a community mental health program can provide its greatest service to the average citizen. People of the community need a better understanding of mental health, and this education can be provided through the various methods and devices available to community health personnel. Some people need the benefit of mental health counseling; some need guidance in special social and economic problems they may encounter; some need social support. The community needs mental health services just as it needs services that promote physical health. As with physical health, early intervention generally helps prevent more serious problems.

EPIDEMIOLOGY OF SOCIAL PATHOLOGY
Mental Disorder and Social Pathology

Many factors contribute to the **social pathology** of a community, but most seem to relate to a failure in human adjustment. In some instances psychosis, in some cases neurosis, and in other cases inadequate adjustment of an otherwise normal individual is fundamental to a particular social pathology. Mental disorder does not account for all crime, delinquency, alcoholism, drug misuse, narcotic addiction, divorce, child abuse, and suicide. Indeed, of these problems the greatest portion is caused by people who are regarded as normal. Yet, these individuals regarded as normal are generally people with explosive tempers, exaggerated feelings of inadequacy, and marked feelings of persecution, or people who are asocial or antisocial, highly suspicious, overly sensitive, impulsive, overly emotional, unstable, or unable to obtain self-gratification through the usual avenues of life.

Epidemiology of Social Disorder

A review of the extent of social pathology gives some indication of the magnitude of the problem in the United States.

- Approximately one out of every two marriages results in divorce.
- The United States has more than 2 million serious crimes each year.
- About 300,000 children between the ages of 11 and 17 appear in court each year.
- Over 30,000 suicides are recorded each year.
- In a 1991 U.S. survey, 82% of those polled indicated that they ''need less stress in their lives.'' Nearly one in five (18%) said they experience great stress almost every day.
- In recent years suicide has ranked as the eighth leading cause of death for all age groups. It ranks as the third leading cause of death among youths ages 15 to 24. Increasingly, it is also an important cause of death among the aged.
- It is estimated that 200,000 to 4 million cases of child abuse occur each year and that 2000 children die each year in circumstances suggesting abuse or neglect (Figure 9-3).
- Hundreds of thousands of cases of violent, but nonfatal, assault occur each year. These in-

clude instances of spouse and child sexual abuse and rape.
- The death rate from homicide among black males ages 15 to 24 more than doubled in two decades. For black males 25 to 44 years the

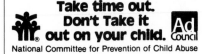

Seven small ways to stop one big problem.

The next time everyday pressures build up to the point where you feel like lashing out—STOP! Here's what to do instead:

1. Take a deep breath. And another. Then remember <u>you</u> are the adult . . .
2. Close your eyes and imagine you're hearing what your child is about to hear.
3. Press your lips together and count to 10. Or, better yet, to 20.
4. Put your child in a time-out chair. (Remember the rule: one time-out minute for each year of age.)
5. Phone a friend.
6. If someone can watch the children, go outside and take a walk.
7. Write for parenting information:
   Parenting
   P.O. Box 2866
   Chicago, IL 60690

Take time out. Don't Take it out on your child.

National Committee for Prevention of Child Abuse

FIGURE 9-3

A national campaign to prevent child abuse provides materials for use in community programs and a national address to which parents can write for parenting information, especially if they do not wish to expose their personal concerns within their own community.

Source: National Committee for Prevention of Child Abuse and Advertising Council.

Technostress and Computers

Computers have contributed enormously to the productivity and efficiency of workers, but they have introduced new sources and symptoms of stress as well. Where they have replaced human contact or provided an excuse to avoid it, computers have added to the alienation or isolation of people from each other. A new syndrome referred to as *technostress* has crept into the world of community health concerns. Some people manifest it as a phobia, fearing the intrusion of computers and related technology in their work. Others manifest technostress as a mania: they become so symbiotically linked to computer technology that they lose a sense of balance about other aspects of their lives. Such obsession or overidentification with the new technology leads to a loss of capacity to feel and relate to others. The importance of these feelings and capacities to community mental health were underlined in a recent campaign by the California Department of Mental Health called "Friends Can Be Good Medicine."

Why should a community health agency concern itself with issues of friendship networks and technostress? Why might these issues be more important in a region such as California than in some other regions?

Objectives for Stress Reduction

- By the year 2000 reduce to less than 35% the proportion of people aged 18 and older who experienced adverse health effects from stress within the past year. Baseline: 42.6% in 1985.

Special target population	1985	2000
People with disabilities	53.5%	40%

- Decrease to no more than 5% the proportion of people aged 18 and older who report experiencing significant levels of stress who do not take steps to reduce or control their stress. Baseline: 21% in 1985.

rate is 12 times the rate for the general population.

Whether these social pathologies are the consequence of many individuals suffering mental disorders, or whether they are causing the mental disorders of individuals can only be conjectured. Causation probably works in both directions, creating a vicious cycle of deteriorating mental and social health in a community.

Control of Stress

Stress is considered an inevitable condition of everyday life. Stress is not necessarily an unhealthy phenomenon; for some people, it may lead to benefits and increased productivity. For others, however, it can have negative consequences by increasing the demands on their emotional resources. Individuals differ in their ability to manage stress. Some people are overwhelmed by trivial crises, yet others are able to maintain their composure even in times of extreme adversity (Figure 9-3).

Excessive and continuous stress can have serious physical and emotional consequences. It contributes to a variety of diseases and conditions, including depression, fatigue, gastrointestinal disorders, coronary heart disease, suicide, homicide, and other violent acts. Stress should be viewed as a risk factor for many health problems—including hypertension, obesity, smoking, and alcohol and drug abuse—and as a direct contributing factor in violent behavior. The many causes of stress and its multitude of health-related outcomes complicate the task of identifying risk factors and reducing the consequences of excessive stress.

Stress and violence control. Stress should be recognized as leading to constructive, self-destructive, and violent health behavior. Individual response to excessive stress is a complex and interactive process. For example, whereas some people react to stress by overeating or drinking too much, others react by abusing members of their family. Unfortunately, many of these coping activities in response to stress do greater damage to health than stress itself. For this reason, stress should be considered a risk factor for many practices of concern to health promotion.

The degree to which stress contributes to most physiological and psychological dysfunctions is largely unknown. There is general agreement, however, that homicide and suicide result from increased levels of stress. In the United States, suicide and homicide account for more than 50,000 deaths annually. Thousands of additional deaths of children are inflicted by parents, usually in response to stress. Mortality statistics, however, reflect only a small proportion of the actual incidence or severity of violent acts in society. For example, the ratio of murders to aggravated assaults is approximately 1 to 17, and estimates of the ratio of suicides to attempted suicides range from 1 to 10 to 1 to 100.

Stress and violence reach all segments of society. In general, however, the economically disadvantaged and certain age groups, such as children, adolescents, young adults, and the elderly, appear to be more vulnerable to violent outcomes of stress. Many of the U.S. national objectives for the year 2000 for control of stress and violent behavior are directed toward these high-risk groups. Other objectives are directed toward a better understanding of the behavioral objectives of stress and increased identification of factors linking stress to health disorders. The boxes in this chapter and in Chapter 13 show high-priority objectives for the control of stress and violent behavior in the United States.

Stress in the workplace. Much of the growing perception of a stressful life in Western countries has been attributed to economic conditions and the pressures these have placed on employers to reduce the work force and demand more productivity and quality control from their smaller work force. Working conditions produce the greatest stress and physical manifestations such as back pain when the worker lacks autonomy or control over the pace of work.

Those whose pace of work is driven by automatic electronic systems or by assembly line machines suffer the most.

Changes in work methods or routines, even when these are intended to increase worker efficiency, can create stress, especially if the workers have not participated in the introduction of the new methods. Computers and new software, for example, create demands for more rapid turnaround of information and expectations of higher productivity. The pressure to produce more work faster becomes a stressful condition. When combined with job uncertainty, poor supervision or relationships with other workers, other automation and robotics controlling the pace of work, or physical aspects of the work area such as poor lighting, temperature, ventilation, furniture, high noise levels, or interruptions, these conditions add up to a stressed worker who likely comes home to a working partner who has suffered similar strains. Parenting responsibilities may then prevent them from taking the time they need to support each other or to look after their own needs.

Divorce and Broken Families

A successful marriage is partly a matter of personality adjustment. The individual who has difficulty adjusting to single life is ill-prepared to adjust to the complexities of married life. One needs only to go over the complaints of wives and husbands in divorce actions to recognize the extent to which inadequate personal adjustment is the basic factor. Husbands' complaints in divorce actions are revealing: wife's feelings are too easily hurt, wife criticizes me, wife is too nervous and emotional, there is a lack of freedom in the home, wife is quick-tempered, wife nags, wife tries to improve me, wife complains too much, wife is not affectionate, wife is too argumentative, we cannot agree on choice of friends. Wives, on the other hand, offer these complaints: husband is nervous and impatient, husband criticizes me, husband is argumentative, husband is quick-tempered, husband doesn't talk things over, husband is selfish and inconsiderate, husband is touchy, husband doesn't show affection, husband is too demanding, our marriage is too confining, husband criticizes my choice of friends. These comments, which were obtained from complaints filed in divorce proceedings, are an indication that personality, maturity, and adjustment are factors in marital stability.

Marriage counselors can provide a valuable service to a community for those individuals who are having difficulty in making an adequate marriage adjustment. More important is a community health service that assists people in problems of mental

health before they are married. Of course, not all people in a community need mental health counseling, and not all married couples need the services of a marriage counselor. However, a community health department that provides mental health counseling for normal people who do need such services will contribute not only to the general level of mental health but also to the prevention of a great deal of social pathology in the form of broken families.

The divorce rate increased steadily from 1958, when it was 2.1 divorces per 1000 population, to 1984 when it was 10.5 per 1000. It has since declined gradually (Figure 9-4). The number of chil-

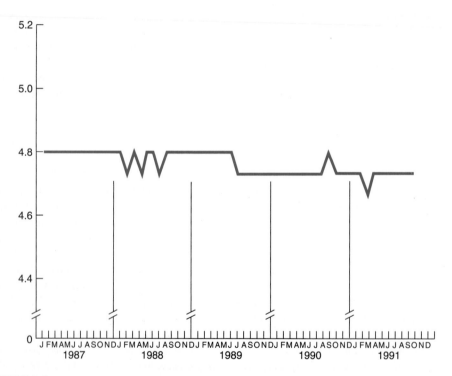

FIGURE 9-4
Divorce rates per 1000 population for the United States, 1987-91, calculated as successive 12-month averages ending with the month indicated, show a slight decrease.
Source: National Center for Health Statistics, *Monthly Vital Statistics Report,* 40(10):4, 1992.

dren involved in divorces also increased from 1953 until recently, when the delays in marriage and in childbirth after marriage, slight reductions in divorce rates, and the reduction in family size reduced the number of children affected by divorce.

Criminal and Antisocial Behavior

Mental illness among prisoners. A study by the National Association for Mental Health in 11 state penitentiaries of 8581 consecutive admissions revealed that 25% of the prisoners were psychotic and that 14% were borderline cases. An early recognition of mental illness might have prevented some of the crimes in which these individuals were involved. In this respect, informed citizens of a community could be of service in recognizing abnormal behavior that could be associated with violence.

Violent and reckless behavior. Individuals who have a tendency toward violent outbursts of temper, who are overly suspicious, who have delusions of persecution, who are antisocial, or who are quarrelsome are more likely to be involved in violent and destructive acts. Behind the wheels of automobiles a community will find people who are frankly psychotic as well as borderline cases. Antisocial drivers have little respect for the rights or welfare of others. Not only will they inconvenience others, but also their recklessness, impatience, carelessness, excitability, and lack of responsibility can be important factors in causing motor vehicle injuries. In terms of injury prevention, the driver's personality is more important than a mechanical ability to handle the car. This situation eventually may force communities to deny motor vehicle operator's licenses because of personality deficiencies as well as because of deficiencies in driving skills.

After a crime has been committed, courts properly refer the prisoner to a psychiatrist for determination of the prisoner's level of mental responsibility. A corollary of this program is the effort to determine irresponsibility in individuals before they become involved in serious crimes. It is not possible to predict all people who may engage in crime, but repeat offenders have identified themselves as possible chronic criminals and have indicated the need to determine whether they are mentally ill. Others who show marked deviation in their behavior should also be examined to determine the degree of mental and emotional competence they possess. Unfortunately, the legal machinery is frequently cumbersome, and threats to civil rights can be so great that people in the professional social work and law enforcement fields are hesitant to initiate any action to provide for the psychiatric examination and counseling of citizens who could be possible threats to the people of the community. A true program of prevention would protect both the rights of the individual whose conduct appears deviant and the welfare of the children and adults in the community.

Suicide

Factors. Most information on the mental state of people who attempt to take their own lives is obtained from those people who failed in a suicide attempt. There is one successful suicide for every 10 attempts, and about 5% of those who fail are repeaters. The rate among men is more than three times that among women. Suicide is now the eighth leading cause of death in the United States. The suicide rate is low among certain groups—for example, among Mormons, Roman Catholics, and blacks. These data would indicate that the suicide rate can be influenced by conditioning in the individual's life. Studies indicate that perhaps 30% of those who take their own lives are actually mentally disordered. The remaining suicides largely result from a decision that death is the best solution to a situation. For many of these situations there were coping possibilities that were not adequately explored. When life has lost its purpose or has resulted in great frustration, loss of self-esteem, or depression, an individual who lacks good personality integration may attempt to escape from reality by self-destruction.

Helping individuals over the immediate crisis, together with counseling to help them see the problem and its solution, will at least prevent a present attempt, and also might prevent further attempts at self-destruction. People who threaten suicide often carry out their threats. Such threats indicate disturbance and the need for assistance. Most suicides can be prevented if people recognize individuals who are disturbed, take action to protect the individuals against themselves, and assist them in understanding and solving the situation. Those who suffer marked depression are particularly in need of guidance during the period of depression. Highly sensitive persons may take their own life to hurt others; these individuals simply are too sensitive for the rugged world in which they live. For these people, mental health counseling is long past due. It can be predicted conservatively that if a community has adequate mental health counseling and a considerable number of citizens who recognize the various factors indicating that a person is likely to attempt to take his or her own life, suicide can be cut to one third of its present rate.

Adolescent suicide. Suicide rates for adolescents 15 to 19 years of age quadrupled from 2.7 per 100,000 in 1950 to 11.3 in 1991. Data from earlier decades are not available to assess similar trends in rates of attempted suicide in this population. Attempted suicide is a potentially lethal health event, a risk factor for future completed suicide, and a potential indicator of other health problems such as substance abuse, depression, or adjustment and stress reactions.

The national school-based Youth Risk Behavior Survey (YRBS) periodically measures the prevalence of priority health-risk behaviors among American youth through comparable national, state, and local surveys. The school-based American YRBS obtains a representative sample of students in grades 9 to 12 in the 50 states, the District of Columbia, Puerto Rico, and the Virgin Islands. Students are asked whether they seriously thought about attempting suicide during the 12 months preceding the survey, whether they made a specific plan about how they would attempt suicide, how many times they had actually made a suicide attempt, and whether their suicide attempt(s) resulted in an injury or poisoning that had to be treated by a doctor or nurse.

For the 12 months preceding the 1990 survey, 27.3% of all students in grades 9 to 12 reported that they had thought seriously about attempting suicide. Fewer students (16.3%) reported that they had made a specific plan to attempt suicide. About half the students who made a specific plan (8.3% of all respondents) reported that they actually attempted suicide. Two percent of the students reported that they made a suicide attempt that resulted in an injury or poisoning requiring medical attention. This systematic decline was noted for both male and female students and for white, black, and Hispanic students (Table 9-2).

Female students were significantly more likely than male students to report that they had thought seriously about attempting suicide, had made a suicide plan, or had attempted suicide one or more times during the 12 months preceding the survey. Similarly, 2.5% of female students and 1.6% of male students indicated they had made a suicide attempt that required medical attention, but this difference was not statistically significant.

Hispanic and white students reported higher levels of suicidal thoughts and behaviors than black students, although these differences were not always statistically significant. Hispanic female students (14.9%) were significantly more likely to have attempted suicide during the 12 months preceding the survey than white female (10.1%) or black female students (8.2%).

Table 9-2 reflects various forms of attempted sui-

TABLE 9-2
Percentage of high school students reporting suicide ideation and suicidal behavior,*
by gender and race/ethnicity—United States, Youth Risk Behavior Survey, 1990†

Category	Suicide ideation %	Made specific suicide plans %	≥1 Suicide attempt(s) %	Suicide attempt requiring medical attention‡ %
		Gender		
Female	33.9	20.2	10.3	2.5
Male	20.5	12.3	6.2	1.6
		Race/ethnicity		
Hispanic	30.4	19.5	12.0	2.4
White	28.1	16.1	7.9	2.1
Black	20.4	13.5	6.5	1.4
Total	**27.3**	**16.3**	**8.3**	**2.1**

*During the 12 months preceding the survey.
†Unweighted sample size = 11,631.
‡Resulted in an injury or poisoning that had to be treated by a doctor or nurse.
Source: Centers for Disease Control: Attempted suicide among high school students—United States, 1990, *MMWR* 40:633, 1991.

cide. Actual (successful) suicides produce the eighth leading cause of death in the United States, but rank third among youth 15 to 24 years and second among white males (including Hispanic) in this age group. The overall suicide rate has not significantly changed since the 1987 baseline of 11.7 per 100,000. In 1991 the suicide rate was 11.5 per 100,000 in the total U.S. population. The year 2000 goal is 10.5 for the total population. Suicide among youths aged 15 to 19, however, has continued to increase from 10.3 per 100,000 in 1987 to 11.3 in 1991. The target is 8.2.

A great number of suicides could be prevented by increased recognition and appropriate treatment of persons with clinical depression and other treatable mental disorders clearly associated with an increased risk of suicide.

Objectives for Suicide Reduction

• By the year 2000, reduce suicide to no more than 10.5 per 100,000 people. Age-adjusted baseline: 11.7 per 100,000 in 1987.

Special Population Targets	1987	2000
Youths aged 15-19	10.3	8.2
Men aged 20-34	25.2	21.4
White men 65+	46.1	39.2
American Indian/Alaska Native Men Reservation State	15	12.8

COMMUNITY RESPONSE TO MENTAL AND SOCIAL DISORDERS

Unfortunately, the physician or psychologist frequently does not see the patient with a mental disorder until the condition is far advanced or some personal, family, or social crisis with serious consequences has occurred. Every community needs to provide the means by which people showing indications of mental disorder will be directed to professional resources for diagnosis, treatment, and care (Figure 9-5).

Citizen Action

Responsible people in the community can be informed about the early indications of mental disturbance or possible mental illness. The popular misconception that a mentally disordered person dresses

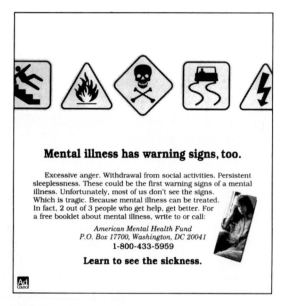

FIGURE 9-5
Recognizing the symptoms or warning signs of mental illness could help people get the help they need earlier and prevent some of the problems that arise from untreated mental illness.
Source: Courtesy American Mental Health Fund.

oddly, has weird mannerisms, is likely to be maniacal, or talks foolishly must be displaced by a more realistic view. People in the parahealth fields, such as teachers and social workers, could be better trained to recognize the early signs of mental disorder. When this nucleus of professional workers coming in daily contact with the public is aided by reliable citizens who understand the early indications of mental disturbance, then a community possesses a valuable means by which individuals likely to need diagnostic services and counsel are directed to services at an early stage when constructive and even preventive measures can be taken. In addition, such a group of informed citizens in a community can be the means by which tragedies such as child abuse and other forms of violence can be prevented.

Informed citizens can give responsible support to programs for providing hospital clinics and other services necessary for the proper care and treatment of the mentally disordered. They can advocate desirable legislation to promote an effective mental health program. They can support the necessary official agencies, including courts, in their programs to deal with the mentally disturbed. Most immediately in their family, work, and friendship circles they can offer understanding and support to those experiencing severe distress, bereavement, depression, anxiety, disorientation, extreme anger, fear, or difficulty with alcohol, drugs, or relationships. Recognizing the warning signs is an essential first step (Figure 9-5).

The most immediate help people can offer a sick relative or friend is compassion, understanding, and support. Pretending that nothing is wrong or blaming the sick person for causing worry, embarrassment, or family problems only makes the problem potentially worse.

Mental illness is a medical condition that requires medical treatment. Willpower alone is not enough. Here are some other steps people can take on behalf of others.

- Seek help from trained professionals and accredited treatment centers.

- Be patient and persistent. After failing to make contact with the right agency or person after one call, try others. Every source offers different services.
- Describe the problem clearly and completely. All information is confidential and privileged.
- Change doctors if not satisfied. A good relationship between doctor and patient is critical.
- Support one another. Do not allow other family relationships to deteriorate. Seek help or counseling if needed for other family members.
- Provide a secure, well-patterned environment for a mentally ill relative or friend. They need love, not stress. ("Tough love" is wrong in this case, because it causes stress.)
- Learn as much as possible about mental illness and its treatments. There is no substitute for becoming well informed.

An example of the mental, emotional, and social health impact of a serious physical illness in the family or immediate friendship network is reflected in Figure 9-6. This shows the relative frequency of problems, identified by partners, family, and friends of people diagnosed with the HIV disease.

A health matter becomes a community health problem when it is amenable to amelioration through collective action. Many aspects of the mental health problem can be dealt with most effectively through public action.

Mental and Social Health Needs of the Community

A community diagnosis of specific mental and social health needs determines what the mental health program should be in that particular community. Certain factors and certain mental health needs are common to most communities, but specific factors that influence the mental health of subpopulations of a community must be recognized and evaluated. Socioeconomic, neighborhood, and ethnic backgrounds, family relationships, child-rearing practices, community norms, and cultural values are such factors affecting the mental health program.

Mental and social health needs include problems

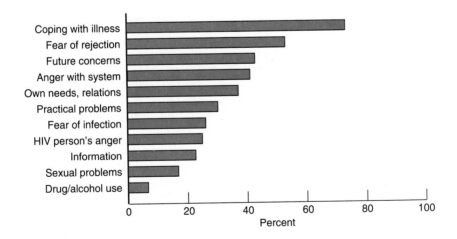

FIGURE 9-6
Problems identified by partners, families, and friends of people infected with HIV, Canada, 1992.
Source: Health and Welfare Canada: *Ending the isolation—HIV disease and mental health in the second decade,* Ottawa, 1992, Minister of Supply and Services Canada, Cat No. H43-53/21-1192E.

for which people have a need for special assistance in the province of normal, everyday adjustment. Individual and family counseling services, marriage counseling, sessions for expectant parents, child study groups, parent discussions, employment services, guidance services for elderly citizens, promotion of cultural interests, recreation programs, and general health information services all address social needs in a community. No one agency will necessarily provide all of the services to satisfy these needs, but by means of an integrated community health and social service program, some agency or individual will provide for each of the various needs. The program will also be concerned with mentally disturbed people in hospitals, patients under physicians' care, patients who have been released from psychiatric hospitals and are in the process of rehabilitation, and individuals who have come to the attention of legal authorities and community agencies and are under the direction of these agencies.

Some of the adults discharged from psychiatric hospitals will be homeless or without employment and resources to care for themselves in the community; they are the special wards of integrated community mental health and social service agencies. The dramatic decline of hospitalized mentally ill has placed a greater burden on communities to provide halfway houses and other facilities to compensate for the **deinstitutionalization** of mental illness.

Child and adolescent mental health services will be provided largely through the schools. In addition, most communities have other agencies that will provide for some of the mental health needs of children and adolescents. These needs include psychological testing and diagnostic services, counseling services for children, consulting services for parents of the youngsters, mental health guidance services for adolescents, remedial programs in the school, an in-service mental health training program for teachers, mental health instruction as a phase of the basic health curriculum, and family life education. An ef-

fective, coordinated community-school mental health program should devote its major attention to the mental health of all youngsters but must also provide for the special mental health needs of the delinquent, the emotionally disturbed, the mentally retarded, the academically handicapped, the homeless (Figure 9-7), and children and adolescents who are having adjustment problems.

Deinstitutionalization and Homelessness

Tales of abuse in large state mental hospitals in the 1950s and concern for the civil rights of the mentally ill in the 1960s led to increasing legislative restrictions making it difficult to commit people to hospitals against their will. At the same time the introduction of new drugs made it possible for more people to be discharged from state hospitals. State cost-cutting measures in the 1970s accelerated the deinstitutionalization trend, which brought the patient count in state institutions from 552,000 in 1955 down to 119,000 in 1990. Many of the deinstitutionalized have not been able to cope with employment or other conditions, leading to financial instability and, for many, homelessness. Up to 30% of the estimated 500,000 homeless and at least 10% of the 1 million people in jail in the United States suffer from serious mental disorders, mostly schizophrenia and manic depression.

Further budget cuts in the 1980s and 1990s resulted in the failure to open halfway houses and other community facilities to help absorb and support the flood of liberated former mental patients. The system of most communities is left capable of responding only to episodic acute care, not chronic care. Some 70% of mental health dollars are spent for hospital rather than clinical or outreach services. Demonstration programs have shown that mentally disturbed people can lead safe, happy, and productive lives outside institutions given community support for monitored medications, specialized training, and stable housing.

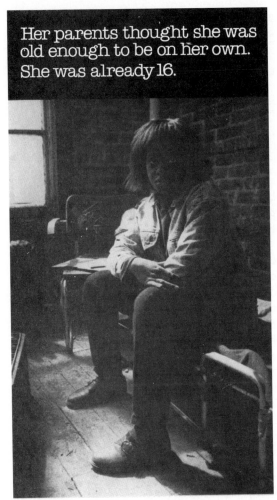

Her parents thought she was old enough to be on her own. She was already 16.

Every year hundreds of thousands of kids are thrown away. Put out onto the streets. With no job, no money and nowhere to go. But now there is a number for kids to call. The Covenant House Nineline helps kids with food, clothing, a place to sleep and, most of all, someone to talk to.

To get help in your hometown call our Nineline 1-800-999-9999. It's free.
Nineline
1-800-999-9999
Anytime.
Anywhere.

FIGURE 9-7
Homeless and runaway teenagers are especially susceptible to a spiral of circumstances that can undermine their mental health. This Covenant House campaign urges communities to seek technical assistance in providing support to this high-risk group.
Source: Covenant House and Advertising Council.

Organization and Administration

Effective community mental health programs require planning, organization, and direction. A community may possess many resources for dealing with its manifold mental health needs, but unless some central agency exists that will assess and coordinate the various services available, many needs that could be fulfilled will be neglected, many services will be inadequately provided, and there will be unnecessary duplication of effort and even conflict in function. Setting up a central administrative agency does not mean that the various individuals, agencies, and services in the community will be hampered or otherwise obstructed in their functioning. Rather, it means a coordination of services available from the various agencies and individuals in the total program that will help reduce duplication and fragmentation of services.

Everyone has a potential contribution to make to the community's mental health program. Unfortunately, individuals with a smattering of knowledge or with a morbid curiosity about mental health may be willing volunteers or even persistent participants, but the public is entitled to protection from the charlatans and the incompetent in mental health as in other areas of health.

Community Mental Health Centers

The U.S. Community Mental Health Centers Act of 1963 authorized the construction of community mental health centers, which form the core of the U.S. national mental health program. Allotments to states continued to rise up to 1980, based on population, financial need, and the need for community mental health centers. Funds were provided on a matching basis. The centers were expected to include the following:

- Inpatient services
- Outpatient services
- Partial hospitalization, including day, night, and weekend care

- Emergency services
- Community services, including consultation with community agencies and professional personnel
- Diagnostic, screening, and follow-up services
- Precare and postcare community services, including foster home placement, home visiting, and halfway houses
- Alcohol and drug problem services
- Training
- Research and evaluation

In 1980 President Jimmy Carter signed into law the Mental Health Systems Act, one of the few health initiatives his administration was able to pry from Congress. The legislation gave states greater authority over mental health grants, allowing funding of programs other than the traditionally defined community mental health centers, targeted certain priority populations, and put greater emphasis on prevention.

Community Health Department Mental Health Programs

Many county, district, and city health departments have had a mental health division or section. Indeed, this was once a standard unit in the local health department. More recently, separate departments of mental health provide this service. Frequently, the mental health program is organized as a clinic with a staff consisting of one or more psychiatrists, clinical psychologists, psychiatric social workers, health educators, and mental health nurse consultants. The staff provides consulting services for children as well as adults. Marriage counseling and family counseling are frequently included in the services.

The community mental health clinic provides diagnosis and recommends treatment. Although a limited amount of treatment may be provided, the program is not designed for complete care. In some instances, the mental health staff advises courts on matters relating to the mental competence of people

---

Objectives for Mental Health Services

- By the year 2000, increase to at least 40% the proportion of work sites employing 50 or more people that provide programs to reduce employee stress. Baseline: 26.6% in 1985.
- By the year 2000, establish mutual-help clearinghouses in at least 25 states. Baseline: 9 states in 1989.

---

before the court. The staff may recommend rehospitalization or may assist in rehabilitation of a patient who has been released from a mental hospital.

The importance of a mental health unit in the community health department lies in its value as a coordinating agency. The community public health department can point out mental health needs in the community that are not being met. It can assume the role of leader in obtaining necessary services to fulfill recognized needs, and it can provide for the fullest use of voluntary services that are available in the community. It can serve as the liaison between segments of the public and the special mental health services they need. Last, it can keep the community informed about matters of mental health, particularly in terms of services available and how these services may be used.

Other Agencies

The value of the service provided by each agency in the community depends on the freedom each agency has to do its best work within the general community mental health program or organized mental health plan. The work of the general medical practitioner or the psychiatrist should be regarded as a part of the total community mental health program. Psychiatric clinics supervised by professional psychiatrists and staffed by other personnel will continue to be vital to the mental health needs of the community.

Medical practitioners. Practicing physicians obviously have an important role in the mental health of the community. About 50% of general medical and surgical patients in the United States are estimated to have some kind of emotional disorder. Serious mental and emotional illnesses are partly responsible for many physical complaints. Individuals who would be classified as having normal mental health often have minor or moderate mental health problems and look to a physician as their consultant in dealing with these mental and emotional disturbances. A citizen with a neurosis—under the supervision of a family physician who understands the patient's total background—can usually adjust reasonably well to his or her situation and live a virtually normal life. In addition, the physician is frequently the first person consulted when a family suspects that one of its members is suffering from mental disturbance. General medical practitioners, although they do not profess to be specialists in psychiatry, nevertheless have an adequate background to be an important resource in the community mental health program if continuing education programs are made available to them.

Other professionals. Nurses, psychologists, health educators, and social workers usually have a background that gives them an understanding of the field of mental health, and their place in and contribution to the field. Working in cooperation with psychiatrists, family physicians, and other medical personnel, nurses, psychologists, health educators, and social workers can make constructive contributions to community mental health through their understanding of various factors operating in the community and of the resources that can be drawn on to help the individual, the family, or the neighborhood.

Regional resources. Many small communities with limited professional mental health resources can draw on the facilities available in a large neighboring community. A reasonably well-organized mental health program, even in a small community, will have complete information on facilities available in nearby communities, so that citizens in the smaller community can benefit from the services of the highly trained psychiatrists and other specialists who are most likely to be practicing in metropolitan areas.

An appraisal of available professional resources in mental health must include clinics and professional personnel available to the general public, as well as psychiatrists, nurses, and other personnel working in psychiatric hospitals. An accurate accounting of all mental health services available to the general public is extremely difficult to make because of the number of human service workers who devote only a limited portion of their practice to the mentally disordered but who nevertheless contribute a very important service. Most studies are limited to those clinics and practitioners concerned primarily with the mentally ill.

Community mental health centers. With the development of effective alkaloids for treating specific types of mental disorder, about one third of the patients currently treated in clinics would have been hospital patients but are now able to remain at home. In addition, many patients hospitalized for chronic disorders can now be released to return to their communities under the supervision of a clinic or a physician. More than one half of these clinics are located in the northeastern United States, which has about one fourth of the population. Qualified authorities maintain that there should be one psychiatric clinic for every 50,000 people, a standard that would require nearly doubling the full-time clinics in the United States.

With more successful treatment of the mentally ill and a declining population in psychiatric hospitals, the need for hospital staff becomes less, but the need for community workers becomes greater.

Citizen Participation in Community Mental Health Programs

Like most of the U.S. health legislation passed during the 1960s, the Community Mental Health Centers Act required "maximum feasible participation" to ensure that they would be responsive to the needs and aspirations of the people. The federal program of Community Mental Health Centers (CMHCs) was based on the premise that to be successful, a CMHC must be responsive to the viewpoints and problems of local communities.

Greater citizen input into the process of making policy-level decisions for a mental health center was expected to improve the delivery of mental health services by making them more responsive, accountable, and flexible. But even though broadly based consensus and support would be beneficial to every health program of the community, many communities have been slow to respond to the particular needs of the people for whom these programs are carried out. Community action groups can work to promote innovative services or programs, to change the goals and priorities of organizations as needed, and to expand the rate and effectiveness of participation by citizens.

How can strong mental health boards develop pressure for action through governments, old and new organizations, lobbying, and advocacy? Steps in an idealized model of community action might answer this question for some boards (see Chapter 3). Face-to-face visits by board members to businessmen have been shown to be an effective activity, but a study of the community must be done before community development by mental health advocacy groups can be very successful.

Typical community awareness surveys address mental health needs and problems in the community, knowledge about community resources, and attitudes toward mental health issues. Data concerning the physical and environmental status of minority groups are important for citizen boards to consider, for these often correlate with mental illness and should influence the selection of priority target ar-

Powerlessness and Stress

Chemophobia, homophobia, fear of airplanes—these special forms of technostress reflect the anxieties generated by news accounts of toxic chemical wastes polluting water supplies, homosexuals contracting HIV infections through unknown channels of transmission, and possible annihilation of the species through nuclear war. The underlying common thread in all such forms of technostress is a sense of helplessness or powerlessness. The antidote to such pervasive feelings in the community is the involvement of people in programs directed at controlling the sources of fear. Community participation in environmental and communicable disease control programs has been the hallmark of success and community pride in developing self-sufficiency and control in relation to health matters.

How does a community health worker go about involving people in health programs? What roles can lay people play in community health programs? Besides their direct contributions to the quality and appropriateness of programs, what other purposes does the participation of people in community health planning and evaluation serve?

eas. The use of, and resistance and accommodation to, mental health services by minority groups in the community are important considerations in programming and delivering services. Alienation from mental health agencies and services must be recognized among minority groups, if it exists; services should be designed to be attractive, responsive, and viable for all groups.

COMMUNITY MENTAL HEALTH PROMOTION

Most communities have provisions for treating the mentally ill, although facilities for early diagnosis and care are frequently inadequate or totally absent. Very few communities have a well-organized, well-functioning program for promoting the mental health of all citizens. Large segments of the community's population have a vital interest in mental health promotion as it relates to their community, their neighborhood, their family, and themselves. Yet, few want to see a mental health facility located in their neighborhood.

Whose Responsibility?

Establishing a community mental health program means developing community support. Leadership can come from the local mental health association, the community health council, United Way, and other sources. Productive action usually requires long-range planning rather than a high-pressure "crash" program. Lay leadership is important, even though primary responsibility must rest with the official community public health agency. Interagency cooperation is necessary for the success of a mental health program and full cooperation can be obtained only with public understanding, interest, and support. These require continuing public education.

Not in My Backyard

Communities recognize the need for treatment facilities and halfway houses for the rehabilitation and reentry of those who have been institutionalized in state mental hospitals. The public now understands that a large number of the homeless on the streets of their communities are people with mental illnesses who should be under care in decent facilities. Yet, the fear of mental illness leads most people to say they want the community mental health facilities located anywhere but in their own neighborhood. "Not in my backyard" has become the rallying cry for neighborhood resistance movements that have blocked not only mental health clinics but also youth centers, drug treatment facilities, halfway houses, and family planning clinics, as well as industrial, transportation, and waste management facilities. The wealthier neighborhoods have the greater power of resistance, so that such facilities too often end up in the poorest neighborhoods. These are sometimes the most dangerous areas of large cities, and the areas least conducive to mental health.

The drive to overcome such public resistance requires public education to demystify mental illness. Some of the earliest mental health education campaigns successfully changed the public's perception of the mentally ill as shameful. This resulted in many people who would not have sought help being more willing to admit they had an emotional problem and going for counseling or psychotherapy. But fear and misunderstanding continue to stigmatize the mentally ill. The American Mental Health Fund has undertaken a national "Anti-Stigma Campaign" to help the public "learn to see the sickness." Part of the campaign seeks to redirect the shame at those who make crude jokes about mental disorders that perpetuate stereotypes rather than seeing them as illnesses (Figure 9-8). Another objective of the campaign is to convince employers to provide more generously for their employees' mental health needs (Figure 9-9).

Education for Mental Health

At the base of the pyramid of community mental health promotion is community education in mental health. Such a program is directed primarily to the mental health needs of the general population and high-risk groups. Its objectives are to promote constructive attitudes toward mental health (Figure 9-8), to help people understand themselves, to show people how to manage and control stress, to keep the community informed of the various mental health services and facilities available and how they are best used, to engage community leaders in support of mental health, and to reduce public prejudice against people who experience mental illness (Figure 9-8).

Workplace Mental Health Promotion

Because of the many ways it influences physical and mental health, the workplace has become an ideal

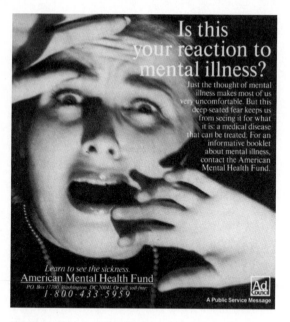

Is this
your reaction to
mental illness?

Just the thought of mental
illness makes most of us
very uncomfortable. But this
deep-seated fear keeps us
from seeing it for what
it is: a medical disease
that can be treated. For an
informative booklet
about mental illness,
contact the American
Mental Health Fund.

Learn to see the sickness.
American Mental Health Fund
P.O. Box 17700, Washington, DC 20041. Or call, toll free:
1·800·433·5959

A Public Service Message

FIGURE 9-8

Reducing the stigma and fear associated with mental illness has
been one of the success stories of mental health education over
several decades, beginning largely in the 1950s.

Source: American Mental Health Fund.

setting for programs to reduce sources of stress, to
prepare and support workers in coping with or managing stress in their work and personal lives, and to
identify early signs of worker problems in coping.
Employers have supported such programs because
they recognize that healthy workers are more productive workers.

Workplace mental health activities include the
reduction of stress in the work setting through work
design (how the work itself is structured), workplace
design (ergonomics), health promotion programs
such as stress management and employee assistance
(Figure 9-9), and surveillance of work-linked risk
factors and psychological disorders in the workplace. Employee assistance programs were for many
years concerned mainly with identifying alcohol
abuse in employees and referring them for professional treatment outside the workplace. If they failed

to heed the referral or to improve, they could then
be disciplined or fired. Increasingly, these programs
have looked to more progressive interventions to
counsel or support workers in managing some of the
work, family, or economic problems that underlie
their alcohol or drug abuse.

A community mental health education program
will function effectively under the direction of an
individual professionally prepared in community
health education. An important function of the program director is to enlist and use the services of all
qualified people or organizations in the community
who can contribute to mental health education. This
means organizing and administering a continuous
program that provides for the mental health education needs of the various segments of the population.
Resourcefulness and ingenuity are demanded, particularly when necessary resource people or organizations are not available.

As in other categorical programs, the function of
health education in community mental health is to
identify behaviors requiring development or change,
to analyze the factors influencing these behaviors,
and then to select or develop communications, community organizations, and training methods to influence these factors. Examples of specific behaviors
to which mental health education can be addressed
are coping and clinic dropouts. It is estimated that
approximately one third of the patients of community mental health centers drop out of treatment
without staff approval or recommendation.

To disseminate information, community mental
health education programs use discussion groups,
pamphlets, radio, television, films, posters, newspapers, journals, and other materials and aids. Personal contacts between the health department and
individual citizens in their homes are usually confined to visits by public health nurses for the purpose
of conveying information or advising the individual
where certain services may be obtained.

The development and use of clinical facilities in
most U.S. communities for temporary hospitalization and care of mentally ill patients require public

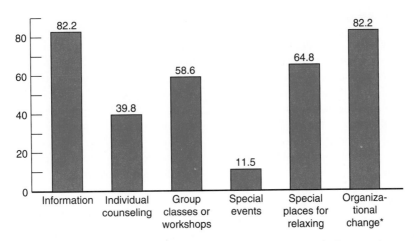

*Respondents were asked: "Does your worksite attempt to change the organization so that the empolyees will experience less stress, such as training supervisors to handle problems more effectively?"

FIGURE 9-9
Types of stress management activities offered by worksites reporting these activities (% of worksites offering any of these activities), United States, 1990.
Source: U.S. Public Health Service: *Prevention report,* March 1991.

education. Acquiring the necessary funds for the construction and maintenance of adequate community facilities depends on the understanding and the interest of the general public. The proper use of such facilities similarly requires public education.

STATE PROGRAMS

In the United States, state governments direct and finance most mental health programs. Unfortunately, psychiatrists are not always receptive to the concept that mental hygiene is a public health responsibility.

Whose Responsibility?

Generally, psychiatric hospitalization is not a function of the state health department but is administered by a separate administrative agency such as a state hospital commission. One debate in the United States is whether state hospital staffs should be responsible for all mental hygiene in the state. The psychiatric hospital is isolated from the community, and the hospital staff has neither the organization nor the experience to deal with integrated community action. If public health departments were to administer hospitals for the mentally disordered, this function would soon dwarf other activities. Mental health promotion is a function of state and local health departments; treatment of severe mental disorders and care of the institutionalized mentally ill are functions of psychiatrists and hospitals for the mentally ill.

Voluntary agencies such as mental health associations play an important role in providing state leadership for those groups and individuals with an understanding of the general problem of mental health and a sincere interest in mental health promotion. Various professional organizations whose members deal with services and problems related to mental health have been of particular value in pointing out the need for greater services in the mental health field and have provided leadership and support necessary for its attainment on a statewide basis. Frequently, it is a movement initiated by groups such as these that gives rise to the establishment of an official mental health agency in the state or province devoted to the promotion of the mental health of the general public.

States that have not enacted a specific mental health services act nevertheless have provided for the establishment of a statewide mental health program. A few states promote mental health as a component of existing programs, such as in the maternal and child health division of the state health department. An identifiable state mental hygiene agency within the state department of public health provides recognition of the importance of mental hygiene as a phase of public health service. For example, Maryland gave prominence to its mental health program by naming the state public health agency the Department of Health and Mental Hygiene.

Population in mental hospitals. From 1880 to 1955 there was a steady increase in the average number of patients in state and county mental hospitals per 100,000 people in the United States. In 1955 the average daily census of the state and county mental hospitals in the United States was 559,000—54% of patients in all hospitals. In 1956 for the first time in the history of the United States, there was a reduction in the number of resident patients in the state and county mental hospitals: on December 31, 1956, there were about 7000 fewer patients in these hospitals than on December 31, 1955. This reduction resulted from the successful use of chemotherapy in treating mental disorder. The decline was particularly significant when one considers that between the years 1945 and 1955 there was an average increase of 10,000 patients per year in these mental hospitals. Each year since 1956

there has been a further decrease in the year-end census of patients in mental hospitals in the United States.

Statistics on the incidence of the various mental disorders of patients in state and county mental hospitals indicate that over 40% are schizophrenic reactions, by far the most prevalent mental hospital diagnosis—four times greater than senility disease, the second most prevalent diagnosis with 10% of all mental hospital patients.

Functions of State Agencies

The division of mental health, or some similarly designated agency, has the primary responsibility for mental health promotion in many states and provinces. This division serves as the coordinating agency for all statewide forces concerned with the promotion of the mental health of the general population. It cooperates with the various voluntary and official agencies in the state or province that are engaged in some phase of mental health. It also cooperates with the state department of education, prisons, law enforcement and social service agencies, hospital commissions, and hospitals. Its major concern is with the mental health of the general population, but it does provide assistance for the maladjusted—the alcoholic, the drug addict, the juvenile delinquent, the criminal—and for the physically handicapped, the aged, and other segments in the population having special mental health risks.

The official division of mental hygiene at the state or provincial level carries out legislation concerning mental health, makes statistical studies, provides library facilities, makes mental health education materials available, provides consulting service to agencies or communities, conducts workshops and seminars for professional personnel, sponsors special programs of mental health promotion, establishes and promotes mental health facilities, and otherwise serves as a general mental health resource for other agencies and for communities.

REHABILITATION

Rehabilitation is the restoration to the fullest degree of physical, mental, social, vocational, and economic usefulness of which an individual is capable. Total rehabilitation of persons who have recovered from mental illness may require only the services of their family physician or may require the well-integrated program of a rehabilitation team consisting of psychiatrist, psychologist, psychiatric social worker, nurse, occupational therapist, rehabilitation therapist, and family counselor.

The success of chemotherapy in the treatment of mental disorders has relieved the overcrowding in mental hospitals in North America but is increasing the need for rehabilitation services. With specific measures for the treatment of mental disorders, a mental hospital has become a place where one can go for a short time for treatment. This revolution in the treatment of mental disease means that custodial care is being replaced by medical treatment and de-institutionalization. A patient who has been hospitalized for several years has a social adjustment to make as well as a medical recovery. When the medication is effective in improving the patient's mental illness, the patient is permitted to visit a neighboring community under the guidance of a hospital attendant. After several escorted visits and observable improvement in adjustment to society, the patient is permitted to visit the community unescorted. When the patient's social adjustment and mental adjustment appear to be sufficiently advanced, the patient is permitted to return to his or her home, but only when adequate supervision is available. This means that both medical and social supervision must be provided.

A family physician may accept responsibility for continuing the treatment the patient has been receiving, or medical supervision may be arranged through a psychiatric clinic in the patient's community. Rehabilitation services also are needed to assist the recovered or recuperating individual in making the necessary social, economic, and other adjustments that normal living requires. Getting a job, finding social groups and interests, adjusting to the tempo of community living, and finding leisure activities may require the services of specially prepared people. Statewide clinic systems are emerging in the United States from the community mental health centers. State hospitals that presently have a rehabilitation service are establishing links with centers throughout the state where former patients in need of assistance may obtain rehabilitation services conveniently and promptly.

RESEARCH

Research has not received the attention in mental health that it has in most other areas of health. The 50 states in the United States, which properly provide millions of dollars for hospitals for the care of the mentally ill, appropriate for research only 1.5% of their total mental hospital budget.

Social and preventive psychiatry is concerned with the mental health of individuals and communities. Researchers in this discipline are investigating the social factors associated with the etiology, prevention, and consequences of mental disorders. Whereas neuropharmacology and psychology are concerned, respectively, with finding a specific drug or psychotherapeutic approach for treatment of a psychiatric disorder, research in social and preventive psychiatry explores the application of these approaches in prevention. These lay the groundwork for the development and assessment of specific psychosocial therapies and types of services apt to improve the mental state and quality of life of individuals with severe psychiatric disorders.

Social psychiatry relies chiefly on the methodologies of evaluative and epidemiological research. The emphasis of evaluative research is on developing tools with which to assess patient care needs. Those tools are subsequently used in epidemiological research to determine whether the assessed needs are being met and to establish policy for the planning of appropriate services.

Despite its enormous impact and cost to society, mental illness has been disgracefully neglected. The United States spent only $9 per patient on mental illness research in 1992. The same amount was spent to study tooth decay. And whereas over one half the money spent on cancer research comes from the private sector, only 10% of the money used for research into mental illness comes from this source.

The most fruitful area of research would be in the prevention of mental illness. One benefit of such research has been the use of alkaloids, enabling many individuals to remain at home who otherwise would be kept in a psychiatric hospital for treatment. As important as preventive medication procedures are in dealing with mental illness, functional or psychological measures for the prevention of mental illness may be an equally productive field of research.

Research is also needed in the mental health of the normal individual. Advances in the health and medical fields in the United States in the past quarter century have included only modest progress in the understanding of the mental health of the normal individual. The motivation of human conduct, the genesis of emotional disturbance, the nature of mild deviations, procedures for improving and fortifying personality attributes, and measures by which a normal individual may cope with stress all warrant intensive study. New methods of research need to be developed, and more behavioral scientists should be prepared to do research in the mental health of the normal individual.

Research on methods of mental health education will become more urgent as other research findings accumulate. Community leaders, particularly those in the health professions, must take the lead in emphasizing the need for research in the field of mental health.

SUMMARY

The essence of community mental health, we have argued in this chapter, is to involve people in collective and mutually supportive efforts to address their quality-of-life concerns. Such concerns will relate to a wider range of issues than health alone. Some will relate to phobias and compulsive behaviors, such as fears of nuclear warfare, overeating, and drug abuse. Some will relate to sources of stress, such as computers, loneliness, bereavement, divorce, and financial difficulties. Mutual self-help groups and institutional arrangements to support people in coping with these fears, compulsions, and stresses represent the best points for intervention for community mental health and the best primary prevention strategies in relation to other health problems, such as alcohol and drug misuse, smoking, obesity, and violence.

Social health is mental health in relation to community criteria of productivity and quality of life. The World Health Organization seeks, as a goal for the year 2000, levels of health so that all people are capable of working productively and participating actively in the social life of their communities.

Such goals are ideals, however; most communities find their mental health programs tied up in medical treatment programs for the psychotic and severely disturbed. Such medical treatment, thanks to modern drugs in particular, has succeeded in returning these mental patients from institutions to their homes and communities. Some of these are homeless or unemployed, or both. These persons become the special wards of integrated community mental health and social service agencies.

The future of community mental health will depend on the success of nations, states, and communities in accomplishing prevention and mental health promotion objectives, such as those for stress and violence control. It will depend on their investment in such programs as employee assistance and student counseling; these programs will permit early intervention in the problems of troubled employees

Objectives for Reducing Mental Health and
Mental Disorders by the Year 2000

Objectives target reducing suicide, suicide attempts among adolescents, mental disorders among children and adolescents, mental disorders among adults, adverse health effects from stress; increasing use of community support programs by people with mental disorders, use of treatment by people with major depressive disorders, the proportion of people who seek help for personal and emotional problems; reducing uncontrolled stress, increasing appropriate suicide-prevention strategies in jails; worksite stress management programs, the number of states with established mutual-help clearinghouses, and routine review of mental functioning by primary care providers for both children and adults.

and students that might lead to alcoholism, drug misuse, suicide, or prolonged depression and isolation. The future of community mental health will also depend on investments in research and evaluation to improve the effectiveness of interventions and support services in the community.

QUESTIONS FOR REVIEW

1. With what phases of mental health should the community mental health program concern itself?

2. Why is social health properly regarded as a dimension of mental health?

3. Why is public health education fundamental to a community mental health program?

4. What can a community mental health program do to assist people in improving their social personalities?

5. Why do citizens with marked aggression represent a special community mental health problem?

6. What are the drawbacks of having the staffs of the states' mental hospitals in charge of the total state mental health program in the United States?

7. Why has a mental health program been slow in developing in your community?

8. What voluntary mental health agencies function in your community, and what are their programs?

9. How would you describe the mental health needs of your community?

10. How can personality maladjustment be the true cause of a divorce?

11. If you had good reason to believe that one member of a family of your close acquaintance was in need of psychiatric service, what measures would you take to bring this about?

12. If you had good reason to believe that one member of a family you did not know was in need of psychiatric service, what measures would you take to bring this about?

13. To what extent is it correct to say that every person has his or her mental measles and emotional chicken pox?

14. How will research in the field of mental disorders create the problem of preparing professional specialists in the field of rehabilitation?

15. What research is needed in mental health?

READINGS

Bui K-VT, Takeuchi DT: Ethnic minority adolescents and the use of community mental health care services, *Am J Community Psychol* 20:403, 1992.
Examines utilization rates, dropout rates, and duration of treatment for minority adolescents in the mental health care system of Los Angeles County. Compares African Americans, Asian Americans, Hispanics, and whites.

Cohen P, Hesselbart CS: Demographic factors in the use of children's mental health services, *Am J Public Health* 83:49, 1993.
Significant lags in mental health service use were found for youths 18 to 21 years of age, for rural and semirural residents, and for those in middle-income families.

Lindstrom B: Children and divorce in the light of salutogenesis—promoting child health in the face of family breakdown, *Health Prom Int* 7:289, 1992.

In Europe, 5.5 million women, children, and men annually face the loss of their intimate relationships, not counting other types of separations besides divorce. This article discusses the epidemiology of divorce and suggests public health approaches to creating healthful social settings for children.

Murrelle L, Ainsworth BE, Bulger JD et al: Computerized mental health risk appraisal for college students: user acceptability and correlation with standard pencil-and-paper questionnaires, *Am J Health Promotion* 7:83, 1992.

Computerized versions of 10 life-style–related mental health appraisal instruments were found to yield comparable results to the pencil-and-paper versions. Students prefered the computerized versions.

Wilson CA: The biospychosocial model: menstrual attitudes, sources of information, and premenstrual symptomatology among mothers with and without PMS and adolescent daughters, *J Health Educ* 23:409, 1992.

This study found that daughters had a high probability of premenstrual symptomatology if their mothers had PMS. Attitudes toward menstruation differed between mothers who had PMS and those who did not.

BIBLIOGRAPHY

Albright CL, Winkleby MA, Ragland DR et al: Job strain and prevalence of hypertension in a biracial population of urban bus drivers, *Am J Public Health* 82:984, 1992.

Bagley C: Changing profiles of a typology of youth suicide in Canada, *Can J Public Health* 83:169, 1992.

Barker PR, Menderscheid RW, Hendershot GE et al: Serious mental illness and disability in the adult household population: United States, 1989. In *Advance data from vital and health statistics,* no 218, Hyattsville, Md, 1992, National Center for Health Statistics.

Bentley KJ, Rosenson MK, Zito JM: Promoting medication compliance: strategies for working with families of mentally ill people, *Social Work* 35:274, 1990.

Dean K: Double burdens of work: the female work and health paradox, *Health Prom Int* 7:17, 1992.

Fahlberg LL, Wolfer J, Fahlberg LA: Personal crisis: growth or pathology? *Am J Health Promotion* 7:45, 1992.

Felts WM, Chenier T, Barnes R: Drug use and suicide ideation and behavior among North Carolina public school students, *Am J Public Health* 82:870, 1992.

Hirsch BJ, DuBois DL: The relation of peer social support and psychological symptomatology during the transition to junior high school: a two-year longitudinal analysis, *Am J Community Psychol* 20:333, 1992.

Homicide among young black males: United States, 1978-1987, *JAMA* 265:183, 1991.

Kelly GR, Scott JE: Medication compliance and health education among outpatients with chronic mental disorders, *Med Care* 28:1181, 1990.

Knight SM, Vail-Smith K, Barnes AM: Children of alcoholics in the classroom: a survey of teacher perceptions and training needs, *J Sch Health* 62:367, 1992.

Leslie M, Mikanowicz CK: The significance of cultural differences and characteristics in program development, *Wellness Perspec* 9:24, 1992.

Levy LH, Derby JF: Bereavement support groups: who joins; who does not; and why? *Am J Community Psychol* 20:649, 1992.

Lustig JL, Wolchik SA, Braver SL: Social support in chumships and adjustment in children of divorce, *Am J Community Psychol* 20:393, 1992.

Martin SL, Burchinal MR: Young women's antisocial behavior and the later emotional and behavioral health of their children, *Am J Public Health* 82:1007, 1992.

Newton J: *Preventing mental illness in practice,* London, 1992, Routledge.

Norris FH, Kaniasty K: A longitudinal study of the effects of various crime prevention strategies on criminal victimization, fear of crime, and psychological distress, *Am J Community Psychol* 20:625, 1992.

Prandoni JR, Wall SM: Effects of mental health and reactance-reducing information on offenders' compliance with court-mandated psychiatric evaluations, *Professional Psychol* 21:204, 1990.

Redman S: Women and body image. In Saltman D, editor: *Women and health,* Sydney, 1991, Harcourt Brace Jovanovich.

Robinson GC, Armstrong RW, Moczuk IB et al: Knowledge of fetal alcohol syndrome among native Indians, *Can J Public Health* 83:337, 1992.

St-Amand N, Clavette H: Self-help and mental health: beyond psychiatry, Ottawa, 1992, Canadian Council on Social Development.

Stein CH, Ward M, Cislo DA: The power of a place: opening the college classroom to people with serious mental illness, *Am J Community Psychol* 20:523, 1992.

Sullivan CM, Tan C, Basta J et al: An advocacy intervention program for women with abusive partners: initial evaluation, *Am J Community Psychol* 20:309, 1992.

Taggart VS, Zuckerman AE, Sly RM et al: You can control asthma: evaluation of an asthma education program for hospitalized inner-city children, *Patient Educ Counsel* 17:35, 1991.

Vega WA: Theoretical and pragmatic implications of cultural diversity for community research, *Am J Community Psychol* 20:375, 1992.

Villeneuve L, Lebel P, Lambert J: Importance du stress et du support social comme variables associées à la détresse psychologique dans une population agée de la région de Montréal, *Can J Public Health* 83:354, 1992.

Walker BR, Wright SM: Whole people: putting personal and social issues into school health curricula—a case study from Australia, *Health Prom Int* 7:99, 1992.

Willms DG, Lange P, Bayfield D et al: A lament by women for ''The People, The Land'' [Nishnawbi-Aski Nation]: an experience of loss, *Can J Public Health* 83:331, 1992.

Ying Y-W, Miller LS: Help-seeking behavior and attitude of Chinese Americans regarding psychological problems, *Am J Community Psychol* 20:549, 1992.

Chapter 10

Community Recreation and Fitness

❖

All parts of the body which have a function, if used in moderation and exercised in labors to which each is accustomed, become thereby well-developed and age slowly; but if unused and left idle, they become liable to disease, defective in growth and age quickly.

HIPPOCRATES

OBJECTIVES

When you finish this chapter, you should be able to:

- Identify the recreational and fitness needs of a community and its subpopulations
- Describe how recreation and fitness contribute to physical, mental, and social health in a community or population
- Identify resources in a community to support the development of recreational and fitness opportunities
- Participate in planning and evaluating recreational and fitness programs

---

The word **recreation** itself implies a health benefit. To recreate means to revive or refresh after toil or exertion, to renew the mind, the spirit, and the body. Amusement serves these purposes, as does exercise. Together, they contribute to the promotion of health, the prevention of certain disorders, and the treatment of certain disabilities. Humor and mirth have healing powers. Most experts believe that the physical and mental benefits of **fitness** combine with the social and emotional benefits of recreation to give individuals, families, and communities a quality of life that produces greater resistance to infection and greater ability to cope with stress.

As an activity pursued during **leisure** time and

273

one that is optional and pleasurable, recreation has its own immediate appeal. It is a behavior available in some degree to everyone. Recreation has come to be viewed also as an emotional state or condition that flows from feelings of mastery, achievement, exhilaration, acceptance, success, personal worth, and pleasure. As such it is not necessarily dependent on any physical or social activity.

Community health is supported by a recreational and fitness program providing for a wide diversity of participation. With the trend toward participation in physical activities, the community finds it necessary to serve citizens who desire to occupy their leisure hours in more stimulating and outdoor pursuits. But recreation includes creative and aesthetic interests as well as those of a predominantly physical nature. The community enhances the quality of life and provides alternatives to drugs and alcohol as leisure pursuits by having an organized recreational program that meets many of the social, creative, aesthetic, communicative, learning, and physical needs of its population.

HISTORY OF RECREATION AND FITNESS IN NORTH AMERICA

The history of recreation and fitness in the United States and Canada provides some insight into the nature of recreation and the roots of its problems. Recreation, as it is recognized today, is largely a reflection of four historical movements: the conservation movement, the urban parks movement, the recreation movement, and the fitness movement. Each has its own particular history.

The Conservation Movement

The conservation movement was based on a belief in the wise and balanced use of natural resources. The U.S. and Canadian governments played a leading role by helping to conserve large areas of open spaces and unique landscapes, beginning with the designation in 1864 of Yosemite Valley as the first national park. The establishment of a national park and national forest system was perhaps the most notable accomplishment of the movement.

The Urban Parks Movement

The urban parks movement was nineteenth-century North American leaders' response to the effects of industrialization and immigration on the rapidly growing urban population. Landscape architects, typified by Frederick Law Olmsted, created a new legacy of public green spaces among the bricks and grime of North America's maturing cities. Beginning with Olmsted's Central Park in New York City, the urban parks movement spread rapidly across the continent. By the early 1900s most big cities had large urban parks, and municipal governments had become well-established parkland providers.

The Recreation Movement

Unlike both the conservation and urban parks movements, initial support for the recreation movement came largely from private and philanthropic sources rather than from government and was specifically aimed at producing social reforms. The movement originated in private settlement houses of major cities where play programs, notably the ''sandgardens'' of Boston in 1885 and Jane Addams' model playground at Hull House in 1892, successfully provided organized recreational opportunities for children of immigrant tenement dwellers.

The recreation movement was also characterized in the 1920s and 1930s by the development of spectator sports and box-office attractions. These were decades that created glamorous films and professional athletics. Leisure time was more plentiful with the 8-hour work day becoming a standard.

The park and recreation efforts expanded rapidly after World War II in response to population growth, large incomes, and new housing developments. By the late 1950s, however, the existing parks and programs could not satisfy the increased demand. In response, the U.S. Congress created the Outdoor Recreation Resources Review Commission in 1958, which stimulated a resurgence of federal interest in parks and recreation.

The 1960s brought expanded protection and development of natural resources and recreational services, as reflected in the creation of the Land and Water Conservation Fund and the National Wilderness, Wild and Scenic Rivers, and Trails Systems.

During the 1970s, recreation expenditures increased at all levels of government. In some cases, however, these funds were unable to keep pace with price escalations affecting recreational land acquisition, capital development, energy supplies, and staffing or programming. The 1980s and 1990s have seen budgetary cutbacks and increased dependence on user fees to finance park and recreation facilities.

The Fitness Movement

The President's Council on Physical Fitness and Sports was established in 1956 by President Dwight D. Eisenhower. The council was an outgrowth of the President's Council on Youth Fitness, established out of concern about the poor performance of American boys and girls on standardized physical fitness tests. Subsequently, it was recognized that the fitness problem permeates all age groups. In 1963 the council was directed to begin promoting adult fitness. Today the Council addresses its efforts to all ages, including the elderly, and its activities are part of national preventive health efforts under the direction of the U.S. Office of Disease Prevention and Health Promotion.

Following the 1974 Lalonde Report on the Health of Canadians in 1974, a new agency was created to oversee the development of physical fitness programs in Canada in cooperation with provincial and municipal governments and with private industry. Fitness Canada makes use of extensive mass media campaigns, materials, and grants in support of local programs, and federal support for na-

tional organizations developing specialized programs in physical fitness.

EPIDEMIOLOGY OF PHYSICAL ACTIVITY

More than half of the U.S. adult population is sedentary and less than 10% exercises at the level recommended by the 1990 National Health Objectives. Just under half of Canadian adults are classified as high on the index of leisure-time physical activity in the 1990 Health Promotion Survey. This is a slight decline from 1985. Most people have little opportunity to be physically active—at a rate great enough and for sufficient duration to accrue health benefits—in routine household or workplace activities during a typical day. Only 22% of people aged 18 years and older engage in at least 30 minutes of activity five or more times per week.

Physical inactivity contributes to several debilitating medical conditions, including coronary heart disease, stroke, hypertension, non-insulin-dependent diabetes mellitus, osteoporosis, colon cancer, obesity, and diminished psychological well-being. Coronary heart disease affects 7 million Americans, causes over 500,000 deaths annually, and costs the United States approximately $43 billion per year in direct and indirect costs.

Hypertension or high blood pressure, a leading risk factor for coronary heart disease, stoke, renal disease, and retinopathy, occurs in 38% of the black population and 29% of the white population (Figure 10-1). Stroke is the third leading cause of death in the United States and a major cause of morbidity with 400,000 to 500,000 Americans suffering nonfatal strokes each year.

Diabetes, also a risk factor for coronary heart disease, has been diagnosed in 7 million people in the United States, and an additional 5 million may unknowingly have the disease.

Physical inactivity contributes to osteoporosis, a bone deficiency characterized by decreased bone mass, that affects 24 million Americans. It is esti-

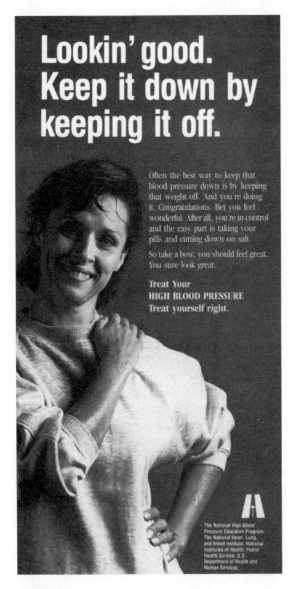

Lookin' good. Keep it down by keeping it off.

Often the best way to keep that blood pressure down is by keeping that weight off. And you're doing it. Congratulations. Bet you feel wonderful. After all, you're in control and the easy part is taking your pills and cutting down on salt.

So take a bow, you should feel great. You sure look great.

Treat Your HIGH BLOOD PRESSURE Treat yourself right.

The National High Blood Pressure Education Program; The National Heart, Lung, and Blood Institute; National Institutes of Health; Public Health Service, U.S. Department of Health and Human Services

FIGURE 10-1

The National High Blood Pressure Education Program provides media materials to support community programs in hypertension control as well as in fitness programs.

Source: National Heart, Lung and Blood Institute, National Institutes of Health, U.S. Department of Health and Human Services.

mated that 50% of women over age 45 years has osteoporosis. Of these, over half will have fractures related to osteoporosis.

Colon cancer is the second leading cause of cancer deaths in the United States. In 1990 nearly 60,000 Americans died from this type of cancer. Obesity affects 24% of men and 27% of women according to the 1976-1980 baseline for the Objectives for the Nation.

An estimated 23 million adults living in communities in the United States are severely incapacitated from mental disorders, not including substance abuse, with almost twice that number having experienced at least one diagnosable disorder at some point in their lives. Many of these disorders can be treated if not prevented with physical activity and recreation as part of the therapy or program.

Efficacy of Risk Reduction

Regular physical exercise has been associated with overall mortality reduction and improved health status in several debilitating medical conditions. For example, more people are at risk for coronary heart disease due to physical inactivity than for any other single risk factor (Figure 10-2). Physically inactive people are almost twice as likely to develop coronary heart disease as people who engage in regular physical activity. If half of those who exercise irregularly became regularly active, the number of cardiovascular deaths would decline about 7% annually, postponing about 35,000 deaths per year. For the inactive, even relatively small increases in activity are associated with measurable health benefits. In addition, light to moderate physical activity is more readily adopted and maintained than vigorous physical activity.

Exercise can reduce the risk of developing hypertension by 35% to 52%, particularly as a result of controlling weight. Regular exercise reduces blood pressure by an average of 10 mm Hg (see Figure 10-1).

Maintaining caloric balance and preventing obesity are notable benefits of exercise. Physical activ-

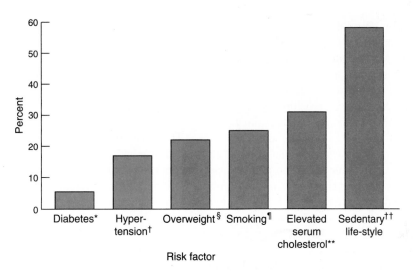

*Respondent self-reported having been told by physician that respondent has diabetes.

†Respondent self-reported having been told by a physician that blood pressure is high on multiple checks, or respondent is on medication for high blood pressure.

§Based on body mass index ≥27.8 men and ≥27.3 for women from self-reported height and weight of respondent.

¶Respondent self-reported currently smoking.

**Measured ≥200 mg/dL by NHANES II.

††Respondent self-reported no physical activity or irregular physical activity (i.e., fewer than three times per week and/or <20 minutes per session).

FIGURE 10-2

Prevalence of modifiable risk factors for coronary heart disease. Increases in physical activity and exercise could reduce the risk for this leading cause of death for more people than any other risk factor change.

Sources: Behavioral Risk Factor Surveillance System and National Health and Nutrition Evaluation Survey. Centers for Disease Control: Coronary heart disease attributable to sedentary lifestyle—selected states, 1988, *MMWR* 39:541, 1990.

ity has been shown to aid in weight control, even after controlling for dietary factors. Physical activity is important at all ages because the fat-to-muscle ratio changes with age. The average person's lean body mass declines with age; about 6.6 pounds of lean muscle mass is lost per decade. For example, in a 20-year-old woman the average fat ratio is 23% to 24%; for a 60- to 70-year-old woman, fat is 44%.

Exercise does not maintain caloric balance by burning a large number of calories. For example, a one-mile walk may amount to only 4% of total daily caloric expenditure. Exercise contributes to the caloric balance by improving and retaining muscle mass. Although a pound of fat and muscle weigh

> ### Objective for Physical Activity and Fitness
>
> - By 2000 increase to at least 50% the proportion of overweight people aged 12 years and older who have adopted sound dietary practices combined with regular physical activity to attain an appropriate body weight. Baseline: 30% of overweight women and 25% of overweight men for people aged 18 years and older in 1985.

the same, muscles burn calories; fat does not. Therefore, the fat-to-muscle ratio is a better way to judge physical fitness than weight alone. Weight gain occurs as a result of small daily differences between caloric intake and expenditure. Thus, reducing the gap with exercise achieves a caloric balance that prevents gradual, cumulative increases in weight (Figure 10-3).

Weight-bearing exercise and regular physical activity may also reduce bone loss in postmenopausal women and lower the number of hip fractures, probably through reduced osteoporosis. These relationships remain to be confirmed by studies showing the effect to be directly attributable to exercise. Research is needed to establish that the increased risk of fractures during exercise is not greater than the reduced risk due to stronger bones and muscles.

Finally, the benefits of exercise on improved affect include positive mood, reduced depression, and lowered anxiety. Physically active individuals report higher levels of self-esteem, possibly because of improved personal appearance and performance. Improvements in strength and flexibility also contribute to improved quality of life.

Specific Forms and Levels of Activity

The relationships between physical activity and health are numerous and complex. The link between exact activity and resulting, precise health benefit is unclear, but several health-related dimensions of physical activity are known to be most important in producing selected health effects.

Exercise cannot lower cardiovascular risk when performed only occasionally or seasonally. High-intensity activity achieves greater benefits than low-intensity activity. Different types of activities vary in intensity (see Table 10-1). High-intensity activities include brisk walking, hiking, stair climbing, aerobic exercise, calisthenics, jogging, running,

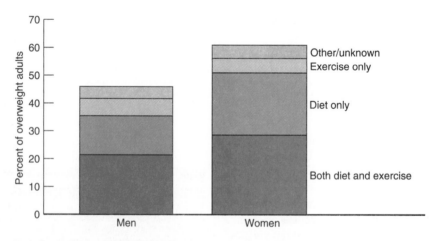

Note: Overweight is defined for men as body mass index greater than or equal to 27.8 kg/m² and for women as 27.3 kg/m². Weights and heights were self-reported.

FIGURE 10-3
Overweight adults who are trying to lose weight, according to method of weight loss and sex, United States, 1990.
Source: National Center for Health Statistics, National Health Interview Survey.

TABLE 10-1
Summary of how seven experts rated 14 sports and exercises

	Jogging	*Bicycling*	*Swimming*	*Skating (Ice or roller)*	*Handball/squash*	*Skiing-nordic*	*Skiing-alpine*	*Basketball*	*Tennis*	*Calisthenics*	*Walking*	*Golf**	*Softball*	*Bowling*
Physical fitness														
Cardiorespiratory endurance (stamina)	21	19	21	18	19	19	16	19	16	10	13	8	6	5
Muscular endurance	20	18	20	17	18	19	18	17	16	13	14	8	8	5
Muscular strength	17	16	14	15	15	15	15	15	14	16	11	9	7	5
Flexibility	9	9	15	13	16	14	14	13	14	19	7	8	9	7
Balance	17	18	12	20	17	16	21	16	16	15	8	8	7	6
General well-being														
Weight control	21	20	15	17	19	17	15	19	16	12	13	6	7	5
Muscle definition	14	15	14	14	11	12	14	13	13	18	11	6	5	5
Digestion	13	12	13	11	13	12	9	10	12	11	11	7	8	7
Sleep	16	15	16	15	12	15	12	12	11	12	14	6	7	6
TOTAL	148	142	140	140	140	139	134	134	128	126	102	66*	64	51

Adapted from President's Council on Physical Fitness and Sports, Public Health Service, U.S. Department of Health and Human Services. Ratings are on a scale of 0 to 3; thus a rating of 21 indicates maximum benefit (a score of 3 by all seven panelists). Ratings were made on the basis of regular (minimum of four times per week), vigorous (duration of 30 minutes to 1 hour per session) participation in each activity.

*Ratings for golf are based on the fact that many North Americans use a golf cart and/or caddy. If one walks the links, the physical fitness value moves up appreciably.

bicycling, rowing, swimming, and sports such as tennis, racquetball, soccer, basketball, and touch football. Low-intensity activities include walking for pleasure, gardening, yardwork, housework, dancing, golf, badminton, croquet, and ping pong.

The greatest risk reductions appear to occur in the most inactive persons who make small increases in their activity levels. For example, increasing fitness through moderate exercise, such as a brisk 30- to 60-min walk daily may reduce an unfit man's risk of early death by approximately 37% and an unfit woman's risk by nearly 50%.

The threshold levels of aerobic intensity that are generally accepted to be necessary to achieve **cardiovascular fitness** include (1) dynamically moving large muscle groups for at least 20 minutes, 3 or more days per week, performed at an intensity of at least 60% of cardiorespiratory capacity; (2) achieving and maintaining a pulse rate equal to the formula $(220 - \text{age}) \times 70\%$; or (3) reaching intensity of 50% to 100% of cardiorespiratory capacity, frequency of two to four times per week, duration of 15 to 45 minutes, and program duration of 5 to 11 weeks. The recommended intensity of exercise, how hard you exercise, can be checked by your pulse rate (see Figure 10-4).

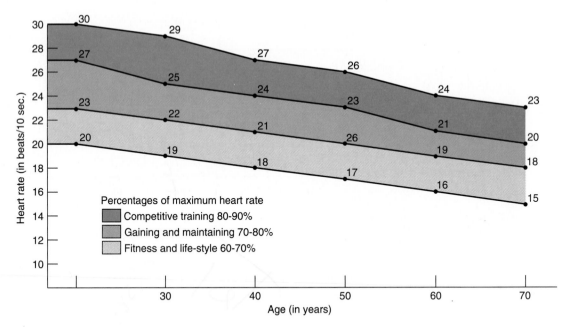

FIGURE 10-4

Pulse rates during exercise in beats per 10 seconds recommended for different ages and levels of training. These levels are shown as percentages of maximum heart rate in the legend.

Source: Fitness Section, Manitoba Health, Winnipeg, Manitoba.

Vigorous exercise may not be advisable for some individuals susceptible to injury or cardiovascular complications. Brisk walking, climbing stairs, gardening, and recreational activities with a modicum of movement now appear to confer more benefits than previously thought, especially in the elderly, the sedentary, those who are hypertensive or obese, and others with low baseline fitness levels. Exercise classes for seniors have been shown to produce physical and mental health benefits.

Prevalence of Physical Inactivity

More than half of the U.S. population is considered sedentary. That is, half the population reports physical activity less than three times a week and/or less than 20 minutes per session. The most active states in the United States are in the west and southwest;

Objective for Physical Activity and Fitness
• By 2000 increase to at least 50% the proportion of children and adolescents in first through twelfth grades who participate in daily school physical education. Baseline: 36% in 1984-1986.

the least active extend throughout the southeast and central United States (see Figure 10-5).

Physical activity varies by population. Black women, the less educated, overweight individuals, and the elderly are most consistently reported as inactive groups in terms of overall physical activity. One study found a significant drop-off in exercise for both men and women after marriage. For women reduced exercise was linked to pregnancy and feelings of overload; for men it was a gradual decrease.

Physical activity five or more times per week of adults aged 18 and over, 1990

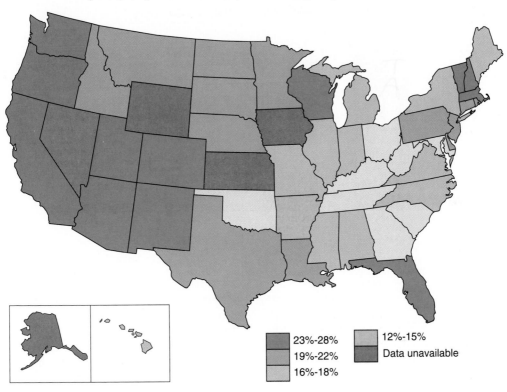

23%-28%
19%-22%
16%-18%
12%-15%
Data unavailable

Source: Behavioral Risk Factor Surveillance System

FIGURE 10-5
Geographic variations in prevalence of physical activity across the United States, 1990.
Source: Centers for Disease Control, Behavioral Risk Factor Surveillance System.

Black men were found to exercise most, then white men, white women, and black women. Women's exercise rose sharply after divorce.

Schools do not emphasize physical education programs. In the 1990 national Youth Risk Behavior Survey of students in grades 9 through 12, 43% of the males and 52% of the females reported that they were not enrolled in physical education classes (Figure 10-6). However, over 80% of children and youths reported participating in physical activities through community organizations.

PROGRESS AND NEEDS

Recreational and fitness attitudes and practices have changed over the past century, mostly in positive ways. More and more public parks, commercial recreational facilities, and home programs for recreation and fitness have materialized. Physicians increasingly prescribe recreation and fitness as ways to maintain and to enhance health and as accepted therapy for many heart patients and other patients.

The United States, Canada, Australia, New Zealand, Japan, China, and some European countries

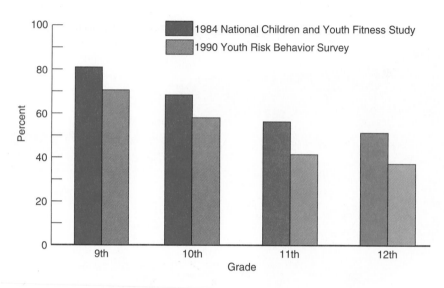

FIGURE 10-6

Percentage of high school students enrolled in physical education classes, by student grade and by survey: United States, 1984 and 1990.

Source: Centers for Disease Control: Participation of high school students in school physical education—United States, 1990, *MMWR* 40:607, 1991.

are in the midst of a genuine exercise boom: more bicycles than automobiles are being bought; sports fashion and athletic footwear have become major industries; and the number of runners, skiers, and tennis players has tripled in the United States. Joggers, backpackers, and bicycling commuters are commonplace in most communities in several Western countries. Commercial fitness centers and worksite fitness facilities have developed rapidly in Canada and the United States.

The increase in the physically active population from 1981 to 1988 in Canada, as measured by energy expenditure or time, was statistically significant and substantial in real terms. In a national survey 90% of the Americans questioned said that there should be physical education programs in elementary and secondary schools.

Despite these advances, public apathy, urban growth, and the modern life-style continually threaten to neutralize physical fitness advances. Daily living no longer provides enough vigorous ex-

ercise to develop and maintain good muscle tone or cardiovascular and respiratory fitness. In homes and factories, and even on farms, machines have virtually eliminated the necessity for walking long distances, climbing stairs, or even bending and stretching. In 1850 human muscles supplied nearly one third of the energy used by workshops, factories, and farms. Today the comparable estimate is less than 1%.

Millions of North Americans and Europeans are willing victims of schemes that promise fitness in a few minutes a day, without sweat or strain. One third of all American children and about 26% of American adults are overweight. The continuing financial crisis of schools and the trend away from required subjects have caused the loss of many physical education programs. A simultaneous trend toward "elective" physical education often results in students taking courses that contribute little to fitness or development of progressive skills.

Objectives for Physical Activity and Fitness

- By 2000 increase to at least 30% the proportion of people aged 6 years and older who engage regularly in light to moderate physical activity for at least 30 minutes per day. Baseline: 22% of people aged 18 years and older were active for at least 30 minutes five or more times per week in 1985.
- By 2000 increase to at least 20% the proportion of people aged 18 years and older and to at least 75% the proportion of children and adolescents aged 6 to 16 years who engage in vigorous physical activity that promotes the development and maintenance of cardiorespiratory fitness 3 or more days per week for 20 or more minutes per occasion. Baseline: 12% for people aged 18 years and older in 1985; 66% for youth aged 10 to 17 years in 1984.
- By 2000 reduce to no more than 15% the proportion of people aged 6 years and older who engage in no leisure-time physical activity. Baseline: 24% for people aged 18 years and older in 1985.

The most pervasive influence on fitness and recreational patterns has been television, which has substituted passive entertainment for creative recreation and sedentary recreation for physical activity. A study by the American Academy of Pediatrics found that from age 2 years on American children watch more than 22 hours of television a week. By the time today's child is 70 years old, he or she will have watched 7 years of television. Statistics Canada reported that Canadians watch on average of 23.3 hours of TV a week now, down from 23.4 hours in 1989. The trend is especially downward among children and teenagers.

RECREATION AS HEALTH PROMOTION

Recreation can contribute to mental, social, and physical health. By breaking the commonplace routine of existence, recreation contributes to a greater realization of the individual's potential for living. Recreation alone cannot produce a high level of health, but combined with other factors affecting health it can elevate health for normal individuals. For some people the contribution of recreation to mental health is its greatest value. For others the physical health values or the social values are recreation's most important attribute. For the individual with a disorder or chronic disability, recreation frequently proves important in restoring health. The rehabilitation value of recreation is universally acknowledged.

Mental Health

Many individuals are able to find self-gratification and self-esteem in their regular vocations, but others derive little gratification from the services they give and will seek some other source of emotional satisfaction. Through recreation an individual can achieve a high level of personal performance, experience mastery, and obtain attention, approval, and praise, all of which arouse emotions of pleasure and elation. Self-esteem, so essential to a high level of mental health, can be enhanced by recreation, which gives the individual an experience in which the self is of importance.

Preventive benefits. Recreation offers many emotional and intellectual benefits. Competitive games can serve as a healthy outlet for aggression, and recent research links physical fitness to high motivation, persistence, learning, achievement, self-confidence, and social acceptance. Cooperative activities can provide a sense of belonging and community. Benefits can be attained through creative, aesthetic, social, communicative, and educational activities as well as through physical activities and performance. For example, relaxation may be achieved through more passive interests such as reading, listening to music, attending lectures, visiting museums, and otherwise serving more the role of the spectator than that of the active participant. Creative urges can be satisfied through programs in crafts, painting, dramatics, music, writing, and other arts.

Therapeutic benefits. As part of the therapeutic procedure in mental health counseling and psychiatric treatment, specific types of recreation may be prescribed for each patient. Dance therapy and music therapy have become professional sub-specialties.

The National Therapeutic Recreation Society, formed in 1982 as a branch of the National Recreation and Park Association, describes the purpose of therapeutic recreation to be the development, maintenance, and expression of an appropriate leisure life-style for individuals with physical, mental, emotional, or social limitations. Therapeutic recreation professionals seek to enhance clients' leisure ability in recognition of the importance and value of leisure in the human experience. Therapy services are applied in various settings, including hospitals and residential and community-based health and human service agencies for people of all ages. Halfway houses, community mental health centers, nursing homes, rehabilitation centers, sheltered workshops, vocational training centers, burn centers, and children's hospitals all use therapeutic recreation specialists.

Social Health

Human interaction should promote a feeling of worth, a feeling of security from group acceptance, approval, and recognition. Social drives include the desire for new experiences, adventure, and identity with others.

Recreation can elevate the feeling of personal worth in those who already enjoy a high level of social health and in those whose social adjustment has been adequate but unsatisfying. It can be a means by which asocial individuals join in social situations. It also can be a means for preventing or correcting antisocial tendencies. Children and adolescents who are vulnerable to delinquency can find both release and wholesome alternatives to drugs,

---

Fitness Controversies

The sudden death of running guru Jim Fixx; news of female runners failing to menstruate; reports of reduced sex drive in male runners; allergic reactions and orthopedic problems following heavy exercise—such adverse publicity has called fitness programs into question in the minds of many people.

Fixx, age 52, died of a heart attack within the first 50 yards of his daily run. At age 39 he had been a two-pack-a-day smoker and weighed 50 pounds more than he should have. He also had a family history of heart disease. He stopped smoking, lost weight, and became a world-famous runner, then died of a heart attack 10 years later.

The menstruation problems reported in runners have been found in women experiencing a dramatic drop in body fat because of low caloric intake and high expenditures of energy.

A Canadian research team compared the levels of male hormones in 18 sedentary men with those in 31 men who regularly run at least 40 miles per week. They found significantly lower testosterone and prolactin levels in the runners, as well as a higher incidence of chronic fatigue.

Allergic reactions to exercise are extremely rare and can be controlled with medication. Orthopedic problems—including fractures, sprains, shin splints, and torn ligaments—are much more common, but their incidence and the risks associated with them must be weighed against the risks of not exercising.

- How do these reports balance out in a community's decision to promote or support fitness programs and activities?
- How would you handle public inquiries about these possible health risks if you were responsible for managing a community fitness program?
- Why are so many of the concerns in community health today issues of relative risk, whereas they once seemed more clear-cut issues of protecting the public's health?

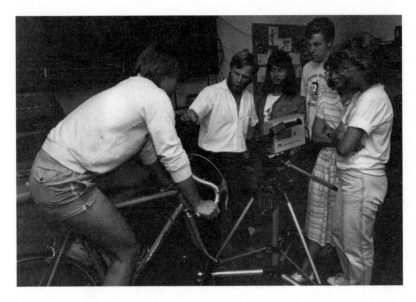

FIGURE 10-7
Cycling laboratories allow exercise physiologists to test physical responses to precise levels of energy expended.
Source: University of British Columbia Community Relations Office and Dr. David Sanderson.

alcohol, and tobacco in recreational participation. Family recreation in particular can be an aid in preventing delinquency. A Detroit study of over 2000 court cases showed that 60% of the juveniles had little or no recreation within the family group, 32% experienced occasional family recreation, and only 8% participated regularly in family recreation. A common recreational interest can bring together a diversity of people and promote a general understanding and appreciation of other human beings, which in turn will improve the individual's ability to adjust socially.

Physical Health

The evidence is mounting that the physically fit live longer, perform better, and participate more fully in life than do those who are not fit. Regular, vigorous exercise adds to vibrant good health and enhances the capacity for enjoying life and **functional health.**

Preventive benefits. The physical exertion inherent in many physical activities creates organic vigor and physiological well-being and increases physiological efficiency. Physical activity develops skills, dexterity, coordination, and stamina. If pursued with enough frequency and intensity, a fitness program will provide sufficient physical exertion to stimulate the body to a higher level of efficiency in its functioning.

The actual amount of exercise that recreation or fitness programs should provide should be determined by the individual's general condition and the exercise he or she gets on the job and from other day-to-day living practices. An individual who adjusts activities to capacity and needs can gain certain established benefits. Metabolism will improve, circulation and respiration will function more efficiently, muscle tone and coordination will improve, greater flexibility may be achieved, and general body efficiency will increase (Figure 10-7).

Therapeutic benefits. Physical rehabilitation programs employ recreational activities as a large part of their occupational therapy. The motivation that a particular activity can give to a rehabilitation patient often makes the difference between inadequate and adequate recovery. Indeed, the mental and physical stimulation that a recreational or fitness activity can give to a normal individual can be even greater for the individual who is recovering from extended illness or a disability. More than one fourth of the hospitals in the United States have organized recreational programs.

SCOPE OF RECREATION AND FITNESS

From the limited philosophy of recreation as sports and competition, the scope of recreation has extended to intellectual pursuits, creative and aesthetic activities, and social events. A specific activity may well be considered as being in all of these categories. For purposes of delineation and convenience, each classification described below will include those activities whose primary function is in that particular category, although secondary functions may serve other purposes (Figure 10-8).

Physical Activities

Activities whose primary purpose is to provide physical exertion, weight control, and exercise include both team and individual events.

The number of calories per minute that might be expended by an individual pursuing a physical activity depends on many variables, such as the activity itself, physical build, age, skill at the activity, and adverse circumstances—for example, a strong

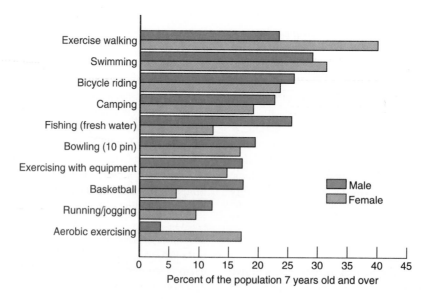

FIGURE 10-8
Participation in 10 most popular sports activities, by sex, United States, 1990.
Source: National Health Interview Survey, National Center for Health Statistics.

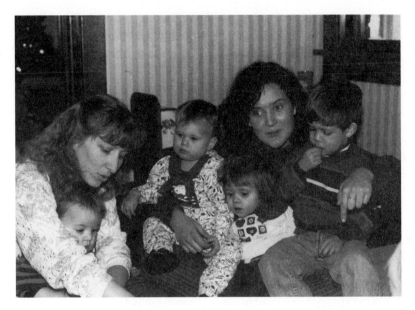

FIGURE 10-9
Children learn social skills, ethics, and manners through social games and organized activities under adult supervision.
Photo courtesy M. Jane Ford, Health Director, Lincoln-Lancaster County Health Department, Lincoln, Nebraska.

wind while running, waves while swimming, or an awkward partner while dancing. Table 10-1 is a comparative guide to the relative benefits of various physical activities in terms of fitness, weight loss, and general well-being and conditioning.

Intellectual Activities

Many recreational activities that are largely intellectual or educational in nature have other values, although their primary attraction is in the intellectual stimulation or the opportunity for learning that they provide. Such activities and interests include astronomy, chess, collecting of scientific materials, computer programming, debates, discussion groups, educational games, educational television, exhibits, fairs, first-aid courses, forums, interest groups and classes, language study, museum visits, ornithology, reading, scouting, stamp collecting, and tours.

Creative and Aesthetic Activities

Most creative and aesthetic activities will have some aspects of a learning experience and will depend on intellectual application. Certain activities particularly satisfy the creative urge of people and provide special opportunities for exercise or aesthetic experiences; among these are aerobic and ballet dancing, clay modeling, dramatics, drawing and painting, group singing, instrumental music, jewelry making, leathercraft, metalcraft, needlework, photography, pottery, puppetry, sculpting, weaving, and woodworking.

Social Activities

Virtually all recreation includes some social aspects. Activities planned primarily for their social value include board games, card games, carnivals, church nights, circuses, concerts, dancing, hobby clubs, holiday parties, and games to teach young children social skills (Figure 10-9).

The array of recreational activities suggests that a person who could not find one such interest would indeed be destitute. Individuals may need help in understanding the broad array of activities possible and in choosing activities that are suitable to their needs, interests, and resources. It is not surprising to find many people with several recreational interests who benefit physically, intellectually, creatively, aesthetically, and socially from these pursuits.

VALUES IN RECREATION AND FITNESS

Many people associate fitness with good physical performance rather than with good health, improved appearance, or better performance on the job and in the classroom. This has been especially true among the poor, the elderly, and the less educated. But perceptions and values are changing.

Vocational and other interests and activities seem to be adequate to provide some people with the necessary motivation for gratification in living. If recreation merely serves to fill time, its value as a positive force and profitable investment of time is lost for the individual, the family, the group, and the community.

According to a Louis Harris survey, Americans have given up an average of 8 hours of leisure time each week over the past decade, devoting 7 of those hours to work in response to economic pressures. Yet the respondents reported seeing television programs, movies, art exhibits, concerts, and dance performances more often than in the previous decade. Three of every four respondents said the arts give them "pure pleasure." Despite the increase in the United States in the total number of hours worked from 1970 to 1989, participation in the arts has increased. During the past year, 78% of Americans attended movies, 67% watched some kindof theater, and 58% visited an art museum.

Bertrand Russell noted how deeply rooted the value attached to exercise is in American tradition: "Unhappy businessmen, I am convinced, would increase their happiness more by walking six miles every day than by any conceivable change of philosophy. This, incidentally, was the opinion of Jefferson, who on this ground deplored the horse. Language would have failed him if he could have foreseen the motor car" (Russell, 1946). The valuing of exercise can be traced at least to Athenian culture, in which the Greek athletic emphasis on health gave rise to the Olympics. But the ancient Greek concept of mind and body gave Western civilization a broader notion of health than mere physical prowess. In 1588 Michel de Montaigne commented on the ability to unbend and be at ease as becoming to a strong and generous soul, and how remarkable it was that Socrates in his old age found time to take lessons in dancing and the playing of musical instruments, and considered it time well spent.

Individual Benefits

Recreation and fitness activities can offer the individual adventure, physical activity, skill development, release of tension, relaxation, participation and a feeling of belonging, challenges, mastery, success, creativity, stimulation, diversion from boring routines, elation, and a fuller life. Doubtless, these benefits can be acquired from pursuits other than recreation, but for people living in a highly organized and mechanized world, it becomes increasingly necessary to satisfy many personal needs through initiatives outside work and normal living habits.

The particular benefits perceived by individuals in relation to their most common physical or athletic pursuits are felt more intensely by those whose level of activity is greater than a minimal or cursory involvement. One study asked reasons for participation in physical recreation; answers included feel better, pleasure, improve flexibility, control weight,

Keeping Fitness in Perspective

A light-hearted but provocative reminder that fitness should not become an end in itself, pursued single-mindedly without connection to deeper or more socially relevant values, is offered by William H. Carlyon's poem "The Healthiest Couple," reprinted with the author's permission:

They brush and they floss
with care every day,
But not before breakfast
of both curds and whey.

He jogs for his heart
she bikes for her nerves;
They assert themselves daily
with appropriate verve.

He is loving and tender
and caring and kind,
Not one chauvinist thought
is allowed in his mind.

They are slim and attractive
well-dressed and just fun.
They are strong and well-immunized
against everything under the sun.

They are sparkling and lively
and having a ball.
Their diet? High fiber
and low cholesterol.

Cocktails are avoided
in favor of juice;
Cigarettes are shunned
as one would the noose.

They drive their car safely
with belts well in place;
at home not one hazard
ever will they face.

1.2 children they raise,
both sharing the job.
One is named Betty,
.2 is named Bob.

And when at the age of
two hundred and three

they jog from this life
to one still more free,

They'll pass through those portals
to claim their reward
and St. Peter will stop them
"just for a word."

"What Ho" he will say,
"You cannot go in.
This place is reserved
for those without sin."

"But we've followed the rules"
she'll say with a fright.
"We're healthy—
"Near perfect—
"And incredibly bright."

"But that's it" will say Peter,
drawing himself tall.
"You've missed the point of living
By thinking so small."

"Life is more than health habits,
Though useful they be,
It is purpose and meaning,
the grand mystery."

"You've discovered a part
of what makes humans whole
and mistaken that part
for the shape of the soul."

"You are fitter than fiddles
and sound as a bell,
Self-righteous, intolerant
and boring as hell."

- What values, besides fitness as an end in itself, might families or couples respond to in participating in community fitness programs?
- By placing fitness in the broader context of recreation and health, how does the community give families and couples broader meaning for their participation?
- By encouraging joint participation of family members in recreational and fitness programs designed for groups, how does the community support values other than fitness as an end in itself?

reduce stress, be with people, learn new things, challenge personal abilities, and respond to advice by others, including a physician.

Family Benefits

Recreation can serve to integrate family action through joint interest. Social changes and new understandings of what constitutes a family have made the promotion of family recreation more complex. The growing tendency has been to disperse the family rather than to consolidate family living. Women, who once devoted their early marriage years to childbearing, formerly had a different set of recreational and fitness needs than those today who seek careers. Neighborhood cohesiveness has been largely supplanted by friendships based on special interests; social groups are not so often formed on a neighborhood basis today. The increasing complexity and overorganization of social services and social structure has had the effect of disrupting the family; children and parents tend not to participate in common events. The child has his or her separate interests and recreational outlets in day-care centers, sports groups, music, art, scouting, and various teenage activities.

Family-centered fun is inclined toward commercialized amusements and sedentary viewing of television. However, there are many other activities in which both children and adults have potential mutual interest and can participate. Some degree of promotion may be necessary (''The family that plays together stays together''), but frequently a common interest already exists that merely needs to be realized. Camping, music, painting, badminton, photography, crafts, picnics, hiking, bicycling, volleyball, motor trips, boating, swimming, fishing, folk dancing, skating, skiing, bowling, tennis, golf, gardening, church activities, walking, jogging, and special family nights suggest the variety of activities that lend themselves to total family participation.

To participate as a group, to enjoy common ex-

periences, to share the gratifications of accomplishment, and to pioneer together in new ventures will promote the physical, mental, emotional, and social well-being of the members of the family. The sense of belonging that recreation cements is important in family integration (and group integration in general). With each member being an individual in his or her own right, joint recreation gives each participant valuable experience in respecting the other members, adjusting to their needs and opinions, and caring about the well-being of the rest of the family.

Surveys show that many adults today want their children to be both concerned and involved with physical fitness. The growing involvement of women in sports has influenced parental attitudes. With the exception of certain competitive or contact sports, parents are almost as eager for their daughters to be involved in athletics as they are for their sons. Collaborative activities for youth and adults are gaining in popularity.

Group Benefits

Recreation is one means by which the gregariousness of the human species is expressed. Association with others who have the same interests and special needs can be made possible through recreation; in fact, recreational and fitness activities often present the best opportunity for such association and group participation. Engaging in common recreational or fitness pursuits rewards members of the group with a richer experience in group participation, in social adjustment, and in understanding people of like interests and needs.

Children, adolescents, adults, and the aging have different recreational and fitness interests and needs (Figure 10-10). Age grouping, however, is not always the pattern on which group recreational or fitness programs are based. The physically challenged and those with impaired vision or hearing often need special group recreational and fitness opportunities. Similarly, the mentally retarded can benefit from

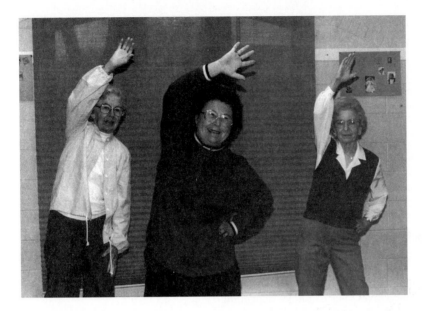

FIGURE 10-10
The benefits derived from increasing physical activity from a minimal (sedentary) level to a moderate level are greatest for the elderly.
Photo courtesy M. Jane Ford, Health Director, Lincoln-Lancaster County Health Department, Lincoln, Nebraska.

special opportunities for group activities. The Special Olympics has demonstrated the value and need for such activities. Intergenerational grouping has benefits for young and old.

Formal groups find recreation an ideal vehicle for the promotion of group solidarity, morale, motivation, and attainment. Informal groups, which retain more individuality, find recreational activities that will permit individual development within group participation. Organized groups, characterized by individual sharing, and unorganized groups, characterized by a lack of cohesiveness, have equal need for recreational activities. Recreation provides both opportunities for cooperative service and a common interest that can hold a group together.

Whether it serves as a primary or ancillary activity of a group, recreation, like mutual self-help in health and fitness, raises the general value and significance of the group to its members. In this respect,

recreation is a means to an end rather than an end in itself.

Community Benefits

The happiness, physical health, character development, and morale of a community are but an expression of these qualities on a composite basis in its citizens. Through its social processes, a community can do much to establish the general standard or pattern of community living. In this highly industrial age, a community that provides opportunities for recreation and fitness makes an investment in community stability and integration.

Economic Benefits

In the United States the amount of personal income available for and spent on recreation has continued to increase from $91 billion in 1970 to $256 billion in 1990. The largest amounts were spent on video and audio products ($53 billion), toys and sport supplies ($28.3 billion), and wheel goods, sports, and photographic equipment ($27.7 billion). In 1990 $19 billion was spent on books, and attendance at major league sports included 55.5 million at baseball games, 17.6 million at football games, and 12.6 million at hockey games.

The stimulus of recreation and fitness affects all levels of the economy. In the United States jobs in the service sector of recreation in particular have been growing at a faster rate than jobs in all other industries, including other service industries. Another significant impact of recreation on the U.S. economy is the generation of federal, state, and local revenues through sales, income, property, amusement, and gasoline taxes. For example, depending on its proximity to private property, parkland can have a positive or negative impact on property values. Generally, however, recreational improvements enhance the monetary value of nearby properties.

Employers and businesses also gain important economic advantages from investments in exercise facilities and recreation for their employees. The assumed benefits include reduced absenteeism, fewer serious health problems, improved worker productivity, reduced insurance premiums or benefits paid, and improved morale, resulting in better recruitment, less turnover, and consequently lower training expenses.

The provision and maintenance of recreational services is a sizable component of local, state, and federal government budgets. Local government spending for recreation tends to be around 2% of county and municipal budgets.

SPONSORS OF RECREATIONAL PROGRAMS

In modern communities planned recreation programs must provide the physical activity that everyday life no longer supplies. The government at all levels, employers, voluntary agencies, schools, and families must join together to provide leadership and facilities for recreation. Programs or activities considered recreational in nature may fall under one or more classifications ranging from commercial entertainment to public recreational and fitness programs.

National Programs and Leadership

In the United States the national physical fitness program sponsored by the U.S. Office of Disease Prevention and Health Promotion and by the President's Council on Physical Fitness and Sports (PCPFS) has the following mission:

- A population committed to physical fitness and possessed of the knowledge and skills to achieve it.
- Acceptance by parents, schools, recreational agencies, and sports organizations of their special responsibilities for fitness (Figure 10-11).
- Recognition by communities and employers that fitness facilities and programs should be a part of the residential and work environments.
- Maximal use of all resources—human and material, public and private—for physical fitness.

Fitness Canada, the federal lead agency for Canadian programs in physical fitness, has a mission similar to that of the lead U.S. agencies.

The task of the federal government in fitness programs is to educate, advise, and encourage. The U.S. government has developed selected Objectives for the Nation related to physical fitness included in this chapter. The responsibility for action usually rests with parents, school administrators, teachers, coaches, recreation supervisors, civic and business leaders, and others at the community level.

National Voluntary Organizations

Hundreds of national organizations in the United States support recreation and fitness activities in local communities. Bikecentennial and the League of

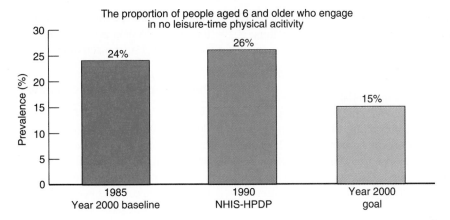

FIGURE 10-11

The proportion of people 6 years and older who engage in no leisure-time physical activity increased slightly between 1985 and 1990. The objectives for the nation in health promotion and disease prevention seek to reverse this trend and reduce the proportion to 15% by the year 2000.

Source: National Health Interview Survey (NHIS), National Center for Health Statistics and U.S. Office of Disease Prevention and Health Promotion (HPDP).

American Wheelmen both promote the use of bicycles. The American Bowling Congress and the Women's International Bowling Congress standardize rules of play and sanction leagues and tournaments. Aerobics Dancing, Inc., and numerous other vendors of health promotion and fitness programs offer tape recordings, videotapes, scripts, or trained instructors to conduct exercise programs. The National Campers and Hikers Association, the Sierra Club, and the U.S. Forest Service all support hiking and camping. Similar organizations for racquetball, running, skating, skiing, swimming, tennis, volleyball, yoga, and even walking (the American Volkssport Association) provide information and guidelines for community organization of programs or events. Directories of these and other resources for **community health events** are available through the Office of Disease Prevention and Health Promotion National Health Information Center (P.O. Box 1133, Washington, D.C., 20013-1133) or from Fitness Canada (506-294 Albert Street, Ottawa K1P 6E6).

Commercial Entertainment

Entertainment is a passive type of recreation in which the individual is a spectator or enjoys the activity vicariously. In recent years it has become fashionable in some circles to condemn entertainment of all kinds. The term *couch potato* has been used to disparage the growing popularity of television. The empathy, exhilaration, and enjoyment that come from watching highly skilled athletes and artists perform can have educational, intellectual, and emotional value. Unfortunately, for some, commercial entertainment is a complete substitution for active recreation. Rather than condemn entertainment as damaging to a community's moral fiber, however, the constructive approach is to prepare people for—and provide the means for—physical recreational activities.

Commercial entertainment is big business. It includes professional sports, high school and collegiate athletics, theatricals, concerts, movies, television and radio programs, horse racing, fairs, circuses, and many other activities in which people derive enjoyment merely from being spectators.

Commercial and Semipublic Recreation

Although certain commercial recreational enterprises actually may be semipublic in nature, the vast majority of them are available to the general public. For example, fitness centers sponsored by hospitals, voluntary health associations, and commercial organizations offer fee-for-service programs in aerobic exercise to individuals and to organizations for their employees.

Semipublic recreation usually is made available through organizations that normally reserve their facilities for their own members, but on occasion make them available to nonmembers. Athletic clubs, golf clubs, tennis clubs, and social clubs may be in this category.

Bowling, roller skating, ice skating, skiing, golf and miniature golf, swimming, canoeing, and horseback riding are examples of commercial and semipublic recreation that can be part of a community's recreational program. Video games are more recent and still dubious entries on the commercial recreation scene, displacing pool halls in many communities.

Private Recreational and Fitness Programs

In providing recreational and fitness opportunities in a community, sports groups and social organizations that limit their facilities and services exclusively to their own members should not be underestimated. Country clubs and private fitness clubs are notable examples of such organizations. From the standpoint of community recreation, members of these groups are privileged to enjoy recreational opportunities that one might hope everyone could enjoy. Even when formed primarily for recreational purposes, most of these private organizations serve more than one function. Private clubs for golf, swimming, dancing, boating, riding, hunting, skeet shooting, tennis, skiing, weight training, bowling, and other physical activities often include creative, social, and aesthetic activities.

Public Recreational and Fitness Programs

Providing opportunities for recreation and fitness does not mean that all recreation must be planned or in any sense formal. Indeed, it is a justifiable apprehension that, particularly for youngsters, there is too little opportunity for self-created recreational activities. Teen centers have been constructed by some communities to provide for unstructured but supervised activity.

Urban areas. Recreational services in urban areas are primarily the responsibility of the local government. Communities generally have the authority to zone and acquire land and to provide public services, including recreation. Political fragmentation too often makes solutions to the problem of providing open space on a regional scale very difficult; it requires a cooperative approach that individual jurisdictions are sometimes reluctant to undertake. The increasing disparity in wealth of communities—poor core cities surrounded by wealthier suburbs—results in inequitable recreational services. Thus local solutions are sometimes impossible and often inadequate. The assistance of higher levels of government is often needed.

State government. States and provinces now are actively providing, or assisting local governments in providing, urban recreational opportunities. Most provinces and states concentrate their park and recreation efforts on acquiring open space of regional or statewide significance. The potential is great for state and provincial governments to identify urban recreational needs, work with local governments in developing comprehensive strategies to alleviate identified deficiencies, and assign priority to urban recreational projects. States and provinces can encourage localities in metropolitan regions to work together to develop regionwide open space strategies; they can also provide technical assistance to local groups.

Community actions. Much can be done locally to improve recreational lands and services without any assistance from state, provincial, and federal governments. The following three objectives are suggested local and state actions. They include actions by both public and private (nonprofit and for-profit) providers. In many cases these suggestions are being carried out successfully in communities, states, and provinces in North America, Europe, Australia, and New Zealand.

1. Conserve open space for its exercise and recreational value. Local governments and private organizations must work together at the community level.

- To develop procedures for multijurisdictional, public-private conservation of open space through mechanisms such as fee acquisition, purchase of easement, management strategies, or establishment of regional resource conservation and recreation authorities with independent taxing and management roles.
- To transfer derelict land, tax-delinquent land, surplus highway rights-of-way, and other land not presently in productive use to park agencies through land exchange, purchase, or long-term, no-fee leases.
- To make maximal use of lands associated with public water supply reservoirs to meet urban recreational needs.
  To adopt regulations for new residential, business, or industrial development and redevelopment that require either the dedication of parklands, provision of recreational facilities, or payment of money to a public recreation fund.

2. Provide financial support for parks and recreation. Accessible facilities, diverse programs, year-round operation, and good maintenance contribute to citizen satisfaction with community recreation. These elements all require substantial numbers of competent staff and a steady source of funds to sustain them. Hiring freezes and staff cutbacks have occurred in a majority of park and recreation departments over the last 12 years in the United States, resulting in reduced program opportunities and facility maintenance.

Communities and state or provincial governments could address these problems in the following ways:

- Evaluate user fee policies and identify ways to increase recreation and fitness revenues through user fees and concession royalties.
- Earmark a portion of local tax revenues for parks and recreational or fitness facilities.
- Hire grants experts to ensure that local governments are taking advantage of all appropriate nonlocal sources of assistance.
- Adopt legislation giving local governments full authority to set tax rates and to issue bonds.
- Adopt legislation authorizing localities to deposit revenues earned from specific park and recreational activities (such as concession stands and golf courses) in accumulated capital outlay funds to be used only for similar park and recreational activities.

Objective for Physical Activity and Fitness

- Increase community availability and accessibility of physical activity and fitness facilities as follows:

Facility	1986 Baseline	2000 Target
Hiking, biking, and fitness trail miles	1 per 71,000 people	1 per 10,000 people
Public swimming pools	1 per 53,000 people	1 per 25,000 people
Acres of park and recreation open space	1.8 per 1000 people (553 people per managed acre)	4 per 1000 people (250 people per managed acre)

- Increase state and local tax incentives for donations of land, easements, and money.
- Create local public trusts and foundations to receive donations that will assist in land preservation or provide programs and services.

3. *Provide close-to-home exercise and recreational opportunities.* Most people, especially in urban areas, want recreational opportunities within walking distance of home. By far the most frequent reason given in most surveys asking people why they are not getting enough exercise is "lack of time" or "inconvenient facilities." For children the problem is often one of transportation.

Many urban neighborhoods lack a variety of year-round programs and facilities that are responsive and available to all residents. About three fourths of the neighborhoods sampled in field studies reported dissatisfaction with neighborhood recreational opportunities.

Recreation in urban areas includes a wide array of programs provided by many organizations in the community: teen and senior citizen centers; service centers and programs of nonprofit, voluntary agencies; bicycle paths; exercise facilities; parks; and other public and private facilities. Indoor recreational facilities and community centers play a critical role in providing recreational services. General purpose community centers serve as neighborhood meeting places, are usable throughout the year, and often have supervised recreational programs not always available at outdoor sites.

Actions that can be taken by local governments and community groups to assure greater accessibility of recreational resources are

- To establish priorities that recognize the location of potential users when considering acquisition of new recreation land.
- To use streets closed to traffic, rooftops, parking lots, utility rights-of-way, water supply reservoirs, and so on, to provide nearby places for exercise and recreation in heavily developed and densely populated areas.

- To use mobile recreation units where appropriate.
- To coordinate park planning and public transit planning to ensure that new parks and fitness facilities are accessible by public transit.
- To improve public transit service to parks and fitness facilities during weekends and evenings, which are times of peak use.
- To plan for maximal pedestrian and bicycle access to new parks as an alternative to automobile access.
- To ensure that transit-dependent people have a real voice in the transportation planning process.
- To develop a comprehensive inventory and plan for all parks and physical improvements as a first step toward removing or modifying architectural barriers to the physically handicapped.
- To provide specialized staff and equipment for the handicapped, senior citizens, and young children to help them make better use of exercise and park facilities and programs.

Public resources for recreation will be expanded very little in the years immediately ahead, with the exception of snow- and water-based facilities. Particular attention must be given to recreation for adolescents and for the elderly in the urban community.

COMMUNITY RESOURCES AND EDUCATION

Organizations having facilities and members who are willing to contribute their services can add appreciably to the community's recreational and fitness resources. It is not just a matter of accepting those who are willing to volunteer, but of recruiting all the individuals who may make a contribution to the program. By enlisting the cooperation and active participation of all such people and organizations in the community, it is possible to have an extensive community-wide recreational program without huge expenditures on the part of any individual or group (Figure 10-12).

Community action can expand the use of existing recreational and physical fitness resources through such methods as the following:

- Use school buildings that have been closed or are underused because of declining enrollment for recreation and fitness.
- Consider the potential for joint recreational use in the planning stages for all new or expanded school and park facilities.
- Develop reciprocal, no-fee policies that encourage both park use by school groups and school use by park groups.
- Assist in providing services required to open school facilities to the public for recreational purposes after school hours; this will overcome present constraints on joint use, such as prohibitive custodial and maintenance costs.
- Encourage joint use for recreation, wherever possible, of lands and facilities committed to other private and public purposes, including federal property, utility rights-of-way, and the property of institutions and private corporations.
- Encourage use of local park and recreational facilities for a wider range of human delivery services, such as health information, consumer protection, and nutrition information.

Relative Strength of the Measures

In the short run, the programs most likely to be successful in recruiting new participants to appropriate physical activity are those that offer services and facilities to individuals and economic incentives to groups and individuals. Programs that can more easily be implemented and are more likely to effect lasting changes include those related to providing public information and education and improving the linkages with other health promotion efforts. The effectiveness of all measures is handicapped by the limitation in knowledge about the relationship between recreation and exercise and physical and emotional health; the optimal types of exercises for various groups of people with special needs; and the appropriate way to measure individual levels of physical fitness.

Official Agencies

Tax-supported organizations are regarded as **official agencies.** The state or provincial conservation department providing park, camping, hunting, and fishing facilities is an example of a governmental agency that serves as a valuable resource in recreation. Official agencies on the county and city level

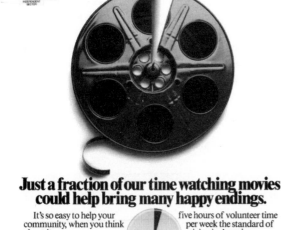

Just a fraction of our time watching movies could help bring many happy endings.

It's so easy to help your community, when you think about it. Millions of people have helped make five percent of their incomes and **Give Five.** five hours of volunteer time per week the standard of giving in America. Get involved with the causes you care about and give five. *What you get back is immeasurable.*

FIGURE 10-12

A national public service campaign sponsored by the Independent Sector and the Advertising Council encourages the American public to give 5% of their income to community charity and 5% of their time as volunteers to help meet community needs.

Source: Advertising Council, New York.

include schools, park boards, and public libraries. A city recreation commission, formally organized by the city council with a staff of full-time professional recreational personnel, should be the nucleus of the entire community recreational program. The recreation commission's program can be financed with only 2% of the city's annual budget. While various recreational activities do produce some revenue for the city, such income is merely an incidental factor in maintaining the program. Cities today accept recreation as a necessary and proper community service and must appropriate funds for its promotion.

Social Groups

People with common interests and needs tend either formally or informally to organize groups to promote their common interests. This is notably true of recreational and fitness interests. These groups usually are limited in their numbers and usually serve only their own members but contribute appreciably to recreation in a community. Dance groups, jogging groups, bridge groups, groups of young married couples, and similar organizations are to be found in most communities. Each group in its own way meets certain recreational needs for its members. Some social groups also undertake to promote recreational activities that will be available to nonmembers. From one social group, many groups may develop to enhance the overall recreational and fitness programs of the community.

Religious Groups

Health and fitness are integral to most religious and philosophical systems. Recreational activities sponsored by religious groups usually are conducted not in competition with official agencies but as supplements to governmental programs. The Young Men's Christian Association (YMCA), the Young Women's Christian Association (YWCA), Boys Clubs of America, B'nai B'rith Hillel Foundations, Jewish Community Centers, Diocesan Youth Councils, the

National Catholic Youth Council, and the Methodist Youth Fellowship are examples of religious groups that promote outstanding recreational and fitness programs. Most of these nationally organized groups have local affiliates or facilities in many communities. For example, in the United States there are nearly two thousand YMCA and YWCA facilities. Similar distributions are found in Canada, Europe, Australia, and most other Western countries. Corresponding groups have been established in African, Asian, and Latin American countries, where religious organizations play an even larger role in community life.

Business and Industry

Apart from their commercial interests in health-related products and facilities, employers have many reasons for contributing to the recreation and fitness of their employees, both at the worksite and in the community. Although existing programs are too new to yield much statistical data, accumulating evidence from research shows that workers taking part in regular physical activity programs miss fewer workdays when they do get sick, are less vulnerable to accidents, have a higher overall work output, and suffer fewer emotional disorders and physical disabilities.

The most extensive research on employee fitness

Objective for Physical Activity and Fitness

• By 2000 increase the proportion of worksites offering employer-sponsored physical activity and fitness programs as follows:

Number of Employees	1985	2000 Target
50-99	14%	20%
100-249	23%	35%
250-749	32%	50%
>750	54%	80%

programs has been carried out in the Soviet Union, where the tangible economic benefits of regular exercise have been repeatedly documented. Russian experts found that working people who exercise regularly produce more, visit physicians less, and seem to be more immune to industrial accidents. Japanese companies also routinely provide for exercise breaks.

National Aeronautic and Space Administration employees who participated in a fitness study in Houston, Texas, reported a general sense of well-being that improved their attitudes about their work and enriched their leisure time. Even more significant was that the results of medical tests bore out the perceived benefits of the program. Those who reported improved stamina, for example, showed marked improvement in cardiovascular performance. Similar results were reported for the employee fitness programs of the New York State Education and Civil Service Department, where risk factors were reduced, health problems eased, and employee absenteeism cut down.

The first true fitness program in a U.S. firm began in 1894 at the National Cash Register Company in Dayton, Ohio, where the president authorized morning and afternoon exercise breaks for employees, then built a gymnasium and a 325-acre park for National Cash Register people and their families. Since then, company-sponsored recreational and fitness facilities have become commonplace.

Today more than half of all companies in the United States with 750 or more employees provide fitness programs for their workers. Some companies, such as IBM, subsidize community facilities such as parks or the programs of the YMCA. Others—for example, Tenneco, Conoco, Pepsico, Johnson & Johnson, and Kimberly-Clark—have developed separate facilities at their own sites.

Some companies hesitate to launch fitness programs because they fear they will be liable for injuries to employees. Studies and on-site experience, however, show that this risk is minimal; where health and fitness programs are properly designed and supervised, the risk of injury is negligible. Anything a company does for its employees—whether a company outing or softball league—involves some liability. A fitness program should be recognized as an integral part of the job, under which the employee is fully protected by workmen's compensation or private insurance.

The experiences of Canada and the United States with employee health promotion and fitness programs have been documented and summarized in guidelines available from Fitness Canada and from the U.S. Public Health Service.

Youth-Serving Agencies

Over 250 organizations in the United States work with children and youth under 25 years of age. The areas in which these organizations serve are so diverse that it would be difficult to imagine any recreational needs left unprovided. Youth-serving organizations include 4-H groups, Future Farmers of America, Future Homemakers of America, Boys Clubs and Girls Clubs of America, Boy Scouts, Girl Scouts, Camp Fire Girls, Big Brothers/Big Sisters of America, and the Junior Red Cross. These and other groups in the United States and worldwide indicate the many agencies created to provide the leisure-time and health activities essential for the best development of the children and youth of the community. Use of school facilities after hours by these groups is an ideal way of maximizing resources and addressing the **latchkey syndrome** of unsupervised youth.

Service Groups

Community service groups sometimes sponsor continuing fitness and recreational programs. Equally important is that these service groups are an ever-present resource that can be called on to support any worthwhile recreational program in the community. Rotary Clubs, Lions Clubs, Kiwanis, Junior League, Exchange Clubs, Soroptimists, Grange, Parent-

Teacher Associations, and similar organizations provide a diversity of services in their communities, not the least of these being the promotion of recreational and fitness programs.

Neighborhoods

Since recreational activities often grow out of group interests, an actual or potential neighborhood interest can serve as a catalyst in initiating and extending recreational activities. Many of these enterprises are self-starting, but others need leadership to crystallize support and to implement the contribution of the group. Interest in building a playground in the neighborhood can be a starting point from which an extensive neighborhood recreational program can be developed. When a playground already exists in the neighborhood, interest can be generated in expanding both the facilities and the activities they accommodate.

Special Interest Groups

The typical community has a number of groups with special recreational interests, such as gardening, music, dramatics, computers, chess, stamp collecting, and photography. Through these groups, others can be encouraged to develop new interests or to enjoy an interest they already have. There is something contagious about an intense interest in some fascinating or challenging hobby. As people become exposed to all possible recreational outlets, they are more likely to find activities that will appeal to their particular abilities and temperament.

Other Community Resources

Labor unions, industrial firms, retail business houses, chambers of commerce, and fraternal groups promote and support various recreational enterprises. Such organizations find that providing recreation is one of the best public relations services

they can contribute to their constituents. In any community it is possible to discover public-spirited organizations that will respond to reasonable requests for support of worthwhile community enterprises. These are the organizations that, with very little fanfare, play an extremely important role in the year-in, year-out promotion of the well-being of the community. They may take an active role and actually administer their own recreational or fitness programs, or their participation may be limited to financial or other support. Resources for the promotion of recreation are rarely more than partially tapped in most communities. To use all possible resources usually requires three things: a worthwhile program, qualified leadership, and an informed community.

Actions that communities can take to strengthen planning, leadership, and public education include the following:

- Employ professionals to do recreational services planning, as well as fitness program and facility planning, on a continuing basis.
- Improve coordination of planning and implementation efforts to ensure realistic plans and responsive action to meet identified needs.
- Coordinate recreational planning with other health and human service planning; coordinate park and facility planning with overall land use planning and physical fitness planning.
- Develop cooperative programs between resource agencies and local education advisors so that park and recreational resources become an instrument for environmental teaching as an extension of school and community health education programs.
- Broaden the scope of interpretive programming to address local environmental issues; sponsor public forums on land use planning, energy conservation, and environmental management programs to involve the public in the decision-making process.
- Encourage residents to assume responsibility

for making neighborhood parks safe by giving them a role in park supervision and maintenance.

- Conduct citizen participation and preference surveys to determine recreation deficiencies.
- Publish information on comparative local recreation preferences and needs throughout the state or province.
- Recruit inner-city personnel through an office of volunteerism to lead recreational and fitness programs.

Physical fitness through recreation will increase in importance with the increase in leisure time and the extension of life expectancy. Many factors enter into the expansion of community fitness and recreational programs. Understanding by the public must be encouraged, qualified professional leadership must be provided, and adequate resources must be distributed more equitably to serve the needs of special populations.

SUMMARY

This chapter has linked recreation and fitness on the premise that recreation serves a variety of physical, mental, and social health purposes, and that a healthful life-style can and should be fun and rewarding. For individuals, families, groups, and communities, fitness should not be seen as an end in itself, but as a means to the achievement of other quality-of-life benefits or social goals. The reasons people gave in the Canadian Fitness Survey for participating in active physical recreation, for example, reveal that to gain pleasure, fun, and excitement are nearly as important as "to feel better." The desire "to be with people" was given as a reason for participation almost as frequently as "to relax or reduce stress."

When approached as a social issue as well as a health issue, fitness falls more clearly into place in the development of community programs for rec-

> **To Increase Physical Activity and Fitness, by the Year 2000 . . .**
>
> Objectives target reducing coronary heart disease deaths and the prevalence of overweight; increasing moderate daily physical activity and cardiorespiratory fitness; reducing sedentary life-styles; increasing muscular strength, endurance, and flexibility; improving diet and physical activity habits among overweight people; increasing daily school physical education participation, physical activity in school physical education, and worksite physical activity and fitness programming; increasing community physical activity and fitness facilities; and increasing physical activity counseling by primary care providers.

reation and health. The history of recreation and fitness reveals the convergence over the past century of natural allies: the conservation movement, the urban parks movement, the recreation movement, and the fitness movement. Today new alliances are emerging with physical educators, recreation professionals, health educators, and others working in schools, in community agencies, and at worksites to develop comprehensive fitness programs with recreational and health benefits.

The health benefits of various sports and exercises include those described in Table 10-1 as criteria for physical fitness and general well-being, as well as various physical, mental, and social health benefits that are less direct.

The scope of recreation and fitness includes physical, intellectual, creative, and social activities. In addition to their health benefits, these activities offer a variety of family, group, and community benefits, including considerable economic value to the community.

Recreational activities can be provided or supported by national programs, commercial entertainment, commercial and semipublic recreation, private recreational and fitness programs, and public recreational programs, including park and open-space programs.

Community resources to support recreational activities include health promotion and educational measures, official agencies, social groups, religious groups, business and industry, service groups, neighborhoods, and special interest groups. Of particular note is the remarkable growth in recent years of corporate sponsorship of health and fitness programs for employees at the worksite.

QUESTIONS FOR REVIEW

1. What is the difference between recreation and fitness?
2. To what extent is recreation a vehicle for health promotion?
3. To what extent is recreation a vehicle for the treatment of disabilities?
4. Why are recreation and fitness growing as community enterprises in the United States?
5. What recreational and fitness activities are available in your community?
6. How can recreation promote social health?
7. Why does the public place so much emphasis on recreation of a physical nature?
8. Why is an intellectual activity recreational for one person but an unenjoyable task for another person?
9. How can group interests in your community be used to expand the community's recreational and fitness program?
10. What alternatives to the tavern and gambling hall does your community offer its citizens?
11. What role does commercial entertainment play in your community?
12. To what extent does commercial recreation contribute to the total recreational program of your community?
13. What recreational and fitness activities are provided publicly in your community?
14. What recreational areas and facilities are available in your community?
15. What additional areas and facilities should be provided?

READINGS

Baranowski T, Bouchard C, Bar-Or O et al: Assessment, prevalence, and cardiovascular benefits of physical activity and fitness in youth, *Med Sci Sports Exerc* 24(suppl 6):S237, 1992.

Reviews the definitions, types, and measurements of physical activity, the regional and national studies on the status of physical fitness and prevalence of physical activity, and the evidence of cardiovascular benefits from physical activity and fitness.

Blair SN, Kohl HW, Gordon NF et al: How much physical activity is good for health? *Annu Rev Public Health* 13:99, 1992.

Reviews the epidemiological evidence and historical analyses of energy expenditures and physical activity, concluding that some exercise is essential to good health but showing that moderate physical activity with regularity is just as good for most people as intensive physical activity.

King AC, Blair SN, Bild DE et al: Determinants of physical activity and interventions in adults, *Med Sci Sports Exerc* 24(suppl 6):S221, 1992.

Reviews the reasons people are more or less inclined to be active or sedentary and suggests program strategies based on these reasons.

Nuessel F: *The image of older adults in the media: an annotated bibliography,* Westport, Conn, 1992, Greenwood.

This bibliography of some 550 books and articles on older adults as they are portrayed in the print and nonprint media offers the student an opportunity to explore how popular conceptions of aging and decline in physical functioning condition public attitudes toward physical activity.

BIBLIOGRAPHY

Astrand P-O: Why exercise? JB Wolffe memorial lecture, *Med Sci Sports Exerc* 24:153, 1992.

Balcazar H, Cobas JA: Overweight among Mexican Americans and its relationship to life style behavioral risk factors, *J Community Health* 18:55, 1993.

Booth M, Bauman A, Oldenburg B et al: Effects of a national mass-media campaign on physical activity participation, *Health Prom Int* 7:241, 1992.

Bouchard C, Shephard R, Stephens T, editors: Physical activity, fitness, and health: consensus statement, Champaign, Ill, 1993, Human Kinetics Press.

Boyce RW, Hiatt AR, Jones GR: Physical fitness of police officers as they progress from supervised recruit to unsupervised sworn officer fitness programs, *Wellness Perspec* 8:31, 1992.

Buchner DM, Beresford SAA, Larson EB et al: Effects of physical activity on health status in older adults. II: Intervention studies, *Annu Rev Public Health* 13:469, 1992.

Cardinal BJ: Readability of printed materials on exercise, *Wellness Perspec: Theory Prac* 9:48, 1993.

Centers for Disease Control: Coronary heart disease attributable to sedentary lifestyle—selected states, 1988, *MMWR* 39:541, 1990.

Centers for Disease Control: Participation of high school students in school physical education—United States, 1990, *MMWR* 40:607, 1991.

Custer SJ, Doty CR: Assessment of self-motivation and selected physiological characteristics as predictors of adherence to exercise in a corporate setting, *J Health Educ* 23:232, 1992.

Edgell D: *Charting a course for international tourism in the '90s.* Washington, DC, 1990, U.S. Department of Commerce.

Eichstaedt CB, Lavay BW: *Physical activity for individuals with mental retardation: infancy through adulthood,* Champaign, Ill, 1992, Human Kinetics Press.

Emery CF, Blumenthal JA: Effects of physical exercise on psychological and cognitive functioning of older adults, *Ann Behav Med* 13:99, 1991.

Field LK, Steinfardt MA: The relationship of internally directed behavior to self-reinforcement, self-esteem, and expectancy values for exercise, *Am J Health Prom* 7:21, 1992.

Fletcher GF, Blair SN, Blumenthal J et al: Statement on exercise: benefits and recommendations for physical activity programs for all Americans, a statement for health professionals by the Committee on Exercise and Cardiac Rehabilitation of the Council on Clinical Cardiology, American Heart Association, *Circulation* 86: 340, 1992.

Jette M, Quenneville J, Sidney K: Fitness testing and counselling in health promotion, *Can J Sport Sci* 17: 194, 1992.

Knapik JJ, Jones BH, Reynolds KL et al: Validity of self-assessed physical fitness, *Am J Prev Med* 8:367, 1992.

Laws A, Reaven GM: Physical activity, glucose tolerance, and diabetes in older adults, *Ann Behav Med* 13:125, 1993.

Lee C: Women and aerobic exercise: directions for research development, *Ann Behav Med* 13:133, 1991.

Leon AS, Connett J, for the MRFIT Research Group: Physical activity and 10.5 year mortality in the multiple risk factor intervention trial (MRFIT), *Int J Epidemiol* 20:690, 1991.

Lissau I, Sorensen TIA: Prospective study of the influence of social factors in childhood on risk of overweight in young adulthood, *Int J Obesity* 16:169, 1992.

Lock JQ, Wister AV: Intentions and changes in exercise and behaviour: a life-style perspective, *Health Prom Int* 7:195, 1992.

Mason JO: Healthy people 2000 goals: How far have we come in physical fitness and activity? *Am Fitness* 10: 29, 1992.

Minor MA: Physical activity and management of arthritis, *Ann Behav Med* 13:117, 1991.

Parcel GS, Simons-Morton BG, O'Hara NM et al: School promotion of healthful diet and physical activity: impact on learning outcomes and self-reported behavior, *Health Educ Q* 16:181, 1989.

Piper MC, Pinnell LE, Darrah J et al: Construction and validation of the Alberta infant motor scale (AIMS), *Can J Public Health* 83(suppl 2):S3, 1992.

Powell KE, Kreuter MW, Stephens T et al: The dimensions of health promotion applied to physical activity, *J Public Health Policy* 12:492, 1991.

Russell B: *History of western philosophy,* London, 1946, George Allen & Unwin.

Russell SJ, Hyndford C, Beaulieu A: *Active living for Canadian children and youth: a statistical profile,* Ottawa, 1992, Canadian Fitness and Lifestyle Research Institute and Active Living Alliance for Children and Youth.

Sidney S, Haskell WL, Crow R et al: Symptom-limited graded treadmill exercise testing in young adults in the CARDIA study, *Med Sci Sports Exerc* 24:177, 1992.

Simons-Morton DG, Parcel GS, Brink SG et al: *Promoting physical activity among adults: a CDC community intervention handbook,* Atlanta, 1988, Centers for Disease Control.

Singer J, Lindsay EA, Wilson DMC: Promoting physical activity in primary care: overcoming the barriers, *Can Fam Phys* 37:2167, 1991.

Smith JA, Scammon DL: A market segment analysis of adult physical activity: exercise beliefs, attitudes, intentions, and behaviors, *Advances in nonprofit marketing,* vol 2, Greenwich, Conn, 1987, JAI.

Stewart AL, King AC: Evaluating the efficacy of physical activity for influencing quality-of-life outcomes in older adults, *Ann Behav Med* 13:108, 1991.

Verhoef MJ, Love EJ: Women's exercise participation: the relevance of social roles compared to non-role-related determinants, *Can J Public Health* 83:367, 1992.

Vertinsky P: Sport and exercise for old women: images of the elderly in the medical and popular literature at the turn of the century, *Int J Hist Sport* 9:83, 1992.

Wagner EH, LaCroix AZ, Buchner DM et al: Effects of physical activity on health status in older adults. I: Observational studies, *Annu Rev Public Health* 13: 451, 1992.

Weller IMR, Thomas SG, Cox MH et al: A study to validate the Canadian Aerobic Fitness Test, *Can J Public Health* 83:120, 1992.

World Health Organization: *Prevention in childhood and youth of adult cardiovascular diseases: time for action,* Geneva, 1990, WHO Technical Report Series, No 792.

YMCA of the USA: *Programs for special populations,* Champaign, Ill, 1992, Human Kinetics Press.

Yesalis CE, editor: *Anabolic steroids in sport and exercise,* Champaign, Ill, 1993, Human Kinetics Press.

Young M, Schuller T: *Life after work: the arrival of the ageless society,* London, 1991, HarperCollins.

Chapter 11

Communicable Disease Control

AIDS has brought fear to the hearts of most Americans—fear of disease and fear of the unknown. . . . Fear can be useful when it helps people avoid behavior that puts them at risk . . . unreasonable fear can be as crippling as the disease itself.

SURGEON GENERAL C. EVERETT KOOP

OBJECTIVES

When you finish this chapter, you should be able to:

- Assess the relative importance of various sources of infection and disease in a community
- Identify the means of transmission of common communicable diseases in a community
- Assess ways to control the spread of an outbreak
- Describe prevention and health promotion methods to reduce the incidence of major communicable diseases by the year 2000

The routine application of immunizations, nutrition, sanitation, and epidemiological principles has caused acute, infectious communicable diseases to give way to chronic diseases as the leading causes of death in the more developed countries. So pervasive are the means of controlling communicable diseases that you probably take most of them for granted in your everyday living. Much of the remaining infection in the community persists because of lapses in the application or enforcement of communicable disease control measures, or because the "host resistance" of individuals has been compromised by poverty, stress, malnutrition, exhaustion, alcohol, or drugs. Hence, major defenses against communicable disease today include economic development and the promotion of physical and mental health.

Why bother to study this aspect of community health if it is so close to being controlled? For one, new communicable diseases seem to emerge to replace the old, eradicated scourges; viral diseases replace bacterial diseases, hepatitis and acquired immunodeficiency syndrome (AIDS) replace gonorrhea, Lyme disease seems to replace Legionnaires' disease. These ''new'' diseases have existed in the past, but their emergence as epidemics seemed to await new social circumstances. This points to a second reason for remaining alert to the communicable diseases—namely, that they are highly sensitive to social conditions; they serve as a barometer of the general status and health of a community or population. The third reason is that much of what is known about health, and most of the concepts and epidemiological methods for community health, derive from the study and experience of communicable diseases.

NATURE OF COMMUNICABLE DISEASE

Disease is defined as a harmful departure from normal. A **communicable disease** is one that can be transmitted from one human being to another or from other animals to humans. Communicable diseases are produced by organisms that are parasitic and **pathogenic,** or disease-producing. Most pathogens of humans are microorganisms, although some, notably the worms, are multicellular forms and can be seen with the unaided eye. **Infectious disease** represents a reaction of the **host** to the invader. The interaction may destroy the pathogen as well as produce abnormalities in the host, even to the point of causing the death of the human host.

Infection and Disinfection

Infection is the successful invasion of the body by pathogens under such conditions as will permit them to multiply and harm the host. The mere presence of pathogenic organisms or toxins in the human body does not constitute disease. A person may be harboring millions of pneumococci in his or her lungs or have billions of streptococcus organisms on the skin without having disease. Only when the pathogens cause harm to the body can the condition be classed as a disease.

Disinfection consists of killing or removing organisms capable of causing infection. Disinfection by the use of chemicals is the usual method. Physical disinfection includes the use of such agents as ultraviolet radiation, sound waves, and electron treatment. The two most common means of chemical disinfection are bacteriostasis and antibiosis.

Bacteriostasis is an arrest in the multiplication or metabolism of pathogens. Thus toxin production by the invading organism is reduced or ceases completely. For example, sulfonamides arrest bacterial action by depriving the organism of the material that it must have to carry on normal metabolic processes. The resulting bacteriostasis enables a person's phagocytes to destroy the pathogen.

Antibiosis, such as produced by penicillin, means antagonism to specific organisms. The antibiotics have had spectacular effects in combating certain pathogens, but they have not proved to be a panacea. Despite their magnificent contribution to the battle against infection, the antibiotics have limitations. Bacteria develop resistant strains in response to antibiotics. This **mutation,** or adaptability, by the bacteria limits the use of antibiotics. Resistant strains of bacteria are found particularly in hospital-acquired (**nosocomial**) infections. An infection with the same organism acquired outside the hospital will more likely be sensitive to the same antibiotics and respond well to treatment. Indiscriminate use of antibiotics, without proper indication, increases the proportion of organisms that can resist that particular antibiotic.

Contamination and Decontamination

Contamination is the presence of toxins or pathogens of humans on inanimate objects, such as needles (Figure 11-1), articles of clothing, furnishings, eating utensils, food, water, or even soil. Because certain organisms, such as *Escherichia coli,* live naturally in the intestines of humans, the presence of these organisms in inanimate matter, including wa-

SHARING NEEDLES CAN GET YOU MORE THAN HIGH.

IT CAN GET YOU AIDS.

You can't tell if someone has the AIDS virus just by looking.
You can't tell if needles or works are infected just by looking.
When you shoot drugs and share needles or works you could get AIDS. Even if you think your drug-sharing partners are clean, if the AIDS virus is present, it could be passed to you.
AIDS is not pretty. It's a long, slow, painful way to die. Do the right thing. Get into treatment. It's the best way to make sure you don't shoot up AIDS.

STOP SHOOTING UP AIDS.
GET INTO DRUG TREATMENT.
CALL 1-800 662 HELP

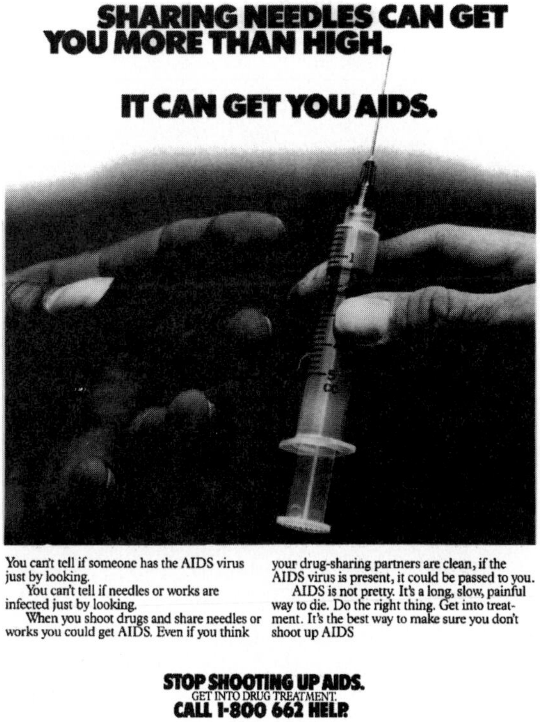

FIGURE 11-1
Intravenous drug (IVD) users are at particular risk of contracting AIDS through sharing of contaminated needles.
Source: National Institute on Drug Abuse, U.S. Department of Health and Human Services.

ter, indicates presence of human discharges. Contact with a possibly contaminated object—and thus with pathogens from the alimentary tract of humans—presents danger. The *E. coli* count is used as a standard in sanitary science and as such is a valuable index of possible danger to people, even though the *E. coli* bacterium itself is not a pathogen.

Decontamination means the killing or removing of toxins or pathogens and *E. coli* in or on *inanimate* objects. More drastic measures can be used here than are used in disinfection, including boiling, the use of steam, pasteurization, high levels of dry heat, long exposure to the sun, highly concentrated chemicals, and radiation.

INCIDENCE OF COMMUNICABLE DISEASES

Dramatic progress has been made in the control of infectious diseases. A comparison of reported cases of selected communicable diseases in the United States in 1900 and 1992 indicates the extent of the gain (Table 11-1). In appraising the general decline in the number of reported cases of these selected diseases, added weight must be given to the increase in population, which is now 180 percent greater than it was in 1900.

More recent gains and setbacks are seen in the comparison of reported cases of communicable diseases in 1976 and 1992 (Table 11-2). These figures indicate that the United States has not reached the point where its citizens can be complacent about communicable disease. Some of the national objectives for 1990 were met, but communicable disease still exists in epidemic, pandemic, and endemic forms.

Epidemic (Greek—*epi,* upon; *demos,* people) refers to a considerable number of more than normally expected cases of a particular disease in a locality such as a city. The number of cases that would classify an outbreak as an epidemic is flexible, depending on the usual frequency of the particular disease,

TABLE 11-1

Reported cases of selected communicable diseases, United States, 1900 and 1992

Disease	1900	1992
Diphtheria	147,991	4
Malaria	184,165	1,004
Smallpox	102,128	0
Typhoid fever	35,994	382

Based on data from National Center for Health Statistics (1900 data); and Centers for Disease Control, *MMWR* 41:979, Jan. 8, 1993.

at the same season of the year, and among the specified population and size of the community. In a city of 12,000 people, 10 cases of chickenpox would not be an epidemic, but in a community of 200, that number might well be regarded as epidemic. Ten cases of cholera or paralytic poliomyelitis in a city of 12,000 would be regarded as an epidemic.

Pandemic (Greek—*pan,* all) indicates a considerable number of cases of a disease in a wide geographical area such as an entire nation, a continent, or the world. Thus the outbreak of influenza in 1918 and 1919 was classed as a pandemic. Despite the advance in communicable disease control, no coun-

TABLE 11-2

Recent progress and setbacks in reported cases of specified notifiable diseases, United States, 1976 and 1992, and objectives for 2000.

Disease	1976	1992	2000 Objective*
AIDS (acquired immunodeficiency syndrome)*	—	46,648	
Botulism (food-borne)	29	19	
Brucellosis	282	88	
Diphtheria	146	4	<50
Encephalitis, infectious	1,616	111	
Gonorrhea (excluding military personnel)	996,468	497,980	300*
Legionellosis*	—	1,267	
Malaria	451	1,004	
Measles (rubeola)	39,585	9,804	0
Meningococcal infections	1,534	2,121	
Mumps	20,964	2,433	500
Pertussis (whooping cough)	925	3,198	<1000
Poliomyelitis	9	4	0
Psittacosis	71	86	
Rubella (German measles)	12,090	147	0
Syphilis (excluding military personnel)	23,499	34,179	10*
Tetanus	68	42	
Toxic shock syndrome*	—	224	
Trichinosis	89	40	
Tuberculosis	32,549	24,073	3.5*
Tularemia	146	157	
Typhoid fever	384	382	
Typhus fever, tick-borne (Rocky Mountain spotted fever)	892	493	

Based on data from Centers for Disease Control, *MMWR* 25:650, Jan. 7, 1977; and 41:979, 1993. *AIDS, legionellosis (Legionnaires' disease), and toxic shock syndrome were not notifiable diseases in 1976. The objectives are expressed as rates per 100,000 for those with an asterisk. Those without an asterisk are numbers of actual cases.

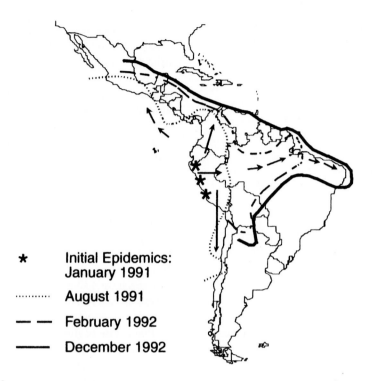

FIGURE 11-2
In January 1991 the initial cases of cholera on the coast of Peru spread quickly, especially in poor communities where water and sanitary facilities were limited, to four neighboring countries by August, and by 1992 had spread across the South American continent and into Mexico.
Source: Centers for Disease Control and Prevention: Update: Cholera—Western Hemisphere, 1992, *MMWR* 42:89, 1993.

Legend:
★ Initial Epidemics: January 1991
·········· August 1991
— — February 1992
———— December 1992

try is completely safe from pandemics. The recent AIDS and cholera epidemics soon became pandemic. The 1991 epidemic of cholera (Figure 11-2), for example, spread from Peru in January to neighboring countries of Ecuador in February, Columbia in March, Brazil and Chile in April, and by 1992 had become pandemic with thousands of cases in Central and North America.

Endemic (Greek—*en,* in) refers to a steady but limited number of cases consistently present in a geographical area. The term is sometimes limited to diseases peculiar to a particular area.

Infectious diseases in the United States still ac-

count for a significant death toll. Table 11-3, however, shows the progress against infectious and parasitic diseases, which accounted for less than 1% of the total deaths in 1990. The increase in some categories such as tuberculosis includes AIDS-related cases.

CLASSIFICATION OF INFECTIOUS DISEASES

For practical purposes of community disease control, the most useful classification of infectious diseases is one that incorporates at least a suggestion

TABLE 11-3
Deaths from selected infectious diseases, United States,
1970, 1983, and 1992

Cause of death	1970	1983	1992
Bacillary dysentery (shigellosis) and amebiasis	89	1	0
Enteritis and other intestinal infections	2567	38	750
Hepatitis, infectious (viral)	1014	89	1720
Measles (rubeola)	89	0	0
Meningococcal infections	550	25	200
Pertussis (whooping cough)	12	0	10
Poliomyelitis	7	0	0
Septicemia	3535	1324	20,150
Streptococcal sore throat and scarlet fever	29	1	0
Syphilis	461	11	100
Tuberculosis	5217	193	1400

Based on data from National Center for Health Statistics: Monthly Vital
Statistics Report 22:721, 1974; 321:8, March 26, 1984, and 41:18, March
18, 1993.

of how the pathogen escapes from the host or reservoir, and how the disease is transmitted. The classification presented in Table 11-4 lists some diseases in more than one category. Thus tuberculosis and smallpox properly can be classed both as respiratory diseases and as open lesion diseases. In these infectious conditions, the avenue of spread from the host to a new host can be either from the respiratory tract or from the open sores that these infections produce.

Respiratory Diseases

Respiratory tract diseases are much more common than the other classes of infectious diseases because the respiratory tract is as exposed as the skin but without the defenses of the skin. Diseases of the respiratory tract are particularly prevalent in the temperate zones. Usually acute, they pose a constant threat to the population.

Infectious diseases of the respiratory tract follow a characteristic cycle of periods—incubation, prodrome, fastigium, defervescence, convalescence, and defection, as defined in Figure 11-3. An understanding of the typical course of a respiratory disease identifies factors operating at a given stage and where and what control measures should be taken.

Incubation starts with the invasion of the causative agent. Although organisms multiply in the host during the incubation period, no symptoms occur. An infectious respiratory disease normally is not communicable during this period, although chickenpox and measles may be transmitted to other hosts during the last two or three days of the incubation period. Duration of the incubation period varies from disease to disease. Generally the more severe diseases have a short incubation period and the less severe diseases have a longer incubation period, although exceptions to this general tendency do exist.

Prodrome begins with the first symptoms in the host and usually lasts about one day. Symptoms during this period are similar for all respiratory infections and resemble those of the common cold; thus, it is difficult to get a definite diagnosis at this stage. From a community health standpoint, there exists a great danger of disease transmission during this highly communicable stage. With the assumption that they ''just have a cold,'' patients continue their normal daily routines and unknowingly expose a considerable number of people.

Fastigium is the period during which the disease is at its height. Differential symptoms and signs appear, making accurate diagnosis possible. Although a highly communicable stage, the fastigium does not represent a serious disease control problem. Because patients are at home or in a hospital, they expose only those who serve their immediate needs.

Defervescence indicates that the disease is declining in the severity of symptoms, although a relapse may occur.

Convalescence represents a recovery period. New problems in preventing disease spread arise because patients feel well enough to be up and about

TABLE 11-4
Classification of infectious diseases by their usual means of escape from one host to reach
another*

Respiratory diseases	*Alvine discharge diseases*	*Vector-borne diseases*	*Open lesion diseases*
Cerebrospinal meningitis	Amebic dysentery	African sleeping sickness	AIDS/HIV
Chickenpox	Cholera	Bilharzia	Anthrax
Coryza	Giardiasis	Encephalitis	Chancroid and chlamydia
Diphtheria	Hookworm	Dracunculiasis	Dracunculiasis
Influenza	Paratyphoid	Lyme disease	Erysipelas
Pertussis (whooping cough)	Poliomyelitis	Malaria	Gonorrhea
Pneumonia	Salmonellosis	Onchocerciasis	Hepatitis B
Poliomyelitis	Schistosomiasis	Plague	Herpes
Rubella (German measles)	Shigellosis (bacillary	Psittacosis	Leprosy
Rubeola (measles)	dysentary)	Rabies	Scarlet fever
Scarlet fever	Typhoid fever	Relapsing fever	Smallpox
Smallpox	Viral hepatitis	Rocky Mountain spotted fever	Syphilis
Streptococcal sore throat		Schistosomiasis	Tuberculosis
Tuberculosis		Tularemia	Tularemia
		Typhus fever	
		Yellow fever	

*In addition to the usual means of transmission, some diseases can be transmitted by hypodermic needles shared by drug users, or by blood transfusions.

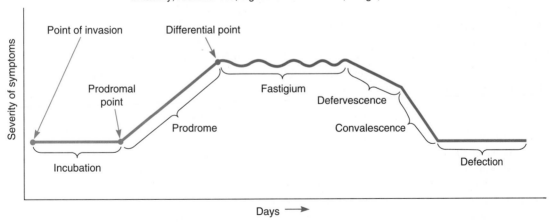

Prodromal symptoms: Nasal discharge, headache, mild fever, general aching,
irritability, restlessness, digestive disturbances, cough, sore throat.

FIGURE 11-3
The natural history of an infectious respiratory disease.

and consequently expose those they come in contact with.

Defection is the stage in which the organisms are being cast off. This occurs through coughing for respiratory diseases, defecating, or urinating for most others. It may run concurrently with the period of convalescence. Termination of defection is the sign for the termination of isolation.

Alvine Discharge Diseases

Control of infections of the alimentary canal, or alvine discharge diseases, is essentially a problem in sanitation. Dysentery, typhoid fever, and other *Salmonella* infections are the principal alvine discharge diseases of consequence in North American and European countries. *Salmonella* infections other than typhoid fever are rarely fatal, but the incidence of such diseases is much higher than is generally recognized. Many cases of digestive disturbances, "intestinal flu," and "summer complaint" technically should be classed as *Salmonella* infections. Environmental control measures for alvine discharge diseases will be covered in Chapters 14, 15, and 16.

Vector-borne Diseases

Vector-borne diseases are normally transmitted to humans by intermediate hosts and **vectors,** such as rodents, bats, dogs, cows, snails, birds, fleas, and ticks. The larger animals are usually intermediate hosts for the pathogen, which is then transferred to humans by vectors such as fleas, ticks, or mosquitoes. These diseases pose a far greater problem in the tropics than in Western countries, where only a few exist and then only in endemic form. Intensive campaigns in these affected geographical regions have brought such vector-borne diseases as malaria, rabies, and Rocky Mountain spotted fever under control. Lyme disease, transmitted by ticks from deer, is now endemic in the northeastern states of the U.S. Community control measures for vector-borne diseases will be discussed in Chapter 16.

Open Lesion Diseases

Syphilis and gonorrhea are the open lesion diseases of primary importance in community health. Infection transfer in this class of disease normally entails direct contact with the open lesion or site of infection. In addition, only certain body tissues, such as the mucous membranes, are specific for the organisms causing these diseases.

Tuberculosis and smallpox, as well as some other diseases producing skin eruptions, technically may be classed as open lesion diseases since the causative agents of these diseases leave their reservoir via the lesions of the infection.

THE CONCEPT OF ERADICATION

The fifteenth through eighteenth centuries saw the New World explored. Transportation and commerce ended the isolation of many remote areas. Smallpox epidemics followed, decimating populations. It is estimated that there were fatalities of 20% to 50% among those who contracted smallpox during the epidemics in the seventeenth and eighteenth centuries. By the middle 1700s smallpox was believed to account for 10% of all deaths in North America and was the leading cause of infant death. Even George Washington bore the scars of smallpox.

Despite the growing widescale use of smallpox vaccination in the 1880s and early 1900s, the disease remained endemic throughout the world, and those who were not immune still ran a high risk of being stricken sometime during their lifetimes.

Strategy for Smallpox Eradication

The concept of worldwide eradication of smallpox gained new supporters as the disease was successfully eliminated from North America, Europe, and a number of other countries following World War II. Travelers without evidence of smallpox vaccination were prohibited from crossing their borders. In 1959 the World Health Assembly passed a resolution directed at smallpox eradication, and the World Health Organization (WHO), UNICEF, and other organizations offered help to those countries willing to undertake mass vaccinations. It was not until 1966, however, that the commitment to worldwide eradication of smallpox was backed up with budget and bilateral agreements sufficient to make feasible the goal of eradication by 1976 (Figure 11-4).

Mass vaccination programs were improved, and costs decreased, with the development of the jet injector gun and the bifurcated needle. Production and quality control of vaccines were also greatly improved. The enlistment of hundreds of thousands of public health workers who educated communities, detected cases, tracked down contacts, and vaccinated entire populations in areas where cases occurred contributed greatly to the success of this effort. A surveillance and containment technique moved these workers rapidly into any area in which a case was detected, sealing off the spread to other areas, isolating and treating the patient, and finding and vaccinating contacts of patients.

Global Victory and New Challenges

The last cases of smallpox in Kenya and Somalia were reported in 1977. A laboratory accident in England in 1978 produced the last verified case of smallpox. The Global Commission for the Certification of Smallpox Eradication required that a 2-year period pass without any reported cases before the disease could be considered to have been eliminated. That period ended in 1980, and the smallpox virus is now considered to be extinct.

The expenditures for smallpox eradication from 1967 to 1979 by the international community are estimated at nearly a third of a billion dollars, a small amount in comparison to the annual costs the disease inflicted only 50 years earlier.

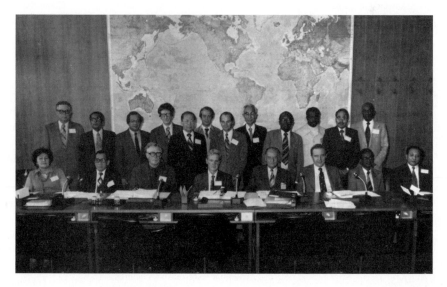

FIGURE 11-4
Members of the Global Commission for the Certification of the Eradication of Smallpox at their historic meeting in Geneva, Switzerland, declaring the smallpox virus extinct in 1980.
Source: Photo courtesy World Health Organization.

Poliomyelitis. Ten years after the eradication of smallpox, enthusiasm began to build about the possibility of achieving the same victory with polio (Table 11-5). The World Health Organization has proposed plans for attempting to eliminate polio from the globe by the year 2000. The effort will succeed only if progress is maintained in building up immunization levels and other health services around the world. The effort of the Pan American Health Organization to eradicate polio in the Americas by 1990 succeeded in the United States and Canada but remains an elusive goal in most Latin American countries. The feature of polio that will make it more

difficult to eradicate is that transmission of polio is far less visible than that of smallpox. Only one in every 200 people who contract the polio virus ever show any major symptoms. Many people can be spreading the disease without anyone realizing contagion is happening. This means that immunization levels must be much closer to 100%.

Measles. Hope of wiping out measles was inspired in the 1980s by the near zero level of reported cases in some countries, including Canada and the United States. Measles is more visible in most cases than polio, and is harbored only in human hosts, so the

TABLE 11-5
Disease eradication

Disease	Current annual toll worldwide	Chief obstacles to eradication	Conclusion
Guinea worm	10 million persons infected; few deaths	Lack of public and political awareness; inadequate funding	Eradicable
Poliomyelitis	250,000 cases of paralytic polio; 25,000 deaths	No insurmountable technical obstacles; increased national/international commitment needed	Eradicable
Onchocerciasis	18 million cases; 340,000 blind	High cost of vector control; no therapy to kill adult worms; restrictions in mass use of ivermectin	Could eliminate associated blindness
Yaws and endemic syphilis	2.5 million cases	Political and financial inertia	Could interrupt transmission*
Rabies	52,000 deaths	No effective way to deliver vaccine to wild animal disease carriers	Could eliminate urban rabies
Measles	2 million deaths, mostly children	Lack of suitably effective vaccine for young infants; cost; public misconception of seriousness	Not now eradicable
Tuberculosis	8-10 million new cases; 2-3 million deaths	Need for improved diagnostic tests, chemotherapy, and vaccine; wider application of current therapy	Not now eradicable
Leprosy	11-12 million cases	Need for improved diagnostic tests and chemotherapy; social stigma; potential reservoir in armadillos	Not now eradicable

*Because persons may be infected for decades and the organisms cannot be distinguished from those that cause venereal syphilis, elimination of transmission—not eradication—is the goal.

Source: International Task Force for Disease Eradication: Report, *MMWR* 39:211, 1990.

isolation and surrounding of cases with a buffer zone of immunized people is possible as it was in the smallpox campaign. Both measles and polio eradication programs, as well as diphtheria and pertussis elimination, will benefit from the global effort to achieve universal childhood immunization in the developing world.

Tuberculosis. After decades of decline in the number and rate of tuberculosis cases, this ancient scourge of communities has risen again in North America. The number of reported TB cases in the United States increased 9.4% between 1989 and 1990 (Figure 11-5). Almost 70% of all TB cases and 86% of those among children up to 15 years old occurred among racial and ethnic minorities. Homeless and low-income persons, and those with HIV or AIDS are particularly susceptible. Adverse social and economic factors have contributed to the rise,

as has the immigration of persons with tuberculous infection.

An Advisory Council for the Elimination of Tuberculosis in the United States (where such a goal is achievable, although it is not achievable on a global level [see Table 11-5]), recommends (1) initiating public awareness campaigns to alert communities about the increasing TB problems; (2) training and educating public and private healthcare providers in the skills needed to relate effectively to the at-risk communities being served, and empowering at-risk populations with knowledge and other resources needed to influence the TB programs directed toward their communities; (3) building coalitions to help design and implement intensified community TB prevention and control efforts; (4) intensifying the screening of at-risk populations for TB and tuberculous infection (skin tests) and providing appropriate treatment; (5) increasing the

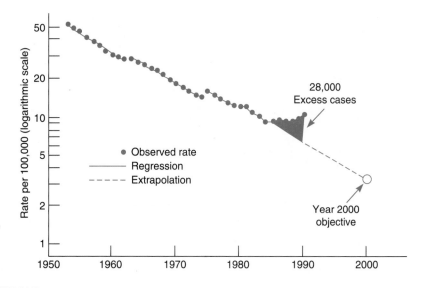

FIGURE 11-5

Trend since 1950 in actual rate of tuberculosis in the United Sttaes shows an excess of 28,000 cases between 1984, when the rate started to rise again, and 1990. The year 2000 objective is based on an extrapolation from the earlier trend (regression) line.

Source: Centers for Disease Control: Prevention and control of tuberculosis in U.S. communities with at-risk minority populations, *MMWR* 41(RR-5):1, 1992.

speed and completeness of reporting suspected cases to health departments; and (6) improving the availability and quality of TB health care services in socioeconomically disadvantaged areas.

Tropical diseases. Some of the other candidates on the list for possible eradication (see Table 11-5) include guinea worm disease (dracunculiasis), river blindness (onchocerciasis), yaws, and leprosy. Guinea worm eradication is feasible if the necessary commitment and resources can be mobilized. Great progress has been made in Africa since WHO declared a goal of eradicating this disease globally, the first such goal since the smallpox campaign. By educating infected villagers who bathe in stream water to keep their open sores out of the water, and others to strain the water they drink from infected streams, the life cycle of the guinea worm can be broken (Figure 11-6).

In considering whether any disease is potentially eradicable, four factors that made smallpox eradication possible must be taken into account: (1) No reservoir of the virus existed except in humans. This makes rabies, for example, a poor candidate. (2) Nearly all persons infected with smallpox had an obvious, distinguishable rash. This is what makes TB most difficult to eradicate. (3) Smallpox made people infectious for a relatively short period. (4) The natural infection, even without vaccination, left most people immune for a lifetime. This is not the case with most other diseases. (5) A safe, effective, and inexpensive vaccine was available. It was also

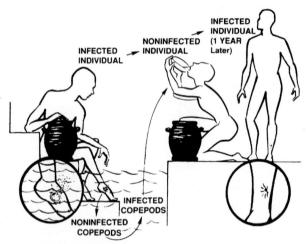

- The mature female worm pierces the skin of the lower leg, causing an ulcer.
- When the ulcer comes in contact with water, the female worm discharges larvae into the water.
- Cyclopoid copepods (small fresh-water crustaceans) become infected by ingesting the larvae.
- Humans drink the water contaminated with the infected copepods.
- The ingested larvae mature in humans in 1 year.

FIGURE 11-6
Life cycle of *Dracunculus medinensis,* the cause of guinea worm disease, which is targeted by WHO for eradication by 1995.

Source: Hopkins DR, Ruiz-Tiben E: Surveillance for Dracunculiasis, 1981-1991. In CDC Surveillance Summaries, *MMWR* 41: 3, 1992.

highly stable in tropical environments. Many vaccines require refrigeration, which is difficult to arrange in many remote areas.

SEXUALLY TRANSMITTED DISEASES

The major sexually transmitted diseases—syphilis, gonorrhea, herpes, chlamydia, and HIV/AIDS— present different clinical and epidemiological patterns. The methodology for syphilis and gonorrhea control has been developed over a long period of time and has been demonstrated to be effective in reducing the incidence of disease when rigorously applied. Control methods for herpes, chlamydia, and AIDS are still in earlier stages of development.

Acquired Immunodeficiency Syndrome (AIDS)

AIDS brought fear and panic with its sudden appearance and spread in North America, its high mortality rate, and its dramatic debilitation and complications in the few years of life following diagnosis. The death rate for cases discovered in the early 1980s was virtually 100%. The full-blown AIDS syndrome includes severe fatigue, persistent cough accompanied often by shortness of breath, persistent diarrhea, persistent white coating or spots inside the mouth or throat, often accompanied by soreness and difficulty of swallowing, purple or brown lumps or spots on the skin, and eventually nervous system impairment including loss of memory, inability to think clearly, and depression.

The devastating statistics, represented in Figure 11-7, are now understood to be the tip of an iceberg. Beneath the 270,000 cases in 1991, 5 to 10 times as many people (up to 2.7 million) have been infected with AIDS-related Complex (ARC). These people suffer some symptoms of AIDS such as enlarged lymph glands, night sweats, and fevers. These may last for years with a general decline in health,

but without developing the full-blown AIDS syndrome.

Deeper still beneath the tip of the iceberg are another 50 to 100 times the number of reported cases, 14 million to 27 million people in 1991, who will have been exposed to the AIDS virus and remain healthy carriers of the virus that causes AIDS, the human immunodeficiency virus (HIV). These people may not know they carry the virus unless they have been tested, and so they continue to spread the disease to other people.

In addition to the sexual transmission of HIV/ AIDS through virus-infected semen, especially during anal intercourse, AIDS is spreading rapidly among drug users who share needles with partners who have infected the needle with virus-infected lymphocytes in their blood (Figure 11-8).

Syphilis and Gonorrhea

Syphilis control involves the reporting of cases, treatment, and follow-up and patient interviews for contact information. Named partners are traced, tested, and treated to interrupt the transmission of disease within the community. The basic technique in syphilis control is contact investigation. Recent decreases in the rates of syphilis and gonorrhea are attributed in part to changing sexual practices, but also to the aging of the baby boom generation.

The major thrust of gonorrhea control programs is screening by bacteriological culture of all females for asymptomatic gonococcal infection, followed by prompt treatment if they are infected.

The examples of syphilis and gonorrhea illustrate the difficulty of prevention and control of sexually transmitted disease, even when the cause is known. The pathogenic organisms are sensitive to drugs, yet behavioral factors are involved that complicate control. Between 1965 and 1975, the number of reported cases of gonorrhea in the United States tripled. Since 1975, however, reported cases have leveled off, with a steady decrease since 1985.

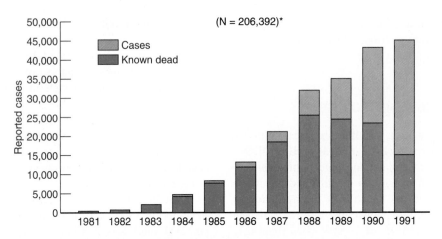

(N = 206,392)*

*Includes Guam, Puerto Rico, the U.S. Pacific Islands, and the U.S. Virgin Islands.

FIGURE 11-7
Acquired immunodeficiency syndrome (AIDS) cases and known deaths, United States, 1981-1991. A large increase in reported cases will show for 1993 in future charts as the result of expanding the definition of AIDS to include a wider range of AIDS-related-complex cases. Deaths as a proportion of cases has declined with improved detection, care, and treatment.
Source: Centers for Disease Control, *MMWR* 40:17, 1992; 42:321, 1993.

Herpes and Genital Warts

Genital herpes infections are very common, with an incidence of one half to one million new cases annually, with several million recurrences each year. For this painful condition, periodic recurrences are the rule. Herpes-complicated pregnancies often result in abortion, stillbirth, or severe neonatal infection; neonatal herpes results in death or permanent disability in two thirds of the cases.

Hepatitis B

Hepatitis B is caused by a virus transmitted by shared needles, sex, and birth. Homosexual males are at very high risk; nearly 60% attending clinics for sexually transmitted disease show evidence of past or present hepatitis B infection. This same population is also at high risk of several other sexually transmitted diseases, including AIDS, amebiasis, and giardiasis.

Prevention-Promotion Measures

Educational measures. The most fundamental component of a community program to control sexually transmitted diseases is education and training. This includes clinical experience in schools for health professionals; education and information about sexually transmitted diseases for school-children before and during the time they are at highest risk; preservice and continuing professional education for both health care providers and health educators to deal with sexually transmitted diseases in a confidential, nonjudgmental fashion; and improved public understanding of sexually transmitted disease risks and confidentiality of treatment through effective and continuous campaigns using mass media. Educational measures may be mass directed or may be targeted to special groups such as women, children, homosexual and bisexual men, adolescents, minorities, populations with special language needs, and specific high-risk groups. They

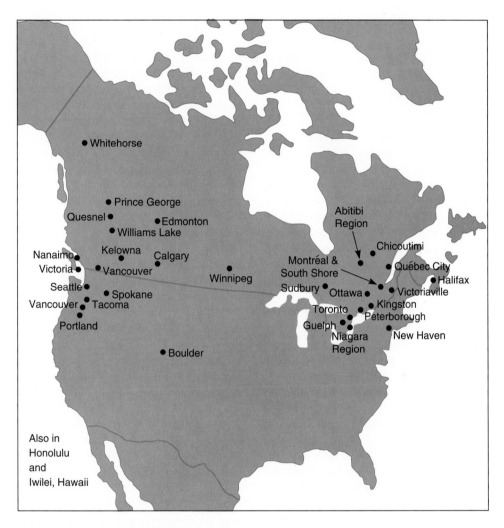

FIGURE 11-8

This map of North America shows those communities in Canada and the United States that had needle exchange programs for intravenous drug users as of July 1992.

Source: *Canadian AIDS News,* 1992.

may include the counseling of patients being treated for sexually transmitted diseases regarding complications and measures to avoid future infection.

Education is all the more critical to the control of viral STDs because the diseases are not curable.

Treatment cannot break the cycle of transmission as it can for syphilis and gonorrhea.

Congress, recognizing the importance of education as the "single most effective means available today to slow the spread of the AIDS epidemic," has approved over $1 billion for AIDS research, education, and control each year since 1989. State health agencies also spent increasing amounts with the largest proportion (26%) going to education.

Service measures. The second level of community strategy is the provision of diagnostic and treatment services for patients with sexually transmitted diseases and their complications. Also included in secondary prevention and control are detection and referral methods, such as counseling infected patients and tracing and treating their contacts; screening for selected sexually transmitted diseases; and encouraging joint availability of services among related programs such as those for sexually transmitted diseases, family planning, and maternal and child health.

A highly controversial but apparently effective service, which has been implemented in many European and Canadian communities but only in nine U.S. communities, is the provision of new, sterile needles to intravenous drug (IVD) users (Figure 11-8). This strategy is referred to as a "harm reduction strategy" because its goal is not the elimination of all harm but rather the reduction of the worst harm. The theory behind needle exchange programs is that IVD users will not be easily stopped from using intravenous drugs, so it is better to protect them and others who might share needles with them by providing sterile needles than to do nothing about the threat of AIDS in this population.

Technological measures. Properly used, condoms are the best known measure for persons engaging in sexual activity to avoid acquiring or transmitting many of the sexually transmitted diseases, including AIDS. A vaccine for hepatitis B is being tested for efficacy; vaccines for gonorrhea and genital herpes are at an earlier stage of development. A vaccine for HIV/AIDS is unlikely to be developed in the near future.

Legislative and regulatory measures. Community agencies need to determine the magnitude of the sexually transmitted disease problem and to establish objectives for inclusion in their annual implementation plans. Health planning agencies need to make certain that the health plan for the community addresses gaps in education and service delivery regarding sexually transmitted diseases.

Other regulatory activities to support community control might include the examination by certifying agencies or other regulatory boards of health professionals' knowledge of sexually transmitted diseases and competency in dealing with such diseases; the repeal of statutes and ordinances that inhibit the advertising, display, sale, or distribution of condoms; and regulations requiring information about sexually transmitted diseases as part of school health education programs.

Economic measures. The two most needed economic supports for sexually transmitted disease services are (1) prevention-related activities that are exempted from coinsurance or deductible provisions of health insurance, and (2) prepaid health plans with financial incentives for sexually transmitted disease prevention activities, including management of persons who have had sexual contact with the affected person and who are not members of the plan.

THE MICROBIOLOGY OF CAUSATIVE AGENTS

A pathogen is a poor parasite because it arouses the host. It is analogous to a burglar awakening the household on which he is preying. The response of the host is usually a defense reaction, basically of a chemical or immunological nature. Host resistance is the key to preventing disease from those pathogens that cannot be eliminated from the environment.

Infecting Organisms

Most organisms pathogenic to the human species belong to the plant kingdom, specifically to the phylum Thallophyta. Bacteria constitute the greatest number of pathogenic organisms. Rickettsiae are small bacteria, and viruses are ultramiscroscopic forms. Certain true funguses, including the molds, are also pathogenic to humans; they may produce infestations (such as athlete's foot) as well as infections (such as valley fever) in that they live *on* the body as well as *in* the body. In the animal kingdom certain protozoa and a few metazoa are pathogens of humans. For the purposes of community health, a classification that can be readily applied to existing conditions, such as Table 11-6, is most useful.

Specificity of infecting organisms. A typhoid bacillus is derived only from a preexisting typhoid bacillus. The virility but not the species may change from generation to generation of a particular type of organism. The severity of the reaction the organism produces in human hosts may rise or subside with subsequent generations of the organism, but the pathogen's action will always be similar in its basic nature. In addition to having specific action, many organisms are harmful only to specific types of human tissue. This basic tendency of all pathogens to be specific accounts both for the manner in which the organism functions and for the reaction it produces in the host. In some respects the diphtheria bacillus may resemble the typhoid bacillus and in some respects they may produce similar reactions in the host, but the two different organisms have definite identities. This specificity of infecting organisms is a universal phenomenon.

Mode of action. Most pathogens injure human tissue by the toxins they produce; in their normal met-

TABLE 11-6
Examples of diseases classified by their means of pathogen transmission

	Indirect contact		Direct contact
Airborne	*Water- and food-borne*	*Vector-borne*	
Anthrax	Dracunculiasis	Dracunculiasis	AIDS*
Cerebrospinal meningitis*‖	Botulism†	Glanders†§	Anthrax†
Chickenpox*	Brucellosis†	Jaundice, infective*	Brucellosis†
Encephalomyelitis, equine†	Cholera*	Lyme disease	Chlamydia*
Influenza*	Diphtheria*	Malaria*	Gonorrhea*
Legionellosis*	Dysentery, bacillary*	Onchocerciasis	Herpes‖
Measles*	Hoof-and-mouth diseases‡§	Plague*	Rabies†
Mumps*	Poliomyelitis*‖	Relapsing fever*	Smallpox*
Pneumonia†	Schistosomiasis	Rocky Mountain spotted fever*§	Syphilis*
Psittacosis†	Streptococcus*	Tularemia*	Tetanus*
Tuberculosis†	Tuberculosis†	Typhus fever*§	Tuberculosis†
Typhus fever*‡	Tularemia*	Yellow fever*§	Tularemia*
	Typhoid fever*		

*Infects humans only.
†Infects humans and animals useful to humans.
‡Infects animals or birds only.

§Artificially transmissible by air in laboratory.
‖Means of transmission unknown.

abolic processes these pathogens generate substances that happen to be injurious to certain human tissues. Some organisms—for example, the diphtheria bacillus—produce toxins that diffuse through the permeable membrane of the bacterium and for this reason are called exotoxins. Other pathogens—for example, the typhoid bacillus—produce toxins that do not diffuse through the impermeable membrane that encloses the organism and for this reason are called endotoxins. When an organism of this type dies, its enclosing membrane undergoes changes that make it permeable to the toxins.

A small proportion of pathogens invade body tissues directly. Some of the protozoa, such as the malaria plasmodium and the spirochete of syphilis, and some viruses and rickettsiae invade human cells, causing cellular change and sometimes destruction. The AIDS virus specifically attacks white blood cells, as shown in Figure 11-9, undermining the body's immune system.

Reservoirs of Infection

Pathogens are relatively fragile organisms that survive only in a highly selective medium. A reported case of a new host for a particular type of organism means that the organism had been harbored in a medium favorable to the organism's survival, multiplication, and functioning. The medium in which organisms are thus harbored usually must have moisture, a relatively high temperature, nutrients, and an absence of light. Most reservoirs of organisms that affect people are living hosts that provide an excellent medium for harboring these pathogens. However, soil can be the reservoir for some pathogens, such as the tetanus bacillus.

Human reservoirs. The human body is the greatest reservoir of organisms pathogenic to other human beings. This is the genesis of the time-tested question asked when a new case of disease is discovered—''Where is the other case?'' Thus the human

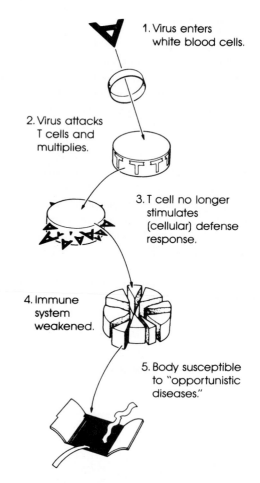

1. Virus enters white blood cells.

2. Virus attacks T cells and multiplies.

3. T cell no longer stimulates (cellular) defense response.

4. Immune system weakened.

5. Body susceptible to "opportunistic diseases."

FIGURE 11-9

The AIDS virus (HIV) causes disease by multiplying inside the productive T cells, leaving them too weak to fight off other diseases and infections.

Source: Public Health Service, U.S. Department of Health and Human Services.

reservoir is the source of the greatest danger of infection. **Frank cases,** or persons obviously ill with a disease, are generally not of much danger to a community. Although the individual who nurses the ill person may be greatly exposed to the disease and thus endangered, the community can be effectively protected by isolation of the identified ill person or other means of preventing transfer of infection from the known reservoir to other possible hosts.

Subclinical infections, variously referred to as missed or ambulatory cases, constitute a reservoir of great danger to the community because the affected individuals usually continue their normal daily routines. An ambulatory patient with diphtheria, scarlet fever, or dysentery could unknowingly infect a considerable number of people before the source of the new cases of the disease was located. **Carriers** are individuals who harbor and disseminate a pathogenic organism without themselves experiencing recognizable symptoms. ''Typhoid Mary'' was a carrier who became infamous because her job as a food handler made her a source of infection for large numbers of people. The longer the

duration of the carrier status, the greater the danger to the community. Chronic or permanent carriers pose the most considerable threat; however, once they are identified, control measures can be instituted that will minimize or virtually remove the danger of communicating the disease to others. A convalescent carrier or transient carrier also can be a serious danger to those in the immediate environment. The distribution of AIDS cases shown in Figure 11-10 reflects the approximate distribution of human reservoirs for spread of the HIV infection.

Lower animal reservoirs. Only a few species of lower animals harbor organisms pathogenic to human beings, and these are principally domestic animals. However, rodents and certain other wild an-

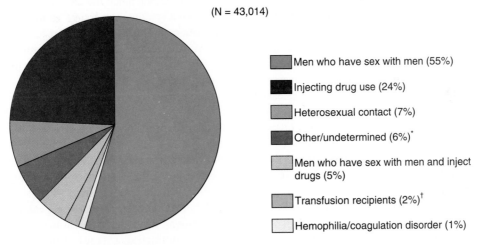

(N = 43,014)

Men who have sex with men (55%)

Injecting drug use (24%)

Heterosexual contact (7%)

Other/undetermined (6%)[*]

Men who have sex with men and inject drugs (5%)

Transfusion recipients (2%)[†]

Hemophilia/coagulation disorder (1%)

[*]"Other" refers to persons who developed AIDS after exposure to HIV-infected blood within the healthcare setting, as documented by evidence of seroconversion or other laboratory studies.
"Undetermined" refers to patients whose mode of exposure to HIV is unknown. This includes patients under investigation; patients who died, were lost to follow-up, or refused interview; and patients whose mode of exposure to HIV remains undetermined after investigation.
[†]Includes transfusion, tissue, and organ recipients from donors who were screened negative for HIV antibody at the time of donation..

FIGURE 11-10
Reservoirs of HIV as reflected by the distribution of reported adult and adolescent cases of AIDS, by patient group, United States, 1991.
Source: Centers for Disease Control: Summary of Notifiable Diseases, United States, 1991, *MMWR* 40:16, 1992.

imals also serve as reservoirs of organisms that produce disease in humans. Society has the necessary means to protect the human species against diseases such as anthrax from sheep and cattle; glanders and tetanus from horses; hoof-and-mouth disease from cattle; brucellosis and tapeworm from cattle, swine, and goats; tuberculosis from cattle; trichinosis from swine; psittacosis from parrots and parakeets; rabies from rodents, canines, and bats; toxoplasmosis from cats; Lyme disease from deer; and Rocky Mountain spotted fever and tularemia from rodents.

Schistosomiasis, the most prevalent of all the serious diseases in this category, is an organ-damaging and sometimes fatal disease. It is caused by a parasitic worm whose life cycle takes it from snail to water to human, during which time it grows to be up to one inch long, lays vast numbers of eggs, and has sexual unions that can last 30 years or more. The eggs of the threadlike parasite hatch in humans, are passed through stools, and often end up in fresh water where they develop into larvae. This preadult form searches out and infects a snail (the disease is sometimes called snail fever), only to be released again into water where it must burrow into a host within 24 hours, or die. Damage to human hosts is caused by the great number of eggs produced by the adult worm. The eggs eventually lodge in the liver, causing a nonalcoholic and reversible form of cirrhosis of the liver. Effects also include infection of the bladder and kidney and a slow sapping of energy.

Prevalent in developing countries where water supplies are not adequately treated by modern purification methods and where life-styles limit hygiene, schistosomiasis is one of the scourges of the Third World: over 200 million people suffer from this disease, and its devastating effects have been felt throughout the Middle East, Africa, Latin America, the Caribbean, and Asia far more than AIDS. Health education campaigns to control schistosomiasis have had to struggle against time-honored cultural and agricultural practices that cannot be eas-

ily challenged, especially in the face of economic hardships.

Escape of organisms from reservoir. The fact that a particular pathogen is harbored in a particular host is important from the standpoint of controlling disease spread, but the organism must escape from the reservoir if other potential hosts are to be endangered. For some diseases, the person harboring the causative agent represents no danger or poses a threat only under most unusual circumstances. For example, a person with trichinosis could endanger only the health of a cannibal, because the causative agent of trichinosis, living in the skeletal muscle of the human, has no avenue of escape. Likewise, under ordinary circumstances a person who has an active case of malaria or who is a carrier does not pose a threat to others, since the causative agent of malaria normally does not escape from the reservoir that harbors it. This pathogen can reach another host only via the female *Anopheles* mosquito, a blood transfusion, or the sharing of a hypodermic needle by drug users.

The avenues by which pathogens escape from the human body are shown in Table 11-4. The avenue of escape depends on the site of infection. The respiratory tract is the most common and most dangerous avenue of escape. While an individual harbors an infection of the respiratory tract, escape of the organism is a continuous process by such means as droplets from coughs and sneezes, eating utensils, or the human hands. Escape via the intestinal tract would be through discharges of the colon and the urinary tract. With AIDS, other body fluids such as semen and blood have been implicated. Open lesions provide an easy means of escape. With tubercle bacilli this is true whether it is a lesion of lung tissue or of the surface of the body. Tiny, imperceptible tears in the delicate tissues of the rectum provide the open lesion for the spread of AIDS from the semen of the host into the blood stream of a new host during anal intercourse. Likewise, the open lesions of syphilis, gonorrhea, and common furunculosis (boils) allow the pathogens that produce the lesion to leave the body. Mechanical escape of organisms from the human body is possible by insects or other animals that bite or suck. Here the organism is aided by a specific vector, or intermediate host.

This is illustrated by Figure 11-11 for schistosomiasis, transmitted by the snail.

Another example is onchocerciasis, carried by the blackfly. It breeds in fast-flowing rivers, hence the name "river blindness." The process begins

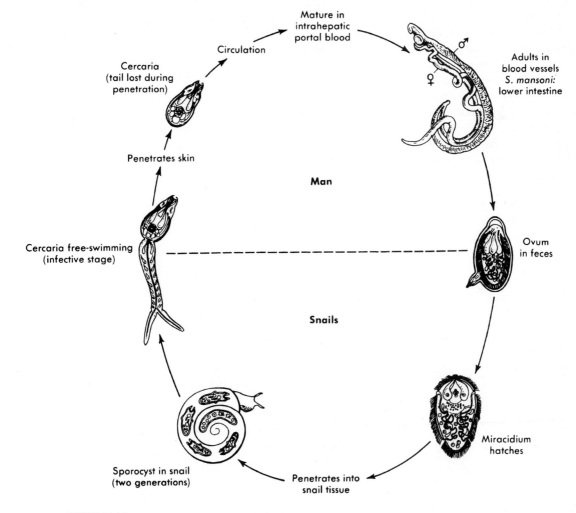

FIGURE 11-11
Life cycle of schistosomes: a complex cycle involving alternate human and water-borne snail hosts. Some 200 million people in 76 countries are affected by schistosomiasis, which can lead to scarring and tissue destruction of internal organs. A patient can be cured for less than $1.00, but the rate of reinfection is high, as people return to the same unsanitary streams and ponds.
Source: Courtesy National Institutes of Health, U.S. Department of Health and Human Services.

when the blackfly bites an infected human and picks up the premature form (microfilariae) of the worm *Onchocerca volvulus.* The premature worm develops inside the blackfly, which then infects another person with the larvae. In the new human host, the infective worm matures, becoming an adult that survives for years and reaches over 2 feet in length while it produces millions of microfilariae. Severely infected people suffer disfiguring skin changes, chronic itching, and various eye lesions that lead eventually to total blindness.

Preventing the organism from escaping from the reservoir obviously provides one means of communicable disease control. Efforts must be based on microbiological knowledge of the nature of the organism and epidemiological knowledge of the specific avenue through which it must escape to spread to a new host.

THE EPIDEMIOLOGY OF INFECTION

Once the organism has escaped from the reservoir it must be transferred to a new host if a new case of the disease is to occur, or if the organism is to survive and spread. The normal pathogens of humans do not walk or run or swim or fly. They must be transported by some vehicle. This transfer can be effected from person to person either directly or indirectly (Table 11-6 and Figure 11-12).

Direct Transmission

Organisms can be transmitted directly from one person to another without an intermediate object. This usually requires intimate association, but not necessarily physical contact. Thus coughing and sneezing can be a direct means of transmitting organisms from one person to another without physical contact

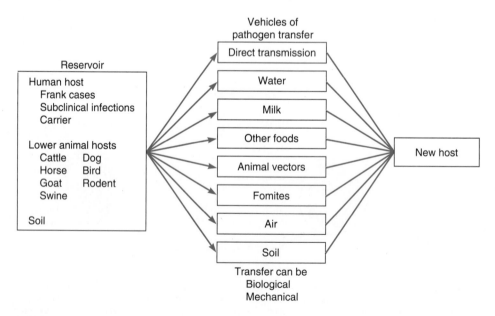

FIGURE 11-12
Routes over which diseases travel. The blocking of routes prevents pathogens from reaching potential susceptible new hosts.

being involved. This accounts for the high incidence of respiratory diseases in crowded living areas. Proper handwashing can reduce the transfer of most respiratory and intestinal diseases.

Indirect Transmission

When an intermediate object is involved in the transmission of disease from the reservoir to a new host, the mechanism is classed as indirect transmission. Such a transfer can occur with no particular close relationship between the reservoir and the new host. There are, however, two basic requirements for indirect transmission. The first is that the organisms involved must be virile enough to survive a long time outside a living body. Thus highly resistant organisms such as those causing typhoid, tetanus, and anthrax are most likely to be transmitted by indirect means. On the other hand, highly fragile organisms such as those causing meningitis, syphilis, and gonorrhea are less likely to be transmitted by an intermediate object except under very unusual survival circumstances. A second requirement for indirect transfer of infection is a favorable vehicle of transmission. It may be a specific living form of life, such as a mosquito, or a highly favorable substance for growth of the pathogen, such as milk. In a high proportion of diseases that can be transmitted by indirect means, the pathogen involved requires a specific medium for its survival.

Vehicles of Transfer

The expression "vehicles of pathogen transfer" refers to the objects that make the transfer from the reservoir to a new host. They might also be referred to as routes of infection insofar as they represent certain pathways by which the organisms are transferred. Vehicles of transfer may be animate or inanimate.

Vectors. Animate vehicles are spoken of as vectors. These intermediate hosts of the organism represent the connecting link between one case of a disease and a susceptible new host. Transfer by vectors can be either biological or mechanical. In a biological transfer the organism spends part of its life cycle in the body of the intermediate host, as illustrated by the Schistosome in Figure 11-11. Biological vectors are specific for specific diseases. Malaria is transmitted only by the female *Anopheles* mosquito, yellow fever by the *Aedes aegypti* mosquito, typhus fever by the louse, plague by the flea, schistosomiasis by the snail, river blindness by the blackfly, and Lyme disease and Rocky Mountain spotted fever by the ticks. When a vector makes possible the mechanical transfer of organisms, such species-specific action does not prevail. In this instance the vector comes in contact with infectious agents that mechanically become attached to the vector's body, legs, or other parts as with the transfer of fleas and ticks by a variety of rodents and other mammals.

A vector that normally produces a biological transfer may also effect a mechanical transfer. Normally, the *Anopheles* mosquito harbors the plasmodium of malaria for about 14 days while the pathogen goes through a life cycle. The resulting young forms are then introduced into a host. This biological transfer, however, can be short-circuited. The *Anopheles* mosquito can get some blood from feeding on a human being with malaria, leave this reservoir, and immediately attach to a new host, where the organisms from the original reservoir can be "mechanically" introduced. HIV has not been found to spread by this means.

Theoretically it would be possible to eliminate all disease transfer via vectors, but it is not practicable. Epidemiology knows how these vectors operate and how they can be destroyed, but given their almost limitless number, public health has to concentrate on their destruction and control in specific geographical areas or populations with a high incidence of vector-borne diseases.

If an inanimate object is to serve as a vehicle of pathogen transfer it must have certain characteristics; otherwise, the organism will not survive the interval between the time it comes into contact with the object and the time it is transmitted to the new host. If the organism is to survive and remain sufficiently virile to set up a new infection, the time interval during which most organisms are carried by the medium must be relatively short. The medium must be moist, bland, warm (near 100° F, or 38° C), and exist in relative darkness. Water, milk, other foods, air, fomites, and soil are the classes of inanimate vehicles of disease transfer (Figure 11-12).

Water. Water serves as a medium for the transfer of organisms from the human alimentary tract. Typhoid, paratyphoid, cholera, and bacillary dysentery are examples of diseases spread via water. Although pathogens normally do not multiply in water, an organism such as the typhoid bacillus can live for 2 or 3 weeks in relatively cool water. Public health has developed the necessary measures to protect communities against disease transmission via water. Filtration and chlorination of community water supplies have been effective in controlling water-borne diseases.

Milk. Milk is an excellent medium for several organisms pathogenic to people. Contamination of milk can come from three sources. The first is infection within the udder from a disease of the cow, such as brucellosis or bovine tuberculosis. The second is infection within the udder by organisms accidentally introduced into the udder by a human being. Septic sore throat and scarlet fever are examples of diseases resulting from this type of contamination. The third type is direct contamination of the milk by a human being after it has left the cow. Thus a milk handler harboring diphtheria, typhoid, or dysentery bacilli may introduce the organism into the milk in the course of milk processing. Through herd testing, dairy sanitation, and pasteurization, public health has been able to prevent the spread of infectious disease via the vehicle of milk.

Other foods. Other foods can be a means of transmitting pathogens but are not offenders as often as the lay public believes. For solid foods to serve as a vehicle of disease transfer, they must be moist, nonacid, not cooked, or handled after cooking. Time is also a factor: if a clerk in a bake shop, through handling, should leave dysentary bacilli on baked goods, the likelihood is remote that these few organisms would survive until the pastries were eaten.

There are three common sources of contamination in food. The first of these is food handlers conveying organisms to food by coughing or by their hands. The second is contamination during growth, as when shellfish develop in a body of water contaminated with typhoid bacilli. The third is when the food comes from infected animals which transmit such diseases as trichinosis and tapeworm. Here, however, proper cooking would destroy pathogens. Indeed, in most cases, this is the key to protection against transfer via the common foods. Boiling or heating to the boiling point for a period of time will destroy the usual pathogens that may be transferred via food. AIDS has never been found to spread by water, milk, or other food vehicles.

Air. The dryness, low temperature, and light of the air are highly unfavorable to most pathogenic organisms. Droplets from sneezing and coughing may give pathogens a moist vehicle that will help them survive long enough to set up an infection if they are inhaled into the respiratory passage of a new host. Measles and chickenpox appear to be more readily transmitted by this means than any of the other known respiratory diseases. Generally, however, air is not a principal vehicle of disease transfer. A cubic foot of air may contain a considerable number of pathogens, but they would be so attenuated before being inhaled into a person's respiratory tract that the likelihood that they could cause an infection in the new host is slight.

Fomites. Inanimate objects other than water, milk, food, air, and soil that might be vehicles of disease transfer are called **fomites.** The term embraces such things as clothing, bed linen, books, toys, handrails, and similar objects. Fomites are no longer regarded as major vehicles of disease transfer because they do not provide a good medium for pathogens. However, disease spread can occur if a susceptible person handles an object immediately after it has been contaminated and then touches his or her mouth, nose, or eyes. Needle punctures following use by an infected person can transmit pathogens from the blood stream of one person directly to the bloodstream of another. Increasing use of disposable items in medical and nursing care minimizes this vehicle of disease transfer, except for drug abusers.

Soil. Soil may harbor the organisms that cause hookworm, tetanus, anthrax, and botulism. Each of these presents a particular type of control problem, but immunization, boiling of food with soil on it, wearing of shoes and clothing, and other procedures can prevent the transmission of disease by soil.

Where an intermediate object is the vehicle for the transmission of disease from a reservoir to a new host, it should be possible to block that route and thus prevent disease spread. Through proper education of the public and the exercise of community control, it is possible to reduce the transfer of disease via animate and inanimate objects. However, public health officials find that control of the social contact (direct) route is a much more difficult task than control of disease transfer by vectors or inanimate vehicles. Human beings, largely because of carelessness or lack of understanding, often do not take sufficient precautions to prevent the spread of disease.

Entry of Organisms into New Host

Arrival and entry are not synonymous. When the organism arrives at the new host, it still must find its proper port of entry and must overcome certain body barriers. Pathogens producing respiratory diseases must arrive at the mouth or nose to enter the respiratory tract. Likewise, the organism causing an infection of the alimentary canal must find its way to the mouth and into the alimentary canal; even then, acid in the stomach may destroy the organism. Direct infection of mucous membranes such as occurs in gonococcal infection requires that the organism come in contact with those membranes. Although hookworms can go through the unbroken skin and mosquitoes and other animals can penetrate the skin sufficiently to introduce pathogenic organisms, percutaneous infections generally require a cut or an abrasion of the skin for the organism to enter the body.

Defenses of the Host

Even after leaving the reservoir, transferring to the new host, and reaching the right port of entry, the pathogen still encounters a series of defenses by the new host. Indeed, usually a large number of viril organisms must enter the new host if all of the host's defenses are to be overcome and infection produced.

Host resistance. Resistance is the ability of the host to ward off pathogens. General resistance against infection is nonspecific in that the various human defenses serve as antagonists to all pathogens. The skin serves as a mechanical barrier, and its natural acid state provides a further defense against those pathogens that require a neutral or alkaline medium. The secretion of mucous tissue serves as a defense against pathogens. The ciliated epithelial tissues of certain passages such as the respiratory tract provide an added defense, as the cilia tend to propel organisms to the exterior of the passageway. The acidity of such structures as the stomach, bladder, urethra, and vagina provides additional resistance to infection. Leukocytes, with their phagocytic action, destroy foreign organisms. Lymph nodes filter out infectious organisms and are capable of destroying them. A highly important defense is the ability of the body to produce an elevated temperature, or fever. The optimum temperature for most pathogens is about 100° F (38° C), which is the approximate normal temperature of the human body. In elevating the temperature by only 2 degrees, the body is able to inactivate the pathogens so that they are unable to multiply and carry on normal metabolism involving toxin production. During this stasis, the phagocytes of the body are able to engulf and destroy the invading organisms.

From time to time pathogens enter the human body without setting up infections. The human body's general resistance is normally able to provide the necessary defenses to prevent infection. This capacity depends on some of the physical fitness, mental health, and social factors discussed in previous chapters.

Immunity and susceptibility. The host with no specific resistance is termed *susceptible* and may be converted to immunity status by a variety of mechanisms. Complete resistance is termed *immunity* and is specific for a particular disease. Immunity is dependent on the presence in the body of specific substances that are most easily identified in the bloodstream but that are present in all tissues. These chemical substances are called antibodies and may be in the form of antitoxin, which neutralizes a particular toxin; agglutinin, which causes organisms to clump together; or precipitin, which produces a disintegration of pathogenic organisms.

Active immunity exists when an individual's own body produces the necessary antibodies. This type of immunity can result either from the actual attack of the disease or from artificial introduction of the necessary antigenic substance into the body by vaccination or immunization (Table 11-7). An **antigen** is a substance (for example, toxin) that, when introduced into the body, causes the formation of antibodies.

Passive immunity is "borrowed" immunity; it exists when antibodies produced in some other individual or animal are introduced into a person. The duration of passive immunity is relatively short because the protective substances tend to disappear, not to be replaced by the individual's own antibody

production. Passive immunity is employed when a susceptible person has been exposed to a disease and there is insufficient time to produce active immunity. For example, the injection of convalescent serum into a susceptible child exposed to measles would give the child temporary immunity or at least limit the case to very mild symptoms. The infantile immunity that a child experiences during the first six months of life is an example of natural passive immunity; antibodies from the mother's bloodstream diffuse through the membranes of the placenta into the bloodstream of the fetus, but the immunity exists only while the mother's antibodies survive in the child. Infantile immunity is extended during breastfeeding through the antibodies contained in the nursing mother's milk.

Natural immunity exists when a species has a genetic immunity to a particular disease to which some other species is susceptible. For example, mammals are immune to many of the microorganisms that cause infection in birds. Domestic animals are susceptible to some diseases, such as distemper, to which humans are immune. Likewise, domestic animals are immune to diphtheria, smallpox, typhoid fever, and other infectious diseases to which humans are heir. Fortunately, the human species possesses natural immunity to a vast number of microorganisms that could be disease-producing but for the human body's distinctive biochemistry. Communities are able to add to this general protection or defense by offering artificial immunity through vaccination.

Acquired immunity is that particular type of active immunity that comes from having an attack of a disease. In humans second attacks are common with such diseases as influenza, pneumonia, gonorrhea, streptococcal sore throat, and the common cold, but are relatively rare with such diseases as chickenpox, diphtheria, measles, poliomyelitis, scarlet fever, smallpox, typhoid fever, and yellow fever. Vaccines to produce artificial active immunity are available for diphtheria, tetanus, pertussis, smallpox, poliomyelitis, typhoid fever, cholera, Rocky Mountain spotted fever, measles, German

TABLE 11-7
Immunization schedules

Disease	Risk group	Primary series	Booster doses	Vaccine
All adults				
Tetanus	All adults	2 doses + 1 dose after 6-12 months	Every 10 years	Combined Td vaccine or
Diphtheria	All adults	2 doses + 1 dose after 6-12 months	Every 10 years	combined Td-Polio
Travel vaccines				
Polio	Travelers to endemic areas, others with occupational risks	2 doses + 1 dose after 6-12 months	Every 10 years*	Salk (IPV) vaccine or combined Td-Polio
Meningococcal	Travelers to epidemic areas	1 dose	Unknown	Meningococcal vaccine
Yellow fever	Travelers to endemic areas	1 dose	Every 10 years	Yellow fever vaccine
Cholera	Where required for foreign travel	2 doses	Every 6 months*	Cholera vaccine
Typhoid	Travelers to endemic areas	3 doses	Every 3 years*	Typhoid vaccine
Japanese encephalitis	Travellers to endemic or epidemic areas	3 doses	Every 4 years*	JEVax
Other adult vaccines				
Influenza	Everyone over 65, others with heart, lung, kidney, or metabolic disorders	1 dose	Every year	Influenza vaccine
Measles	All born after 1956 who are susceptible	1 dose	None	Measles vaccine or combined MMR
Mumps	All young adults with no history of mumps	1 dose	None	Mumps vaccine or combined MMR
Rubella	All susceptible women of childbearing age	1 dose	None	Rubella vaccine or combined MMR
Hepatitis B	Patients on renal dialysis, repeated use of blood or blood products, health care workers exposed to blood, staff and residents of mental institutions, household contacts of carriers, homosexually active males, some travelers	3 doses	Every 5 years*	Hepatitis B vaccine
Rabies	Veterinarians, trappers, animal technicians, animal control, zoo keepers, conservation officers, wildlife biologists, travelers to endemic areas, and others at high risk of exposure	3 doses	Every 2 years*	HDC rabies vaccine
Pneumococcal	Everyone over 65, others with medical conditions that increase risk	1 dose	None	Pneumococcal vaccine

*While risk or travel requirement lasts.
Source: National Advisory Committee on Immigration, U.S. Department of Health and Human Services.

measles, mumps, and influenza. Various immunization schedules apply to these vaccines (see Chapter 5 and Table 11-7).

Smallpox vaccination has been discontinued because there is now a greater threat to human health in possible complication from smallpox vaccination than in not being immunized. The spread of an epidemic through a population is determined by the immune/susceptible ratio. When the supply of susceptibles is exhausted, the epidemic ceases. In the case of smallpox, the pathogen itself was isolated from susceptible populations until the agent-host chain was broken with the isolation of the last case in Somalia.

Agent–Host–Environment

The outcome of disease in the individual is determined by the interaction of agent, host, and environment. The agent may be of high virulence or present in high concentrations. The host's defenses may be compromised by age, exhaustion, or concomitant disease, or the immune system may be affected by drugs or radiation given for chronic disease. The environment may be unfavorable, as in the case of air pollution. Community action can be applied at any of the three points. Resistance of the host can be enhanced by better nutrition or by vaccination, for example. The agent may be directly attacked by chemicals or antibiotics, and the environment may be altered by sanitation or housing reforms.

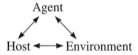

This interactive model may also be used to consider conditions other than infectious diseases, such as automobile injuries, where the agent is the automobile, the host is the driver, and the environment is the highway.

EPIDEMIOLOGICAL PRINCIPLES OF DISEASE CONTROL

Epidemiology is the study of the distribution and determinants of disease in a population. The unit of study is not the individual, as in microbiology and clinical medicine, but the community. Epidemiology compares and contrasts, studying both sick and well groups. Variables such as age, sex, race, and occupation are analyzed in an attempt to determine which are found frequently in the sick but rarely in the well. The validity of the conclusions reached is subject to statistical tests.

Disease in the community is first categorized by time, place, and person. By studying the time or place of onset in an epidemic, a shared event, such as a meal, may be identified. It can then be determined if this particular meal was attended by many of the sick persons but by few of a comparison group of well people. Food histories may then be assembled and a suspect vehicle identified. The place of the epidemic may help to identify the offending vehicle, as when there is a density of cases in an area with a common water supply, or when the cases are predominantly on the route of a mobile food vendor. The personal characteristics of those afflicted in an epidemic may point to its cause. For example, the sick people might share a common exposure to toxic inhalants in an industrial plant or to asbestos fibers in construction work.

Legal Authority

Communicable diseases are legally controlled through the exercise of police power, which is the authority or power of the people, represented by government, to protect the general well-being of the public. Basically, sovereignty or ultimate authority rests with the people, who vest it in the state or province to exercise for them. The state or province may in turn delegate police power to counties or parishes to exercise disease control measures within their geographical boundaries. Municipalities may be granted a charter that gives broad authority, including police power, to protect the well-being of the people within the political limits of the borough, village, town, or city. Municipalities and counties usually assign some authority to schools to carry out certain control measures.

In practice the state or province enters into communicable disease control practice in a broad advisory capacity to the community governmental units and by direct action when communicable diseases spread beyond a single locality. The state or province usually does not step in and take action unless local authorities request assistance or are unable to cope with the situation.

In the exercise of police power the one governing principle recognized by the courts is that whatever action is taken must be reasonable. Thus it may be reasonable for health authorities to isolate an indi-

vidual in his home for a period of five days when he suffers from a diagnosed case of a certain communicable disease, but a court might rule that it would not be reasonable to require that patient to be removed to a hospital and isolated there for two weeks. The science of epidemiology has advanced to a point where the action taken is usually reasonable because it is based on sound statistical probability, microbiology, and medical science. People today are spared a great deal of the inconvenience suffered by their grandparents because modern public health science has displaced much of the arbitrary police action based on guesswork once involved in disease control.

Health authorities cannot ignore the personal and religious rights of the individual, but courts have been reluctant to censure official public health ac-

The AIDS Controversy

The pressure on governmental agencies to exercise their police power in matters of health grows intense when the community feels threatened by a new, mysterious, socially stigmatized or frightening disease. Such was the case with the enforced isolation of lepers in the Middle Ages. Such has been the case in the 1970s and 1980s with the fear concerning Legionnaires' disease, herpes, and most recently, AIDS.

More than 76% of the AIDS patients diagnosed before July 1982 had died by mid-1984. Homosexual or bisexual men continue to be, by far, the group at highest risk for the disorder, with 72% of the cases occurring in this group. Intravenous drug users make up 17% of the cases. The disease evokes more fear and punitive reaction than sympathy, at least in conservative communities.

But even in progressive San Francisco, the controversy over the closing of bathhouses—meeting places for homosexual encounters—led to the resignation of the city and county health officer. In Houston, the city council was forced to place a referendum on the ballot, which allowed the public to vote down a controversial ordinance protecting homosexuals from discrimination

in city hiring. An antihomosexual psychologist has suggested that homosexuals be required to stay in their homes until a cure or a vaccine for AIDS is found. Many states have laws that would empower public health officials to quarantine people who have been exposed to a communicable disease, and even to force them to undergo treatment. These laws, however, have seldom been used to quarantine entire groups, only individuals known to have been exposed. Large-scale quarantines would raise constitutional questions concerning an individual's right to due process and hearings before being placed in custody.

Quarantines are more common in institutions such as prisons or boarding schools where many people live in close proximity. The only instances in recent years of entire groups being quarantined have been on ships arriving in port with passengers discovered to have cholera.

If homosexuals were to be quarantined, what about hemophiliacs and other minority groups with higher-than-average rates of AIDS? Where would you draw the line in evoking the police power of the state in controlling communicable diseases?

tion exercised reasonably in the interest of the general population. Courts have ruled that while official health boards cannot require a person to be immunized in opposition to religious beliefs, imposing quarantine on susceptible nonimmunized people when an epidemic threatens the community is just and reasonable. In the present era, however, control measures are so highly effective that if a relatively small percentage of the population is not immunized against a disease, the fact that most of the people are immune virtually eliminates the spread of the particular disease. This is sometimes referred to as "herd immunity." In the final analysis, the exercise of police power often reflects a failure of public health education and other means of communicable disease control.

Segregation of Reservoir

Theoretically, perfect prevention of spread would mean perfect control of communicable diseases. It is possible to establish certain barriers around a reservoir of infection and thus block the spread of the disease.

Isolation. The oldest communicable disease control measure is the segregation of an infected person or lower animal until danger of conveying infection has passed. **Isolation** can be a highly effective control measure, but in practice it occasionally fails because of subclinical cases, variability in the duration of the communicable state, and human failures in observing regulations.

Bacteriological methods can determine the required interval of isolation with precision. Laboratory examination of the secretions of a patient with tuberculosis will establish the presence or absence of the tubercle bacillus and thus determine the continuance or termination of isolation. Likewise, examination of secretions from the nose and throat of a patient with diphtheria will provide an accurate bacteriological determination of whether isolation should be terminated.

The longer the period of isolation, the greater the safety—but also the greater the injustice, because many patients reach a noncommunicable or at least relatively safe state long before the maximum isolation period is reached. No definite rule applies; for this reason, great variation is found from community to community. To set an inflexible isolation period would make no provision for individual variation. For this reason, the usual practice is to set a minimum time that experience has demonstrated will be ample in perhaps 80% to 90% of the cases, and then leave to the discretion of the attending physician the need for extending the isolation in individual cases. An arbitrary period of isolation can be quite satisfactory for diseases such as measles and chickenpox where no convalescent carriers occur.

Isolation has certain limitations. Hidden cases—those never reported by patients or parents—are not technically under isolation. Carriers of a disease usually do not have overt symptoms and thus are not identified as potential hazards. In addition, during the early or prodrome stage of a respiratory disease, individuals may not be ill enough to remain home, yet they are in a highly communicable state and capable of spreading the disease to others.

Quarantine. The detention of susceptible individuals who have been exposed to a communicable disease is called **quarantine.** These individuals are often spoken of as "contacts." Nonsusceptible people who have been exposed are not included as contacts. Quarantine is used infrequently in disease control at present because the individual is rarely in a communicable state during the incubation period of a disease. As a consequence, not until first symptoms appear does the individual present a danger, and, at this point, isolation can be imposed. Measles and chickenpox are exceptions in that they may be communicable during the last two or three days of the incubation period. Even in the case of these two diseases, however, quarantine is of questionable value in controlling spread.

Quarantine time is based on laboratory findings, the maximum incubation period, or both. Thus if several laboratory specimens are negative, the person is released from quarantine; or if the usual incubation period for the disease in question is seven days, then after the seventh day following exposure to the disease the subject is released from quarantine if he or she exhibits no symptoms.

Reducing communicability. Treatment of a patient limits the reservoir and therefore represents an important procedure in communicable disease control. Medical treatment of patients can be highly effective in reducing communicability of certain diseases. For example, through the use of chemotherapy and antibiotics, a case of syphilis can be rendered noncommunicable, although some symptoms may persist in the patient.

Reservoir Eradication

Logically the most permanent and thus the most desirable measure of communicable disease control would be the complete elimination of the reservoir. This is possible when lower animals serve as reservoirs of organisms pathogenic to humans. Bovine tuberculosis and brucellosis have been eliminated by an orderly, widespread program of testing cattle and then slaughtering those that are reactors.

The principle of reservoir eradication can sometimes be applied to the human organs harboring infectious organisms. This procedure has been directed to the carriers of disease. Some typhoid carriers, for example, have been rendered noncarriers by the removal of the gallbladder.

Environmental Measures

Sanitation measures usually are directed toward the vehicles of disease transfer and are effective in limiting the spread of such diseases of the intestinal tract as hepatitis, typhoid, paratyphoid, dysentery, salmonellosis, staphylococcus infection, and chol-

era. Application of the principles of sanitation to water supplies, processing of milk and other foods, and sewage disposal has played an important role in reducing the incidence of these alvine discharge diseases since the beginning of the century. Sanitation has been effective also as a measure in controlling vector-borne diseases such as malaria and yellow fever. By destroying the breeding places of the vectors and by using effective insecticides, sanitation programs can effectively control the spread of insect-borne diseases.

Environmental measures are of little value in the control of such respiratory diseases as measles, chickenpox, scarlet fever, streptococcal sore throat, diphtheria, smallpox, and pertussis. Although decontamination measures may be of some value in preventing the spread of respiratory diseases, their effectiveness has never been scientifically established.

Increasing Resistance of New Host

Even when organisms of sufficient number and virility to establish infection invade a new host, measures still may be taken to protect the host and to prevent further spread of the disease.

Passive immunization can give transient emergency protection. Before this procedure is employed, it must be ascertained that the person actually was exposed and is susceptible to the disease. Because passive immunization lasts but a few weeks, it provides only a stopgap for a particular situation when no other measures are feasible. Passive immunization has one marked disadvantage in that the serum usually used may sensitize the individual so as to set up the future danger of anaphylaxis—extreme reaction to a second exposure to the foreign serum. For this reason, passive immunization is not regarded as a good community measure to be used on a widespread basis.

Limiting the severity of a disease should be regarded as a control measure. Diseases such as diphtheria and scarlet fever can be modified by treatment, and by this procedure communicability can be reduced.

Immunization of children and adults has provided the most dramatic examples of epidemiological control of infectious diseases, as in the case of smallpox eradication, which combined immunization with isolation and quarantine. More exclusive use of immunization has accounted for the spectacular drops in poliomyelitis and measles in the past 20 years, as illustrated for measles in the United States in Figure 11-13. Measles is now a candidate for possible eradication, at least in some countries.

Personal hygiene and health behavior. Individual behavior continues to be a factor in the control of

infectious diseases, particularly among those spread by person-to-person contact. Evidence for the continuing importance of proper hygienic measures is illustrated by outbreaks of illness associated with improper food handling both in private homes and institutions. Correct use of condoms is an effective measure in the prevention of sexually transmitted diseases. Similarly, simple handwashing techniques will prevent the transmission of many bacterial illnesses in both the hospital and the home.

Certain factors such as smoking, alcohol consumption, poor nutrition, drug misuse, and stress place people at increased risk for infectious diseases and subsequent morbidity and mortality. Alcoholics are known to be at higher risk for several infectious

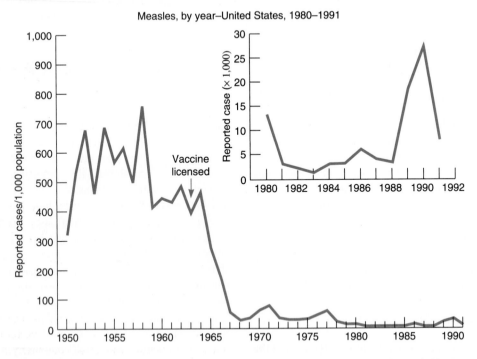

FIGURE 11-13
The decline in reported measles (rubeola) incidence since the measles vaccine was licensed in the United States. The jump in 1989 and 1990 rates was the result of widespread slippage in state and local immunization efforts.
Source: Centers for Disease Control: Measles surveillance—United States, 1991, *MMWR* 41(SS-6):1, 1992.

diseases, including pneumonia. Smokers are at risk, in particular, for pulmonary diseases such as bronchitis and pneumonia. Intravenous drug users are at risk for AIDS (Figure 11-4), hepatitis B, and endocarditis (most commonly caused by staphylococcal infection). Poor nutrition, particularly in children, puts the individual at risk for gastroenteritis and respiratory illnesses, secondary to infectious pathogens. Finally, studies indicate that stress can increase people's susceptibility to many kinds of illness, including infectious diseases.

Community education measures. Community health education and health promotion programs directed at these health practices and life-styles will contribute to the control of infectious diseases, even though this may not be the primary objective of such programs. Community health education interventions designed to support behavior conducive to infectious disease control could occur at any of the following five steps when people (1) become more susceptible (life-style behavior), (2) become exposed (hygienic behavior), (3) become infected (protective or prophylactic behavior), (4) become symptomatic (appropriate medical care), or (5) suffer complications or relapses (adherence to prescribed medical regimens). The first three points of intervention are primary prevention steps to build host resistance; the last two are secondary and tertiary prevention steps.

In addition a well-informed public will not be stampeded by scare rumors or fantastic reports such as fatal reactions to immunization. Further, a good community health education program will assist in obtaining funds for the promotion of immunization and other control measures.

Community health education should provide useful immunization information to all mothers and new parents through hospitals, physicians, and others; aim educational programs at members of the health care professions; include discussion of immunization and preventive measures in school health curricula; enlist daycare centers, senior citi-

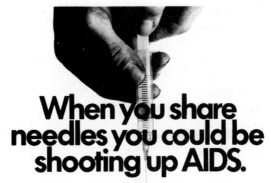

When you share needles you could be shooting up AIDS.

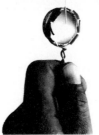

People who shoot drugs can get AIDS from sharing needles.

If the needle or cooker has been contaminated you could be infected.

You can't tell if the AIDS virus is on the needle just by looking.

You can't tell a person has the AIDS virus just by looking.

There is no cure for AIDS. It's a slow, painful, ugly way to die.

If you can't stop shooting up, get into treatment before you shoot up AIDS.

STOP SHOOTING UP AIDS.
GET INTO DRUG TREATMENT.
CALL 1-800 662 HELP.

FIGURE 11-14
Public service magazine advertisements and posters alert high-risk groups to the dangers of infection with the HIV virus if they are sharing needles.
Source: National Institute on Drug Abuse, Department of Health and Human Services.

zen centers, and churches to provide immunization information to parents and to older people; use the mass media for immunization activities; and continue the use of volunteers.

Service measures. Community health centers and other medical care settings can contribute to the control of diseases for which vaccines are available by adopting standardized official immunization records; developing and using tickler files and recall systems to ensure that children return for immuni-

---

Objectives for Immunization
By 2000 at least 95% of children attending licensed day-care centers and kindergarten through twelfth grade should be fully immunized. (In 1988 the immunization level was about 94% for licensed child care, 97% for first school entrants.)

By 1990 all mothers of newborns should receive instruction prior to leaving the hospital on immunization schedules for their babies.

What would you set as corresponding objectives for your community for the year 2000? |

zations on schedule; making immunizations available and affordable in all health care settings as a part of comprehensive health services; and using local volunteers who know the population at risk.

Legislative and regulatory measures. Further organizational supports should include the following legislative and regulatory steps: enforcing existing school immunization requirements and extending them to include children at all grade levels in both public and private schools, as well as in organized preschool settings; including coverage of immunization as a health insurance benefit not subject to deductible provisions; requiring carriers under any national health insurance plan to reimburse for immunization services; requiring immunization as a condition of employment (for example, in health care institutions); and including rubella immunization as a service routinely offered in family planning clinics, primary care clinics, hospitals, and HMOs.

Economic measures. Related economic supports for immunization programs include reimbursing for immunizations under public and private health insurance plans; supplying vaccines free to all health care providers as long as they do not charge for vaccinations; and offering economic incentives to health care providers and vaccine recipients.

DISEASE CONTROL RESOURCES

Official health agencies require the cooperation and assistance of individuals and other agencies competent to assist in the general problem of disease control. Health education of the public is fundamental to effective communicable disease control measures, and official health agencies recognize that the supplementary health education contributed by other organizations is highly valuable in the general control program. Indeed, education of the public is the primary approach of the official and voluntary health agencies in controlling diseases. In the philosophy of modern community health, a department of health that must rely continually on its legal authority for an effective program would be regarded as an outdated and ineffective agency. Schools, voluntary agencies, hospitals, and medical practitioners should be expected to contribute their resources to the communicable disease control efforts. (See Chapters 18 to 21 for descriptions of these resources.)

SUMMARY

The dramatic decline in the relative importance of communicable diseases as causes of death since the beginning of this century might lead one to believe that little more needs to be done. The inspiring story of the eradication of smallpox might encourage the conclusion that the other communicable diseases are on their way out also. Diphtheria, malaria, poliomyelitis, trichinosis, and typhoid fever all seem near extinction, and measles has been targeted for eradication. However if further reduction in any of these diseases is to be accomplished, existing control measures cannot be taken for granted or relaxed. Maintaining high levels of immunization requires persistent effort on the part of community health agencies, schools, and other cooperating institutions. The importance of vigilance was seen in the 1970s and again in 1989 through 1990, when immunization levels in the United States dipped perilously below the 90% standard, resulting in the resurgence of measles and certain other diseases.

The distinct modes of transfer for respiratory diseases, alvine-discharge diseases, vector-borne diseases, and open lesion diseases have divided the strategies for control into broad classes of intervention. For respiratory diseases the main control measure has been the strengthening of host resistance, primarily through immunization, but also significantly through improved nutrition and general health promotion. This approach has succeeded where any other hope of controlling airborne transmission would be limited by the realities of social contact and indoor living.

The alvine-discharge diseases are transmitted primarily by water and food contaminated through unsanitary conditions. The major interventions, therefore, have been environmental control measures directed at water purification, sewage disposal and treatment, food protection, and personal hygiene. These means of control also have been aided by more general improvements in housing, urban design, and economic conditions, and by promoting public understanding of disease control.

Vector-borne diseases have been controlled largely through the killing or containment of vectors such as rodents, mosquitoes, flies, ticks, and fleas. Some vectors carry other vectors as part of the life cycle of the pathogenic organism. The vehicles of transfer from reservoir to new host can thus be both mechanical and biological.

The diseases most difficult to control have been those transmitted by direct contact, particularly open lesion diseases. The obstacles here seem to be related to the value-laden, socially and politically controversial aspects and implications of governmental or other third-party intervention in people's intimate relations. The sexually transmitted diseases illustrate the problem most poignantly today, as tuberculosis and leprosy have in the past. For this reason public health education has proved to be the most durable and essential intervention for the ultimate control of these diseases.

QUESTIONS FOR REVIEW

1. What distinction can be made between infectious disease and communicable disease?

2. If effective methods of immunization were developed for all of the communicable diseases, would humankind eliminate all existing communicable diseases?

3. Of recent outbreaks of communicable disease you have observed or otherwise were acquainted with, do you class these outbreaks as endemic, epidemic, or pandemic?

4. What communicable respiratory diseases are most likely to appear in epidemic form in your community?

5. What disease do you predict will cause the next worldwide pandemic?

6. To what extent is there justification for saying that an epidemic is evidence of an inadequate public health education program?

7. Is pasteurization of the community milk supply less necessary today than it was 30 years ago?

8. What services does your health department provide in its communicable disease control program?

9. What organizations or agencies in your community contribute to communicable disease control?

10. What steps should an ordinary citizen take when he or she has evidence that a case of communicable disease may exist in a household where no physician has been called and no precautions are being taken to prevent possible spread of the disease?

11. What is being done and what further should be done in your community to prevent the spread of communicable diseases via foods other than milk or water?

12. From the standpoint of public health education, how would you change this prevailing attitude: ''It's just a cold''?

13. Why should passive immunization be rejected as a community-wide procedure?

14. What disadvantages in respect to communicable disease control does a democracy have that a dictatorship does not have?

15. Is there any evidence that new infectious diseases are appearing?

READINGS

Aral SO, Holmes KK: Sexually transmitted diseases in the AIDS era, *Sci Am* 264:62, 1991.

Gonorrhea, syphilis, and new viral STDs follow different epidemic paths. This article examines the social conditions that help to fuel the new epidemics, especially the changing demographics and economic conditions affecting young people and minorities or transient workers. Only a combination of social and health programs can defeat these diseases.

Freudenberg N: *Preventing AIDS: a guide to effective education for the prevention of HIV infection,* Washington, DC, 1990, American Public Health Association.

Using case histories of successful and unsuccessful community programs, this book summarizes the experience of the 1980s in educating people about AIDS, with attention to the social and political forces that shape AIDS educators.

Hopkins DR, Ruiz-Tiben E: Surveillance for dracunculiasis, 1981-1991. In CDC surveillance summaries, Special focus I: public health surveillance and international health, *MMWR* 41:1, 1992.

After successfully eradicating smallpox, WHO designated dracunculiasis (guinea worm disease) as the next disease scheduled to be eradicated (by 1995). This article reports progress on this goal, emphasizing the importance of epidemiological methods of surveillance.

Jereb JA, Kelly GD, Dooley SW Jr et al: Tuberculosis morbidity in the United States: final data, 1990. In CDC surveillance summaries, *MMWR* 40(SS-3):23, 1991.

After a long historic decline, the number of tuberculosis cases increased between 1988 and 1990. The 1989 through 1990 increase of 9.4% was the largest annual increase since 1953. Shows the ethnic group, age, and origin of cases.

Smith LL, Lathrop LM: AIDS and human sexuality, *Can J Public Health* 84(suppl 1):14, 1993.

Specific strategies for a comprehensive approach to AIDS is outlined using the PRECEDE-PROCEED model introduced in Chapter 4 of this book. This whole issue of the *Canadian Journal of Public Health* is devoted to AIDS.

BIBLIOGRAPHY

Alteneder RR, Price JH, Telljohann SK et al: Using the PRECEDE model to determine junior high school students' knowledge, attitudes, and beliefs about AIDS, *J School Health* 62:464, 1992.

Aruffo JF, Coverdale JH, Pavlik VN et al: AIDS knowledge in minorities: significance of locus of control, *Am J Prev Med* 9:15, 1993.

Barua D, Greenough WB III: *Cholera,* New York, 1992, Plenum.

Benenson AS, editor: *Control of communicable diseases in man,* ed 15, Washington, DC, 1990, American Public Health Association.

Centers for Disease Control: Health information for international travel, 1992, Pub No (CDC) 92-8280, Washington, DC, 1992, U.S. Government Printing Office.

Chen LC, Amor JS, Segal SJ, editors: *AIDS and women's reproductive health,* New York, 1991, Plenum.

Ciesielski SD, Seed JR, Esposito DH et al: The epidemiology of tuberculosis among North Carolina migrant farm workers, *JAMA* 265:1715, 1991.

Committee for the Study on Malaria Prevention and Control: *Status review and alternative strategies,* Washington, DC, 1991, National Academy Press.

Coverdale JH, Aruffo JF, Laux LF et al: AIDS, minority patients, and doctors—what's the risk? Who's talking, *South Med J* 83:1380, 1990.

Coyle SL, Boruch RF, Turner CF, editors: *Evaluating AIDS prevention programs,* Washington, DC, 1991, National Academy Press.

Cundy KR, Kleger B, Hinks E et al, editors: *Infection control: dilemmas and practical solutions,* New York, 1990, Plenum.

Cutts FT, Orenstein WA, Bernier RH: Causes of low preschool immunization coverage in the United States, *Annu Rev Public Health* 13:385, 1992.

Dabbagh L, Green LW, Walker GM: Case study: application of PRECEDE and PROCEED as a framework for designing culturally sensitive diarrhea prevention programs and policy in Arab countries, *Int Q Commun Health Educ* 12:293, 1991-92.

Decosas J, Pedneault V: Women and AIDS in Africa: demographic implications for health promotion, *Health Pol & Planning* 7:227, 1992.

Donowitz LG, editor: *Infection control in the child care center and preschool,* Baltimore, 1991, Williams & Wilkins.

Ellerbrock TV, Bush TJ, Chamberland ME et al: Epidemiology of women with AIDS in the United States, 1981 through 1990: a comparison with heterosexual men with AIDS, *JAMA* 265:2971, 1991.

Evans AS: *Viral infections of humans: epidemiology and control,* ed 3, New York, 1991, Plenum.

Evans AS, Brachman PS, editors: *Bacterial infections of humans: epidemiology and control,* ed 8, New York, 1991, Plenum.

Germain A, Holmes KK, Piot P et al, editors: *Reproductive tract infections: global impact and priorities for women's reproductive health,* New York, 1992, Plenum.

Gorman M, Mallon D: The role of a community-based health education program in the prevention of AIDS, *Med Anthropol* 10:159, 1989.

Hope-Simpson RE: *The transmission of epidemic influenza,* New York, 1992, Plenum.

Horowitz LG, Kehoe L: Fear and AIDS: educating the public about dental office infection control, *Dent Age of AIDS,* Special issue: Spring 1992.

Kim-Farley R, the Expanded Programme on Immunization Team: Global immunization, *Annu Rev Public Health* 13:223, 1992.

LeBaron CW, Lew J, Glass RI et al: Annual rotavirus epidemic patterns in North America: results of a 5-year retrospective survey of 88 centers in Canada, Mexico, and the United States, *JAMA* 264:983, 1990.

Lederberg J, Shope RE, Oaks SC Jr, editors: *Emerging infections: microbial threats to health,* Washington, DC, 1992, National Academy Press.

Lupton DA: From complacency to panic: AIDS and heterosexuals in the Australian press, July 1986 to June 1988, *Health Educ Res* 7:9, 1992.

Miller HG, Turner CF, Moses LE, editors: *AIDS: the second decade,* Washington, DC, 1990, National Academy Press.

National Institute of Allergy and Infectious Diseases: PID: guidelines for prevention, detection and management, *Clin Courier* 10:1, 1992.

National Institute of Allergy and Infectious Diseases: *Toxoplasmosis,* Bethesda, 1992, NIAID, National Institutes of Health.

Oaks SC Jr, Mitchell VS, Pearson GW et al, editors: *Malaria,* Washington, DC, 1991, National Academy Press.

de Quadros CA, Andrus JK, Olive J-M et al: Polio eradication from the Western Hemisphere, *Annu Rev Public Health* 13:239, 1992.

Quinn TC, Ruff A, Modlin J: HIV infection and AIDS in children, *Annu Rev Public Health* 13:1, 1992.

Rhodes T, Holland J: Outreach as a strategy for HIV prevention: aims and practice, *Health Educ Res* 7:533, 1992.

Roberts L: Zebra mussel invasion threatens U.S. waters, *Science* 249:1370, 1990.

Rozovsky LE, Rozovsky FA: *AIDS and Canadian law,* Ottawa, 1992, Canadian Public Health Association.

Simon PM, Morse EV, Balson PM et al: Barriers to human immunodeficiency virus related risk reduction among male street prostitutes, *Health Educ Q* 20:261, 1993.

Snider DE, Roper WL: The new tuberculosis, *N Engl J Med* 326:703, 1992.

U.S. Department of Health and Human Services: *Healthy people 2000: national health promotion and disease prevention objectives,* Boston, 1992, Jones & Bartlett.

Zapka JG, Marrocco GR, Lewis B et al: Inter-organizational responses to AIDS: a case study of the Worcester AIDS consortium, *Health Educ Res* 7:31, 1992.

Chapter 12

Life-Style and Community Health Promotion

Good health is a major resource for social, economic and personal development and an important dimension of quality of life.
   Ottawa Charter for Health Promotion

OBJECTIVES

When you finish this chapter, you should be able to:

- Identify the behavioral risk factors that account for more than half of the leading causes of death and disability

- Describe the epidemiological patterns and trends associated with these risk factors

- Propose health promotion strategies combining educational, organizational, economic, and environmental supports for behavior and conditions of living conducive to health

- Apply the model of community health promotion to the planning of a large-scale program to support life-styles conducive to health

---

Life-style, a concept describing value-laden, socially conditioned behavioral patterns, has a rich history of study in anthropology and sociology. Only recently has it taken on special significance in epidemiology and community health. With the mid-century shift from acute infectious diseases to chronic, degenerative diseases as the leading causes of death in Western societies came a new perspective in epidemiology. No longer could the predominant diseases be controlled by the isolation and suppression of a single germ or agent. The causes of most chronic diseases tend to be multiple and elusive. They defy simple environmental control measures because they involve people's pleasures and rewards, their social relationships and physical needs and ultimately, for some, their habits and addictions.

In this chapter we will examine four kinds of behavior or health-related habits that are or can be harmful: alcohol use, smoking, eating patterns, and drug use. All involve physiological changes and may involve a compulsive or dependency component in behavior. Each results in widespread mortality (Table 12-1), morbidity, and social pathology in the community. These four patterns of behavior, together with physical activity or exercise, stress management or recreation, and safety practices, constitute the set of personal actions that are termed life-style. They are health related but not necessarily health directed.

EPIDEMIOLOGY OF LIFE-STYLE RISK FACTORS

The health field concept described in Chapter 2 has four elements: health services, environment, human biology, and life-style. Of these, life-style is responsible for most (over half) of the years of life prematurely lost in the more developed nations (Figure 12-1). To put this revealing statistic in more positive terms, the greatest gains in preventing premature death and disability can be achieved today through community supports for more healthful life-styles.

TABLE 12-1

The five leading causes of death in North America and their associated risk factors or precursors

Cause of death	Risk factors
Cardiovascular disease	Tobacco use
	Elevated serum cholesterol
	High blood pressure
	Obesity
	Diabetes
	Sedentary life-style
Cancer	Tobacco use
	Improper diet
	Alcohol
	Occupational/environmental exposures
Cerebrovascular disease	High blood pressure
	Tobacco use
	Elevated serum cholesterol
Unintentional injuries	Safety belt noncompliance
	Alcohol/substance abuse
	Reckless driving
	Occupational hazards
	Stress/fatigue
Chronic lung disease	Tobacco use
	Occupational/environmental exposures

Source: National Center for Health Statistics, and Health and Welfare Canada.

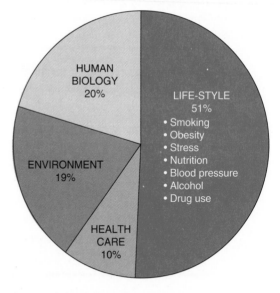

Source: U.S. Public Health Service

FIGURE 12-1

Life-style risk factors contribute more than the combination of health care, environment, and human biology to the years of life lost prematurely (before age 75). Nutrition includes overnutrition, obesity, anorexia, bulimia, undernutrition, and control of diabetes.

Source: Centers for Disease Control and Prevention, Public Health Service, U.S. Department of Health and Human Services.

Reducing risk means that chances of developing a disease are lowered. It does not guarantee that a disease will be prevented. Because several factors are involved in the development of disease, risk reduction usually involves several strategies or approaches.

The entire burden for improved health or reducing risk must not be placed on the individual alone. The responsibility must be shared between individuals and their families; between families and their communities; and between communities and their state, provincial, and national governments. Each level of organizational influence on behavior must assume some responsibility for setting the economic and environmental conditions that will support healthful life-styles. Families, for example, must set examples for children. Communities must provide facilities and pass local ordinances to encourage, enable, and reinforce healthful behavior. State and national governments and private organizations must assume responsibility for the production, sale, and advertising of foods and other substances that can be either helpful or harmful to health.

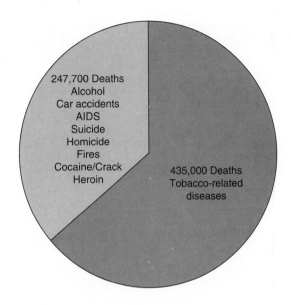

FIGURE 12-2

Smoking kills more Americans every year than alcohol, automobile crashes, AIDS, suicides, homicides, fires, and drugs combined.

Source: Centers for Disease Control and Prevention, Public Health Service, U.S. Department of Health and Human Services.

TOBACCO MISUSE

Tobacco use is the single most preventable cause of death in North America (Figure 12-2). It is responsible for more than one in six deaths in the United States. In 1988 approximately 430,000 deaths in adults aged 35 and older were attributed to the intentional inhalation of tobacco smoke. Included in these deaths are 201,000 deaths from cardiovascular disease, 112,000 from lung cancers, 83,000 from chronic lung disease, and 31,000 from other cancers.

Evidence on the effects of unintentional inhalation of tobacco smoke were presented in a 1992 position statement by the American Heart Association. Two types of smoke are emitted from cigarettes: mainstream smoke, which is directly inhaled into the smoker's lungs, and sidestream smoke, which is emitted into the air between puffs. Environmental

smoke is estimated to be 85% sidestream and 15% mainstream smoke. Contained in this environmental smoke are more than 4,000 chemicals collectively called "tar," including at least 40 carcinogens.

In 1988 it was estimated that 3,800 lung cancer deaths and 37,000 cardiovascular deaths occurred in nonsmokers who had been exposed to environmental tobacco smoke. An additional 2500 perinatal deaths were estimated to have been caused by smoking among pregnant women, and another 1300 deaths resulted from burns related to smoking.

Epidemiology of Tobacco and Health

Although cigarette smokers suffer the highest **relative risk** with respect to cancer, the community impact of smoking is greatest in cardiovascular disease because the latter is so prevalent.

Objectives for Tobacco Use Reduction

- By 2000 reduce cigarette smoking to a prevalence of no more than 15% among people aged 20 and older. Baseline: 29% in 1987, 32% for men, and 27% for women.

Special Target Populations	1987	2000
People with high school education	34%	20%
Lower socioeconomic youth	40%	18%
Military personnel	42%	20%
Hispanics	33%	18%
American Indian/Alaska native	42-70%	20%
Pregnant women	25%	10%

- By 2000 reduce smokeless tobacco use by males aged 12 to 24 to a prevalence of not more than 4%. Baseline: 6.6% among males aged 12-17 in 1988; 8.9% among males aged 18 to 24 in 1987.

Cigarette smoking accounts for 21% of all coronary heart disease deaths and 30% of cancer deaths. Selected sites where the **attributable risk** from smoking is high include lung cancer (87%) and larynx cancer (82%). Attributable risk (AR) is the percentage of total cases that can be ascribed to a particular risk factor—in this case, cigarette smoking.

Smoking trends. The first decline in cigarette consumption in the United States came in 1954 after more than 40 years of increases. This was the year that the first American Cancer Society report was published showing that the death rate for cigarette smokers from all causes was much higher than for nonsmokers and that the lung cancer mortality of cigarette smokers was 10 times that of nonsmokers. The second decline in consumption came in 1964, when the first Surgeon General's Report on Smoking and Health was published.

The third reduction in smoking prevalence rates occurred between 1968 and 1970, when the "fair-ness rule" in broadcasting required television networks to provide air time for thousands of antismoking messages in response to cigarette advertisements. The more steady decline since 1973 is attributed to the cumulative effects of federal, state, and local action; the growing influence of the nonsmokers' rights movement; and the rising cost of cigarettes, including the U.S. federal excise tax increase in 1983 from 8 cents to 16 cents per package, the first increase since 1952. Several communities and states undertook aggressive antismoking campaigns in the 1980s and 1990s.

The overall prevalence of smoking in the United States has been falling in recent decades at a rate of approximately 0.5 percentage points per year. The smoking rate among adults has declined from 40% in 1965 to 26% in 1990, toward a target of 15% by the year 2000. Nearly half of all living adults who ever smoked have quit. The smoking rate remains disproportionately high among blacks, blue-collar workers, and people with fewer years of education. The declines have also been substantially slower among women than among men. By the late 1980s women's death rate from lung cancer surpassed their death rate from breast cancer. The smoking epidemic had caught up with them full force. Although smoking rates for women have fallen again to 27%, the rise in the number of women smokers has not escaped the attention of cigarette manufacturers. They have stepped up advertising campaigns for new brands of cigarettes designed expressly for women.

Smokeless tobacco. As smoking decreased in the 1970s, a fourfold increase in chewing tobacco users and a fifteenfold increase in snuff users between 1970 and 1986 have prompted new national, state, and community campaigns directed at teenagers. Most smokeless tobacco users begin their use before age 21; 37% begin before age 16. Smokeless tobacco use declined among males aged 12 to 17 from 6.6% in 1988 to 5.3% in 1991. It also declined among males aged 18 to 23 from 12.3% in 1987 to 11.6% in 1991.

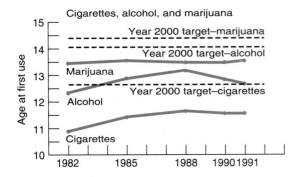

FIGURE 12-3

Average age of first use of cigarettes, alcohol, and marijuana among 12- to 17-year-olds, relative to objectives for first use of these substances by the year 2000.

Source: Office of Disease Prevention and Health Promotion, Public Health Service, U.S. Department of Health and Human Services.

Age and sex. Tobacco use habits established in the teens (Figure 12-3), in the great majority of cases, will persist into adulthood. Teenage girls, who in the past never smoked to the extent that teenage boys did, have now caught up. In 1968 only about half as many teenage girls smoked as boys, but by 1979 girls had surpassed boys in teenage smoking. Smoking declines with age after early adulthood.

Smoking parents set the example for children. Studies show that youngsters whose parents smoke are more likely to adopt the habit than are children of nonsmoking parents.

International Smoking Rates

Cigarettes are projected to kill one in five people in industrialized countries over the next 30 years. The lag time between smoking prevalence and related morbidity and mortality is seen in different patterns around the globe. Most industrialized countries are now experiencing the incongruous combination of declining prevalence and increasing morbidity and mortality from smoking. Less-industrialized countries are entering a period of high prevalence and are beginning to experience some of the disease

and disability associated with smoking. The least-industrialized countries have low prevalence of smoking and related mortality but have other public health issues to contend with.

Eventually, smoking may kill even more in the currently less industrialized countries. In China, with almost one third of the world's population, more than 60% of the men smoke. Half of all Polish men who die between the ages of 35 and 69, die of smoking-related causes.

Prevention of Tobacco Use

A national strategy to reduce tobacco use requires multiple kinds and levels of strategies that are economic, legal, educational, and pharmacological in nature.

The eventual demise of smoking as a socially acceptable habit will be achieved by persistent action and a variety of concerted approaches. Realistic achievement of goals should be expected in a time frame of several years, perhaps of decades.

Increased life expectancies and concomitant changes in health statistics that would result from a successful national program of smoking prevention would lead to changes in various economic indicators and consequently in legislative attitudes. For example, it is estimated that the gross national product for the United States would increase by 0.6%, or almost $15 billion in constant dollars greater than otherwise projected, by the year 2000. Private housing starts would be projected to increase by 4%, and unemployment would decrease by nearly 4% with the reductions in smoking. These estimates assume that efforts to eliminate the adverse health effects of tobacco usage will gradually become fully effective by the year 2000. Even if a "smoke-free" society or a "smoke-free class of 2000" is a realistic goal, the fact remains that millions still smoke and will continue to do so, at least for the immediate future. The projected improvements in economic indicators could be used to justify legislative support for smoking prevention programs in communities.

Economics. Tobacco has been a major economic factor in the first 200 years of the development of North America. The profitability of its industry has been legendary and has resulted in lavish promotional efforts. With the invention of automatic manufacturing equipment, the use of cigarettes has increased dramatically during the past 100 years, aided by astute advertising through the press, the cinema, and later through the electronic media. The two major wars and the minor wars of this century have also contributed to the diffusion of cigarettes and to their image as cultural symbols of sophistication and machismo.

From a few hundred cigarettes per adult citizen at the turn of the century, annual consumption has skyrocketed to about 3500 per adult. Cigarettes have indeed reached an unprecedented position in the mythology of Western culture, a condition that is rapidly spreading to other cultures as well.

Governments, of course, have not been indifferent to this potential source of revenue. The tobacco industry contributes, from the tobacco field to the vending machine, some $18 billion to the gross national product of the United States and gives livelihood to a well-publicized segment of the population in several states (Figure 12-4).

Naturally, these economic activities are protected and fostered by the U.S. Department of Agriculture

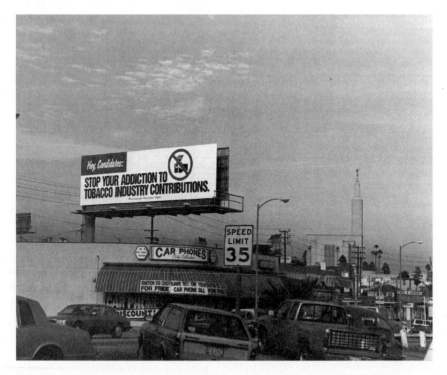

FIGURE 12-4
Billboard political action messages such as this one in Los Angeles seek to alert the public to the tobacco lobby's influence on legislators and to embarrass legislators and other political candidates into not accepting contributions from the tobacco lobby.

Source: Americans for Nonsmokers' Rights.

and the Department of Commerce and add some billion dollars annually to a precarious balance of payments. With billions in cigarette advertising, the media tend to defend the tobacco industry and resist constraints on advertising on the grounds of First Amendment rights to free press. As the North American and European markets for tobacco products decline, U.S. and European manufacturers of cigarettes are advertising and selling more aggressively in the less-developed nations where smoking is regarded as a symbol of modern living.

Federal, state and local governments collected about $11 billion in cigarette excise taxes in 1991. Still, the United States lags behind other countries in collecting tax on tobacco products (Figure 12-5).

The economic revenue from smoking is offset by the compensation for the burden of death, disease, health care, fires, and lost productivity. The U.S. population of civilian, noninstitutionalized persons aged 25 years or older who ever smoked cigarettes will incur lifetime excess medical care costs of $501 billion. The estimated average lifetime medical costs for a smoker exceed those for a nonsmoker by over $6000. The number grows approximately $9 to $10 billion annually because of the additional excess lifetime health care costs of the 1 million teenagers who take up smoking each year.

Legal and legislative. The tort law in the United States exposes manufacturers to class action suits if they express doubt about the safety of their products. Thus the cigarette industry can be expected to continue to deny any association of tobacco and disease, even to the point of not engaging in research toward less hazardous products; indeed, this would presume an admission of hazard. Moreover, the cigarette industry has little incentive to develop products that are less habit-forming or that facilitate habit cessation in the smoker. Because of this situation, demonstrating the feasibility of less hazardous cigarettes is unlikely to happen.

Traditionally, legislatures have been more sensitive to the immediacy of economic issues and thus have given only token attention to funding public health needs in smoking.

Increasingly local and state legislatures have been passing laws that limit or prohibit smoking in public places such as public buildings, transit, worksites, and restaurants. In 1992 the New York City Council overwhelmingly passed a landmark antitobacco law that makes it more difficult for minors to buy cigarettes, expands antismoking messages, bans smoking in public and private schools, outlaws the sale of loose cigarettes, and requires store owners to ask for proof of age to buy cigarettes. Similar legislation is pending in other communities. In 1988 California voters approved Proposition 99, which raised the state cigarette taxes from 10 to 35 cents per pack, the second-highest in the nation at the time. Health and economics benefits included a 17% decline in smoking between 1989 and 1991, twice the U.S. average. Revenues raised by the tobacco tax have been used to fund medical care for the poor, tobacco control programs and research, parks and wildlife programs, and firefighting services.

Canada has raised federal and provincial per pack cigarette taxes from 46 cents in 1980 to $3.27 in 1991 (Figure 12-6). During the time period, teen smoking has been reduced by approximately two thirds and total cigarette consumption is falling faster than in any major industrialized nation. Cigarette tax revenue has grown from about $1 billion in 1981 to $7 billion in 1991.

Health education. Communities can mount antismoking campaigns, and local groups can reinforce national leadership on this issue. People must be made aware of the hazards of cigarette smoking. This awareness results in (1) individuals being motivated not to smoke, and (2) smoking becoming less socially acceptable, which will reinforce decisions not to smoke. Such awareness is very important in the young because advertising presently directed at youth depicts smoking as being socially acceptable and desirable.

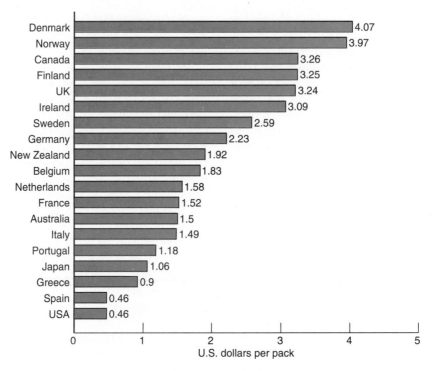

Notes: 1. Foreign taxes expressed in U.S. dollars are approximate due to
currency fluctuations.

2. Data provided by the Non-Smokers' Rights Association of Canada;
analysis by Public Citizens' Health Research Group; chart produced
by the Coalition on Smoking OR Health.

FIGURE 12-5
The United States lagged behind most other Western countries in taxing cigarettes in 1991 and 1992.
Source: Coalition on Smoking OR Health.

In the young, it is also necessary to negate peer influence, which often emphasizes risk taking. During the **socialization** process, nonsmoking must be instilled. Role models—persons teenagers admire—may prove effective. The difficulty is that not smoking is a "nonaction" rather than a dynamic force easy to associate with hero figures. To teenagers, smoking may also be a symbol of independence and rebellion against the **norms** of the family or group to which they belong.

The educational approach requires identification of, and provision for assistance to, those individuals at an increased risk of tobacco-related diseases (Figure 12-7). Epidemiological surveys are conducted to determine the environmental, social, and psychological characteristics of the population at risk. The main thrust in this component of smoking education has been in the development of epidemiological methods for identifying groups at high risk of tobacco-related disease; analysis of smoking patterns

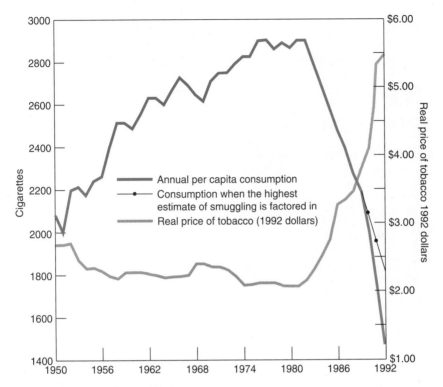

Note: Cigarettes include fine-cut equivalents

FIGURE 12-6
Annual per capita consumption of cigarettes in Canada went down dramatically with the increase since 1981 in taxes that increased the real price of tobacco (per 20 cigarettes). The large discrepancy in prices between the low U.S. cost for a carton of cigarettes and the high Canadian price has resulted in smuggling of cigarettes across the U.S.-Canadian border for illegal profiteering. An adjustment for black market consumption is shown in the most recent year.
Source: Non-Smokers' Rights Association, Ottawa, Ontario, Canada.

and behavior; research in smoking cessation techniques; and evaluation of smoking education programs.

Pharmacological approaches. Cigarette smoking is a form of drug dependence on nicotine. In 1988 the Surgeon General of the U.S. Public Health Service declared tobacco an addictive substance. Nicotine is recognized as a potent drug eliciting pharmacological effects on the central nervous system and playing an important role in controlling smoking behavior. Consequently, pharmacological intervention is a possible method for controlling smoking behavior. Such activities are directed at reducing relapse in smoking cessation programs through combined pharmacological, physiological, and psychological approaches; improving and maintaining initial quitting rates; improving people's understanding of the physicochemical properties of nicotine and its metabolites; and identifying substances that taste, smell, or react like nicotine to use as substitutes for cigarette smoking.

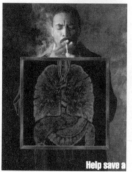

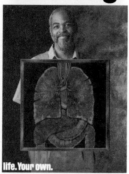

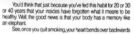

You'd think that just because you've fed this habit for 20 or 30 or 40 years that your insides have forgotten what it means to be healthy. Well, the good news is that your body has a memory like an elephant.

See, once you quit smoking, your heart bends over backwards

to repair itself. After a while, it actually starts working better. In a number of years, it's almost as if you've never lit up. And, to some extent, the same can be true for your lungs.

So even if you can't forgive yourself for all the time you wasted on smoking, your body can. You just have to give it the chance.

 CDC

FIGURE 12-7
This federal campaign ad targets those who have continued to smoke for long periods of their adulthood, thinking that they have already done irreparable damage and that it is therefore too late to quit. In fact, statistics show that most of those who quit after many years of smoking return to normal cardiovascular and respiratory functioning over a period of 2 to 5 years.

Source: Centers for Disease Control and Prevention and National Heart, Lung, and Blood Institute, Public Health Service, U.S. Department of Health and Human Services.

Another pharmacological approach is to produce a less hazardous type of cigarette. The genetics and agricultural practices of tobacco growing and curing are analyzed to reduce precursors of tobacco smoke toxicity. This entails the following sequence of events: (1) tobacco blends are analyzed to determine their chemical constituents; (2) cigarette smoke condensate, whole smoke, and chemical constituents are bioassayed by use of several animal models; (3) flavor components are identified; (4) bio-

assays are conducted to assess whether toxicity results from the reintroduction of flavor components; and (5) chemical, bioassay, and flavor results are correlated to identify the characteristics of less hazardous cigarettes. Average tar and nicotine content of cigarettes sold in the United States have declined by more than 50% since 1954 as a result of these efforts, although a truly "safe" cigarette does not exist. Labeling the cigarette package with the amounts of each hazardous substance and with a general health warning has helped remind smokers of the specific risks.

Schools and worksites. The foregoing approaches address the host and the agent of cigarette-induced diseases. The environment in which smoking occurs

---

Environmental Objectives for Tobacco

- By 2000 establish tobacco-free environments and include tobacco use prevention in the curricula of all elementary, middle, and secondary schools. Baseline: antismoking education was provided by 78% of school districts at the high school level, 81% at the middle school level, and 75% at the elementary school level in 1988.
- By 2000 increase to at least 75% the proportion of worksites with a formal smoking policy that prohibits or severely restricts smoking at the workplace. Baseline: 27% of worksites with 50 or more employees in 1985; 54% of medium and large companies in 1987.
- By 2000 enact and enforce in 50 states laws prohibiting the sale and distribution of tobacco products to youth younger than age 19. Baseline: 44 states had, but rarely enforced, laws regulating the sale and/or distribution of cigarettes or tobacco product to minors in 1990; only 3 set the age of majority at 19, and only 6 prohibited cigarette vending machines accessible to minors.
- By 2000 eliminate or severely restrict all forms of tobacco product advertising to which youth under 18 are exposed.

or is encouraged is the third essential point of intervention in the community. The school classroom is most frequently regarded as the setting in which antismoking education should take place. Unfortunately, this curriculum focus on schools often ignores the even greater problems and opportunities outside the classroom where children and youth gather, observe, and are exposed to smoking influences. Some of the most promising health education programs in relation to smoking are those addressing the total school environment and "inoculating" pupils against the social pressures they may encounter in that environment. Role playing by re-

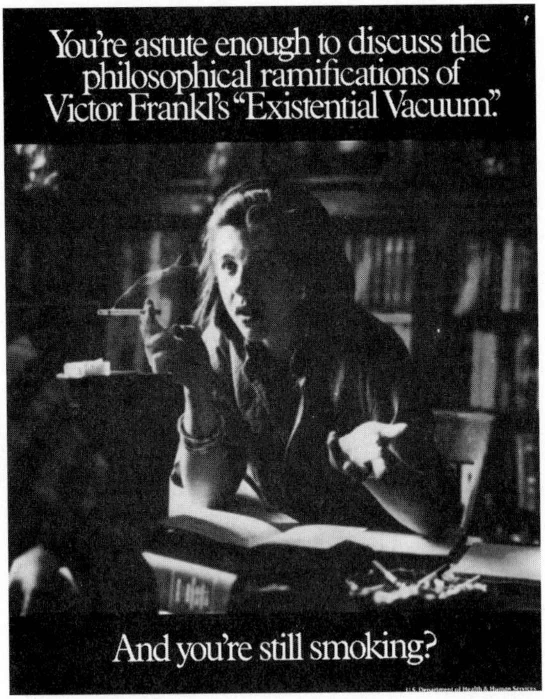

FIGURE 12-8
This CDC poster targets college and university students expected to be the leaders and role models in the workplace in future years, challenging the thinking of those who smoke and reinforcing the decision of those who do not.

Source: Office on Smoking and Health, Center for Chronic Disease Control and Health Promotion, Centers for Disease Control and Prevention, Public Health Service, U.S. Department of Health and Human Services.

hearsing in the classroom how to decline a cigarette offer from a peer has proved effective in delaying the uptake of smoking.

Worksites represent the other environment where people gather, observe, and are influenced by their social and physical surroundings for the greater part of their waking hours (Figure 12-8).

Increasing numbers of businesses in the United States have programs to help their employees stop smoking. A significant number have policies to restrict or prohibit smoking in the workplace, most frequently in areas where smoking poses the greatest health hazard. Antismoking programs are the third most common health education program sponsored by companies, after hypertension control and diet-weight management.

ALCOHOL MISUSE

After smoking, alcohol is the most important known cause of mortality and morbidity in most Western countries. The American experience with Prohibition and the longer history of alcohol in civilization indicate that alcohol is a drug that society cannot entirely eradicate. Like most of the life-style **risk factors,** the use of alcohol in moderation (with possible exceptions, such as by alcoholics and by women during pregnancy) can be tolerated and even can be beneficial.

Epidemiology of Alcohol Misuse

Alcohol is undoubtedly the most abused drug in North America, Europe, Australia, and New Zealand today. Four to six million Americans have been diagnosed as alcoholics, and 10% of the U.S. adult population is believed to have a serious drinking problem. One in four adolescents is at very high risk of alcohol and other drug problems, school failure, early unwanted pregnancy, and/or delinquency. Adolescents have been using alcohol at increasingly early ages since 1988, setting the stage for early and

Objectives for Alcohol and Other Drugs

- By 2000 reduce deaths caused by alcohol-related motor vehicle crashes to no more than 8.5 per 100,000. Baseline: 9.8 in 1987.
- By 2000 reduce cirrhosis deaths to no more than 6 per 100,000. Baseline: 9.1 in 1987.
- By 2000 reduce drug-related deaths to no more than 3 per 100,000. Baseline: 3.8 in 1987.
- By 2000 increase by at least 1 year the average age of first use of cigarettes, alcohol, and marijuana by adolescents aged 12 to 17. Baseline: age 11.6 for cigarettes, age 13.1 for alcohol, and age 13.4 for marijuana in 1988.
- By 2000 reduce alcohol consumption by people aged 14 and older to an annual average of no more than 2 gallons of ethanol per person. Baseline: 2.54 gallons of ethanol in 1987.

potentially sustained use of alcohol as an indicator of chronic lifelong mental and physical health problems, as well as social maladjustment (Figure 12-3).

It is estimated that 50% of all traffic fatalities and fatal intentional injures such as suicides and homicides are alcohol-related. Nearly 20,000 people were killed in 1991 in alcohol-related traffic crashes. Overall, such fatalities have declined from 9.8% in 1987 to 7.9% in 1991. Approximately one third of all victims are intoxicated in homicides, drowning, and boating deaths. In addition to lives lost, more than 10,000 infants are compromised at birth each year by Fetal Alcohol Syndrome due to alcohol consumption by their mothers during pregnancy.

Epidemiological, clinical, and laboratory evidence have made it clear that cirrhosis of the liver, one of the 10 leading causes of death in most Western countries, is caused primarily by alcohol consumption. The cirrhosis death rate has shown a significant decline from 9.1 per 100,000 in 1987 to 8.3 in 1990. Other diseases and conditions associated with alcohol include acute poisoning and chronic intoxication; toxic psychoses; gastritis; pancreatitis; hypertension; cardiomyopathy; peripheral neuropathy; home, recreational and occupational fires; and

cancer of the mouth, pharynx, larynx, esophagus, and liver. Alcohol can lower resistance and increase risk of infectious disease. Alcohol contributes to ill health, crime, poverty, broken homes, unintended pregnancy, divorce, social conflicts, loss of earning power, loss of productivity, social degradation, and other social pathology.

Low socioeconomic groups have a higher prevalence of cirrhosis than do high socioeconomic groups. There is a relationship to occupation: those handling alcohol show higher rates of hepatic cirrhosis. Mortality from injuries and hepatic disease drops suddenly when alcohol is removed from the community or when supply or demand is restricted by an **excise tax.**

Costs related to alcohol problems are estimated to exceed $70 billion per year in the United States, with the majority of those costs attributed to low productivity. Approximately 1.4 million persons in 41 states and the District of Columbia receive alcohol and other drug treatment services annually from publicly funded agencies. In Canada heavy federal and provincial taxes are placed on alcohol, raising about $4 billion annually in revenue. Still, the costs of abuse, estimated at $5 billion annually, exceed the revenues generated by alcohol.

Prevention of Alcohol Misuse

Like tobacco use prevention, the prevention of problems related to alcohol consists of interventions on agent, host, and environment levels.

Agent. Alcohol is the agent, an anesthetic that is toxic in overdose. The healthy adult liver can oxidize about ¼ ounce of absolute alcohol per hour. The alcohol content is half the proofage, so ¼ ounce is equal to 0.6 ounce of 86 proof alcohol. Because the absorption of alcohol into the bloodstream is delayed by food in the stomach, peak blood levels are not reached so quickly after eating.

Defining ''moderate'' drinking is difficult because the size of a standard drink varies among countries, the percentage of alcohol by volume varies among cultures, and the methods of conversion of known quantities of beverage alcohol to absolute alcohol vary. The American Heart Association recommends that daily intake of alcohol should be limited to 1 to 2 ounces of ethanol. (One ounce of ethanol is contained in two ounces of 100 proof whiskey, eight ounces of wine, or 24 ounces of beer.) The U.S. Dietary Guidelines for Americans suggests that women should limit drinks to one per day and men limit themselves to two drinks. (A drink is counted as 12 ounces of regular beer, 5 ounces of wine, 1½ ounces of distilled spirits, 80 proof.) The U.S. Department of Health and Human Services and the National Research Council warn that with the consumption of three or more drinks per day, harmful effects such as high blood pressure, cirrhosis of the liver, and even heart attacks begin.

Host. Altering the behavior of the host is the most popular intervention. Exhortation, coupled with deprivation, is usually tried. Group therapy and mutual self-help groups using behavioral modification techniques have the best success records. Alcoholics Anonymous is the leading exponent of this approach. Counselors are frequently former alcoholics, who are better able to appreciate the difficulties of abstinence than are those who have never overcome such a problem. A nonjudgmental, supportive, understanding relationship must be established.

Environment. Most medical treatment merely results in rendering the alcoholic fit enough to resume drinking. Surviving cirrhosis depends on cessation of alcohol consumption. If the alcoholic persists in drinking, medical and surgical measures are to no avail. Worksite and other social networks to help alcoholics, such as Alcoholics Anonymous and the help of family and friends, should be supported in the community.

Public Education and Action

The communication of effective alcohol-related health messages is particularly challenging and dif-

Legislative (Environmental) Supports for Alcohol Abuse Prevention

Public outrage with drunk driving and alarm about the rates of teenage drinking and alcohol-related crimes have led to recent collective action in many U.S. States and communities. For example, in 1984 Massachusetts passed a ban on "happy hours." In 1985 Texas banned "two-for-one" drink promotions during happy hours. In 1988 the Omnibus Drug Act of the federal government required a warning label on every bottle of liquor. Model legislation has been drafted to encourage more states and communities to adopt these and other measures to restrict availability of alcohol and to curtail economic incentives related to alcohol promotion. Perhaps the most controversial of these legislative bills was one that required states to raise the legal drinking age to 21 or face a loss of federal highway funds amounting to 5% in 1987 and 10% in 1988.

Controversy about such legislation centers on the issue of states' rights when the measures are federal initiatives, and on infringement of civil liberties when they are proposed at any level of government. Communities and college campuses have struggled with these issues. What do you consider the difference, if any, between these issues and laws to protect the public's health through compulsory immunization or quarantine? What hazards would you foresee in failing to involve the community in understanding and supporting the passage of such laws?

ficult. Few products can match alcohol in the ability to evoke strong sentiments—both positive and negative. Most people already have firm opinions concerning the appropriate role of alcoholic beverages in their personal lives, and such beliefs, whether based on accurate information or not, are highly resistant to change.

Perceptions about alcohol use may be acquired through personal experience with alcoholic beverages or through the experiences and influence of associates, friends, and family members. Perceptions may also be acquired vicariously from the depiction of alcohol use in publications and in film, radio, and television dramatizations. Unfortunately, some of these perceptions are incorrect or incomplete. Many people do not know how alcohol is metabolized in the body and have only partial knowledge about the effect that food or time can have on this process; they also assume, incorrectly, that coffee can have a mitigating effect. People are insufficiently aware that consumption of large amounts of alcohol in a short period of time, such as may occur in a drinking contest, can cause death. Often, they are also unaware that drinking can cause or contribute to many health hazards.

Advertising and counteradvertising. An important source of perceptions is alcoholic beverage advertising, particularly for young people. For example, the favorable image alcohol users are given in television advertising and programming creates a barrier to be overcome in alcohol education efforts. The alcoholic beverage industry commits over a billion dollars annually to an extensive array of product advertising in the print and broadcast media.

Considering the pervasiveness of positive images concerning alcohol use, communication techniques that could be effective in carrying appropriate health-related messages about alcohol use to current or potential users must include mass media campaigns and product labeling to inform, to raise awareness levels, or to reinforce old knowledge, and to change potentially harmful responses to social situations in which alcohol use is encouraged (Figure 12-9). Education should be used to inform people of the methods of advertising alcohol.

Organizational and environmental supports. Altering the environment is the most effective way of reducing alcoholism in the community. In many instances the social environment of schools, colleges, worksites, and public gathering places creates pressure on the individual to drink. Social ambience must be altered so that alcohol is not regarded as a reward, as a status symbol, or as something that is glamorous.

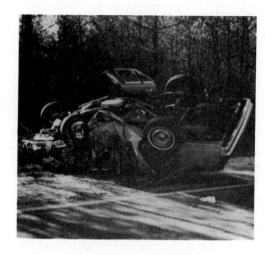

Ever Get Somebody Totally Wasted?

TAKE THE KEYS.
CALL A CAB.
TAKE A STAND.

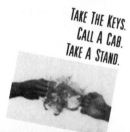

FRIENDS DON'T LET FRIENDS DRIVE DRUNK

U.S. Department of Transportation

FIGURE 12-9
This public service ad from the Drunk Driving Prevention Campaign of the U.S. Department of Transportation encourages and reinforces new norms of social behavior and life-style in which people take greater responsibility for protecting the safety of friends who have had too much to drink to be able to drive home safely.
Source: U.S. Department of Transportation and Advertising Council.

Objectives for Services and Protection for Alcohol and Other Drugs

- By 2000 establish and monitor in 50 states comprehensive plans to ensure access to alcohol and drug treatment programs for the traditionally underserved.
- By 2000 provide to all school children educational programs on alcohol and other drugs.
- By 2000 extend adoption of alcohol and drug policies for the work environment to at least 60% of worksites with 50 or more employees.
- By 2000 extend to 50 states administrative driver's license suspension or revocation laws for people determined to have been driving under the influence of intoxicants. Baseline: 28 states in 1990.
- By 2000 increase to at least 20 states that have enacted statutes to restrict promotion of alcoholic beverages focused principally on young audiences.
- By 2000 extend to 50 states legal blood alcohol concentration tolerance levels of 0.04% for motor vehicle drivers aged 21 and older and 0% for those younger than age 21. Baseline: 0 states in 1990.
- By 2000 increase to at least 75% the proportion of primary care providers who screen for alcohol and other drug use problems and provide counseling and referral as needed.

Economic supports. The cost of alcohol has increased much less than other beverages. It can be greatly increased by taxation, so that a more significant part of discretionary income must be expended to buy alcohol. This economic approach works best with teenagers, but it penalizes the poor. It has an effect on overall community consumption, but not necessarily on the most addicted and heaviest drinkers.

Warning labels. The 100th Congress passed an Omnibus Drug Bill with provisions for a new label on all alcoholic beverages that would read: "Government Warning: (1) According to the Surgeon General, women should not drink alcoholic beverages during pregnancy because of the risk of birth defects. (2) Consumption of alcoholic beverages impairs your ability to drive a car or operate machinery and may cause health problems."

OBESITY, OVERNUTRITION, AND UNDERNUTRITION

Nutrition has improved in the United States, but the mean body weight of Americans has steadily increased. Overnutrition and **obesity** are now major health problems in the United States and in many other Western countries, especially the consumption of dietary fats. Food intake is a paradox within the United States. On one hand, 26% of adult Americans and as many as one out of every three children is overweight. On the other hand, it is estimated that one out of eight American children under age 12 suffers from hunger and that many homeless and poor adults experience the same. Both overnutrition and undernutrition reflect environmental, cultural, and socioeconomic conditions. Overnutrition, in addition, may involve hereditary and psychological conditions.

Epidemiology of Nutrition

Status and trends. The prevalence of overweight has not declined among adults for more than two decades (Figure 12-10). In the United States 1976-1980 baseline figures indicate that 24% of men, 27% of women, and 15% of adolescents are overweight (that is, at least 120% of desirable body weight). Current levels exceed the 1990 objective of no more than 10% among men and 17% among women. A more recent survey found an increase from 24% in 1984 to 34% in 1991 in the number of children ages 3 through 17 considered overweight. Canada's Health Promotion Survey in 1990 found approximately 22% of Canadians were overweight.

The burdens of overweight are more often carried by women, the poor, and members of certain ethnic

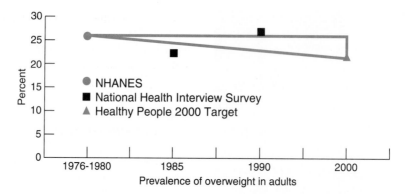

FIGURE 12-10

The National Health and Nutrition Examination Survey (NHANES) and the National Health Interview Surveys show no improvement in prevalence of overweight (120% of ideal weight for height) in U.S. adults since the 1976-1980 baseline; indeed, there appears to have been an increase in recent years.

Source: National Center for Health Statistics, Centers for Disease Control and Prevention, Public Health Service, U.S. Department of Health and Human Services.

groups. The rates of significant overweight for black men and white men differ very little, but black women are about a third more likely to be obese than are white women. Among children, overweight was found in boys more than in girls, lower income children more than higher income, African American and Hispanic children more than white, and older children more than younger.

The economic costs of obesity are reflected in premature morbidity and mortality as well as reduced productivity. In addition, consumers spend billions of dollars annually on weight loss and exercise programs. The top five diet companies in the United States had revenues near $4 billion in 1992. The costs of nutrition fraud, which remain unmeasurable and unquantifiable at this time, deserve attention during the next decade.

Throughout the 1980s people in developed countries appeared to be increasingly concerned not only with the amounts of food they eat but also with its content. Although the average number of calories consumed per person per day in the United States increased between 1963 and 1983 from 3180 to 3450, the source of those calories improved. Annual consumption of vegetables increased from 187 pounds to 207 pounds per person; of fruits, from 120 to 143 pounds; and of flour and cereals, from 144 to 150 pounds. Not since the Great Depression of the early 1930s have animal products such as meat, milk, and eggs made up a smaller share of the diet of Americans than they did in the 1980s. Although consumption of animal fats has declined in general, fish and poultry consumption has increased. Economic factors have influenced some of these choices, but most analysts concur that health concerns have motivated much of the shift in diet. By the 1990s consumers were bombarded with contradictory messages to stay fit and eat lean, yet enjoy gourmet ice cream, smell warm cinnamon buns baking at the mall, and return to old-fashioned cooking. The commercial assault on dietary concerns of the public influences future dietary trends.

Consumer attention to diet is undoubtedly responsible for the fact that average cholesterol levels in the U.S. population have declined nearly 10% in the past 20 years. Most of this decrease has occurred in higher educational and occupational groups, but it does reflect the potential for change in the populations reachable through community health programs.

Health effects. Nutrition and food consumption involve complex interactions of social, cultural, economic, behavioral, and physiological factors. Adequate intakes of sources of energy and of essential nutrients are necessary for satisfactory rates of growth and development, reproduction, lactation, and maintenance of health. The consensus of the National Research Council and the Surgeon General's 1988 Report on Nutrition and Health is that the U.S. population needs to reduce its percentage of calories derived from fat.

There are basically two kinds of fat: saturated and unsaturated. Saturated fat is found in food from animals and some vegetable oils, such as coconut and palm oils. Unsaturated fat (monosaturated or polyunsaturated) is found in foods from plants and is considered better for health than saturated fat. Hydrogenated oils are vegetable oils that have been changed into a more solid, saturated fat, such as

margarine and shortening. In 1989 both U.S. adults and children received 36% of their calories from fat; 13% was from saturated fat. That is a decrease from 40% of calories from fat in 1977, but above the 30% year 2000 target (Figure 12-11).

Deficiencies of essential nutrients or energy sources can lead to several specific diseases or disabilities and increased susceptibility to others. Excessive or inappropriate consumption of some foods may contribute to adverse conditions, such as obesity, or may increase the risk for certain diseases, such as heart disease, adult-onset diabetes, high blood pressure, gall bladder, osteoarthritis of weight-bearing joints, dental caries, and possibly some types of cancer. Such chronic diseases are clearly of complex cause, with substantial variation in individual susceptibility to the several risk factors. The role of nutrients in some of these diseases is not definitively established, but epidemiological

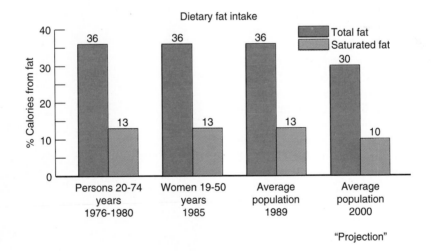

FIGURE 12-11

By all measures available, the percentage of calories consumed from fat by the American population had not declined as of 1989 (latest data available) since the initial drop in the early 1970s from 40%. Other surveys indicate that the U.S. population in the early 1990s was trying to consume lower-fat foods, but recent indications suggest a softening of even this positive trend, which will make the year 2000 objectives of 30% calories from any fat and 10% from saturated fat difficult to achieve.

Source: Office of Disease Prevention and Health Promotion, Public Health Service, U.S. Department of Health and Human Services.

and laboratory studies offer important insights that may help people in making food choices that will enhance their prospects of maintaining health. Diet plays a part in five of the ten leading causes of death in the United States.

Anorexia nervosa and **bulimia** are compulsive disorders with consequences similar to those of malnutrition. Both disorders involve depletion of nutrients, and both are considered epidemic in adolescent and young women in the United States. The fixation on slimness as a necessity causes the anorexic to starve herself, the bulimic to "binge and purge"—eating compulsively, then regurgitating. The bulimic person also suffers from upper intestinal and oral tissue damage from the frequent exposure of the throat and mouth to stomach acids. Dentists are often the first to detect the bulimic, recognizing their pattern of tooth erosion.

Frequent consumption of highly cariogenic (decay-producing) foods (those containing fermentable or orally retentive carbohydrates), especially between meals, can nullify some of the caries-preventive benefits of adequate fluoride intake and can cause rampant caries in children with a fluoride deficiency. No consistent or independent relationship has been shown, however, between sugar consumption and the onset of heart disease or diabetes. Once diagnosed, of course, a diabetic person must control sugar intake.

Inadequate nutrition may be associated with poor pregnancy outcome, including low-birth weight deliveries and suboptimum mental and physical development. Excessive sodium intake has been associated with high blood pressure in susceptible individuals. Dietary fat, especially saturated fat and cholesterol, are risk factors for heart disease, along with smoking and high blood pressure. Dietary fat has also been associated epidemiologically with some types of cancer. Indeed, the National Cancer Institute estimates that 35% of all cancer deaths are attributable to diet. Eating more foods high in fiber may reduce the risk of colon cancer and may alleviate the symptoms of chronic constipation, diver-

ticulosis, and some types of "irritable bowel" in some individuals. Finally, poor nutrition may increase susceptibility to infections, fatigue, and stress.

Overweight infants and children tend to become obese adults. Prevention must begin early, before learned patterns of compulsive overeating are established (Figure 12-12). Obesity and overnutrition are

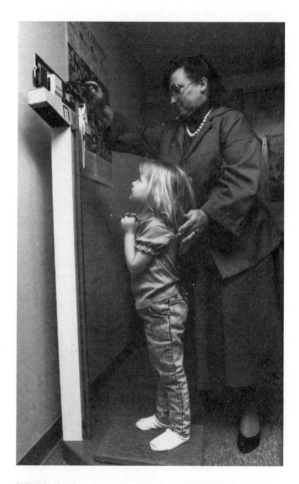

FIGURE 12-12
Weight control needs to begin early, but with care, to ensure that balanced nutrition is achieved, not a compulsive preoccupation with weight or body shape.
Source: Missouri Department of Health.

associated with increased rates of coronary heart disease, adult-onset diabetes, hypertension, stroke, and accidents, and the combined toll on community health is very large.

Prevention and Nutrition Promotion Measures

Education. Nutrition education measures directed at the community should emphasize safe weight control and reduction strategies based on energy balance concepts. Most important, these programs need to move the community away from quick-fix schemes that may be successful in the short term but most often lead to weight regain in the long term. Repeated weight gain and loss may have harmful physiological, psychological, and economic effects. The public needs support to set reasonable and achievable goals in making lifetime commitment to dietary and life-style changes.

Educational programs can also include awareness of nutrition principles and areas of scientific controversy about the relation of diet to heart disease, high blood pressure, certain cancers, diabetes, dental caries, and other conditions. They can provide information and teach behavioral skills to enable people to select and prepare more healthful diets. More effective means of communicating nutrition information to people in different age and ethnic groups are needed. Nutrition information and education about food choices can be imparted in the home (via the media and outreach services), in schools, at the worksite, by and to health care providers, at the point of purchase (supermarkets and restaurants), as a part of government food service programs (such as the Head Start, school lunch, and Women, Infant, and Child programs in the United States), and by appropriate advertising of food products (Figure 12-13).

Service measures. The provision of food and nutrition services in the community should include nutritious breakfast and lunch programs for school-

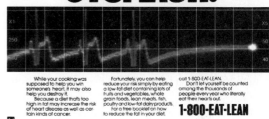

FIGURE 12-13
High-fat foods contribute both to heart disease and colon cancer as well as obesity, which contributes to diabetes and high blood pressure. This public service ad was sponsored by a national coalition of agencies organized by the Kaiser Family Foundation as part of Project LEAN (Low-Fat Eating for America Now).
Source: Henry J. Kaiser Family Foundation and Advertising Council.

children and meals for senior citizens at congregate sites; food stamps for low-income populations; food supplements for low-income women, infants, and children; nutritious food offered in business and institutional settings; dietary counseling routinely offered to high-risk individuals by health care providers, schools, and employers; and psychosocial support groups focused on weight control and weight maintenance.

Technological measures. Most of the technological means of improving nutrition must be exercised

- By 2000 reduce overweight to a prevalence of no more than 20% among people over 20 and no more than 15% among adolescents aged 12 to 19. Baseline: 26% for people aged 20 to 74 in 1976-1980, 24% for men and 27% for women; 15% for adolescents aged 12 to 19 in 1976-1980.

Special Target Populations	*1976-1980*	*2000*
Low-income women	37%	25%
Black women	44%	30%
Hispanic women	37%-39%	25%
American Indians/Alaska natives	29%-75%	30%
People with disabilities	36%	25%
Women with high blood pressure	50%	41%
Men with high blood pressure	39%	35%

at the national or state or provincial level, but some community action is possible in ensuring nutritional quality and content of manufactured foodstuffs, from production through consumption. Communities can support changing livestock practices to produce leaner meat; fortifying certain foodstuffs, such as bread; developing and making readily available new products lower in fat, saturated fat, cholesterol, sodium, and sugar; and positioning products in supermarkets and restaurants so that key information on caloric, cholesterol, fat, sodium, and sugar contents is readily apparent.

Legislative and regulatory measures. Again, national or state or provincial action is often required to obtain legislation or regulatory changes to maintain or improve the nutritional quality of the food supply; to require nutrition labeling on foods about which nutrition claims are made or to which nutrients are added; to include information on calories, fat, carbohydrate, protein, cholesterol, sugars, sodium, and other nutrients of public health concern; and to control fortification of foods when this control is of public health significance. One example of

such legislation is the Nutrition Labeling and Education Act of 1990. It calls for activities that educate consumers about the availability of nutrition information on the food label and the importance of using that information to maintain healthful dietary practices. For their part, communities can control food vending practices in schools to reduce or eliminate highly cariogenic foods and snacks; adjust school lunch standards to give greater emphasis to low-fat products; and regulate local televised advertisements directed at young children that promote cariogenic and nonnutritious foods and snacks.

Economic measures. Possible economic incentives or sanctions include adjusting insurance premiums for corporations offering employee health promotion programs with a nutrition component; assessing feasibility and cost benefits of reimbursement by third-party payers of nutrition counseling services that meet appropriate standards; and decreasing local sales taxes on staple foods.

Appraisal of the measures. Service programs are likely to be effective in improving the nutritional status of pregnant women and children and in reducing the incidence of low-birthweight infants. Certain segments of the public in the United States have responded to educational messages about fats and cholesterol by reducing intake. On the other

Dietary Guidelines for Americans

1. Eat a variety of foods
2. Maintain healthy weight
3. Choose a diet low in fat, saturated fat, and cholesterol
4. Choose a diet with plenty of vegetables, fruits, and grain products
5. Use sugars only in moderation
6. Use salt and sodium in moderation
7. If you drink alcoholic beverages, do so in moderation

Canada's Guidelines for Healthy Eating
• Enjoy a variety of foods.
• Emphasize cereals, breads, other grain products, vegetables, and fruit.
• Choose lower-fat dairy products, leaner meats and foods prepared with little or no fat.
• Achieve and maintain a healthy body weight by enjoying regular physical activity and healthy eating.
• Limit salt, alcohol, and caffeine intake.

hand, some government messages have been mixed and contradictory, leaving the public confused. Technological measures hold real promise, particularly if governmental policies could be generated in support of such measures and if resultant products are acceptable to consumers. With the exception of food sanitation and labeling, regulation and economic incentives have not been employed and are therefore of uncertain potential.

World Hunger and Nutrition

Although the developed countries are preoccupied with the problems of obesity and nutritional content, Third World countries and some populations within developed countries have a more compelling problem of malnutrition and hunger. Developed nations have a special capability and special responsibility to lead the campaign against world hunger. The United States is by far the most powerful member of the world's increasingly interdependent food system. It harvests more than half the grain that crosses international borders, and its grain reserves are the world's largest. Because of its agricultural productivity, its advanced food technology, and its market power, the United States automatically exerts a major influence, intended or not, on all aspects of the international food system. These resources and those of the other developed nations must be deployed to address nutrition and health on a global scale.

The epidemiology of world hunger today. The major world hunger problem today is not periodic famine, but chronic undernutrition, which results when people consume fewer calories and less protein than their bodies require to lead active, healthy lives. Although chronic or repeated shortages of calories may appear less newsworthy than outright starvation, they steadily take a greater toll in human lives. For example, the much-publicized Ethiopian famine in the mid-1980s and the Somalian famine in the early 1990s are only the tip of a pyramid of some 40,000 deaths monthly from undernutrition in 27 African nations. More than three quarters of the world's inadequately nourished people live on the Indian subcontinent, in Southeast Asia, and in sub-Saharan Africa. Many also live in parts of Latin America and the Middle East. Pockets of the poorly nourished persist in the United States and other rich countries as well.

In the United States hunger is particularly common among migrant and seasonal farmworkers, Native Americans, the elderly, and the 32 million Americans with incomes below the poverty level. In the 1970s the number below the poverty line never exceeded 28 million. Federal programs to alleviate hunger were greatly expanded during the 1960s, and there is evidence that the nutrition of the American poor participating in the programs improved. Today, subtler forms of hunger and the malnutrition inevitably associated with poverty persist, exacerbated by economic trends increasing the gap between the haves and the have-nots. Cuts in the federal budget during the 1980s for poverty programs in general and food programs in particular have strained the resources of church and other private or voluntary relief programs.

Children under the age of 5 make up over half of the world's malnourished population. A survey by the Food Research and Action center found that 5.5 million children in the United States under age 12 are hungry. Significantly more women are affected by malnutrition than men. Despite its magnitude, moral aspects, and high social and economic costs, world hunger seldom captures widespread public attention except in times of catastrophe. World hunger is at least as much a political, economic, educational, and social challenge as it is a scientific, technical, or logistical one.

Public education. A broad-base plan of action to eliminate world hunger calls for a major reordering of global and national priorities. For such a marked shift in established policies and practices to occur, public support must be mobilized. The public is only dimly aware of what Western as well as Third World nations could gain if people in all nations could afford to feed themselves. A successful effort to end hunger will require long-term economic and political support, and this support can exist only if the Australian, North American, and European publics understand the realities of world hunger. Rock concerts such as "We are the World" and local food drives have helped increase public awareness and arouse public concern.

The issue of ending world hunger comes down to a question of political choice—a factor that is no more predictable than the weather, but far more subject to human control. The quantities of food and money needed to eliminate hunger are very small in relation to available global resources. Political will is the missing ingredient; it is required in abundance

at community and national levels to channel the necessary food resources to those in need.

Nutrition is the foundation on which other aspects of health and life-style develop. Without attending first to issues of hunger, community health programs may gain the attention of the affluent at the expense of the poor and disadvantaged populations who have the most to gain from health promotion.

DRUG MISUSE

Drugs have been used throughout the ages for various medicinal, recreational, and religious purposes. At the end of the nineteenth century, drug abuse was largely concentrated in opium dens (Figure 12-14). As recently as the close of World War II, the term *problem drugs* generally meant only morphine or its derivative, heroin. This limited concept of problem drugs has expanded to the point where opium and morphine use now are the lesser drug problems. As more and more people become dependent on drugs, there has arisen an alarming misuse of stimulants, depressants, hallucinogens, and narcotics, cutting across all social strata.

Epidemiology of Drug Misuse

Although the use of drugs has declined in some populations, it remains a persistent and increasing problem in others. In the nation's inner cities, the problem seems to be worsening and is related to violent crimes and injuries. There is evidence that youth are trying drugs at later ages, but drug-related deaths increased from 3.8 per 100,000 in 1987 to 4.1 in 1989. Although there are recent declines in their use, an estimated 66 million Americans have tried marijuana at least once, and 22 million have tried cocaine. Highly addictive crack cocaine use is increasing, especially in some urban centers, and has led to an increase in the birth of crack-addicted babies.

Service and Protection Objectives for Nutrition

- By 2000 achieve labeling for virtually all processed foods and at least 40% of fresh meats, poultry, fish, fruits, vegetables, baked goods, and ready-to-eat foods. Baseline: 60% of sales of processed food in 1988.
- By 2000 increase to at least 90% the proportion of restaurants and institutional food service operations that offer identifiable low-fat, low-calorie food choices, consistent with the Dietary Guidelines for Americans.

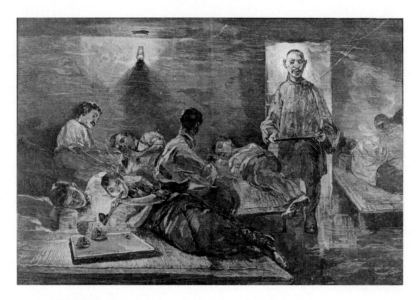

FIGURE 12-14
American opium smokers in a New York City opium den in the early 1900s.
Source: Photo of drawing by J.W. Alexander, courtesy National Library of Medicine.

The abuse of illicit drugs drained the U.S. economy of $76 billion in 1991, double the figure for 1985, according to one study. The figure included $49 billion in lost resources and $27 billion in drug control, prevention, and treatment. In 1990 70% of the U.S. drug control budget went to law enforcement.

Adverse Drug Reactions

In addition to purposeful misuse, the uninformed or misguided mixing of prescription drugs, over-the-counter drugs, alcohol, and certain foods leads to adverse reactions, including hormonal imbalances, digestive disturbances, mood alterations, and other problems that interfere with normal functioning, productivity, and safety. To say that we are a ''pill-happy'' society is not an exaggeration, and reliance on pills is the genesis of much drug misuse and abuse.

The elderly. The elderly, who make up 10% of the U.S. population, spend an estimated 20% of the national total for drugs. The per capita expenditure by the elderly for prescribed drugs exceeds that for other age groups. The average elderly person spent over $500 in 1990 for prescription and over-the-counter drugs and average more than 13 prescriptions (including renewals) a year.

It is now well recognized that older patients are more likely than younger patients to have adverse drug reactions. In a study of 700 hospitalized patients at the Johns Hopkins Hospital, 25% of those over age 80 had adverse drug reactions, compared with 12% in the 41- to 50-year-old age group. Similar data have been obtained in England.

In the United States hearings in the House Select Committee on Aging revealed that patients in nursing homes take an average of 7 to 10 different drugs a day, drugs often administered by unlicensed, untrained personnel. As a result, there have been reports of adverse reactions and serious side effects.

Drug information. There is no readily accessible, single source of information on drugs, their uses, and their monitoring. The most frequently used source is the labeling on each drug approved by the Food and Drug Administration.

Drug misuse is a complex social and health problem. Its solution must come through education and social change, not punishment. Sometimes there is a place for a "crash" program of education, but the problems of drug misuse call for a long-term, continuing program of education and related organizational, economic, and environmental change.

Addiction and Habituation

Drug **addiction** is a state in which an altered state of the body tissue produces a physical dependence that becomes known only after discontinuation of the drug; this dependence is masked while the drug is being taken. The World Health Organization's criteria for addiction are (1) a compulsion to use and to obtain a substance by any means; (2) a need to increase the dosage to obtain the desired effects; (3) a physiological as well as a psychological dependence on the effects of the substance; and (4) a detrimental effect not only on the individual but also on the community.

Levels of use. The U.S. National Commission on Marijuana and Drug Abuse has divided the entire spectrum of drug-using behavior into the following five patterns:

1. *Experimental.* The most common type of drug-using behavior—a short, nonpatterned trial of one or more drugs, motivated primarily by the individual's curiosity or desire to experience an altered mood state.
2. *Recreational.* Voluntary or patterned use of a drug, usually in social settings; behavior is not sustained because the user is not dependent on the drug.
3. *Circumstantial.* Behavior generally motivated by the user's perceived need or desire to achieve a new and anticipated effect to cope with a specific problem or situation (for example, amphetamine use by students preparing for examinations or long-distance truckers).
4. *Intensified drug-using behavior.* Drug use that occurs daily and is motivated by an individual's problem or stressful situation or a desire to maintain a certain self-prescribed level of performance (for example, housewives regularly using barbiturates or other sedatives, business executives regularly using tranquilizers, youth turning to drugs as sources of excitement or meaning); the salient feature of this group is that the individual still remains integrated within the larger social and economic structure.
5. *Compulsive use.* Patterned behavior at a high frequency and high level of interest, characterized by a high degree of psychological dependence and perhaps physical dependence as well. This category encompasses the smallest number of drug users. The distinguishing feature of this behavior is that drug use dominates the individual's existence, and preoccupation with drug taking precludes other social functioning (such users include chronic alcoholics and heroin-dependent persons).

Habituation means the customary use of some substance or practice that a person finds pleasurable, either as relaxation or activation. Habituation to a drug differs from addiction in that the drug has not produced a physical or psychological dependence; the individual can terminate the use of the drug without discernible side effects. For example, habituation to coffee, tea, and cola drinks is widespread, but little evidence exists that addiction occurs.

Epidemiological Approach to Drug Misuse

If drug misuse, as other life-style issues, is seen as a practice that is transmitted from one person to another, it may be considered for operational purposes as a contagious illness. This approach makes it possible to continue to apply the methods and terminology used in the epidemiology of infectious disease. (See Chapters 3 and 11.)

In epidemiological terms, the infectious *agent* is the drug, the host and reservoir are both the human, the environment is the community, and the vector is the drug-using peer. The conventional notion of the ''pusher'' as the vector is effectively dispelled by a careful review of studies in which an effort was made to trace the spread of drug use from person to person. These studies establish that, in the vast majority of instances, the addict or abuser is introduced to the use of the drug by a well-meaning friend, usually in the environment of previously established peer group activity. Beginners must learn snorting or intravenous injection techniques from other addicts or users.

Drug misuse presents all the well-known characteristics of epidemics, including rapid spread, clear geographical bounds, and certain age groups and strata of the population being more affected than others.

THE COMMUNITY HEALTH PROMOTION MODEL APPLIED TO DRUG ABUSE

Misuse and abuse of drugs, like smoking, alcohol abuse, obesity, and stress management, are intertwined social and health problems. Any program to deal with such complex problems must address the social, environmental, economic, psychological, cultural, and psysiological factors encompassed by the life-style in question. Communities and health officials alike recognize the importance of the drug misuse problem, yet only sporadic attempts have been made by communities to deal with it.

Health education traditionally has been called on to alert the public to complex community health problems, but health education by itself can hardly be expected to solve such problems. The life-styles in question are too embedded in organizational, socioeconomic, and environmental circumstances for people to be able to change their own behavior without concomitant changes in these circumstances. **Health promotion** combines health education with organizational, economic, and environmental supports for behavior and conditions of living conducive to health.

As this chapter concludes Part Three of this book, the models and concepts introduced in Part One can be reviewed as they apply to community health promotion and more specifically to the difficult problems of life-style exemplified by drug misuse and drug misuse prevention. In Chapter 4 a model of health *education* was introduced and applied to problems of maternal and child health. That model will now be expanded to include the additional elements of economic, organizational, and environmental supports for behavior that is conducive to health and applied as a model of health *promotion* for drug misuse prevention. The PROCEED model has been applied to health promotion programs at international, national and local levels.

Drug Misuse Prevention

Health professionals sometimes employ a taxonomy of three levels of prevention: primary, secondary, and tertiary.* Primary prevention is accomplished by activities that promote optimum health and provide specific protection against the onset or incidence of a health problem (for example, proper nutrition, genetic counseling, fluoridation, disease inoculation). In drug misuse prevention, the goal of primary prevention activities is to decrease the rate

*The authors acknowledge the assistance of Dr. Donald Iverson in developing this section.

at which new cases of drug misuse appear in a population by counteracting circumstances conducive to the development of drug misuse before they have a chance to produce drug misuse behavior.

Secondary prevention refers to activities concerned with the early diagnosis and prompt treatment of health problems (for example, the Papanicolaou [Pap] smear, regular physical examination, referral programs for troubled employees, neonatal metabolic screening). The goal of secondary drug misuse prevention activities is to reduce the disability rate caused by drug misuse by early treatment of such cases in the community.

Tertiary prevention refers to minimizing the disability from existing illness through treatment and rehabilitation efforts (for example, treatment for persons with lung cancer, alcoholism rehabilitation, treatment of sexually transmitted diseases). The goal of tertiary drug misuse prevention efforts is to reduce the complications and social pathology in the affected population by reducing or eliminating the addiction to drugs. Whereas primary prevention may reduce the *incidence* of drug misuse, secondary and tertiary prevention can reduce its *prevalence*.

Prevention strategies. Three types of strategies can be used in each of the three prevention levels to accomplish health promotion goals:

- *Educational strategies*—inform and educate the public about issues of concern, such as the dangers of drug misuse, the benefits of automobile restraints, or the relationship of maternal alcohol consumption to fetal alcohol syndrome.
- *Automatic-protective strategies*—directed at controlling environmental variables, such as public health measures providing for milk pasteurization, fluoridation, infant immunizations, and burning or chemical killing of marijuana crops
- *Coercive strategies*—employ legal and other formal sanctions to control individual behavior, such as required immunizations for school

entry, mandatory tuberculosis testing of hospital employees, compulsory use of automobile restraints, and arrests for drug possession or use

Table 12-2 gives examples of community health programs and measures classified by level of prevention and category of prevention strategy. The examples illustrate traditional public health strategies and new strategies in community health promotion and drug misuse prevention.

Prevention programs in public health can also be classified by the site where the program occurs. Although the community has been the primary site for most prevention programs, increasingly such programs can be found in the work, school, and medical care settings. **Employee assistance programs** to detect and refer alcohol and drug misuse problems among workers have become fixtures of most large companies.

Health education methods and theories. Regardless of the setting in which the community health promotion program occurs, there are three basic types of educational strategies:

- Direct communications with the target population to *predispose* behavior conducive to health. These include lecture-discussion, individual counseling or instruction, mass media campaigns, audiovisual aids, educational television, and programmed learning.
- Training methods to *enable* or *reinforce* behavior conducive to health. These include skills development, simulations and games, inquiry learning, small group discussion, modeling, and behavior modification.
- Organizational methods to *support* behavior conducive to health. These include community development, social action, social planning, and economic and organizational development. Such methods usually go beyond health education in supporting behavior.

One of the most noticeable changes in prevention and health promotion programs in community

TABLE 12-2
Examples of interventional strategies for each level of prevention of health problems, including those associated with drug misuse

Type of Strategy	Levels of prevention		
	Primary	*Secondary*	*Tertiary*
Educational	Genetic counseling School health education Public education about drugs	Community hypertension screening education programs Teacher training in recognition of drug problems	Drug education programs for patients in coronary care
Automatic-protective	Fluoridation of community drinking water systems Legal control of prescription drugs	Neonatal metabolic screening Requiring medical prescription for drug refills	Referral to community mental health center for counseling following discharge from drug treatment center
Coercive	Immunization requirements for schoolchildren Arrests of drug traffickers	Mandatory classes for persons convicted of drinking while intoxicated or using illicit drugs	Mandatory treatment for persons having an addiction or a sexually transmitted disease

health in recent years has been the increasing integration of behavioral theory into health education and other phases of program development. Insofar as health behavior is only partially understood (the level of understanding varies with the complexity of the health behavior), multiple theories have been used in planning for prevention programs. The most successful programs consult relevant theory in their planning to clarify the assumptions about the causes of behavior on the basis of which strategies are selected or developed.

Historical differences. The prevention approach of public health has differed from that frequently found in past drug misuse prevention efforts, but the two fields are converging. Drug misuse programs have differed from traditional public health programs in their educational and behavioral theories and models. The bases of earlier drug misuse programs were drawn primarily from personality, cognitive, and sociological theories. However, taking its cue from the

public health field, the drug misuse field is increasingly incorporating principles from developmental and social learning theories.

Another important distinction between the theoretical orientation and underpinning of program development efforts in the two fields is the level of understanding of the target behaviors. Many of the target behaviors of traditional public health programs are relatively simple and easily understood (for example, immunization and proper infant feeding), whereas drug misuse behavior is far more complex.

A third distinction has been in recognizing the role of ethnicity and racial background in influencing health behavior. Public health professionals have always been cognizant of the ethnic and racial influences in health behaviors, such as public use of health practitioners, and have designed prevention programs to account for these influences. People in the drug misuse field have taken increasing notice of ethnicity and racial background as powerful influences on the causes of drug misuse, so major as to alter the nature of the problem and subsequently the prevention techniques that may be effective. For example, the information on drug misuse among black populations has indicated that prevention efforts must focus on social and environmental factors rather than on individual factors, as they often do with white populations.

The drug abuse field and the more traditional public health field are increasingly using similar approaches, as both address social problems involving life-style. Strategies for intervention differ; but there are some common elements. They include prevention through education that starts early and extends throughout life; altering the social climate of acceptability; reducing individual and social stress factors; and legal enforcement. The National Institute on Drug Abuse now refers to four modalities of prevention: information, education, alternatives, and intervention. Similar to the public health approach, drug misuse prevention programs are targeted at populations (demographically defined groups, families, peer groups) and settings (community, school, workplace) and usually employ multiple educational methods.

National strategies. Lengthy and detailed examinations of the public health problems facing the United States, Great Britain, Canada, and Australia were initiated by their respective legislatures and national administrations in the 1970s. A framework similar to the Canadian health field concept described in Chapter 2 was useful in devising strategy in both the United States and Canada to affect public health problems. The framework included three points of intervention:

1. *Human life-style*—recognizing that the choices an individual makes about personal life-style behaviors can increase risk of health problems
2. *Human environment*—recognizing that environmental settings and other external sources of hazards can increase health problems

3. *Human services*—recognizing that preventive services can influence the incidence and effects of preventable diseases and conditions

It is the thesis of both the Canadian and the American initiatives in disease prevention and health promotion that programs or interventions in all three areas—life-style, environment, and services—are required to combat the leading causes of death and disability. A drug misuse prevention program would include program components, as shown in Table 12-3, intended to affect individual behavior (life-style), to provide medical treatment of drug misuse and drug dependence as early as possible to prevent permanent damage (human services), and to modify the environmental factors influencing the misuse of drugs (economics and the social environment). The balance of these areas in a community drug misuse

TABLE 12-3

Priorities for drug misuse prevention activities within the three spheres of the health field concept

Framework areas from the health field concept	*Activities—goals*
Life-style	Inclusion of drug misuse prevention as a major component of a comprehensive school health education program
	Public and physician education programs to reduce the number of sleeping pill prescriptions, emphasizing problems of cross-addiction
Services	Education of health care providers on the taking of a drug history for adolescents and preadolescents
	Promotion of involvement of national and local youth-serving agencies in drug misuse prevention
	Strengthened drug misuse prevention research
Environment	Encouragement of parent groups to provide supportive networks to help youths resist drug misuse
	Improved enforcement of legal and economic regulations of drug market

prevention program has seldom, if ever, been attained.

Objectives. The U.S. initiative in disease prevention and health promotion developed a consensus on specific measurable objectives for each of the 15 high-priority problems related to the goals identified in *Healthy People.* A national panel of experts was convened for each of the 15 priorities to formulate measurable objectives.

The U.S. expert panel on drug misuse prevention reviewed information on the status and trends of drug use, the health implications of drug use, and the potential drug-related prevention-promotion measures available, including the strength and feasibility of each measure. The panel then identified two major objectives and 11 measurable objectives to be achieved by 1990. These objectives were circulated to more than 3000 organizations and additional experts for comment and review. This process resulted in the closest that one can expect to come to consensus on U.S. national goals to be achieved in 10 years. The objectives for drug misuse were published in the final document of *Promoting Health, Preventing Disease: Objectives for the Nation* in 1980. The objectives for the year 2000, published in 1990, followed a similar development process.

Planning Framework Applied to Drug Misuse

Drug misuse prevention efforts have too often been based on fear-arousal strategies. Although such strategies have valid uses, their applicability to community health programs is limited. To maximize the effectiveness of a community drug misuse prevention program, concurrent efforts should be initiated in the three health field categories described in *A New Perspective on the Health of Canadians* and in *Healthy People:* human life-style, human environment, and human services. In all three, attention must be given to factors that predispose, enable, and reinforce behavior conducive to health.

Prevention programs, whether they be directed at drug misuse, communicable disease, teenage pregnancy, or some other health problem, have as a base health education activities. Health education is defined in Chapter 4 as any combination of learning opportunities designed to facilitate voluntary adaptations of behavior conducive to health. Well-planned drug education programs have been shown to be effective for some people, but they have not demonstrated an ability to resolve a community drug misuse problem. Perhaps no single effort will be able to resolve such problems totally. But drug misuse prevention programs incorporating the integrated health promotion approach of educational, organizational, and economic supports for life-style conducive to health have a much greater chance of success than programs directed at only one of these categories.

Health education versus health promotion. Health promotion has been defined as any combination of educational, organizational, environmental, and economic supports for behavior and conditions of living conducive to health. With health education as an integral part of all health promotion interventions it follows that the interventions should be directed toward voluntary behavior at all levels—individuals, organizations, and communities. At the community, state or provincial, or national level, additional interventions may be legal, regulatory, political, or economic, and therefore potentially coercive. Nevertheless, such interventions to be successful must be supported by an informed and consenting public. Such informed consent requires health education. Ideally, the coercive measures are directed at the behavior of those whose actions may affect the health of others, such as the manufacturers, distributors, and advertisers of hazardous products. Even then, public health education is required to ensure the support of an informed public because taxes, prices, availability of services and products, and jobs may be affected by such regulations of health- or drug-related industries and sources.

For example, one part of a health promotion program for drug misuse prevention could target organizational change. Health education could be combined with various incentives (such as free program consultation services) and persuasion techniques (such as program promotion by local public leaders) in an attempt to increase the number of schools offering peer counseling programs for those who misuse drugs. If the program also targeted political change, community organization techniques could be combined with health education activities to develop "concerned parent groups" in neighborhoods and to apply political pressure on local school, law enforcement, and government officials to support drug misuse prevention efforts. If the program directed other efforts toward economic change, health professionals and others could work with representatives of insurance carriers to initiate health insurance reimbursements for counseling and rehabilitation services. The point is simple: when health education activities are combined with appropriate changes in organizations, political systems, and environmental and economic supports for behavior, the end result is more likely to be favorable than is the result achieved by a series of single, uncoordinated changes. Indeed, uncoordinated changes sometimes make things worse by throwing a community system out of balance and forcing an overreaction or overcompensation by the wrong elements in the community.

The relationships of health education and health promotion activities to the three prevention targets and the relationships of these targets to the health or drug misuse objectives set for the community and the nation are depicted in Figure 12-15. The three prevention targets are not isolated. Life-style is continually affected by the human environment and the organization of services (as seen in Chapter 4). Furthermore, a successful program must effectively integrate and coordinate activities in relation to each of these targets. To facilitate the integration of activities within and between the prevention strategies, a planning framework is needed. The planning framework proposed in Chapter 4 forces an encompassing and systematic analysis of public health problems in the context of social problems or quality-of-life concerns.

Phases in Planning

When using the framework in Figure 12-15 to plan community drug prevention programs, one starts with the final consequences—namely, social problems usually defined as community drug-related problems but not necessarily as health concerns. One works back from there to the original causes—that is, the causes of the behavior, which influenced the health problem or community drug-related social problem. The following is an application of the phases, corresponding to those in Chapter 4, in this process to prevention of drug misuse.

Phase 1: social diagnosis. The first phase involves a consideration of the quality of life in a community by assessing the social problems of concern to the various segments of the population. This has the effect of forcing planners to consider the desirable social outcomes of a program before setting priorities on health or selecting program approaches. It also helps justify a program to the community. This is especially important in the planning of community drug prevention programs because of the relationship between drug-related health problems and the social problems of a community. For example, when a community has a large number of drug-dependent persons, it is likely that there will be high rates of violent and nonviolent crime, school truancy, early dropouts from school, juvenile delinquency, and unemployment (all social problems). Conversely, when a community is experiencing such social problems as high unemployment, inadequate housing, inadequate private and public school programs, or discrimination, a serious drug dependence problem will be present, because the use of drugs for some will be a method of coping with the social problems. By identifying the major social problems of concern

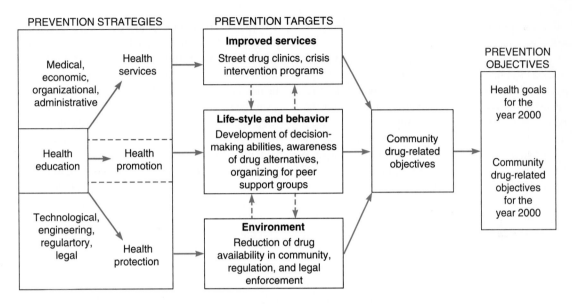

PREVENTION STRATEGIES   PREVENTION TARGETS

FIGURE 12-15
The structure of the objectives for the nation in health promotion are seen here as applied to drug abuse prevention. The relationship of community health education and health promotion also is shown as part of the prevention strategies box to the left. Health promotion, however, can serve community development needs other than the prevention of specific diseases or life-style problems.

to the community, one can select potential outcome evaluation measures and gain an understanding of the community's concerns as they relate to the particular health problem that is the target of the prevention program.

A community's social problems can be diagnosed from analyses of existing records, files, publications, and informal interviews and discussions with leaders, key informants, and representatives of various community populations. This is an important first step that should not be undertaken too hastily, because its outcome may well affect program scope and quality as well as the extent of community support.

Phase 2: epidemiological diagnosis. The objective of the epidemiological diagnostic phase is to identify the specific health problems that appear to be contributing to the social problems noted in phase

1. By using data from community surveys, hospital admissions, city and county health departments, health systems agencies, and selected state or provincial and national data, the drug-related morbidity, mortality, and disability trends can be identified. The incidence, prevalence, distribution, intensity, and duration of each identified health problem should be described (see Chapter 3). These data can be analyzed to determine the populations most affected by the health problem. This process will often reveal and locate a variety of existing health problems such as drug dependence, drug-related psychoses, drug-related depression or anxiety, injuries, and other drug-related problems such as AIDS, serum hepatitis, and endocarditis. The use of spatial maps to depict the distribution of the identified health problems within the city or county is an effective way of presenting data if there is reason to believe that the problems vary by geographical location.

By use of the results of epidemiological analyses, program objectives should be developed. The objectives should be stated in epidemiological terms and answer the following: Who will be the recipients of the program? What benefit should they receive? How much of that benefit should they receive? By when or for how long? For example, it has been estimated that in a 6-month period, approximately 1000 persons die of drug overdose in New York City. Therefore, a program objective for a drug prevention program in New York City could be stated as follows: ''To reduce the number of drug overdose deaths in New York City by 25% within 1 year and an additional 25% within the next year, until the national average is reached.'' The major drug-related health problem for most communities would not be death or drug overdose; rather, it would be physiological or psychological dependence.

Phase 3: behavioral and environmental diagnosis. The behavioral diagnosis phase requires the systematic identification of health behaviors that appear to be causally linked to each of the health problems identified in the epidemiological diagnosis. The outcome of the behavioral diagnosis is the generation of a ranked list of specific behaviors to be used as the basis for specifying the behavioral objectives of the program.

The process of identifying the health behaviors linked to the health problems usually relies on the professional literature. The review of the literature can be combined with structured and unstructured interviews of persons familiar with the health problem (such as drug treatment personnel), data from observations, and intuition based on personal experiences. In the case of drug dependence, the behavioral *causes* leading to the health problem are drug use and drug misuse. These should be perceived not as distinct behaviors but, rather, as a continuum of drug use to drug misuse with varying types and amounts of drugs used. Distinct behaviors

within the continuum could be specified, such as misuse of prescription medications, use of illicit drugs such as marijuana and cocaine, and use of illicit drugs in a manner that predisposes the user to health problems. To take another example, if the identified health problem was cardiovascular disease, the behavioral problems would include smoking, high intake of saturated fats, heavy alcohol consumption, and a sedentary life-style.

A second part of this phase is the identification of environmental factors that contribute to the health problem. These are the organizational and environmental conditions that influence the health problem and the behavior but that are not controlled directly by the behavior of the target population. Nonbehavioral causes of drug dependence include such factors as the housing situation in the community, the school environment, and the law enforcement activity in the community. Identification of these factors is important, because it provides the planners with direction for health promotion activity other than educational measures, such as organizational and economic interventions directed at the regulation of the environment and the availability of services.

Phase 4: educational diagnosis. The educational diagnosis phase assesses the relative influence of various predisposing, enabling, and reinforcing factors on each of the identified behavioral causes of the health problem. Figure 12-16 focuses attention on the order of causation of behavior, as indicated by the numbered arrows: (1) an initial motivation to act, (2) a deployment of resources and skills to enable the action, (3) a reaction to the behavior from someone else (or in the case of drug use, the drug effects themselves), (4) the reinforcement and strengthening or the punishment and discouragement of the behavior, (5) the reinforcement or punishment of the behavior as it affects the predisposing factors by strengthening or extinguishing the motivation to act, and finally, (6) the increased ability

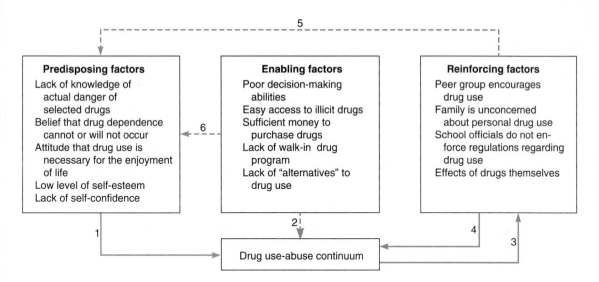

FIGURE 12-16

The three categories of factors influencing life-style are shown here as related to drug use and abuse. The numbered arrows indicate the approximate order of expected cause and effect.

to take certain actions, which tends to increase the predisposition or motivation to take such actions.

In the process of identifying and listing factors in the three areas, one may include factors that seem to encourage the behavior as well as those that seem to discourage the behavior. Consider the data in Figure 12-17 and their implications for the relative importance of predisposing factors (perceived risk) and enabling factors (perceived availability) for cocaine use.

After completing the list, the next step is to select from among the predisposing, enabling, and reinforcing factors those that will be most likely to bring about the behavior desired. The factors that should be selected as targets for the program are those that are most changeable and most important. Importance is determined by answers to the following questions:

- How widespread or frequent is the factor?

(For example, low self-esteem, use of drugs by peer group members, easy availability of drugs.)
- How compelling or urgent is the factor? (For example, alternatives to drugs, fear of effects of drugs.)
- How close is the connection between the factor and the behavior? (For example, lack of decision-making skills and drug use, availability of drugs and drug use.)

Changeability is assessed from data or professional judgments addressing the following questions:

- Does the literature suggest that the factor can be changed? (For example, can self-esteem levels be changed? Can decision-making skills be taught? Can school officials be encouraged to enforce regulations?)
- Does the experience of previous programs indicate that the factor can be changed? (For ex-

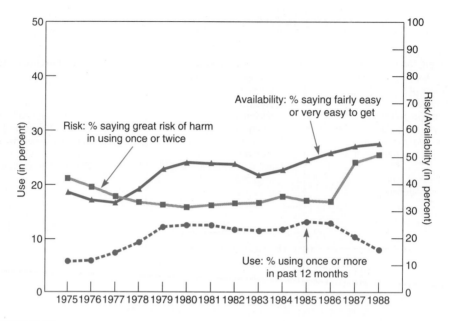

FIGURE 12-17

Trends in high school seniors' perceptions of cocaine availability and risk associated with the use of cocaine, and their actual (self-reported) use in the past year, United States.

Source: National Institute on Drug Abuse. Data from O'Malley in Gerstein DR, Green LW, editors: *Preventing drug abuse: what do we know?* Washington, DC, 1993, National Academy Press.

ample, have programs been successful in changing parental attitudes and behaviors? Have community organization efforts been successful in stimulating development of drug alternatives programs?)

The factors determined to be both important and changeable form the basis of the prevention program. This level of specificity helps to use scarce resources in the most appropriate manner as well as to increase the chances of the program being successful. Difficult choices will be made in this phase of the planning process, but in the decision-making process the level of understanding of the nature of the problem usually increases.

Phase 5: program development. The program development phase selects the right combination of strategies to affect the selected predisposing, en-

abling, and reinforcing factors. As a general rule, selected communication methods are effective in altering predisposing factors (Figure 12-18); organizing resources and training are effective in altering enabling factors; and strategies such as consultation, training, feedback, and group development are effective in altering reinforcing factors. Refer to Table 12-2 for an example of considerations in selecting appropriate educational and other strategies according to the level of prevention.

Phase 6: administrative diagnosis. The administrative diagnosis phase assesses resources available and organizational problems likely to be encountered as the program becomes operational. Factors such as interagency cooperation, staffing patterns, and budgeting should be thoroughly discussed. This phase of planning analyzes the potential problems

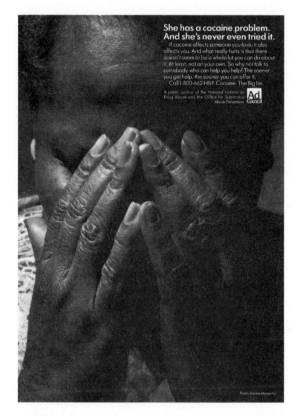

She has a cocaine problem. And she's never even tried it.
If cocaine affects someone you love, it also affects you. And what really hurts is that there doesn't seem to be a whole lot you can do about it. At least, not on your own. So why not talk to somebody who can help you help? The sooner you get help, the sooner you can offer it.
Call 1-800-662-HELP. Cocaine. The Big Lie.
A public service of the National Institute on Drug Abuse and the Office for Substance Abuse Prevention.

FIGURE 12-18
Appealing to family solidarity and the desire of most youth to make their parents proud rather than disappointed is one strategy; getting help to parents is another.
Source: National Institute on Drug Abuse and the Advertising Council.

within programs, within organizations, and between organizations. A well-conceived program is seldom effective without an implementation plan.

SUMMARY

There is no simple solution to such health-related life-style problems as drug misuse, alcohol misuse, obesity, and smoking. Problems as complex as these may defy even well-planned preventive efforts. Nevertheless, the effects of well-planned and sys-

tematically implemented preventive efforts are more likely to be successful than the single-focused, uncoordinated efforts that have typified many of the early attempts to address life-style, particularly those at the local level.

The Canadian Ministry of Health and Welfare and the U.S. Public Health Service have proposed that their prevention efforts focus on three areas: life-style, environment, and services. Specific measurable objectives for the United States were set, which, if met by 2000, will have the effect of substantially reducing the scope and intensity of health problems attributable to life-style, the environment, and inadequate health services. These objectives can serve to concentrate the limited resources of communities where they can be most productive. To illustrate community health programs to work toward the objectives, a planning framework encompassing the three areas of life-style, environment, and services has been presented.

Efforts should be directed at individuals and environments, as well as at organizational, political,

---

Objectives for Reducing Use of Tobacco by the Year 2000

Objectives target reducing coronary heart disease deaths; slowing the rise in lung cancer deaths and deaths from chronic obstructive pulmonary disease; reducing cigarette smoking and the initiation of cigarette smoking by children and youth; increasing the proportion of cigarette smokers who stopped smoking and smoking cessation during pregnancy; reducing smokeless tobacco use and the proportion of children who are regularly exposed to tobacco smoke at home; establishing tobacco use prevention in schools; increasing nonsmoking policies in worksites and state plans to reduce tobacco use; enacting clean indoor air laws; enacting and enforcing laws prohibiting the sale of tobacco products to minors; eliminating or restricting tobacco advertising directed at minors; and increasing primary care and oral health providers who advise smoking cessation.

> ### Objectives for Improving Nutrition by the Year 2000
>
> Objectives target reducing coronary heart disease deaths, dietary fat intake, overweight prevalence, and growth retardation among low-income children; reversing the rise in cancer deaths; increasing complex carbohydrate and fiber-containing foods in adult diets and the proportion of overweight people who have adopted sound dietary practices combined with regular physical activity to attain an appropriate body weight; increasing calcium intake and breastfeeding; decreasing salt and sodium intake and iron deficiency; increasing the proportion of parents and caregivers who use feeding practices that prevent baby bottle tooth decay; achieving useful nutrition labeling and increasing the proportion of people who use food labels to make nutritious food selections; increasing the availability of low-fat products and of food service operations that offer low-fat, low-calorie food choices; increasing the proportion of schools that provide nutrition education and of school and child care food services with menus consistent with the *Dietary Guidelines for Americans;* increasing receipt of home food services by people in need of home-delivered meals and the proportion of worksites that offer nutrition education and/or weight management programs; and increasing the proportion of primary care providers who provide nutrition assessment, counseling, and/or referral to qualified nutritionists or dietitians.

and economic systems. Applying the latest findings from the rapidly developing research in designing and evaluating prevention programs and ensuring the necessary quality and quantity of resources for programs will not guarantee success but will increase the probability of reaching the objectives set for a community.

QUESTIONS FOR REVIEW

1. What do alcohol misuse, smoking, overeating, and drug misuse have in common?

2. Why is alcohol misuse so costly for the community, beyond the direct health effects on the individual?

3. What is the distinction between addiction and habituation?

4. Using the model for drug misuse prevention, how would you design a community program for prevention of alcohol misuse or smoking?

5. How can alcohol misuse, smoking, overeating, anorexia nervosa, bulimia, world hunger, and drug misuse be characterized as epidemics?

6. What should the school teach children about alcohol, smoking, drugs, and nutrition?

7. What does your community have to offer as alternatives to alcohol and drugs for recreation and coping?

8. What can be done in worksites to reduce the prevalence of smoking?

9. Why should women in reproductive ages be singled out as a priority for smoking and alcohol reduction?

10. How does health promotion go beyond health education?

11. When are coercive strategies justified in disease prevention and health promotion?

12. What has public health added to the traditional approach to drug misuse prevention?

13. What are some predisposing, enabling, and reinforcing factors in marijuana use?

READINGS

Bracht N, editor: *Health promotion at the community level,* Newbury Park, Calif, 1990, Sage.

This compilation of community health promotion perspectives features chapters by authors who have planned or evaluated programs in heart disease prevention, smoking reduction, cancer prevention, and other aspects of life-style change to identify the essential elements in successful community-based programs.

Gerstein DR, Green LW, editors: *Preventing drug abuse: what do we know?* Washington, DC, 1993, National Academy Press.

This report of the Committee on Drug Abuse Prevention Research of the National Research Council summarizes the studies assessing the causes of drug abuse and health promotion strategies to prevent drug abuse.

Green LW, Kreuter MW: *Health promotion planning: an educational and environmental approach,* Mountain View, Calif, 1991, Mayfield.

This book presents the PRECEDE-PROCEED model for planning, implementation, and evaluation of health promotion, with references to some 300 published applications of the model in various community settings, including schools, workplaces, medical care, and community-wide programs.

Kaiserman MJ, Rogers B: Forty-year trends in Canadian tobacco sales, *Can J Public Health* 83:404, 1992.

Even with high taxes relative to the United States, the price of tobacco products continues to be a bargain for smokers in Canada based on analyses of trends since 1950 in real tobacco price index, per capita disposable income, smoking prevalence, and sales of cigarettes.

Rodin J: Determinants of body fat localization and its implications for health, *Ann Behav Med* 14:275, 1992.

Abdominally localized fat increases risk for cardiovascular disease, diabetes, hypertension, and some cancers. This review examines genetics, the aging process, gender, and environmental/life-style variables influencing fat deposits to the intraabdominal depots. Life-style factors are given particular importance.

BIBLIOGRAPHY

Bulger R, Reiser S, editors: *The role of academic health centers in disease prevention and health promotion,* Washington, DC, 1993, Association of Academic Health Centers.

Carruthe S, James R: Evaluation of the Western Australian school development in health education project, *J Sch Health* 63:165, 1993.

Chapman S, Wong WL, Smith W: Self-exempting beliefs about smoking and health: differences between smokers and ex-smokers, *Am J Public Health* 83:215, 1993.

Chen M Jr, Zaharlick A, Kuun P et al: Implementation of the indigenous model for health education programming among Asian minorities: beyond theory and into practice, *J Health Educ* 23:400, 1992.

Contento IR, Basch C, Shea S et al: Relationship of mothers' food choice criteria to food intake of preschool children: identification of family subgroups, *Health Educ Q* 20:243, 1993.

Ellickson PL, Bell RM, Harrison ER: Changing adolescent propensities to use drugs: results from project ALERT, *Health Educ Q* 20:227, 1993.

Environmental Health Directorate, Health Protection Branch: *Smoking by-laws in Canada—1991,* H46-1-26-1991E, Ottawa, 1993, Health and Welfare Canada.

Frank E, Winkleby M, Fortmann SP et al: Cardiovascular disease risk factors: improvements in knowledge and behavior in the 1980s, *Am J Public Health* 83:590, 1993.

Glanz K, Rimer B, Lewis FM, editors: *Health education theory and research,* San Francisco, 1991, Jossey-Bass.

Goodman RM, McLeroy KR, Steckler AB et al: Development of level of institutionalization scales for health promotion programs, *Health Educ Q* 20:161, 1993.

Gottlieb NH, Lovato CY, Weinstein RP et al: The implementation of a restrictive worksite smoking policy in a large decentralized organization, *Health Educ Q* 19:77, 1992.

Green LW: Preface. In *Healthy people 2000: national health promotion and disease prevention objectives,* Boston, 1990, Jones and Bartlett.

Green LW: Health promotion research agenda revisited, *Am J Health Prom* 6:411, 1992.

Green LW, Kreuter MW: CDC's planned approach to community health as an application of PRECEDE and an inspiration for PROCEED, *J Health Educ* 23:140, 1992.

Health and Welfare Canada Scientific Review Committee: *Nutrition recommendations,* H49-42-1990E, Ottawa, 1990, Health and Welfare Canada.

Katcher BS: Benjamin Rush's educational campaign against hard drinking, *Am J Public Health* 83:273, 1993.

Klein BEK, Klein R, Linton KLP et al: Cigarette smoking and lens opacities: the Beaver Dam Eye Study, *Am J Prev Med* 9:27, 1993.

Kok GJ: Quality of planning as a decisive determinant of health education effectiveness, *Hygiene* 11:5, 1992.

Lank NH, Vickery CE, Cotugna N et al: Food commercials during television soap operas: what is the nutrition message? *J Community Health* 17:377, 1992.

Lewit EM, Botsko M, Shapiro S: Workplace smoking policies in New Jersey businesses, *Am J Public Health* 83:254, 1993.

Long KA: The concept of health—rural perspectives, *Nurs Clin North Am* 28:123, 1993.

Mackinnon DP, Pentz MA, Stacy AW: The alcohol warning label and adolescents: the first year, *Am J Public Health* 83:585, 1993.

Marin G: Defining culturally appropriate community interventions: Hispanics as a case study, *J Comm Psych* 21:149, 1993.

Nutbeam D, Smith C, Murphy S et al: Maintaining evaluation designs in long-term community-based health promotion programs: Heartbeat Wales case study, *J Epidemiol Community Health* 47:127, 1993.

O'Donnell M, editor: *Health promotion in the workplace,* ed 2, Albany, NY, 1993, Delmar.

Palank CL: Determinants of health promotive behavior: a review of current research, *Nurs Clin North Am* 26:815, 1991.

Pederson LL, Bull SB, Ashley MJ et al: Restrictions on smoking: changes in knowledge, attitudes and predicted behaviour in metropolitan Toronto from 1983 to 1988, *Can J Public Health* 83:408, 1993.

Perry CL, Williams CL, Forster JL et al: Background, conceptualization and design of a community-wide research program on adolescent alcohol use: Project Northland, *Health Educ Research* 8:81, 1993.

Pill R, Peters TJ, Robling MR: Factors associated with health behavior among mothers of lower socioeconomic status: a British example, *Soc Sci Med* 36:1137, 1993.

Price JH, Telljohann SK, Roberts SM et al: Effects of incentives in an inner city junior high school smoking prevention program, *J Health Educ* 23:388, 1992.

Reynolds DL, Chambers LW, DeVillaer MR: Measuring alcohol abuse in the community: consumption, binge-drinking, and alcohol-related consequences (''alcoholism''), *Can J Public Health* 83:441, 1992.

Rigotti NA, Stoto MA, Bierer MF et al: Retail stores' compliance with a city no-smoking law, *Am J Public Health* 83:227, 1993.

Robbins AS: Pharmacological approaches to smoking cessation, *Am J Prev Med* 9:31, 1993.

St Pierre TL, Kaltreider DL, Mark MM et al: Drug prevention in a community setting: a longitudinal study of the relative effectiveness of a three-year primary prevention program in boys and girls clubs across the nation, *Am J Community Psychol* 20:673, 1992.

Waldrop K: A framework for health promotion . . . a framework for AIDS, *Can J Public Health* 84:S9, 1993.

Wickizer TM, Von Korff M, Cheadle A et al: Activating communities for health promotion: a process evaluation method, *Am J Public Health* 83:561, 1993.

PART FOUR

. . . .

Environmental Health Protection

Ecology and *environment* are convenient terms for everyday discussion, but they are concepts mainly of theoretical value to the health scientist. They represent bodies of scientific knowledge. They suggest ways of organizing reality and ideas so as to keep sight of the whole while trying to analyze and solve problems that represent only parts of the whole. Effective community health practice requires the concentration of efforts and actions on specific parts of the environment. Health personnel deal with particular conditions in the environment. Even within categories of environmental conditions, such as water or air pollution, more specific problems must be identified before useful action can be taken. In Part Four, you will see how the environment makes up a complementary part of the larger health field concept, but you will also delve more deeply into the specific aspects of the environment that must be addressed in community health protection.

Chapter 13

Community Injury Control

❖

If a disease were killing our children in the proportions that injuries are, people would be outraged and demand that this killer be stopped.
—former SURGEON GENERAL C. EVERETT KOOP, M.D.

OBJECTIVES

When you finish this chapter, you should be able to:

- Describe the relative importance of injuries as causes of death in various age groups in a community

- Identify the major causes of injury subject to community intervention

- Propose appropriate combinations of educational, technological, legal, and environmental interventions to prevent injuries and violent deaths

- Propose realistic objectives for the reduction of injuries and violent deaths in a community

---

Injury prevention and control deserve the first chapter in the environmental health protection section of this book because injuries are the leading cause of death among environmentally induced and controllable causes of death. Most of the preventive measures for cardiovascular disease and cancer depend more heavily on behavioral or life-style changes such as smoking and diet. Injury prevention does have a large behavioral component, but great progress has been made through legislative and regulatory control of the environment, such as with improved automobiles and roads. Control of behavior, as with enforcement of seat-belt laws, has also had greater effect than attempts to persuade people to be more vigilant and cautious in protecting their own safety. As with other areas of health promotion covered in the previous section, injury prevention programs require a combination of environmental, social, and behavioral components. But the attention to the physical and regulatory environment has been greater in injury control and other issues in the chapters to follow.

Those concerned with safety in a community often specialize in one aspect, such as occupational, recreational, motor vehicle, school, or fire safety. These agencies make their most effective contribution when the community has a well-organized, well-integrated safety program. Such organization and integration depend on a clear understanding of the epidemiology of injuries and the science of preventing them.

EPIDEMIOLOGY OF INJURIES

Like health promotion and disease prevention, injuries and traumatic death are subject to definition, research, and intervention. They are not, as the term *accidents* implies, acts of providence or random events over which individuals or communities can exert no control.

Definition

In times past accidents were considered outside the purview of public health. The preferred term today is **injury control** rather than accident prevention. This semantic shift was needed for several reasons.

First, an **accident** is a sudden, unanticipated, unintentional occurrence that may or may not produce a human injury. Many accidents occur with no human involvement at all. Community health is concerned with the prevention of threats to the health of human populations, not primarily with property damage, liability, or other consequences of accidents that are essentially moral, legal, or economic. Thus, human *injury* is the health problem rather than *accidents* per se.

Second, some injuries and deaths are inflicted intentionally rather than accidentally, as in the case of homicide, rape, assault, battery, child abuse, and suicide. Community health is concerned with **intentional injury** as well as **unintentional injury.**

Some of the issues in intentional injury have been addressed in Chapters 5, 6, and 9.

Third, it is not always necessary to prevent accidents to prevent human injury. Some of the most effective community safety programs are those that limit the impact of accidents rather than prevent them, as in campaigns promoting the use of automobile seat restraints. Some accidents, such as hurricanes and earthquakes, remain unpreventable, but the resulting injuries can be minimized through planning, organization, public education, training, rescue operations, and preparation.

Finally, shifting the focus from accident prevention to injury control has worked to the advantage of public health education. It emphasizes ways in which people can exert control, either directly in their personal actions and environment or indirectly through legislative support for such measures as safe speed limits, enforcing use of child restraints in vehicles, handgun controls, and drunk-driving laws. It emphasizes training and organization, such as the first aid and disaster preparedness programs of the Red Cross, to enable families and communities to manage injuries. Yet it also encompasses injury prevention through such proven strategies as swimming instruction, lowering speed limits, child-proof containers, lowered thermostats on water heaters to prevent scalding, better construction of buildings and highways, lowering blood-alcohol limits permitted in drivers, modifying potentially dangerous products to incorporate safety features (as in fire-safe or self-extinguishing cigarettes, training wheels on bicycles, and shatterproof glass), and design of toys, tools, machinery guards, and sports equipment to prevent or minimize injuries.

Injury control indicates not only the prevention of injury but also the control of damage that might result from injury. This is accomplished through 911 telephone systems (Figure 13-1), **emergency medical services** (EMS), and rehabilitation programs.

A community health definition of **injury** then is an event in which tissue damage is caused, either unintentionally or intentionally, by a rapid transfer (less than minutes) of excessive amounts of energy.

LEARN TO USE THIS LIFE-SAVING DEVICE.
KNOW YOUR LOCAL EMERGENCY NUMBERS.

There's been a crash. Someone is hurt. Do you know how to call for help?

Keep emergency numbers by your phone for medical help, police and fire services. The right number gets help on the way *faster*.

For medical emergencies, contact

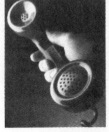

EMS, Emergency Medical Services. One call connects you to a whole emergency medical team—ambulance, paramedics, physicians and nurses—who are specially trained to help people who are hurt or sick.

Your phone can help save time, and lives, in an emergency. Know how to use it.

United States Fire Administration

the right EMS **call** *...when seconds count.*

National Highway Traffic Safety Administration

FIGURE 13-1
Injury control goes beyond injury prevention to include the community's capacity to limit the damage of injuries through rapid response with 911 telephone systems, disaster preparedness, first aid and CPR training to resuscitate injury victims, ambulance and helicopter transport systems, acute trauma care, and rehabilitation programs.
Source: United States Fire Administration and National Highway Traffic Safety Administration.

The energy may be one of five types: (1) kinetic or mechanical, (2) chemical, (3) thermal, (4) electrical, or (5) radiation. Injuries may result also from the absence of such essentials as heat or oxygen.

Relative Importance

The place of injury control strategies in relation to other health concerns in a community health program can be assessed by considering the mortality and morbidity statistics presented in previous chapters, as well as the various classes and causes of injuries.

Years of life lost. As seen in previous chapters, **fatal accidents** are the fourth leading cause of death for all ages combined. Suicides are the eighth lead-

ing cause of death. Both intentional and unintentional injuries are higher in the younger groups (Figure 13-2). Consequently, injuries gain in significance relative to other community health concerns when total years of potential life lost from each cause of death is calculated. Because they tend to occur at younger ages than deaths from chronic disease, unintentional injuries rank ahead of heart disease and cancer in years of potential life lost. Suicides and homicides rank fourth ahead of other leading conditions causing death. Alcohol is implicated in nearly half of these years of potential life lost.

Classification. Seven specific causes of injuries— falls, burns, poisonings, vehicle crashes, firearms, sports, and drownings—have been demonstrated to

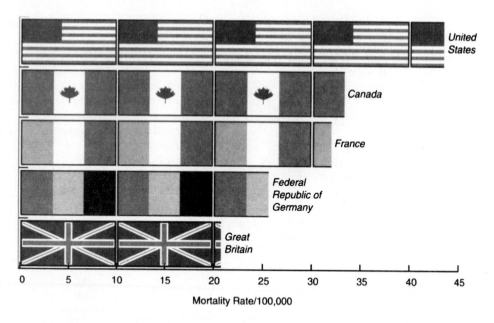

Mortality Rate/100,000

FIGURE 13-2

Injury mortality rates per 100,000 population, including violence, for ages 0 to 24 in five countries. About 75% of U.S. child injury mortality is caused by unintentional injury; the other 25% by violence, including homicide and suicide.

Source: World Health Organization: *World health statistics annual 1990*, Geneva, 1991, World Health Organization. Chart by Children's Safety Network: *A data book of child and adolescent injury*, Washington, DC, 1991, National Center for Education in Maternal and Child Health.

be preventable. Six settings—highway, home, farm, occupational, school, and recreational environments—are useful areas in which to concentrate preventive efforts.

Injuries and violent deaths in home, recreational, and farm environments, as well as those associated with motor vehicles, represent a public health problem of cardinal significance for which no strong national preventive focus exists in many countries. As with disease control problems, morbidity and mortality from injuries are amenable to reduction through epidemiological, environmental, and educational approaches. In addition, injuries can be reduced through changes in engineering and technology. A community approach to the prevention and control of unintentional injuries in residential and

recreational environments, on farms and at other worksites, on the highways, and in schools will focus on those groups at high risk, most particularly those exposed to behavior and environments that increase the risk of injury.

Components of a community injury control program should include a surveillance system, epidemiological investigations, standards setting, public education, environmental reforms, and professional training. The primary national role should be one of providing leadership, direction, technical and financial assistance, and information to support injury prevention actions undertaken by state or provincial and local health agencies. State or provincial health agencies can serve to coordinate the flow of resources and expertise. The local community role is

Objectives for Motor Vehicle Injury Control

- By 2000, reduce deaths caused by motor vehicle crashes to no more than 1.9 per 100 million vehicle-miles traveled; the motor vehicle death rate should be reduced to no greater than 16.8 per 100,000 population. (In 1989, when this objective was drafted, there were 2.4 deaths per 100 million vehicle-miles traveled, and the death rate was about 19 per 100,000 population.)
- By 2000 deaths from motor vehicle injuries involving drivers with blood alcohol levels of 0.01% or more should be reduced to fewer than 8.5 per 100,000 population per year. (In 1987 the rate was 9.7 deaths per 100,000 population.)
- By 2000 the motor vehicle death rate for children under 15 years of age should be reduced to no greater than 5.5 per 100,000 children. (In 1987 the rate was 6.2 per 100,000 children.)
- Reduce deaths of youth aged 15 to 24 years caused by motor vehicle crashes to no more than 33 per 100,000 people. (Baseline: 36.9 per 100,000 people in 1987.)
- Reduce deaths of people aged 70 years and older caused by motor vehicle crashes to no more than 20 per 100,000 people. (Baseline: 22.6 per 100,000 people in 1987.)
- Reduce deaths of motorcyclists to no more than 33 per 100 million vehicle-miles traveled and 1.5 per 100,000 people. (Baseline: 40.9 per 100 million vehicle-miles traveled and 1.7 per 100,000 people in 1987.)
- Reduce deaths of pedestrians to no more than 2.7 per 100,000 people. (Baseline: 3.1 per 100,000 people in 1987.)

Judging from the most recent statistics you can obtain for the United States, how much progress has been made toward achieving these objectives? How does your country, state, province, or community compare? How can greater progress be achieved?

one of innovation and implementation of injury prevention strategies.

Community health priorities might appropriately be based on the relative frequency of fatal injuries. Based on national data, these would include the following types of injuries: (1) motor vehicle injuries, (2) falls, (3) industrial injuries, (4) drownings, (5) burns, and (6) poisonings. Injuries disproportionately affect certain age groups, particularly children, adolescents (Figure 13-3), young adults, and the elderly. Males suffer a much higher death rate from injuries than do females, and the poor suffer a higher proportion of injuries than do other income groups. Among people aged 1 to 44 years, unintentional injuries are the leading cause of death.

Even more relevant as a criterion for community priorities might be the impact of morbidity. Hospital and emergency room (ER) data can measure morbidity better than state or national surveillance systems if the community uses **E-codes** to identify causes. For every death from injury, there are many more hospitalizations or ER visits (Figure 13-4).

Motor Vehicle Injuries

Automobile crashes and motor vehicle mileage have continued to increase, but the death rates have decreased sporadically since 1977 and the death rate per 100 million vehicle-miles has decreased steadily since 1935 (see Figure 13-5 for 1966-1991 rates). The reduction is generally attributed to increased use of seat belts, child restraints, and the renewed popularity of larger cars following the emphasis on compact models during the fuel shortages of the 1970s. Nevertheless, automobile crashes still account for more than 42,000 deaths and nearly 3.4 million injuries every year in the United States. Furthermore, the cost of crashes—including wage loss, **permanent disability** medical expenses, administrative and claims settlement costs, and property damage—amounted to over $69 billion in 1984.

Age, sex, alcohol consumption, and vehicle size

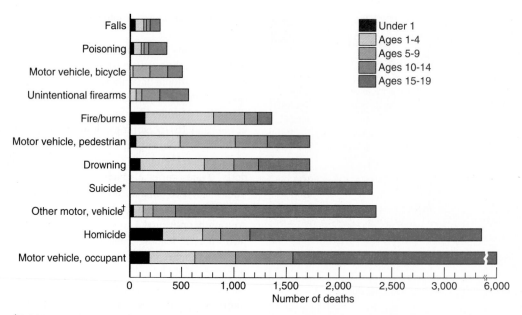

* Suicide statistics are only tabulated for persons 10 and older.
† "Other motor vehicle" includes deaths involving motorcycles, mopeds, snowmobiles, and all-terrain vehicles.

FIGURE 13-3
Annual numbers of deaths by cause and age group for American children 0 to 19 years.
Source: Children's Safety Network: *A data book of child and adolescent injury,* Washington, DC, 1991, National Center for Education in Maternal and Child Health. Data from Fingerhut and National Center for Health Statistics, unpublished, for 1988.

are significant variables in vehicle injuries. Although psychological factors may also play a role, they are very difficult to separate from cultural and social components of behavior.

Age and sex. Male motor vehicle occupants in the 15- to 24-year age group have an exceptionally high death-to-injury ratio. Half of all deaths of white males aged 20 to 24 years are caused by injuries, and over one third of all deaths in this age group result from automobile crashes alone. The influence of age is demonstrated by comparing this distribution with that in the 50- to 54-year age group, where less than 3% of deaths are the result of automobile crashes.

Age differences in resistance to injury and in the ability to survive a given injury influence the age distribution of injuries and deaths. As a result, decreased ability to survive crashes is a major factor causing older persons to be overrepresented among fatally injured drivers. It is important to separate the effect of age on the initiation of an event from the effect of age on the outcome of the event.

Alcohol. Consumption of alcohol is the most important human element known to be causally related to all types of injuries and is a contributing factor in over half of all fatal injuries (see box and Figure 13-6). Consumption of alcohol is a factor that tends to increase the severity of the outcome. A drinking driver, for example, will be less capable of escaping from a burning or submerging car. Alcohol impair-

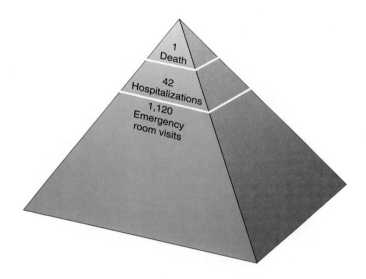

FIGURE 13-4
Mortality is but the tip of the iceberg or pyramid of childhood injury. Based on a study in Massachusetts, 42 hospitalizations and 1120 emergency room visits can be found for every death due to unintentional or intentional injury. The costs of hospitalization, emergency room care, and disability could be more compelling to a community in giving priority to injury control programs than the number of deaths.

Source: Attributed to Gallagher, unpublished, by Children's Safety Network: *A data book of child and adolescent injury*, Washington, DC, 1991, National Center for Education in Maternal and Child Health.

Year 2000 Safety Objectives Related to Alcohol and Other Drugs

- Reduce deaths caused by alcohol-related motor vehicle crashes to no more than 8.5 per 100,000 people. (Baseline: 9.8 per 100,000 people in 1987.)
- Reduce deaths of people aged 15 to 24 years caused by alcohol-related motor vehicle crashes to no more than 18 per 100,000 people. (Baseline: 21.5 per 100,000 people in 1987.)
- Extend to 50 states administrative driver's license suspension/revocation laws or programs of equal effectiveness for people determined to have been driving under the influence of intoxicants. (Baseline: 28 states and Washington, D.C., in 1990.)

ment makes emergency treatment difficult and can obscure diagnosis.

Size of vehicle. Drivers under age 25 run an 87% greater risk of being injured in a subcompact car than in a full-size one. Nearly two thirds of the drivers under age 25 in the United States drive small cars in the compact and subcompact classes. About 44% of older drivers do also. All age groups in the United States are expected to suffer increased motor vehicle fatalities with increased use of foreign import cars and as car manufacturers trim automobile weight to meet progressively tougher federal gas mileage requirements and consumer preferences. The nation may well pay for these fuel economies with thousands of additional deaths and injuries, un-

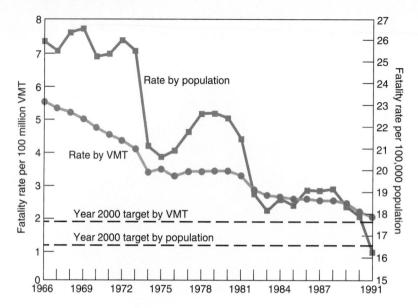

FIGURE 13-5

Motor vehicle fatality rate by vehicle miles traveled (VMT) and by population, 1966-1991.

Source: Fatal Accident Reporting System (FARS) data tapes, National Highway Traffic Safety Administration, U.S. Department of Transportation.

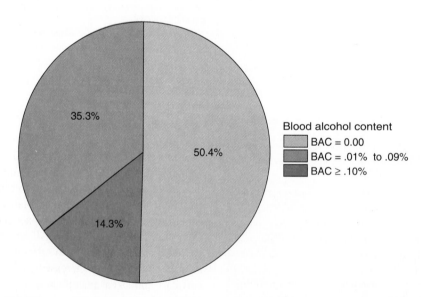

FIGURE 13-6

Alcohol use in fatal motor vehicle crashes, April to June 1990, U.S. adolescents aged 15 to 20. The proportion of intoxicated drivers has decreased in all age groups, but during this 3-month period in 1990 nearly half of these adolescent fatalities involved alcohol. More than one third had a blood-alcohol concentration greater than or equal to 0.1%, the legal limit for driving in most states.

Source: Centers for Disease Control: Quarterly table reporting alcohol involvement in fatal motor-vehicle crashes, *MMWR* 40: 24, 1991

less people drive less often and for shorter distances. Particularly dangerous is the combination of small cars and inexperienced young drivers. Small, light-weight cars do not provide nearly as much crash protection as heavier vehicles.

Heavy trucks contribute to about one fourth of fatal motor vehicle crashes in the United States; passenger cars are involved in over two thirds of such crashes. Many of these fatalities result from collisions of large trucks with passenger vehicles. Two-wheeled vehicle and tractor crashes account for the remaining deaths.

Interaction with other factors. The interaction of age and alcohol with interpersonal and situational factors predisposes adolescents to injuries on two-wheeled vehicles, including bicycles, motor scooters, motorbikes, and motorcycles. The interaction of various factors in bicycle injuries is shown in Figure 13-7. This analytical framework applies the PRE-CEDE framework introduced in Chapter 5. It identifies the psychological, social, and environmental factors amenable to modification through various combinations of educational, legal, and engineering interventions. This kind of epidemiological and behavioral diagnosis provides the framework for a coordinated community program of safety interventions. A similar analysis and framework could be drawn for each of the following types of injury.

Burn Injuries

More than 1 million Americans are burned each year, over 60,000 severely enough to be admitted to a hospital. Of those admitted to a hospital, about 15% are likely candidates for intensive burn care. The annual cost of providing intensive burn treatment is about $11,000 per patient. Projection of those figures would place total annual patient costs of specialized burn treatment in the United States at about $100 million.

Of burn injuries resulting in hospitalization, about two thirds occur in the home and about one fifth occur in the workplace. The first decade of life is a period of high risk for both injuries and deaths from burns (Figure 13-8 and box). Other high-risk periods are the early working years and the years after age 50. Older people are especially susceptible to scalding from bath water because their skin is less sensitive to the heat. Burn injuries occur about twice as frequently in males, and the rate of occurrence for blacks is about three times that for whites.

Each year about 3500 deaths and 21,275 injuries in the United States result from burns from fires—preponderantly house fires—and an additional 1300 Americans die from other kinds of burns such as scalds and electrical burns. Scalds cause about 40% of hospital admissions for burns. A simple environmental intervention effective in reducing scalding is to lower the temperature on hot water heaters to 120° F or below. This can be accomplished both through regulation of manufacturers and through community health education (Figure 13-8).

About half of the fatal fires and a substantial number of burn injuries are cigarette related, frequently from people falling asleep while smoking in bed. Painful recovery, permanent disability, and disfigurement can be among the tragic consequences for injured survivors. About 40% of the victims of residential fires who have been studied have had blood alcohol concentrations above .10%.

When the statistics from the United States are compared with those from other industrialized countries, fire incidents and the resulting casualties and income loss per capita for Americans rank among the highest in the world. In terms of years of life lost, fire burns rank second only to traffic injuries among all unintentional injuries causing death. It is estimated that the years of life lost from burns in the United States each year approach 225,000.

Fall Injuries

Falls account for about 12% of all deaths related to unintentional injuries. Fortunately, the mortality from falls has been declining in recent years, but

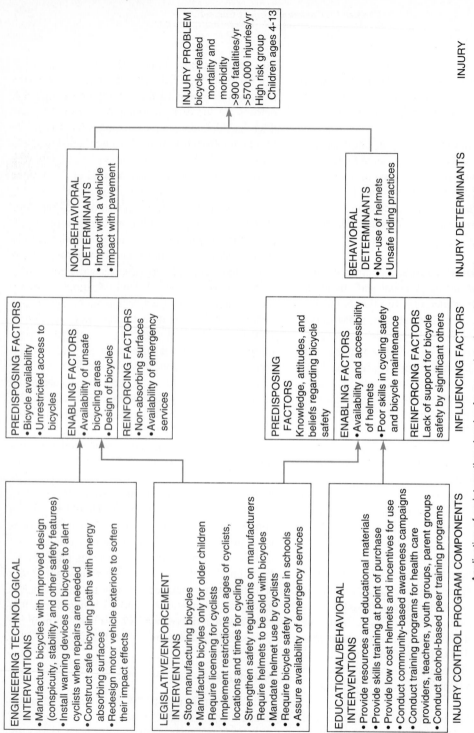

ENGINEERING TECHNOLOGICAL
INTERVENTIONS
• Manufacture bicycles with improved design
  (conspicuity, stability, and other safety features)
• Install warning devices on bicycles to alert
  cyclists when repairs are needed
• Construct safe bicycling paths with energy
  absorbing surfaces
• Redesign motor vehicle exteriors to soften
  their impact effects

LEGISLATIVE/ENFORCEMENT
INTERVENTIONS
• Stop manufacturing bicycles
• Manufacture bicycles only for older children
• Require licensing for cyclists
• Implement restrictions on ages of cyclists,
  locations and times for cycling
• Strengthen safety regulations on manufacturers
• Require helmets to be sold with bicycles
• Mandate helmet use by cyclists
• Require bicycle safety course in schools
• Assure availability of emergency services

EDUCATIONAL/BEHAVIORAL
INTERVENTIONS
• Provide resources and educational materials
• Provide skills training at point of purchase
• Provide low cost helmets and incentives for use
• Conduct community-based awareness campaigns
• Conduct training programs for health care
  providers, teachers, youth groups, parent groups
• Conduct alcohol-based peer training programs

INJURY CONTROL PROGRAM COMPONENTS

PREDISPOSING FACTORS
• Bicycle availability
• Unrestricted access to
  bicycles

ENABLING FACTORS
• Availability of unsafe
  bicycling areas
• Design of bicycles

REINFORCING FACTORS
• Non-absorbing surfaces
• Availability of emergency
  services

PREDISPOSING
FACTORS
Knowledge, attitudes, and
beliefs regarding bicycle
safety

ENABLING FACTORS
• Availability and accessibility
  of helmets
• Poor skills in cycling safety
  and bicycle maintenance

REINFORCING FACTORS
Lack of support for bicycle
safety by significant others

INFLUENCING FACTORS

NON-BEHAVIORAL
DETERMINANTS
• Impact with a vehicle
• Impact with pavement

BEHAVIORAL
DETERMINANTS
• Non-use of helmets
• Unsafe riding practices

INJURY DETERMINANTS

INJURY PROBLEM
bicycle-related
mortality and
morbidity
>900 fatalities/yr
>570,000 injuries/yr
High risk group
  Children ages 4-13

INJURY

FIGURE 13-7
This integration of the PRECEDE framework with epidemiological and planning models from the injury prevention field illustrates the interaction of various factors in bicycle-related injuries and the strategies available to address them.

Application of an integrative planning framework to the problem of bicycle-related injuries.

Source: Gielen AC: Health education and injury control: integrating approaches, *Health Educ Q* 19:203, 1992. Reproduced with permission of the author and the Society for Public Health Education.

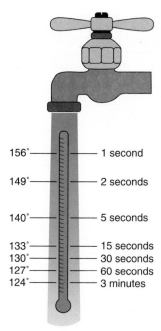

Length of time to receive a severe burn

FIGURE 13-8
The simple lowering of the temperature setting on a hot water heater to 120° F can prevent a large proportion of scald injuries (see box).

Source: The Trauma Foundation: *Injury prevention network newsletter* 9: 13, 1992.

falls still cause more deaths than any other type of unintentional injury, except motor vehicle crashes.

Nearly half of the people treated in emergency rooms with injuries resulting from falls have at least one preexisting health problem (for example, obesity, cardiovascular disease, or arthritis) known to predispose people to falls. Nearly half of children's emergency room visits related to injuries are for those caused by falls, mostly in the home.

Over half of fatal falls occur in the home, and 57% of fatal falls involve people over 75 years of age. Older people who survive falls are more likely to sustain fractures than are younger people. Alcohol impairment is implicated in many falls.

"We're always cautious as far as our children go. Never in my wildest dreams did I think something like this could happen. . . . I thought 'how serious can a hot tap-water burn be?' But when I saw him I just started to cry. It looked like somebody had just blow-torched his back."

Karen O'Connor had just filled a bucket with hot tap-water and had turned around to grab the mop to clean the kitchen floor when she heard a splash and a scream. Her two-year-old son had fallen into the steaming water. Though he was only in it for two seconds, it was long enough to scald his back and buttocks. Five months later (when this article was written), his injuries were still healing with the help of three daily medicated cream rubdowns, a nightly bath and a pressure garment—elasticized shorts he wears under his pants.

Toronto Star, 6/17/90

Intentional Injury

Intentional injury includes homicide, suicide, rape, and family violence and child abuse. Preventive measures have not yet succeeded in reducing the rates of intentional injuries in the United States (Figure 13-10). The U.S. Centers for Disease Control has established a Violence Epidemiology Branch to examine the epidemic character, if not the contagion, of violence.

Homicide. Next to motor vehicle crashes, injuries from firearms cause the greatest number of violent deaths in the United States. Alcohol, again, is often implicated. The U.S. death rate from firearm injuries is 23 times greater than that of England and Wales.

Homicides are the fourth leading cause of years of potential life lost in the United States and the second among persons aged 15 to 24 years. In the United States someone is murdered every 23 minutes. More than 50% of violent crime goes unreported.

Homicide is more common among the poor and among minority groups. Although homicide rates

Objective for the Reduction of Deaths in Residential Fires

Reduce residential fire deaths to no more than 1.2 per 100,000 people by the year 2000. (Age-adjusted baseline: 1.5 per 100,000 in 1987.)

Special Population Targets

Residential Fire Deaths (per 100,000)	*1987 Baseline*	*2000 Target*	*Percent Change*
Children aged 4 years and younger	4.4	3.3	
People aged 65 years and older	4.4	3.3	
Black males	5.7	4.3	
Black females	3.4	2.6	

Type-Specific Target

	1983 Baseline	*2000 Target*
Residential fire deaths caused by smoking	17%	5%

Baseline data sources: National Vital Statistics System; National Fire Incident Reporting System (NFIRS).

Objectives for Reduction of Fall Injuries

By 2000 the death rate from falls should be reduced to no more than 2.3 per 100,000 population.

With a sheet of graph paper, plot the possible trend lines from the following rates: 6.2 per 100,000 in 1978, 5.9 per 100,000 in 1979, and 5.9 per 100,000 in 1980. How would these points project trend lines to 1990, one assuming a continuation of the declining rates between 1978 and 1979, the other assuming that the rates leveled off between 1979 and 1980 and will remain constant through the 1980s? Compare your projections with actual data in Figure 13-9.

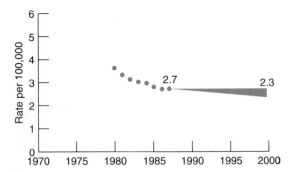

FIGURE 13-9

The reduction of age-adjusted death rates from falls and fall-related injuries for 1979 to 1987 were projected to set an objective of 2.3 deaths per 100,000 population by the year 2000, assuming a further 20% reduction in age-adjusted rates.

Source: *Healthy people 2000: national health promotion and disease prevention objectives,* Washington, DC, 1991, U.S. Department of Health and Human Services.

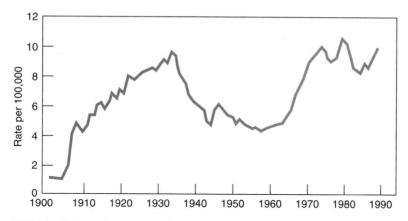

*1933 is the first year all states reported.
Data source: National Center for Health Statistics Mortality Tapes.

FIGURE 13-10
Homicide rate, United States, 1900-1990.
Source: Centers for Disease Control: Homicide surveillance, *MMWR* 41(suppl 3):29, 1992.

for white males and white females have increased the most in recent years, young black males are about five times more likely to become victims of homicide than are young white males, and young black females are more than four times as likely to become victims as are young white females. The opposite is true for suicide.

Suicide. White males are at much higher risk of suicide than other males of the same age. The suicide rates in most Western countries increase with age and are highest for the oldest men and for northern European and Japanese men. As is true for homicides, females are at consistently lower risk of suicide. The increase in the rate of suicide has also been much greater among young males than among young females. Firearm use as a method of committing suicide has been increasing at a much faster rate than other means. Over half of the deaths from gunshot wounds in the United States (Figure 13-11) are suicides. The regions where firearms are most prevalent are also the regions with the highest suicide rates. In various countries, high suicide, ho-

micide, and unintentional injury rates occur where highly lethal methods are available (Figure 13-12).

Rape. Rape has been called the fastest growing violent crime in the United States. There were 81,500 *reported* cases in 1981. Criminologists estimate that 10 times as many sexual assaults are committed as are reported. The President's Task Force on Victims of Crime reported that in the United States, on the average, a rape occurs every 6 minutes. One woman in 10 will be the victim of attempted or actual rape during her lifetime; in 85% of these cases the woman will be beaten or intimidated with life-threatening force. One in four victims is subjected to group rape. Only 50% of the accused are brought to trial, and few trials end in the conviction of the assailant.

Some of the more prevalent myths about rape are that rape is the result of spontaneous, uncontrollable sex drive in the male; that only young, physically attractive women are targets of rapists; and that women invite rape by going out alone or by provocative attire or seductive behavior. The myth

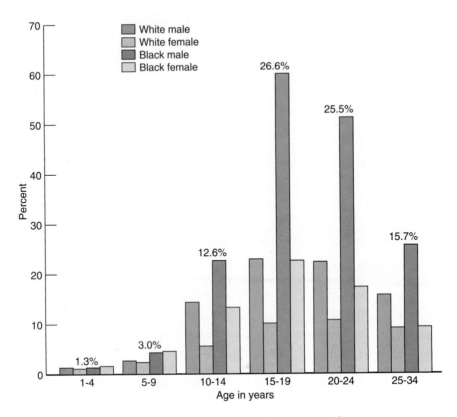

Note: Total percent (at top of bars) includes races not shown separately.

FIGURE 13-11
Percent of deaths (homicides, suicides, and unintentional deaths) due to firearms for persons 1 to 34 years of age, by age, race, and sex, United States, 1990.

Source: Fingerhut LA: Firearm mortality among children, youth, and young adults 1-34 years of age, trends and current status: United States, 1985-1990. Advance data from vital and health statistics, no 231, Hyattsville, Md, 1993, National Center for Health Statistics.

about the "uncontrollability" of the male sex drive is like the attribution of accidents to the uncontrollable fates. In fact, 70% of rapes are premeditated, and 50% of all rapists have committed violent crimes before. The second myth is refuted by the fact that the incidence of rapes of women over 60 years old increased by 800% between 1971 and 1981. The myth concerning women inviting rape, especially in strange company or places, is refuted by the fact that only 4.4% of rapes are found to have

been even partly provoked by the victim's behavior. Furthermore, some 60% of rapes occur in the victim's own home (Figure 13-13). This touches on the subject of family violence.

Family violence and child abuse. About 16 million Americans each year are affected by **family violence,** ranging from a simple slap across the face to murder. In 1985 a federal task force recommended that police should not need formal com-

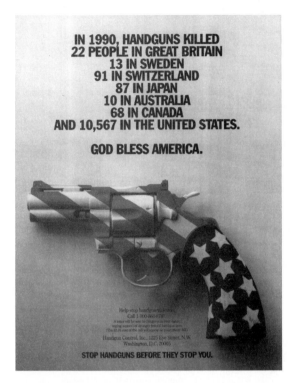

IN 1990, HANDGUNS KILLED
22 PEOPLE IN GREAT BRITAIN
13 IN SWEDEN
91 IN SWITZERLAND
87 IN JAPAN
10 IN AUSTRALIA
68 IN CANADA
AND 10,567 IN THE UNITED STATES.

GOD BLESS AMERICA.

STOP HANDGUNS BEFORE THEY STOP YOU.

FIGURE 13-12
Handguns have proliferated in their availability to the point that children bring them to school. Approximately 60% of the homicides each year in the United States involve firearms. Canada and the other countries listed in this poster have much stricter gun control laws.

Source: Handgun Control, Inc., Washington, DC.

Risk Factors

Child Abuse

- Family history of abuse (parent or spouse abuse)
- Parental mental illness and/or substance abuse
- Family dysfunction or disruption (absent parent or inadequate parenting skills)
- Socioeconomic stress (poverty, homelessness)
- Child characteristics (overactive, difficult, or disabled)

Suicide

- Psychiatric disorders
- Alcohol and other drug abuse by the adolescent or family members
- Family history of suicide, violence, and/or disruption
- Biochemical (decreased serotonin levels)
- Prior attempts
- Close relationship with a suicide victim
- Incarceration
- Ready access to firearms

Homicide

- Poverty
- Violence in the family and community
- Effects of substance abuse
- Buying and selling illicit drugs
- Ready access to firearms

plaints from victims before pressing charges. Some regard such police intrusion as interference with family life; others argue that family violence is so prevalent that it must be treated as criminal behavior. Others view family violence as a medical or psychiatric problem to be treated as an illness. The epidemiological or community health approach seeks ways to identify patterns of family violence and to intervene in the antecedent stage to prevent injury (see box for risk factors).

Based on incidents that come to official attention, the National Center on Child Abuse and Neglect estimates that some 250,000 children are physically abused each year. National survey data suggest a rate of 14 child abuse cases out of every 100 children aged 3 to 17 years; this rate would place the number of cases at 6.5 million per year. The average number of assaults for these children was 10.5. The only type of family violence to exceed parent-to-child violence is child-to-child violence. The annual incidents of severe violence (kicking, biting, punching, hitting with an object, beating, threatening to use or using a knife or gun) is 14.2 per 100 families for parent-to-child violence, but 53.2 per 100 fam-

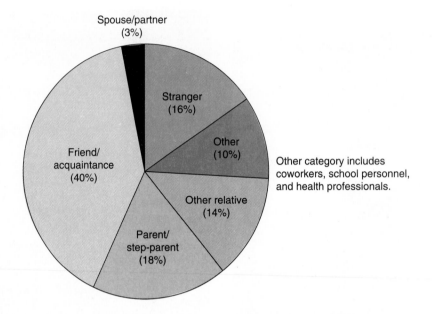

Other category includes
coworkers, school personnel,
and health professionals.

FIGURE 13-13
Relationship between rape victim (ages 13 to 17) and assailant. Accurate rates of sexual assault among adolescents are extremely difficult to obtain because the vast majority occur between two people who know each other.

Source: Massachusetts Department of Public Health: *Shattering the myths: sexual assault in Massachusetts 1985-1987,* Boston, 1990, Women's Health Division, Bureau of Community Health Services. Chart courtesy National Center for Education in Maternal and Child Health.

ilies for child-to-child violence. The comparable rate for child-to-parent abuse is 9.2 per 100 families, and for spouse abuse only 6.1 per 100 couples.

INTERVENTION TO REDUCE INJURY

Intervention may be directed at the agent, host, or environment. Most effort is directed at the host, for the urge to reform and alter other people's behavior is strong. Although investigation frequently reveals the cause of injury to be human error, this approach to injury control is the least efficient of the three available. Consideration of automobile-related injuries illustrates this point. Three classes of people—young males, alcoholics, and elderly people—are most likely to be involved in automobile

accidents, and these three groups are particularly difficult targets of educational programs.

More efficient is intervention to modify the **agent** so that the product is made safer and the potential harm lessened. This has been done to a limited extent in the automobile. Other examples are medication containers designed so that children cannot open them and poison themselves, and children's pajamas made of flameproof fabric. Safety is now built into the design of many products. The doctrine of manufacturers' liability for harm resulting from faulty design or operation has done much to accelerate this trend; legal accountability for products used by the public has forced companies to incorporate safety features. Ralph Nader is recognized for his early crusading efforts on behalf of consumer safety in the United States.

The most effective site of intervention is the environment. The environment should be designed or modified so that accidents will rarely happen and will result in little harm when they do occur.

Highway Environment

Intervention can make the highway environment substantially safer. Construction of a wide median strip featuring a sturdy guardrail can immediately and permanently reduce fatal accidents. Safe access and exit ramps, clear signs, lighted junctions, and rest areas contribute to safe driving. Other safety methods well known to highway engineers and now available, such as covering frequently struck highway structures with compressible materials and using oil drums filled with sawdust as barriers, also reduce injuries. Pedestrian areas may be made safe by nonslip surfaces, grading, and lighting. The environment in industrial areas may be modified to increase safety by reducing air and noise pollution and installing guardrails.

The environmental changes necessary for safety frequently involve enforcement of existing regulations (for example, the speed limit) or enactment of new legislation. Such radical changes need to be preceded by information campaigns to educate the public about the advantages of the change proposed. Even after a measure has been successfully enacted, people may not appreciate the ensuing benefit to public health; such laws are sometimes rescinded. For example, laws requiring the wearing of helmets by motorcyclists have been reversed in many states in the United States.

Seat belts are effective in preventing injury and death, but only about 60% of automobile occupants in the United States use them (Figure 13-14). This represents an annual 10% increase since 1982. The U.S. Transportation Department requires automobile manufacturers to install shoulder harnesses in the front and back seats of all new cars. Lap-belted drivers have 43% fewer serious and fatal injuries than their unbelted counterparts in frontal impact crashes. Some communities and states in the United States have reduced crash injuries substantially with the enforcement of mandatory seat belt use (Figure 13-14). In 13 cities in states with seat belt laws more than 51% of drivers used their belts compared with only 36% of the drivers in 6 cities located in states that do not have seat belt laws. England achieves 90% wearing of seat belts; Canada, Germany, and Australia 80%; France 70%.

The relationship between the public health and traffic safety fields and their differences are reflected in Table 13-1.

Mandatory Use of Seat Belts versus Passive Restraints (Air Bags)

Seat belt laws were once resisted by the American automobile industry because they were considered costly and inconvenient. Now the industry favors laws for mandatory use of seat belts to avoid the impending requirement for more costly installation of air bags that inflate automatically on impact and seat belts that lock automatically when the car door closes. Such passive restraints would save an estimated 8000 lives per year and $2 billion in health care costs, lost wages, and lowered productivity from injuries. The Reagan administration deferred mandatory passive restraints with a provision to suspend the rules in 1989 if two thirds of the population was covered by state laws requiring use of seat belts.

The quandary for community health professionals was whether to work for passage of the seat belt requirements, which could prevent thousands of deaths and disabling injuries, or to hold out for the passive restraints which would be installed in new cars if the seat belt laws were not passed by enough states. Passive restraints built into cars would be more effective in the long run only if used with seat belts and shoulder belts, but the experience of some states and other countries has shown that increased use of ordinary seat belts under penalty of law is a guaranteed life-saver in the short run. Which course of action would you support, and why?

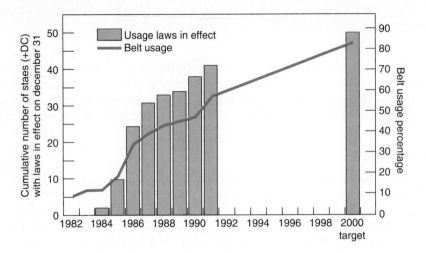

FIGURE 13-14

Safety belt use laws and estimated percentage of the U.S. population using safety belts regularly.

Source: Office of Disease Prevention and Health Promotion and National Highway Traffic Safety Administration, survey of legislative activity through February 1, 1991, and public usage rates based on 19-city survey.

TABLE 13-1

A comparison of the roles of state public health and traffic safety agencies in injury prevention and how they work together

Public health		Traffic safety
• Periodic federal funding via grants (frequent sources for traffic-injury prevention programs include Section 402, Maternal and Child Health, Preventative Health Services, Centers for Disease Control and Prevention) • Occasional state funding	← Funding source →	• National Highway Traffic Safety Administration • State
• Single-focus coordinator housed in one of many public health offices	← Administration →	• State highway safety office
• Problem identification • Prevention • Targeted education • Use of safety devices • Training of local agencies • Intervention at social and individual levels	← Focus →	• Problem identification • Legislation • Enforcement • Education • Public information/awareness • Intervention • Training • Prevention
• Local health departments • Local agencies • Community groups • Universities	← Links between states and local communities →	• Cooperation with community agencies involved in traffic safety activities • Local government agency/grantees

Source: Natural Highway Traffic Safety Administration: *Commitment, communication, cooperation: traffic safety and public health working together to prevent traffic injury,* Washington, DC, 1993, U.S. Department of Transportation.

Passive restraint systems have the ability to cushion and protect people, including children, during crashes. The U.S. Congress mandated passive restraint systems to be placed on all new automobiles sold in the United States by 1983, but repeated deadline extensions obtained by the automobile industry have delayed universal implementation.

For over 30 years motorcycle helmets have been known to reduce head injuries and death, but the repeal in most states of laws that require helmet use produced an increase in motorcycle rider fatalities of one third in those states. Enlightened legislators can pass laws, but unless the public is also enlightened to support them, the laws will often be repealed or fail to be enforced. Motorcycle deaths in the United States in 1992 dropped to less than one half what they were in 1980.

Tractor fatalities have been reduced in those areas where large farms regulated by the Occupational Safety and Health Administration (**OSHA**) are required to have rollover protective structures on tractors. But most farms do not fall under OSHA's jurisdiction. Tractors have been associated with 40% of the work- and non-work-related injuries on farms. More than one half of these deaths occur when tractors overturn and crush the operator.

Other objectives for traffic safety and strategies proposed by four national consensus groups are summarized in the appendix at the end of this chapter.

Home Environment

Each year about 22,000 people in the United States require medical attention or restricted activity as the result of an injury in the home. Indeed, the home is the leading site for disabling injuries. The most dangerous area for accidents is the bedroom, because it is most often the site of falls, chiefly among older people. The second most dangerous area is the kitchen. These two sites also produce the majority of fires in homes.

Community home safety programs. The combination of residential burns, falls, poisoning, cuts, drowning, and violence means that more people are injured in the home than in motor vehicle crashes, yet few communities have organized more than fire prevention programs. Such efforts are laudable even though limited to one aspect of home safety. In the United States, for example, Cincinnati has a "Target System" of fire inspections supported by a Tactical Inspection and Educational Unit. Inspections of structures are made by assigned members of each fire company. Frequency of inspections is determined by the "target" or category of the structure, and the five categories are determined by the inspectors based on the nature of the occupancy and the past inspection record. For buildings in the poorest category, inspections are made as frequently as every 2 weeks. When persuasion does not result in hazards being corrected, court action may be taken to fight noncompliance with fire department orders. In some communities the fire department encourages citizens to request fire inspection by the department staff. This is often associated with Fire Prevention Week.

These fire prevention plans are not to be discouraged, but obviously such piecemeal home safety programs are not adequate. A community-wide home safety program spanning all aspects of home injury prevention is the goal.

Because education is a basic ingredient of home safety promotion, the health education division of the community health department can provide the leadership for a community program to prevent injuries in the home. With the health department spearheading the program, safety activities and contributions of organizations (for example, the fire department) and individuals can be integrated with the efforts of the health department. A community-wide home safety coalition can serve as a sounding board and as a means of access to the public and their homes.

Most home injuries are caused by some combination of improper practices and unsafe conditions.

Objective for Home Safety

• By 2000 each inhabitable floor of all residential units should have a properly placed and functioning smoke detector. (In 1990 86% of inhabited dwellings had systems installed.)

How would you proceed to accomplish this objective in your community?

Promotion of home safety must focus on the correction of these practices and conditions. Efforts to educate the public should precede any action directed to improvement of private property. This means the use of all possible communication media and the promotion of special measures for alerting the public to the need for home safety.

Once the interest of the public has been aroused, the next step should be a **home safety survey** conducted by householders themselves. Such a survey can identify unsafe conditions and practices and is especially applicable to older homes.

A survey is a means to an end, not an end in itself. Follow-up action to correct unsafe conditions and practices is the logical corollary to the survey. Through the various communication media, continual emphasis must be placed on the importance of corrections if this approach is to yield tangible results. Projects in Denver, Philadelphia, and San Francisco have demonstrated new approaches to home injury prevention in elderly people and in inner-city black populations.

Objective data may be obtained on injuries and how they occur in the home by providing all households with a form for reporting the time, place, and nature of the injury and the factors involved. These collective data can be highly meaningful in pinpointing where emphasis should be placed in the home safety program.

Fires. Nearly 8 out of 10 U.S. fire deaths happen at home, and more than half of them occur in one- and two-family homes. More than half of the home fires in the United States occur between midnight and 6 AM. Cigarettes, cigars, and pipes are still the major culprits, most often igniting in living rooms and bedrooms. They may smolder for several hours, but it takes only 2 to 4 minutes after ignition for combustible materials to go up in roaring flames that release poisonous gases. Unfortunately, all this can happen undetected by a sleeping family.

Smoke detectors can often mean the difference between life and death. Recent technology has produced a ready assortment of low-cost alarms. These devices are particularly effective in detecting fires in their early stages. As their name implies, smoke detectors are designed to detect the presence of smoke particles in the atmosphere. In the early stages of fires, smoke often develops before there is any appreciable increase in temperature, and smoke inhalation is a major cause of fire deaths.

The distribution of fire locations in houses that have burned shows that the majority of fires start in the three rooms where people spend most of their time—living room, bedroom, and kitchen—in that order of frequency.

Poisoning. A community health definition of **poisoning** is the ingestion, inhalation, injection, or absorption of a chemical agent that results in illness or death. Poisoning is the fifth leading cause of unintentional injury deaths in the United States. Childhood poisoning deaths have declined markedly in recent years with the manufacture and enforcement of special child-proof lids on medicine bottles and household chemical containers.

Homicidal and suicidal poisonings are rare by comparison with unintentional poisoning, through the increases in drug-related unintentional poisonings might be interpreted as a form of homicide or suicide in many cases. The leading causes of fatal unintentional drug poisonings are opiates and related narcotics and local anesthetics including cocaine. Most of the deaths from other solids and liquids are due to alcohol ingestion. Motor vehicle exhaust (carbon monoxide fumes) accounted for nearly half the deaths attributed to unintentional poisoning by gases and vapors.

The unintentional poisoning mortality rate for males tends to run more than twice as high as that for females. The rates for blacks of both sexes are consistently higher than those for whites.

The annual observance of National Poison Prevention week in mid-March gives communities an opportunity to cooperate with over 30 national organizations representing industry, consumer groups, poison control centers, health professionals, government, and the media. The community **poison control centers** play a pivotal role in preventing poisonings among children by providing public information, expert consultation, and specialized diagnostic and treatment recommendations within their respective communities.

Other residential or home environment safety issues will be addressed in Chapter 15.

Family violence. Most preventive programs for child abuse and spouse abuse assume that the source of the problem is the legitimization over time of physical force as an acceptable way to control family members and to express dissatisfaction or frustration. For example, in one survey, nearly 72% of the respondents did not consider shaking a child as abusive, yet medical authorities consider shaking an infant or small child to be extremely dangerous. The mass media tend to reinforce attitudes that violence is necessary, legitimate, and effective to maintain family control and to punish transgressions of authority. Thus violence is perpetuated from generation to generation.

Interventions are designed to break into this cycle. The detection of abusive parents or spouses is a first step. A federal task force on family violence recommended in 1985 that police should be allowed to intervene in violent domestic situations without formal complaints from victims; that schools and hospitals now required to report child abuse should also be required to report abuse of the elderly; and that broadcasters should voluntarily limit violence

on television programs. Progress has been noted in 33 states that have given police more power in responding to family violence. Illinois has rules to keep victims from being harassed, and Brooklyn, San Antonio, Los Angeles, and Westchester County, New York, have special units for family violence and sexual abuse cases.

After detection of such cases, group psychotherapy with a heavy emphasis on coping skills can be an effective intervention. Identification of alcohol abuse is often a starting point (Figure 13-15). Primary prevention strategies include training in parenting skills, emphasis on early bonding between newborns and their mothers (especially important if the baby is born prematurely), and public education to recognize signs of family violence tendencies.

Other violence. In the past, murder, suicide, and rape have been the concern primarily of law enforcement agencies, but increasingly health organizations are involved in finding effective interventions. A case in point is prevention of teenage suicides, which sometimes occur in clusters within communities, suggesting a pattern of contagion. Following an outbreak of teenage suicides, officials may develop a countywide suicide prevention program. Such programs usually include suicide prevention training for teachers, guidance counselors, parents, and students. Telephone hot lines provide a crisis-counseling resource for potential suicide victims who wish to maintain their anonymity.

Rape prevention programs have emphasized public education and security programs for safe transportation for women at night. Other approaches have included the development of more humanitarian, structured assistance for rape victims in the hospital emergency room, at police headquarters, and in the courts; better informed, more sympathetic police officers, physicians, and nurses to interview and treat rape victims; standardized kits in hospital emergency rooms for collection of evidence; and public education to alter community attitudes to-

Over 60% of all violent crimes begin and end behind bars.

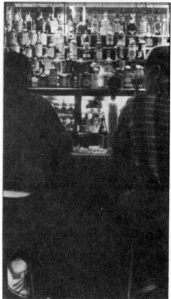

We hear about assault, rape and murder everyday.

What we don't hear about is how often alcohol is involved.

Most of us don't realize that well over half of all violent offenders were drinking when they committed their crimes.

When problem drinkers don't get help, their problem eventually affects all of us. One way or another.

The Responsibility is Yours.

1-800-663-1441

Alcohol and Drug Programs
Ministry of Labour and Consumer Services
The Honourable Lyall Hanson, Minister

FIGURE 13-15
Alcohol abuse contributes to large proportions of the various forms of violence and intentional injury. Alcohol counseling and treatment for problem drinking depend on self-referral or referral by concerned family members or health professionals and employers.

Source: Alcohol and Drug Programs, British Columbia Ministry of Health and Ministry of Labour and Consumer Services.

ward rape and to gain community support for preventive and control measures.

Handgun control laws could help reduce several forms of violence and the lethality of resulting injuries. Morton Grove, Illinois, was the first community in the United States to ban the possession of handguns by anyone except law enforcement officers. The citizens of Maryland waged a pitched political battle with the National Rifle Association to pass a statewide gun control measure on the ballot.

Polls indicate that most Americans now favor stiffer gun control. Most other countries are more restrictive in the possession of handguns than is the United States, and most Western countries have lower rates of violent injuries (see Figure 13-12).

Farm Environment

Safety on the farm encompasses aspects of occupational, home, motor vehicle, and recreational safety. From the standpoint of occupation, about one fifth of all industrial accident deaths in the United States occur in farming. The rate of accidental deaths in farming, which is higher than that in any other industry, also has shown the least improvement over recent years.

Agricultural work covers a wide variety of jobs depending on the farm's size, its location, its agricultural products, and availability of help. The work is seasonal and often demands long hours, physical strength, and quick execution. Farm workers usually perform multiple job functions, frequently without adequate safety instruction. Many times children, young adults, and uneducated laborers perform urgent work on family farms using a wide variety of heavy equipment, dangerous machinery, and intricate production methods. Farm families and workers are often exposed to the elements and may become vulnerable to sun, heat, and cold. Rural living and farm work also expose these persons to dangerous animals, toxic plants and insects, pesticides, and hazardous and volatile chemical compounds.

Departments of agriculture and federal extension services carry on programs for promoting farm safety. Farm organizations such as the Farmers Union and the Grange also have continuing and special farm safety programs. These efforts are commonly supported by a variety of statewide safety education programs that include farm safety education. The state department of education usually promotes safety education in the schools, and farm safety is included in the program, particularly in rural areas.

Farm injuries. Farm life places the agricultural family in a variety of situations with unique problems in safety. Machinery poses a special hazard. Fatal injuries from machines and firearms on farms occur three to five times more frequently than fatal injuries from the same implements in other environments. Data on farm injuries can identify where the greatest emphasis should be placed in safety promotion on the farm. Injuries pose a special problem for the farm population, calling for more effective action than has been expended thus far.

Prevention of farm injuries. Preventing farm injuries involves the farm families through self-direction as an outgrowth of an extensive program of farm safety education. Correlated with safety education should be a **farm safety survey** that farm families themselves can use profitably.

Combined with the home safety survey, a farm safety survey can be used as the basis for an evaluation of hazards and safety in farm life. All farm families should be encouraged through health education to take the time necessary for safety surveys and to follow up by correcting any hazardous conditions and practices revealed by the survey.

In some communities a farm safety committee under the aegis of the community safety council coordinates the efforts of organizations and individuals in farm health promotion. More than 20 organizations participate in farm safety on the local level in the United States; these include the Cooperative Extension Service, Grange, Farmers Union, American Farm Bureau Federation, Future Farmers of America, 4-H clubs, and Future Homemakers of America. Meetings, campaigns, contests, demonstrations, and studies are the channels through which these organizations promote safety on the farm.

In the United States most states have full-time or part-time farm safety specialists. With a professional safety expert working with a farm safety council, statewide programs serve to bolster local efforts as well as to promote special safety programs.

Occupational Environment

Industrial safety refers to injury control in a branch of trade or production on a wide geographic basis, such as in the steel industry or automobile industry. Occupational safety refers to injury control within the confines of a single operational unit, such as the safety program in a specific chemical plant. Industrial safety is of value because of the pooling of experience and know-how among the various units within an industry. Yet it is on the local operational level where accidents must be prevented and where a safety program will yield the greatest results in **occupational injury** control.

Of the major safety programs, occupational safety appears to have made the greatest progress in injury control in the United States. Although the enactment of Workmen's Compensation laws beginning in 1912 made safety economically profitable, management and labor have more than a business interest in safety promotion; they are interested in protecting the lives and health of employees. The effectiveness of safety programs is attested to by the drop in the injury frequency rate for companies reporting to the National Safety Council. Occupational injury deaths per 100,000 workers dropped 71% from 1912 to 1980. This remarkable accomplishment was matched by an additional 23% reduction from 1980 to 1986. The average rate for 1983 through 1987 was 5.9 deaths per 100,000 workers.

The Occupational Safety and Health Act mandates the reporting of occupational injuries and illnesses by employers. A new system of uniform reporting and recording has resulted in more complete reporting. Between 1970 and 1980, the number of work-related fatal injuries decreased by 28%. Because of deregulation since 1981, however, some of the OSHA standards now are not being enforced.

Generally speaking, industries with the highest injury frequency rates (disabling injuries per 100,000 work hours) also have the highest severity rates (days lost per 1 million work hours). By their very nature, certain industries such as mining, marine transportation, quarrying, and construction tend to be hazardous. Other industries have a minor degree of hazard. Data for a total industry are of value to a local operation, but each plant or place of employment must deal with the hazards it has in its own operation.

In any consideration of occupational injuries, it must be pointed out that workers suffer more than three times as many accidental deaths off the job than they do on the job. Further, the probability of an injury incurred at work being fatal is only half that of injuries incurred away from work.

Prevention of occupational injuries. Organization, a planned program, expert direction, and the enlistment of all personnel are the ingredients of an effective occupational injury control program. Usually such a program consists of the following eight aspects:

1. Leadership by management and labor unions
2. Assignment of responsibility
3. Safe working conditions
4. Safety training of all personnel
5. Accident and injury records
6. Analysis of accidents and research in safety measures
7. Employee and employer acceptance of responsibility for safety
8. First aid and medical services

Industry employs safety experts who are usually designated as safety engineers. This concept could well be applied to other provinces of human activity where injuries are even more prevalent. More will be discussed on occupational health and safety in Chapter 15.

School Environment

For school-age youngsters, injuries loom as a greater threat to life and limb than do diseases. In the United States in the 5- to 15-year age group, accidents other than automobile injuries are the leading cause of death.

School injuries. About 43% of accidental deaths among school-aged children in the United States are connected with school life—about 6% occur on the way to or from school, about 20% in school buildings, and about 17% on school grounds. Youngsters between the ages of 5 and 14 years have the highest injury rate. Their vigor and abandon lead to many of their injuries with recreational equipment (Figure 13-16).

Prevention of school injuries. Schools can prevent accidental deaths and injuries among students and faculty with a systematic, vigorous, and sustained program. Leadership, vision, organization, and teamwork bridging school and community are the ingredients of an effective school safety program, which is one facet of the total community safety program. A school-based driver education training program, for example, can do more harm than good if the community uses it to license youth to drive too early.

A safety council composed of students and faculty supports the school safety program. A school safety patrol can have subdivisions such as a traffic patrol, a building and grounds patrol, and a fire patrol. Student participation under teacher guidance is the working pattern, ideally using school safety checklists both as a survey tool and as a safety education opportunity. Involving students actively in the planning and execution of programs helps give the students a sense of ownership and commitment to the programs.

Surveys of conditions and practices affecting safety in the school environment point up hazards and indicate preventive measures that must be taken. These surveys properly include conditions between the school and children's homes, as well as school playgrounds.

A system for reporting accidents and injuries is of legal significance as well as of preventive value. This is particularly true when a systematic investigation and follow-up is tied in with the reporting system.

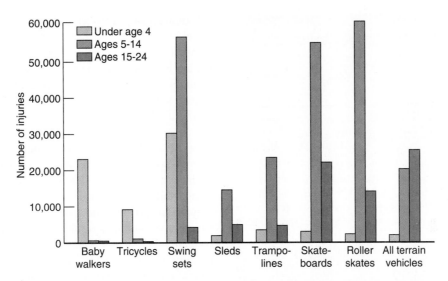

Because of their far greater magnitude, bicycle injuries are not included in this graph.

FIGURE 13-16
National estimates of injury associated with child and youth recreational equipment, United States, 1990.
Source: U.S. Consumer Product Safety Commission: Product summary report, Washington, DC, 1990, National Electronic Injury Surveillance System, National Injury Information Clearinghouse. Chart courtesy National Center for Education in Maternal and Child Health.

Safety education as an integral phase of early health education has been effective in developing good safety attitudes and practices among children. It is in the early, formative years of life that good safety habits are most readily acquired.

Recreational Environment

Europeans, Canadians, Australians, Japanese, and Americans have gained increased vacation time and early retirement as work benefits from business and industry. Accordingly, the population at risk from various recreational activities has steadily increased. Because complete figures on recreational morbidity and mortality are not available, however, injuries from recreational pursuits have not been identified specifically as a major problem except in sports medicine.

It would be unrealistic to restrain recreation for the purpose of preventing all injuries. It would be equally unrealistic to think that recreation could be injury-free, but past experience has demonstrated that safety promotion can go hand in hand with the expansion of recreation.

Injuries in recreation. Public accidents, other than those related to home, noncommercial motor vehicle, and employment accidents, caused 17.1 million personal injuries and approximately 19,000 deaths in the United States during 1985. Most occurred in recreational and leisure settings. Disabling injuries numbered approximately 2.4 million.

Most drownings involve water sports such as swimming and boating. The annual number of deaths from drowning has declined over the past 20 years despite the increasing numbers of people par-

---

Objective for Reduction of Drowning

By 2000 the death rate from drowning should be reduced to no more than 1.3 per 100,000 population. (In 1987 it was 2.1 per 100,000 population.)

During the last decade, boating activities, which have increased greatly, have exposed more people to the risk of drowning. Nonetheless, boating-related drownings declined between 1978 and 1987, and the rate decreased from 0.6 per 100,000 to 0.4 per 100,000 population, nearly a 29% reduction in the rate of such fatalities. Alcohol use by boat operators is increasingly recognized as contributing to boating fatalities. From 1978 to 1984, nonboating drownings decreased from 5784 to 4444, and the rate of such drownings decreased nearly 27%, from 2.6 per 100,000 to 1.9 per 100,000 population. Despite improved safety in residential swimming pools and spas, approximately 300 children under 5 years of age drown each year in this setting.

How would you attempt to reduce fatalities from drowning in your community?

---

ticipating in water sports. About one third of adults who drown have high levels of alcohol in their blood.

Some 50.5 million boaters use 10 million boats in the waters of the United States. Recreational boating now accounts for fewer than 1000 fatalities each year in the United States. Although few by comparison with the number of motor vehicle deaths, this figure represents a rate of approximately 44 fatalities per 100 million exposure hours compared to the automobile rate of about 55 fatalities per 100 million exposure hours. Hypothermia (exposure) fatalities appear to be increasing with the growing interest in cold weather activities and the increasing numbers of individuals participating in winter recreation.

The yearly death toll in recreation has increased in recent years. Yet when considered in terms of the increased number of participants in recreation, the *rate* of fatal accidents has declined. Furthermore, not all of these deaths are strictly chargeable to recreation. Flying and railway fatalities can occur in commercial travel as well as in recreational travel.

Most of the people who lose their lives in recreation injuries are in the prime of life. This is particularly true for injuries in boating and other water sports, with firearms, and in airplane or balloon crashes.

Prevention of injuries in recreation. On the community level, organized, supervised recreation is usually safe recreation. Trained personnel, definite responsibilities, enforced codes and regulations, regular supervision, safety surveys, and safety education have produced results. It is in unsupervised recreation that action is most needed, and here the primary approach is safety education. This is not a simple matter because education in one area, such as the safe use of firearms, does not carry over into other areas, such as safe conduct in swimming or boating.

Part of the safety education in recreation is provided by such organizations as rifle clubs, boating clubs, camping groups, and other sports clubs. The Red Cross, the YMCA, and similar organizations have contributed greatly to the promotion of safe recreation with such activities as swimming instruction and cardiopulmonary resuscitation (CPR) training. Despite these efforts, an organized community program of safety education in this sphere of activity is a difficult assignment. The efforts of agencies and individuals promoting safety education in other areas make an indirect contribution to recreational safety.

The reductions in drowning deaths during the 1980s could represent an increased number of near-drowning victims saved by CPR and other emergency response capabilities in the community. This has produced an unknown number of near-drowning victims with neurological damage and disabilities.

Regulations governing recreational activities have a considerable effect on the promotion of safety. This is particularly true of regulations designed to prevent the inexperienced from participating in activities for which they are not prepared or

qualified. The inexperienced or unskillful participant is most likely to suffer injuries, and the reckless
participant is most likely to cause injuries to others.

Each community can survey the recreational
safety needs of its people and formulate a program
accordingly. The cooperation of all groups sponsoring recreational activities or programs will add assurance for the success of the safety program. Recreational safety promotion should be coordinated
with other safety programs in the community.

COMMUNITY SAFETY PROGRAM

The coordination of community safety poses a problem because safety in a community is the province
of many organizations and individuals. These include the health department, fire department, police
department, recreation department, schools, industry, chamber of commerce, service clubs, Red Cross,
civil defense, medical profession, other health and
recreation professionals, and news media. The need
is to integrate the contributions of all agencies into
one unified, effective community safety program.

Organization

The community health department is the most logical agency to bring together the various forces influencing injury prevention in the community.
While the official health department can be the catalyst, a basic ingredient is a coalition of community
groups that have an interest in and a contribution to
make to safety. This voluntary, nonofficial body is
at one and the same time a sounding board, a source
of information, an expression of community thinking, and a supporter of the various safety programs
operating within the community.

Community Safety Promotion

Each agency will continue its ongoing program, expanding as conditions and the council indicate. Unnecessary duplication can be eliminated, but some

---

Elements of Successful Community Injury Control

Planning and Prioritizing

- A broad-based coalition representing the community
  of interest;
- surveillance tools and methods to identify and monitor the number of injuries:
- the use of E codes to aid in the ascertainment of
  injury causes; and
- selection of priority areas for injury control.

Comprehensive Multifaceted Approach

- Evaluation of prevention strategies to determine effectiveness;
- dissemination and universal implementation of effective strategies;
- targeting of high-risk groups, such as low income;
  and
- incorporation of prevention messages and efforts
  into service systems for children and adolescents.

Institutionalization and Acceptance

- Coordination of local, state and federal efforts;
- institutionalization of injury prevention programming;
- enforcement of existing legislation protecting children; and
- development of a societal norm of a ''safe childhood
  and adolescence.''

---

duplication is highly desirable. Unmet needs will be
recognized, and an understanding will be reached
on which agency will deal with a recognized need.

A poison control center is a valuable segment of
the community safety program. It is the place where
people can call for help in case of unintentional or
intentional poisoning. Properly, such a center is
open 24 hours a day and is staffed by a person who
knows how to use the standard references on poisons and who can recommend countermeasures. He
or she needs to know both the physiology and toxicology involved. In small communities a hospital
is the logical location for such a center. In larger

communities a poison control center may be located elsewhere and staffed with pharmacists.

Safety surveys may be sponsored by health or safety councils or initiated by member organizations. The two essential factors are to discover where injuries occur and where hazards exist in the community. Once hazards are located and the causes of injuries identified, measures can be initiated within the community to reduce or even eliminate them.

Safety education by various community agencies must be coordinated and integrated to be extensive enough to be fully effective. Safety consciousness in a community can be developed, but it takes a clear focus on specific, attainable objectives.

SUMMARY

In Canada and the United States unintentional injuries—once referred to as accidents—account for the largest number of potential years of life lost among all causes of death. Deaths from intentional injuries account for the fourth largest number of potential years of life lost. These facts have turned public health attention to injuries as a health problem subject to epidemiological study and preventive intervention. The term *accident* has fallen into disfavor because the scientific study of injuries has largely displaced the tendency to think of accidents as uncontrollable events attributable to fate.

Public health leadership has provided a map for community action with national objectives for injury control. The following box summarizes those objectives for the year 2000.

Although many injuries can be traced to human error, the frequency of such errors can be reduced most efficiently by structuring the environment or products involved to minimize the need for human decisions or preventive actions. Safety education remains an essential component of community injury control, but for those dangerous events that occur most unexpectedly or suddenly, the limited oppor-

Objectives to Reduce Unintentional Injuries by the Year 2000

Objectives target reducing unintentional injury deaths, nonfatal unintentional injuries, motor vehicle crash deaths, fall-related deaths, drowning deaths, and residential fire deaths; reducing hip fractures among people aged 65 years and older; reducing nonfatal poisonings, head injuries, spinal cord injuries, and secondary disabilities associated with head and spinal cord injuries; increasing use of occupant protection systems, and use of motorcycle and bicycle helmets; increasing laws requiring safety belt and motorcycle helmet use; enacting laws on handgun design; increasing installation of fire sprinklers and functional smoke detectors; providing injury prevention instruction in schools; extending the requirement of the use of protective headgear at sporting and recreation events; increasing roadway safety design standards and counseling on safety precautions by primary care providers; and extending emergency medical services and trauma systems.

tunity to exercise judgment or take split-second action renders education and training relatively ineffective.

Legal controls on products, structures, and practices that tend to cause injuries help limit the damage that might otherwise result. But the passage, retention, and enforcement of such laws still depends on an informed and committed public, which in turn depends on effective health education and the work of community action groups.

The advantages of environmental approaches to injury control lead to intervention strategies aimed at settings where hazards can be analyzed and injuries prevented. These include the home, highway, farm, occupational, recreational, and school environments. Interventions to reduce injuries and deaths from fires, scalds, vehicle crashes, falls, poisonings, drownings, and some types of family violence have gained in effectiveness in recent years. Most types of intentional injury, including homi-

> ### Objectives to Reduce Violent and Abusive Behavior by the Year 2000
>
> Objectives target reducing homicides, suicides, and weapon-related deaths; reversing the rising incidence of child abuse; reducing physical abuse of women by male partners, assault injuries, rape and attempted rape, and adolescent suicide attempts; reducing physical fighting among youth, weapon-carrying by youth, and inappropriate storage of weapons; improve emergency room protocols to identify, treat, and refer suicide attempters and survivors of sexual assault and of child, partner, and elder abuse; improve child death review systems; improve evaluation and follow-up of abused children; improve emergency housing for battered women and their children; improve school programs for conflict resolution; and increase violence prevention programs and suicide prevention in jails.

cide, suicide, child abuse, and rape, however, have not yielded to comparable interventions. These represent new frontiers for community health. The objectives for intentional injury reductions are summarized in the box above.

QUESTIONS FOR REVIEW

1. To study the epidemiology of injuries in your community, what factors would receive your attention?
2. How would you account for a high injury rate in a community that had a much better safety program than that of another community with a lower injury rate?
3. The death rate from injuries in the United States has declined since the turn of the century, yet injuries now rank as the fourth leading cause of death. How do you explain this apparent contradiction?
4. How is your state or provincial highway injury control program organized and administered?
5. In the United States, why are the state industrial safety programs generally more effective than the state traffic safety or firearm control programs?
6. On the state or provincial level, who has responsibility for the promotion of home safety?
7. What agencies in your locality promote farm injury control?
8. If a car traveling 55 mph crashes into a fixed concrete abutment, with how much force will a person of 160 pounds be thrown forward? Use the equation $MV = Ft$, in which M = mass, V = velocity, F = force, and t = time (1 second).
9. How would you draw an organizational chart for a model motor vehicle safety program for some community?
10. What agencies in your community are engaged in the promotion of poison control?
11. How would you evaluate the safety record and the injury control program of one of the industrial firms in your community or in another community?
12. How effectively have your community's schools taken advantage of their opportunity to promote safety?
13. What obstacles are there to the promotion of recreational safety?
14. If you were to set up a safety council for your community, who would be on the council and what would be the specific provinces of its program?
15. What is the greatest safety need in your community?

READINGS

DeBruyn LM, Lujan CC, May PA: A comparative study of abused and neglected American Indian children in the Southwest, *Soc Sci Med* 35:305, 1992.
Native populations of the United States and Canada have the highest rates of injury among all major ethnic groups; child abuse accounts for some of this, and alcohol abuse is present in virtually all families that abuse children.
Gallaher MM, Fleming DW, Berger LR et al: Pedestrian and hypothermia deaths among Native Americans in New Mexico: between bar and home, *JAMA* 267:1345, 1992.

Over half of the unintentional injuries among Native North Americans result from hypothermia and pedestrian–motor vehicle crashes. At death 90% of those Native Americans tested were highly intoxicated. Most deaths occurred at off-reservation sites in border towns and on roads leading back to the reservation.

Gielen AC: Health education and injury control: integrating approaches, *Health Educ Q* 19:203, 1992.

This article integrates the PRECEDE model with Haddon's host–agent–environment model of injury prevention to offer a single planning model for this area of community health.

Hsu JS, Williams SD: Injury prevention awareness in an urban Native American population, *Am J Public Health* 81:1466, 1991.

Injury-related mortality rate for Native American children 1 to 4 years old is nearly three times that of the same ages in the general U.S. population. Survey responses revealed that Native American families are less likely to keep small objects, household products, and medicines out of the reach of their children or to possess and understand the use of ipecac in the case of poisoning.

Johnston I: Action to reduce road casualties, *World Health Forum* 13:154, 1992.

Progress in road safety is reviewed with particular reference to radical measures that have proved beneficial in Australia. Community involvement in decision making is vital if gains are to be made and sustained in road safety.

BIBLIOGRAPHY

Aldridge D, St John K: Adolescent and pre-adolescent suicide in Newfoundland and Labrador, *Can J Psychiatry* 36:432, 1991.

Alexander CS, Ensminger ME, Somerfield MR et al: Behavioral risk factors for injury among rural adolescents, *Am J Epidemiol* 136:673, 1992.

Bagley C: Poverty and suicide among native Canadians: a replication, *Psychol Rep* 69:149, 1991.

Balanda KP, Spinks D, Ring I et al: The Brisbane home safety survey and its role in the Queensland pool safety campaign: domestic swimming pool fencing characteristics, compliance and attitudes, *Health Prom J Austral* 1:37, 1991.

Becker TM, Wiggins CL, Key CR et al: Changing trends in mortality among New Mexico's American Indians, 1958-1987, *Int J Epidemiol* 21:690, 1992.

Bijur P, Durzon M, Overpeck MD et al: Parental alcohol use, problem drinking, and children's injuries, *JAMA* 267:3166, 1992.

Bjaras G: The potential of community diagnosis as a tool in planning an intervention programme aimed at preventing injuries, *Accid Anal Prev* 25:3, 1993.

Boruch RF, Coleman D, Doria-Ortiz C et al: Violence prevention strategies targeted at the general population of minority youth, *Public Health Rep* 106:247, 1991.

Brent DA, Perper JA, Allman CJ et al: The presence and accessibility of firearms in the homes of adolescent suicides, *JAMA* 266:2989, 1991.

Callahan CM, Rivara FP: Urban high school youth and hanguns, *JAMA* 267:3038, 1992.

Centers for Disease Control: Safety-belt use and motor-vehicle related injuries—Navajo Nation, 1988-1991, *MMWR* 41:705, 1992.

Centers for Disease Control: Toddler deaths resulting from ingestion of iron supplements—Los Angeles, 1992-1993, *MMWR* 42:111, 1993.

Gielen AC, Radius S: Project KISS (Kids in Safety Belts): educational approaches and evaluation measures, *Health Educ* 15:43, 1984.

Grossman DC, Milligan BC, Deyo RA: Risk factors for suicide attempts among Navajo adolescents, *Am J Public Health* 81:870, 1991.

Howard-Pitney B, Johnson MD, Altman DG et al: Responsible alcohol service: a study of server, manager, and environmental impact, *Am J Public Health* 81:197, 1991.

Hull C: *Gender and childhood injury,* Victoria, British Columbia, 1991, Ministry of Health and Ministry Responsible for Seniors.

Hunter EM: An examination of recent suicides in remote Australia: further information from the Kimberley, *Austral NZ J Psychol* 25:197, 1991.

Iverson DC: Homicide prevention from the perspective of the Office of Health Promotion, *Public Health Rep* 95:559, 1980.

Johnson KC, Ford DE, Smith GS: The current practices of internists in prevention of residential fire injury, *Am J Prev Med* 9:39, 1993.

Jones CS, Macrina D: Using the PRECEDE model to design and implement a bicycle helmet campaign, *Wellness Perspec Res Theory Prac* 9:68, 1993.

Kent D: How to manage poisoning in pediatric patients: preventing accidental deaths, *Can Fam Phys* 37:1979, 1991.

Krishman R: Safe travel—a worthwhile destination, *World Health Forum* 13:163, 1992.

Maxwell EK, Maxwell RJ: Insults to the body civil: mistreatment of elderly in two Plains Indian tribes, *J Cross-Cul Gerontol* 7:3, 1992.

May PA: Alcohol policy considerations for Indian reservations and border-town communities, *Am Indian Alas Native Men Health Res* 4:5, 1992.

National Committee for Injury Prevention and Control: *Injury prevention: meeting the challenge,* New York, 1989, Oxford University Press, as a supplement to the *Am J Prev Med,* vol 5, no 3, 1989 (whole issue).

Nelson D, Sklar D, Skipper B et al: Motorcycle fatalities in New Mexico: the association of helmet nonuse with alcohol intoxication, *Ann Emerg Med* 21:279, 1992.

Newberger EH: The helping hand strikes again: unintended consequences of child abuse reporting, *Clin Child Psychol* 12:309, 1992.

O'Carroll PW, Loftin C, Waller JB Jr et al: Preventing homicide: an evaluation of the efficacy of a Detroit gun ordinance, *Am J Public Health* 81:576, 1991.

Occupational Safety and Health: *Occupational injuries and their cost: Canada 1988-1990,* Ottawa, 1992, Labour Canada.

Ontario Public Health Association: *Report of the Injury Prevention Priorities Consultation,* Toronto, 1992, Ontario Ministry of Health.

Pekkarinen A, Anttonen H: Safety in the use of four-wheeled all terrain vehicles in Finland, *Arctic Med Res* 51(suppl 7):77, 1992.

Runyan CW, Gray DE, Kotch JB et al: Analysis of U.S. child care safety regulations, *Am J Public Health* 81: 981, 1991.

Sabey B: *The scientific basis of childhood injury prevention,* London, 1993, Child Accident Prevention Trust.

Sleet DA: Health education approaches to motor vehicle injury prevention, *Public Health Rep* 102:606, 1900.

Stevenson T, Lennie J: Empowering school students in developing strategies to increase bicycle helmet wearing, *Health Educ Res* 7:555, 1992.

Waters C, Gibbons L, Semenciw R et al: Motor vehicle traffic accidents in Canada, 1978-87 by time of occurrence, *Can J Public Health* 84:58, 1993.

Traffic safety goals and strategies: federal policy statements

	2000	NHTSA	TS SUM	SG DD
Overall fatality rates				

Goals

	2000	NHTSA	TS SUM	SG DD
Per 100,000 people	17			
Per 100 million VMT	1.9	2.2 by 1992		

Occupant protection

Goals

	2000	NHTSA	TS SUM	SG DD
Occupant restraint use	85%	70% by '92	70% by '92	
Number of states with laws	45	All states		

Legislation/enforcement

	2000	NHTSA	TS SUM	SG DD
Mandatory seat belt laws	•	•		•
Enforce seat belt laws		•		•
Law enforcement officials be required to wear seat belts		•	•	

Education/information

	2000	NHTSA	TS SUM	SG DD
Educate law enforcement officials & parents that restraints are important	•			
Educate parents on need for car seats up to age 5	•			
Support child passenger safety coalitions		•		
Coordinate education campaigns of Depts. of Educ. & HHS and AMA			•	
Encourage MV Dept. to include info on seat belts in their programs			•	
Public information campaigns by local police agencies		•		
Recognize organizations achieving 70% usage		•		
Target groups such as rural & minority			•	
National media campaign: occupant protection		•	•	
Involve insurance industry in education efforts		•	•	
Provide training and technical assistance to corporations implementing safety belt programs		•		
Assist OSHA to implement worksite safety belt programs		•		

Other

	2000	NHTSA	TS SUM	SG DD
Develop belt use survey method guidelines		•		
Provide data on seat belt use to law enforcement officials			•	

2000: Year 2000 Objectives for the Nation, U.S. Department of Health and Human Services, 1989.
NHTSA: Moving America Safely—NHTSA's Priority Plan 1990-1992, August, 1990.
TS SUM: Traffic Safety Summit, U.S. Department of Transportation, 1990.
SG DD: Surgeon General's Workshop on Drunk Driving, U.S. Department of Health and Human Services, 1988.
Source: Education Development Center, Inc: Building bridges between traffic safety and public health. Newton, MA, 1991, EDC and Natl. Highway Traffic Safety Admin. Region I.

Traffic safety goals and strategies: federal policy statements—cont'd

	2000	NHTSA	TS SUM	SG DD
Amend FARS to include seat belt use info			•	
Establish seat belt coalitions in each state			•	
Assist service organizations & medical communities in providing car seats			•	
Improve technology of restraint systems	•	•		•-airbags
Fund 3 statewide programs to educate public about automatic crash protection devices		•		

Drinking & driving

Goals

	2000	NHTSA	TS SUM	SG DD
Alcohol-related motor vehicle crash deaths per 100,000 people	8.5	Reduce		
Alcohol-related motor vehicle crash deaths per 100 million VMT	0.9	by 10% by '92		

Legislation/enforcement

	2000	NHTSA	TS SUM	SG DD
Passage of admin. per se	•	•	•	•
Lower legal BAC to .08			•	•
Test all drivers in serious crashes	•		•	•
National Registry of problem drivers		•		
Roadsite checkpoints		•		
Provisional entry system for <21 yr. olds				•
.00 BAC for drivers <21 yrs. old				•
Enforce restrictions on youths obtaining alcohol	•			•
Prohibit TV & radio ads for alcohol			•	
Provide technical assistance to communities to develop and improve effective enforcement of underage drinking and driving		•		

Information/education

	2000	NHTSA	TS SUM	SG DD
Increase funds for education				•
Increase public awareness of impact of DUI		•	•	•
Work with media on ongoing basis	•		•	•
National media campaign		•		
Train judges, prosecutors, and police on DUI issues		•		
Info on drinking & driving in schools			•	•
Encourage drug-free events in schools				•
Guidelines and education for communities on alcohol & recreation		•		•
Professional education on drinking & driving: teachers, healthcare providers, elected officials, parents				•
Provide training and technical assistance to corporations implementing impaired driving initiatives		•		
Involve insurance industry in education efforts		•		

	2000	NHTSA	TS SUM	SG DD
Data/evaluation				
Establish committee to collect databases, assess validity and completeness				•
Evaluate DD countermeasures for effectiveness, acceptability, cost				•
Determine characteristics of drunk drivers				•
Other				
Establish coalitions in each community to develop programs, advocate for legislation				•
Cooperate with community organizations (e.g., MADD)	•		•	•
Speeding				
Gather data on effects of 65 MPH			•	
Prohibit use of radar detectors	•		•	
Prohibit ads depicting speeding			•	
PSAs & news items about speeding	•	•	•	
Awareness campaign for legislators & other policymakers			•	
Evaluate effectiveness of new speed measuring technology		•		
Motorcycle helmets				
Goals				
Fatalities per 100,000	1.5			
Usage rates	80%			
Number of states with mandatory helmet laws			All, by '92	
Legislation/enforcement				
Mandatory helmet laws	•	•		•
Pedestrian safety				
Goals				
Pedestrian fatalities	2.4/100,000			

2000: Year 2000 Objectives for the Nation, U.S. Department of Health and Human Services, 1989.
NHTSA: Moving America Safely—NHTSA's Priority Plan 1990-1992, August, 1990.
TS SUM: Traffic Safety Summit, U.S. Department of Transportation, 1990.
SG DD: Surgeon General's Workshop on Drunk Driving, U.S. Department of Health and Human Services, 1988.
Source: Education Development Center, Inc: Building bridges between traffic safety and public health. Newton, MA, 1991, EDC and Natl. Highway Traffic Safety Admin. Region I.

Traffic safety goals and strategies: federal policy statements—cont'd

	2000	NHTSA	TS SUM	SG DD
Other				
Public information	•	•		
Crosswalk design/sidewalks		•		
Signaling			•	
Grants to community traffic safety programs		•		
Bike safety				
Bike helmets encouraged	•			
Highway design & maintenance				
Promote safer design & maintain	•	•		
Data collection: general				
Develop a common set of data elements to be collected in state police reports		•		
Integrate injury-related data collected by law enforcement, transportation, fire safety, health departments, EMS, hospital records, and others	•			

• •

Chapter 14

Community Water and Waste Control

❖

If you consider the contribution of plumbing to human life, the other sciences fade into insignificance.
JAMES GORMAN

OBJECTIVES

When you finish this chapter, you should be able to:

• Identify the sources and contaminants of community water supplies

• Describe the major procedures for sewage and solid waste disposal, including toxic agent controls

• Plan for the improvement and enforcement of environmental protection measures directed at water and waste control

From the introductory chapters you will recall that community health consists of strategies under three broad headings: health promotion, health protection, and health services. Health protection measures consist primarily of environmental controls, including those directed at water, waste, food supplies, vectors, housing, work environments, air, noise, and radiation. Among these, water and waste management have had the most direct, pervasive, and continuous relationship to health. Most of the other factors have much to do with esthetics, comfort, and quality of life but usually threaten health less directly, less immediately, or less frequently. This could change in the future, with growing pollution of the atmosphere and of food supplies. These issues will be addressed in subsequent chapters in this section. This chapter will address water supply, and liquid and solid waste control.

SOCIAL AND ECONOMIC IMPORTANCE OF WATER TO THE COMMUNITY

The life and the economy of virtually every community depend on water supply and quality. With 80% of water consumption going for irrigation, an

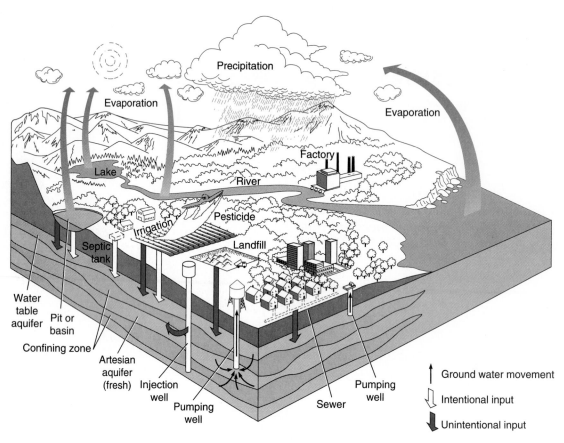

FIGURE 14-1
The recycling of water through the air and soil includes the contamination of streams and groundwater sources in the water table aquifers and the lower artesian aquifer.
Source: U.S. Environmental Protection Agency.

average of 7% is left for municipal use, and the remainder is divided almost equally among manufacturing, mining, livestock watering, and steam-electric generation. Greater congestion of people in urban areas, concentration of industry, population mobility, and sheer increases in numbers have made control and distribution of the water supply more efficient but more vulnerable to crisis.

Metropolitan centers, which have usually developed near waterways or lakes (**surface water**) for historical and economic reasons, actually have fewer problems in maintaining an adequate, safe water supply than do rural areas with dispersed populations and small towns. On the other hand, the heavy planting of trees, each of which consumes some 300 gallons of water per day, and the paving of surfaces that once absorbed water have caused the reservoirs and water tables of some cities to subside. Thus, there are many trade-offs between quality of life (as determined by such things as trees, paved streets, manufactured goods, irrigated and fertilized foods) and the resulting depletion and pollution of the water supply.

Fortunately, most of society's uses of water allow

it to be used over and over—recycled through soil, retrieved as surface water from lakes, streams, rivers, and as **groundwater** from **aquifers,** then redistributed through evaporation and rain or snow (Figure 14-1). The growing populations and the runoff conditions of some regions, however, place an increasing burden on communities, states or provinces, and national governments to negotiate the control and distribution of water supplies.

EPIDEMIOLOGY OF INFECTIOUS AND TOXIC AGENTS IN WATER

Health problems attributed to infectious and toxic agents in water include acute effects such as infection and poisoning, teratogenesis (abnormality pro-

duced in the fetus during pregnancy), developmental abnormalities, mutagenesis (damage to genes), oncogenesis (including cancer), neurological and behavioral impairment, immunological damage, and chronic degenerative diseases involving the lungs, joints, digestive and vascular systems, kidneys, liver, and endocrine organs.

Distribution and Trends

Infectious and toxic agents affect people differently, depending on their sex, age, history of past exposures, and possible predisposing genetic conditions. Similarly, the genetic and chronic disease effects of infectious and toxic agents may be manifested in varying ways in future years or future generations. For these reasons, the current incidence and prevalence rates of diseases associated with waterborne agents do not accurately measure either the true potency of some of these agents or the effectiveness of current control and protection measures.

These uncertainties make the tasks of risk identification and risk reduction enormously difficult, particularly since more than 60,000 chemical compounds are produced commercially and more than 1000 new compounds appear on the market each year. Over 13,000 substances currently in use have been identified as being toxic; many of these find their way into water systems. Most of the infectious agents of greatest concern were mentioned in Chapter 11 (for example, see Tables 11-2, 11-3, and 11-4 for information about the alvine discharge diseases). This chapter will address the control of both infectious and toxic agents in the water supply.

Control Measures

Current evidence builds a convincing case for the carcinogenicity in humans of 20 chemicals and compounds; over 2300 specific chemicals are suspected carcinogens. Also, more than 20 agents are known to be associated with birth defects in humans, and many times this number are associated with birth defects in animals.

Regulation and surveillance. Current contamination of drinking water supplies in the United States range from 1% to 2%. This may expose as much as 10% of the population. The U.S. Environmental Protection Agency (**EPA**) operates a series of programs to prevent new contamination. If EPA guidelines are followed, there should be almost no preventable contamination of water associated with wastewater management. A related goal is to develop a plan to protect communities from the consequences of toxic agents in existing sites of toxic solid waste disposal, as from the Love Canal in upstate New York. Approximately 30,000 solid waste disposal sites may be involved.

There is as yet no comprehensive surveillance system in any country to monitor new or continuing environmental threats to health. The development of

such a system to assess and reduce the risks from infectious and toxic agent exposures is a particularly important objective for communities.

Health education. Access to information and education about hazardous exposures is an essential goal. Objectives include informing managers of industrial firms; increasing the ability of consumers and health professionals to detect, control, and deal with the effects of hazardous exposures; and increasing the capabilities of community health agencies and hospitals to respond appropriately.

Water Uses

Communities need water for recreation, irrigation, industry, and domestic use. The population increases, industry expands, and other water uses multiply, yet the quantity of water remains fixed. Water must be reused because the supply is finite. Society's ingenuity is economically and technically challenged by the task of maintaining the quality of water.

At the beginning of the twentieth century communities used water that people assumed was safe for household purposes as long as it was clear. Not until residents recognized that water was a vehicle for disease transmission was preventive action taken. It took years of community education before citizens understood what had to be done to safeguard the water supply. In some communities officials took the lead in providing the people with a safe and adequate water supply, whereas in other communities the people had to push the officials to take necessary action.

Today the concern is as much with toxic agents in the water as with infectious agents. Contamination by chemicals and nuclear wastes threatens community water supplies in ways that worry citizens now as much as organic pollution ever worried their parents and grandparents. It is not known what the additive effects of these chemicals will be on the total incidence of cancer. As water resources be-

---

Objectives for Regulation of Contaminants by the Year 2000

- Reduce human exposure to toxic agents by confining total pounds of toxic agents released into the air, water, and soil to no more than 0.24 billion pounds of those toxic agents included on the Department of Health and Human Services list of carcinogens. Baseline: 0.32 billion pounds in 1988.
- Reduce human exposure to solid waste-related water, air, and soil contamination, as measured by a reduction in average pounds of municipal solid waste produced per person each day to no more than 3.6 pounds. Baseline: 4 pounds per person each day in 1988.
- Increase to at least 85% the proportion of people who receive a supply of drinking water that meets the safe drinking water standards established by the EPA. Baseline: 74% of 58,099 community water systems serving approximately 80% of the U.S. population in 1988.

come in shorter supply, more and more surface water used for drinking water will be recycled or reprocessed, continuing the recycling of chemical pollutants.

Water is the most important commodity humans consume, and the consumption of water has increased steadily, so that today in the United States the average daily use for domestic purposes is 150 gallons per person. Communities with industries requiring vast amounts of water may have a total use that reaches 2000 gallons per person per day. Community leaders tend to be too conservative in estimating future water requirements. Many areas in the United States will experience an increasing shortage for the rest of this century unless low-cost desalinization of sea water is employed or the harnessing of runoff from glaciers is successful. The cost of water may double or triple in the future, especially if desalinization remains an expensive procedure.

Etiology and Effects of Toxic Agents

Substances found naturally in water or occurring as industrial pollutants can be harmful when they reach concentrations above levels established by the Safe

Drinking Water Act in the United States, by the Federal-Provincial Advisory Committee on Environmental and Occupational Health of Canada, or by the guidelines of the World Health Organization.

The primary drinking water contaminants and the sources and possible health effects of each contaminant are shown in Table 14-1. Maximum levels permitted are usually stated in milligrams per liter of water. In 1989, dozens of new contaminants were added to the EPA list, requiring more extensive testing. The significance of selected chemical elements and compounds in water are discussed in the following sections.

Pesticides. Various insecticides, fungicides, rodenticides, and herbicides, present in water primarily as a result of agricultural runoff and spills, pose increasing problems because they are environmentally persistent and cumulative in the water and food chains. These chlorinated hydrocarbons are neuropoisons that can cause symptoms ranging from dizziness to convulsions and even to death by either cardiac or respiratory arrest. Some pesticides may be teratogenic or mutagenic (causing species abnormalities or species alterations). Endrin, a pesticide

TABLE 14-1
Primary drinking water contaminants and the source and possible health risks associated with each

Substance	Source	Health risk
Chlorinated solvents	Industrial pollution. Used for chemical degreasing, machine maintenance and as intermediaries in the manufacture of other chemicals	Cancer
Trihalomethanes	Produced by chemical reactions in water that has been disinfected with chlorine	Liver and kidney damage, possibly cancer
Lead	Old piping and solder in public water distribution systems, homes, and other buildings	Nerve problems, learning disabilities in children, birth defects, possibly cancer
PCBs	Wastes from many outmoded manufacturing operations	Liver damage, possibly cancer
Pathogenic bacteria and viruses	Leaking septic tanks, overflowing sewer lines	Acute gastrointestinal illness, more serious diseases such as meningitis

Source: U.S. Environmental Protection Agency.

commonly used on field crops, is the most toxic, with a standard limit of 0.0002 mg/L. Lindane, used to control cotton insects and grasshoppers, must be limited to 0.004 mg/L in the drinking water supply. Herbicides used in weed control may cause muscular tenseness, paralysis, and coma and may trigger mutations and teratogenic effects.

Radionuclides. Uranium, radon, and radium occur naturally in groundwater and to a lesser degree in surface water, as a result of leaching from rock deposits. These radiochemicals are proven carcinogens. The standard limits in drinking water are somewhat arbitrary; for radium, the limit is 5 pCi/L (Picocurie per liter of water).

Selenium. A chemical element obtained as a by-product of copper mining, selenium (Se) is normally found in groundwater and occasionally in surface water as a natural occurrence. Selenium attacks the central nervous system and can be fatal in extreme cases. Minor amounts, however, may be beneficial to health. There is some evidence of lower cancer rates in areas where the level of selenium in the water supply exceeds the 0.01 mg/L standard.

Other standards. Most other chemical agents in water are not toxic but need to be restricted in drinking water resources for other reasons. **Turbidity** refers to cloudiness of water caused by a variety of suspended materials, sometimes organic, but usually inorganic. Turbidity makes disinfection and proper bacteriological analysis more difficult, so a standard limit has been established as 1 turbidity unit (tu). Turbidity can also harbor viruses and cause tastes and odors.

Corrosivity is the tendency of water to corrode metals. It is related to pH, alkalinity, hardness, and dissolved oxygen. Chloride (Cl) in drinking water produces a salty taste when combined with sodium (Na) and may cause corrosiveness, so a 300 mg/L limit has been set. The presence of color makes water objectionable primarily for visual reasons but

may also indicate organic contamination from decaying vegetation.

Waterborne Infectious Diseases

Pathogens of humans do not normally multiply in water, yet they can survive in water and remain virulent enough to set up an infection in a new host. Water serves as a vehicle of transfer of diseases of the alimentary canal and of transfer of certain worms, notably the schistosomes. Evidence is conclusive that five infectious diseases—typhoid, paratyphoid, giardiasis, cholera, and bacillary dysentery—are transmitted by water. The contention that AIDS, viral hepatitis, amebic dysentery, and poliomyelitis are transmitted by water is not substantiated. Likewise, no evidence exists that respiratory diseases of humans are conveyed via water.

Since 1975, *Giardia lamblia* has been the most commonly identified pathogen in waterborne disease outbreaks in the United States and Canada (Figure 14-2, *A*). Giardiasis, an intestinal infestation by a single-celled protozoan, is transmitted more frequently in day care centers where frequent diaper changes carry the organism, than in drinking water. Most water outbreaks occur where sewers and people pollute surface water and backpackers, hikers, and others drink untreated water from lakes and streams (Figure 14-2, *B* and *C*). Public water supplies can become infected by upstream human and animal feces deposited in or near waterways.

Less than 2% of all reported cases of typhoid fever, salmonellosis, shigellosis, or infectious hepatitis since 1951 have been traced to water. In contrast, more than one fourth of all reported cases of giardiasis were attributable to water. One reason *Giardia* slip by community water systems (Figure 14-2, *B*) is that in small communities, especially recreational communities, the treatment of water is limited to disinfection with chlorine. Standard chlorine treatment may kill coliform bacteria, but *Giardia* cysts survive, especially when the water is unfiltered so that other turbid matter absorbs much of the chlo-

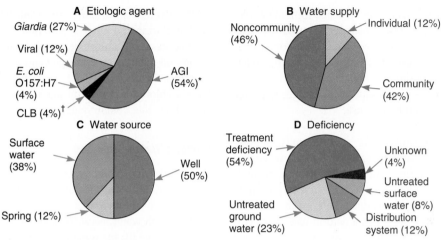

A Etiologic agent

Giardia (27%)

Viral (12%)

E. coli
O157:H7
(4%)

CLB (4%)[†]

AGI
(54%)*

B Water supply

Noncommunity
(46%)

Individual (12%)

Community
(42%)

C Water source

Surface
water
(38%)

Well
(50%)

Spring (12%)

D Deficiency

Treatment
deficiency
(54%)

Unknown
(4%)

Untreated
surface
water (8%)

Untreated
ground
water (23%)

Distribution
system (12%)

*AGI = acute gastrointestinal illness of unknown etiology.
†CLB = cyanobacteria (blue-green algae)-like bodies.

FIGURE 14-2
Outbreaks associated with water intended for drinking, United States, 1989-1990.
Source: *MMWR* 40:SS-3, 1991.

rine. Filtration is the key to stopping *Giardia* cysts from surviving chemical treatment of water (Figure 14-2, *D*).

SOURCES OF WATER

For community purposes, water must be in sufficient supply and free from contamination, pollution, and turbidity. Water that may be suitable for household purposes may not be satisfactory for individual use if it is high in mineral content.

Rainfall is the primary source of water, whether it is surface water in a river, lake, pond, or reservoir created by a dam, or whether it is groundwater that has percolated through the ground to a stratum of gravel. In nature there is no pure water. All untreated water contains dissolved gases, minerals, and organic matter from the decay of algae, funguses, and other life forms.

Hardness of water is caused by the presence of calcium and magnesium salts. Water with a hardness of 100 parts per million (ppm) or less of calcium carbonate is soft enough for household use. Softening can be done at the time of filtration by adding lime and soda; the calcium carbonate formed will precipitate out and leave a residual hardness of less than 100 ppm. To reduce alkalinity, the effluent from the softening process may be carbonated with carbon dioxide.

Drinking water containing too much sulfate (2000 ppm), chloride (1000 ppm), or calcium carbonate (300 ppm) will cause digestive disturbances in most people. Osmotic balance in the human colon can be upset by water high in mineral content, and severe diarrhea can result.

Groundwater Supplies

Groundwater from shallow wells and deep wells is usually the preferred source for communities with populations of under 50,000. Rarely will a larger city locate sufficient groundwater for its needs, although San Antonio, Texas, the tenth largest city in the United States with more than one million people, depends on a groundwater supply. Groundwater has certain merits. It is relatively free from contamination, pollution, turbidity, and color. Its disadvantages are its scarcity, its high mineral content, and the threat of sinking property when groundwater levels are lowered by overuse.

Underground source. As a community supply, groundwater is usually safe, and the low capital funds and operating costs involved make groundwater an economical source. The first requirement is to find an adequate supply. This means locating a gravel bed that serves as a natural reservoir. Test wells are drilled to outline the reservoir. The object is to locate a yard-thick gravel bed below an impervious layer 60 feet or more beneath the surface. At least one more gravel stratum should be located to ensure an uninterrupted flow of water by having a second source. The rate of underground flow can be measured by putting dye or an electrical current into one hole and timing the interval required for it to reach another hole that is being pumped.

Wells. Wells are cased with pipe that has a brass intake screen where the pipe is embedded in the gravel. Spacing of wells depends on the underground flow and community needs. Electrically operated centrifugal pumps raise the water into a concrete receiving reservoir. A second set of pumps forces the water up into a large storage or pressure tank.

Bacteria attach to sand grains and secrete a sticky covering that causes other bacteria to adhere to this biological film. As water percolates into the ground, bacteria are filtered out by the sticky film. This natural process purifies groundwater. However, groundwater may be contaminated by seepage along the well casing, by limestone, by other previous material above the groundwater supply that does not intercept bacteria, by sea water near the seacoast, and by direct surface contamination into the groundwater stratum (see Figure 14-1).

Well water is normally free from turbidity and can be chlorinated without filtration. Frequently, it is unnecessary to chlorinate groundwater, although it may be done as an extra precaution. Some communities do not chlorinate their groundwater but have a chlorination unit on hand in case the water should become contaminated.

Surface Water Supplies

New York City requires more than 1 billion gallons of water a day. Multiply this by 365 and one gets some idea of the task that city has in supplying its citizens with water. New York gets only 10% of its water from wells; the remainder comes from surface water and necessitates a number of protected storage reservoirs and flumes. Cities such as Chicago and Milwaukee are fortunate in having Lake Michigan as an excellent water source. The Mississippi River serves as both a water source and a sewage disposal receptacle for a long string of cities, including Minneapolis, St. Louis, Memphis, and New Orleans. Surface water has certain merits. It is more abundant, more easily measured, and softer than groundwater. However, it is frequently polluted by shore wash, transportation waste, industrial waste, and human waste. It is usually contaminated, is highly colored, and is often turbid.

Treatment. With the increasing population and the high mobility of people today, virtually all surface water must be treated before it is safe for human consumption. Some lakes and streams have clear water, so no filtration is necessary; however, chlorination may be required. Most surface water is so turbid, polluted, and contaminated that both filtration and chlorination are necessary.

Rapid sand filtration was developed in the United States and is designed to filter out particles and bacteria. If the water contains considerable **sediment,** a preliminary settling chamber may be used to precede the treatment process. Otherwise, the water is pumped directly from the intake in the river or lake into the series of tanks comprising the treatment plant. These tanks are usually of concrete construction; frequently, surplus tanks will be constructed so that some tanks may be shut off and cleaned or repaired while the rest of the tanks carry on the treatment process. The treatment usually consists of five steps: **flash mix, flocculation, sedimentation, filtration,** and **chlorination,** as shown in Figure 14-3.

Flash mix is done in a relatively small tank. Aluminum sulfate is fed into the incoming water and forms a flaky hydrate, or floc. At the same time, chlorine is added.

Flocculation consists of trapping particles by the mechanical process of adsorption of suspended solids. Because flocculation causes an increase in the density and size of coagulated particles, floc particles settle at a fast rate. Flocculation tanks are fitted with slowly rotating wooden paddles to ensure an even and continuous water-chemical mixture.

Sedimentation is the settling of the floc and is carried out in sedimentation tanks connected directly to the flocculation tanks (Figure 14-4). Water is retained here for about 2 hours to allow the floc to settle to the bottom of the tanks, where it will be scraped into troughs. Other troughs around the top of the tanks collect the upper layer of water, which is relatively free of floc.

If the water has an odor, activated carbon may be added to the water in the sedimentation tank or may be added at some other stage of treatment. The activated carbon is effective in removing odor and objectionable taste.

Filtration removes whatever turbidity may remain after the flocculation and settling. At the bottom of a filtration tank is a layer of gravel, topped

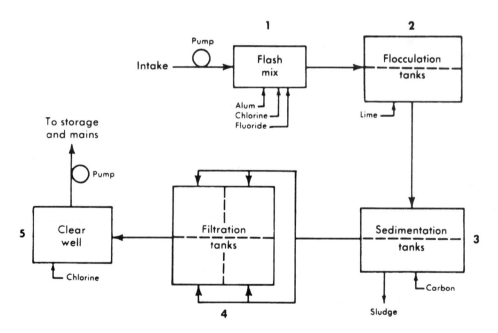

FIGURE 14-3
Flow diagram of water treatment, beginning with the introduction of the floc material, then through flocculation, sedimentation, and filtering. The clear water is then ready for final chlorination to assure potability.

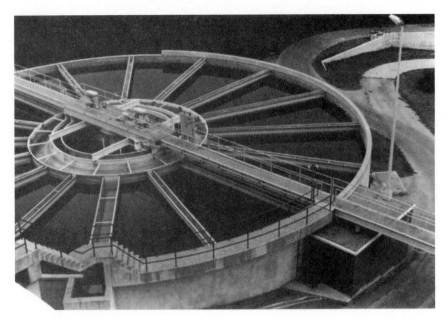

FIGURE 14-4
Flocculation tanks in a series. The separation of tanks allows for cleaning and repairing some tanks while others remain in use.
Source: Texas Department of Health.

by either sand or anthracite coal. Water percolates through this medium and goes out via drains at the bottom of the tank. To clean floc that accumulates on the anthracite coal or sand, the water level is lowered to the top of the troughs just above the coal level. The water flow is then reversed so that the accumulated floc is flushed into the troughs and carried off as waste.

Chlorination, the final step, decontaminates the water and is a simple, effective method for destroying bacteria. Postchlorination is designed to bring the residual chlorine to a level between 0.25 and 0.7 ppm. The chlorine residual level is determined for water in the distribution system as well as at the plant of origin. Two samples a day at the plant and one from the system are recommended. A chlorine residual between 0.2 and 0.3 ppm will destroy all

bacterial pathogens of humans; at this concentration, the chlorine cannot be detected by either taste or smell. In emergencies a chlorine residual of 0.7 ppm may be maintained. Although chlorine can be detected at this concentration, it is not harmful to humans.

The *slow sand* (European) method of filtration uses instead of an artificial gelatinous layer, a film produced by bacteria as the interceptive medium. The rapid sand method is 40 times faster and generally more reliable; thus, it is preferred in most communities establishing new water systems.

Addition of Fluorides

Based on available knowledge, the most effective, inexpensive, and simple method of preventing dental caries is the fluoridation of the public water supply. By studying local areas where people had a low incidence of dental caries, scientists discovered that these areas had water that naturally contained about 1 ppm of fluorides. Where the fluoride content of water was much lower than this, the incidence of caries was high.

Distribution. On the recommendation of dentists and public health scientists, U.S. municipalities began adding fluorides to water supplies as a preventive measure against dental caries. Most water supplies contain a small amount of fluorides; the need is simply to add enough fluorides to bring the concentration up to 1 ppm. Northern cities in the United States raise the fluoride content slightly above this level, and southern cities hold the fluoride content just a little below 1 ppm. This is an adjustment to the difference in water consumption and average water temperatures.

One national health objective for the year 2000 is to increase to at least 75% the proportion of persons served by community water systems providing optimal levels of fluoride—a goal already achieved by 20 states and the District of Columbia (Figure 14-5). To achieve this objective nationally, an additional 30 million persons must receive optimally fluoridated water from public water systems. People in more than 5860 communities have public water supplies containing an adequate concentration of fluorides.

New York City, San Francisco, Baltimore, Chicago, Philadelphia, Pittsburgh, Milwaukee, St. Louis, and Washington, D.C., have fluoridated wa-

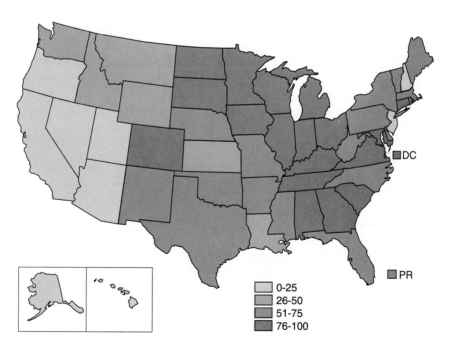

FIGURE 14-5

Percentage of states' population on public water who receive fluoridated drinking water, United States, 1989.
Source: *MMWR* 41:375, 1992.

ter supplies. It has been the history of public health that the small communities are the last to adopt new health measures, and this has held true for fluoridation. Only about 40% of U.S. cities with populations between 2500 and 10,000 have adopted fluoridation, and less than 20% of communities under 2500 fluoridate their water supplies. Canada, Sweden, the Netherlands, West Germany, Japan, and many other nations are making fluoridation available to their populations.

Opposition. Public health people are not surprised by the opposition to fluoridation, because health innovations have always been opposed. Vaccination, pasteurization of milk, chlorination of water supplies, and even indoor plumbing were initially opposed by the easily frightened, the uninformed, and those who resisted change. Fortunately, fluoridation is gradually gaining acceptance, and this is repeating public health history. Courts in the United States have ruled that fluoridation is a reasonable legal exercise of the local police power in the interest of the public health and is not a violation of individual rights.

Some communities have water supplies with a high natural fluoride content of 8 ppm. This concentration prevents caries but causes mottling of the teeth. The only other suspected harm to the human body from such a high fluoride content is possible orthopedic problems for the elderly. These communities add phosphate to the water to reduce fluorides to a level of 1 ppm. In communities having a water supply with a natural fluoride content of 2 ppm, people have health histories showing no deviation from that of the population at large.

Alternatives. In communities that do not fluoridate their municipal water supply, some citizens have their family dentist or physician brush their children's teeth with a covering of fluoride at each visit. As a similar preventive measure, some elementary

schools have their children retain fluoridated water in their mouths for about 40 to 60 seconds.

TESTING OF WATER

As a community health measure, bacteriological and chemical examination of a municipal water supply can be of great importance to industry and to the general public. Radiological examination of water is of more recent vintage and not usually a concern, but in specific instances the possibility of radioactive contaminants in water can be significant. **Bioassays** are necessary to evaluate toxicity in fish, and biological examinations are used to determine the extent of plankton and other life forms in the water.

The Coliform Test

For some 70 years the standard test of drinking water safety was the **coliform** determination. Coliform organisms are not pathogenic, but because they are always present in the human intestinal tract their presence in water is a sure indicator of fecal contamination. Unfortunately, the test for coliform bacteria (*E. coli*) is tedious and time-consuming, providing results too late to prevent the ingestion of water from the supply being checked. For quality control purposes, the quicker chlorine test is used.

The Chlorine Test

The chlorine residual determination is a simple test to ensure that a sufficient level of chlorine is being maintained, given the temperature and pH of the water, to destroy organisms of the coliform group and organisms pathogenic to man. Because turbidity may interfere with the effectiveness of chlorine, the turbidity limit was lowered from 5 tu in the 1962 standards of the EPA to 1 tu in the 1976 standard. Water purveyors are still required to take bacteriologic samples at regular intervals. The number of samples required ranges from 1 sample per month for communities with fewer than 2500 residents to 3000 samples per month for communities with populations greater than 1 million.

Other Tests

Virological techniques have barely advanced to the point that efficient tests can be used for routine monitoring of water quality. Viral agents of infection for man occur in a ratio of 1 per 50,000 to 100,000 coliform organisms, suggesting that it should be possible to estimate the frequency of enteric viruses by using the coliform test. Unfortunately, viruses are more resistant than are coliform organisms to water treatments, including chlorination; thus the ratio of viruses to coliform organisms might be much higher during an outbreak of a viral disease, such as hepatitis type A.

Chemical examination of water varies, depending on the specific chemical one wishes to detect. Tests for hardness are most frequent. A test for chlorine residual is used to determine the decontamination effect of chlorination.

REGULATION OF WATER SUPPLIES

Providing water to a community is a recognized function of local government in most countries. The city government usually constructs and manages the water system as a corporate function. This is not a responsibility of the health department. In most communities a special water department or the department of public works operates the water system. A few communities grant a franchise to a private corporation to sell water as a commodity to the public.

Although providing water to the community is a local government function, the regulation of public water supplies is the legal responsibility of the state, which usually delegates this authority to the state or

provincial department of health. A public water system is one that provides piped water for human consumption and has at least 15 service connections or regularly serves at least 25 people. If a city wishes to build a water plant, the plans must be approved by engineers from the state department of health. In practice, these engineers serve as advisors for the city in developing the plans. This advisory service is without cost to the city. Even though the city pays to have plans drawn and the water system constructed, it is the state that ensures the adequacy of the plans and the construction.

Once the plant is in operation, the state continues its supervisory authority. Plant operators must be certified by the state. Regular reports on water analysis must be submitted to the state as the state department of health decrees. The state representative serves as a consultant should the community encounter a problem in the operation of its water system. This service is free of charge to the community.

Safe Drinking Water Legislation

A 1970 national community water supply study in the United States revealed that the quality of household water was declining. Part of this decline was attributed to the careless use of various chemical substances and other toxic wastes. As an outgrowth of this study by the EPA and growing public concern, Congress enacted the Water Pollution Act of 1971 and the Safe Drinking Water Act of 1974. This provided for the periodic updating of water standards. Congress also authorized the EPA to support state and local community drinking water programs by providing financial and technical assistance. It is recognized that the federal government, through the EPA, has the authority and responsibility for setting and enforcing standards and otherwise supervising public water systems, overriding state authority.

Standards. The EPA establishes standards for drinking water quality. These standards represent the Maximum Contaminant Levels (MCLs) allowable and consist of numerical criteria for specified contaminants.

Treatment and monitoring. Local water supply systems are required to monitor their drinking water periodically for contaminants with MCLs and for a broad range of other contaminants as specified by EPA. Additionally, to protect underground sources of drinking water, the EPA requires periodic monitoring of wells used for underground injection of hazardous waste, including monitoring of the ground water above the wells.

Enforcement. States have the primary responsibility for the enforcement of drinking water standards, monitoring, and reporting requirements. States also determine requirements for environmentally sound underground injection of wastes.

Grants. The Safe Drinking Water Act authorizes the EPA to award grants to states for developing and implementing programs to protect drinking water at the tap and groundwater resources. These several grant programs may be for supporting state public water supply, wellhead protection, and underground injection programs, including compliance and enforcement.

Thus a vigorous, organized program was authorized by Congress to ensure the nation's people safe drinking water. Standards include maximum contaminant levels and general criteria for operation, maintenance, and intake water quality. Secondary standards relating only to taste, odor, and appearance of drinking water are enforced only when the individual states want to.

A state can continue to enforce its own laws and regulations governing drinking water supplies if it complies with certain requirements such as the following:

1. Adoption of regulations at least equal to federal regulations

2. Adoption and implementation of adequate enforcement procedures
3. Provision for emergency circumstances
4. Keeping adequate records and providing reports for the EPA

Recent controversies. The Clean Water Act, as the Water Pollution Act of 1971 came to be known, must be reauthorized every 5 years. The debates leading up to the 1994 bills to reauthorize the act set the stage for struggles over enforcement and administration of this legislation in the years ahead. According to national surveys, public support for clean water has increased. This support, however, is countered by the Chemical Manufacturers Association that emphasizes deregulation. They have suggested amendments to the act that would (1) delay or abandon the act's cleanup goals for toxic waste sites; (2) roll back deadlines for industries to clean up their own toxic wastes; (3) weaken or eliminate the national standards for limiting toxic agents in drinking water (described earlier in this chapter); (4) curtail the EPA's budget, strength, and authority; and (5) revert to regulatory policies that Congress rejected as unworkable in 1972.

One of the central strategies in the nationwide cleanup of water would control "nonpoint" sources of water pollution; these involve toxic agents that do not come out of a specific drainpipe but run off from fields. Although these nonpoint sources of water pollution have been given less attention than the industrial-point sources, they account for over half of all water pollution (Table 14-2).

DRINKING WATER IN DEVELOPING COUNTRIES

The World Health Organization (WHO) declared 1981 to 1990 the International Drinking Water Supply and Sanitation Decade. This represented an essential first stage in the global strategy of "Health for All by the Year 2000." Only 43% of the people

TABLE 14-2
Pollutants and their sources

	Common pollutant categories							
	BOD	Bacteria	Nutrients	Ammonia	Turbidity	TDS	Acids	Toxics
Point sources								
Municipal sewage treatment plants	•	•	•	•				•
Industrial facilities	•							•
Combined sewer overflows	•	•	•	•	•	•		•
Nonpoint sources								
Agricultural runoff	•	•	•		•	•		•
Urban runoff	•	•	•		•	•		•
Construction runoff			•		•			•
Mining runoff					•	•	•	•
Septic systems	•	•	•					•
Landfills/Spills	•							•
Silviculture runoff	•		•		•			•

Source: U.S. Environmental Protection Agency.
Abbreviations: BOD, Biological Oxygen Demand, TDS, Total Dissolved Solids.

in developing countries had access to safe drinking water. In rural areas of these countries only 29% had such access. By increasing the quantity and quality of water supplied to these 3 million people, WHO's ''Decade'' program helped reduce the incidence of many diseases among the people most at risk. The estimates now are that one-half billion rural residents and several hundred million city dwellers in the developing world lack safe drinking water (Figure 14-6).

New technologies are sought to provide higher standards of service at lower unit cost to large numbers of relatively dispersed and isolated villages and towns. Local community and external resources must be increased to provide for the construction and maintenance of public and private water supplies. A Japanese citizens' movement has provided a model of such a new technology, in which fresh water and sanitation systems are being provided in-expensively to poorer neighborhoods through a combination of simple technology, decentralized systems, and community organization. The Jishu-Koza Citizen's Movement has helped communities build backyard ponds to recycle sewage and has installed waste disposal systems that require little water, unlike the large, centralized public systems of urban communities in both developing and industrialized countries.

COMMUNITY WASTES

Household, commercial, recreational, and industrial wastes are the general sources of community wastes. These are in the form of garbage, refuse, street cleanings, human and animal discharges, kitchen, scavenger, and commercial wastes, and wastes from manufacturing and processing plants. The sheer vol-

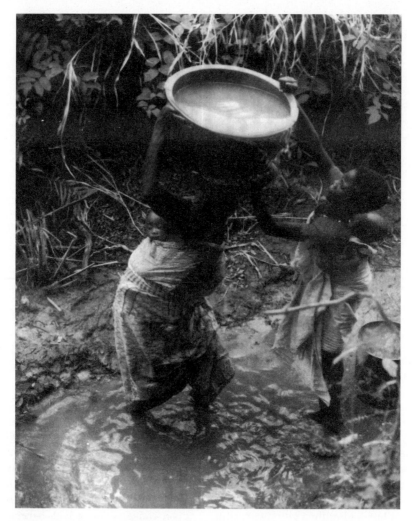

FIGURE 14-6
Bringing water from streams and wells has been the burden of women in many developing countries, as in this typical waterhole scene in Nigeria.
Source: Photo by W. Brieger, courtesy World Health Organization.

ume in a year would run into millions of tons and would make a mountainous stockpile. If each year's wastes accumulated, in a period of 20 years a community would be buried by its own waste products. Fortunately, the lowly bacteria, by decomposing an-imal proteins, not only reduce the great mass of wastes to a negligible volume but also make invaluable nitrogen available for reuse. This process is customarily referred to as the **nitrogen cycle,** as shown in Figure 14-7.

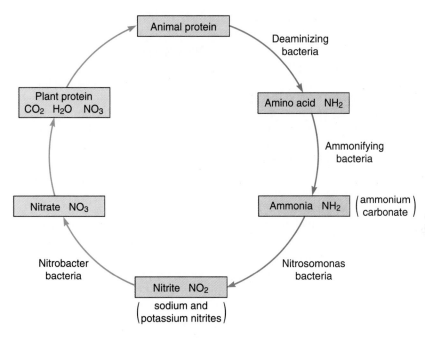

FIGURE 14-7
The nitrogen cycle explains the decomposition of organic material in the soil, which goes on continuously thanks to four varieties of bacteria that save communities from burying themselves in their own waste.

Nitrogen Cycle

Animal proteins begin decomposing by the action of bacteria that convert the proteins to amino acids. Another set of bacteria next converts the amino acids to ammonia. The ammonia combines with carbon dioxide to form ammonium carbonate, which in turn is converted to nitrites by a third type of bacteria. Nitrites combine with sodium and potassium, and the resulting nitrites are converted into nitrates by yet another group of bacteria—*Nitrobacter* organisms. Nitrates dissolved in soil water diffuse into the root hairs of plants, where they combine with carbon dioxide and water to form plant proteins. The plant proteins are consumed by animals and converted into animal proteins, thus completing the nitrogen cycle.

Communities aid nature in this process of waste disposal by providing the beneficial bacteria with a favorable environment and by the dilution, chemical treatment, burning, and recycling of wastes. The task of disposing of wastes is a continual one that is both important and costly. Processes involved in getting rid of human wastes are also processes for destroying or removing pathogens that can cause disease and death. Perhaps the most important of these processes is sewage disposal.

SEWAGE DISPOSAL

Sewage consists of the liquid wastes from household effluents, commercial effluents, and industrial liquid wastes. It is carried in a system of pipes and other means of conveyance called a *sewage system.* In some communities storm water also is carried in the *sewerage* system; in other communities a separate system of pipes carries off storm water, saving the wastewater treatment plant from having to treat large volumes of rain water.

Generally, community sewage will be about 99% water containing animal, plant, and mineral matter in solution and in suspension. Bacteria of many types, mostly nonpathogenic, are always present. Paper, sticks, grease, and other materials are in suspension.

The strength of sewage is measured by its biochemical oxygen demand **(BOD),** which is the quantity of oxygen required in a given time to satisfy the chemical and biological oxidation demands of the sewage. A high BOD means that an excessive quantity of oxygen is being used up by the biochemical action in the sewage, indicating a high sewage concentration.

The primary purpose of sewage treatment is to prevent the spread of disease among human beings. For additional reasons the proper disposal of sewage is imperative in any community or nation, particularly one with a high population concentration. Sewage treatment protects water supplies, protects fish and other aquatic life, protects food by preventing soil pollution, protects livestock, and renders water fit for industrial use. Thus, in addition to preventing disease spread, sewage treatment returns water to a condition such that it can be reused with safety and with its general condition unimpaired.

Sewage Treatment

Treatment of community sewage addresses five factors: solids in suspension, organic matter in suspension, inorganic matter in suspension, organic matter in solution, and bacteria. A properly designed and efficiently operated sewage disposal plant will eliminate all five of these undesirable factors and leave an end product of clear, uncontaminated water that can be safely consumed.

Even before discharging wastewater, industries may be required to provide for *pretreatment* to remove pollutants from their wastewater (Figure 14-8).

A community sewage disposal plant that does the complete job of treatment involves the following six steps: preliminary treatment, primary treatment, secondary treatment, tertiary treatment, chlorination, and final disposal.

Preliminary treatment. A series of parallel screens set at an angle permit sewage to flow through but intercept large suspended objects (Figure 14-9). Mechanically or manually operated rakes clean the debris and dump it into receptacles, where it is burned. Some community sewage plants use shredders or comminutors, which cut coarse material into fine enough particles to pass through with the effluent for further treatment.

Grit chambers for preliminary treatment cause gravel, sand, and other heavy materials to settle to the bottom. At least two grit chambers allow one to be in operation while the other is being cleaned.

Primary treatment. Sedimentation or clarifier tanks are about 10 feet deep. The effluent flows into the center of the circular tank through a pipe coming up from the bottom. This prevents agitation of the effluent in the tank and ensures that particles will settle to the bottom. To aid this sedimentation, chemicals are added to form a gelatinous floc that settles, carries suspended solids to the bottom, and forms sludge.

Digestion of the sludge by anaerobic bacteria takes place in the sedimentation tank or in separate sludge tanks. Undigested sludge is pumped out and hauled away to be used as fertilizer because it is rich in nitrogen. Sludge-drying beds are used to dehydrate this sludge before it is used, since fresh sludge is contaminated and thus unsafe for immediate use in vegetable farming.

Bacterial action is slow. Scientists have been ex-

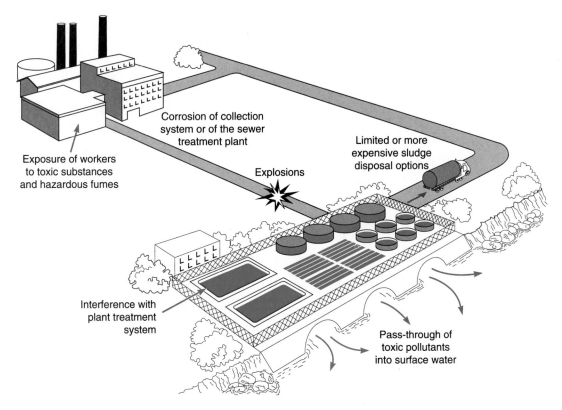

Exposure of workers to toxic substances and hazardous fumes

Corrosion of collection system or of the sewer treatment plant

Explosions

Limited or more expensive sludge disposal options

Interference with plant treatment system

Pass-through of toxic pollutants into surface water

FIGURE 14-8

Problems that may occur when industrial wastewaters are discharged into sewage treatment systems can be controlled through pretreatment of pollutants by the industry source before discharging its wastes.

Source: U.S. Environmental Protection Agency.

perimenting with chemicals as a replacement for bacteria. Their efforts have been fruitful: although some expense is involved and the precipitate has to be disposed of, chemical digestion is fast-acting and will likely become the standard method of primary treatment.

Secondary treatment. To reduce the oxygen demand of the sewage, the secondary treatment requires aeration so that organisms can convert the organic matter in the effluent into stable nitrogenous products. Trickling filters are constructed of con-

crete with a bed of gravel, crushed stone, or similar material, which provides good ventilation of the bed.

Effluent comes from the clarifiers, or primary tanks, in pipes. Connected to these pipes is a series of equally spaced nozzles or rotary spray heads, 1 or 2 feet above the surface of the stone bed.

A gelatinous film that intercepts bacteria, algae, protozoa, worms, and molds forms on the stones as the effluent sprays over the stone bed. The organisms in this film convert dissolved, suspended, and colloidal materials into stable nitrogenous material.

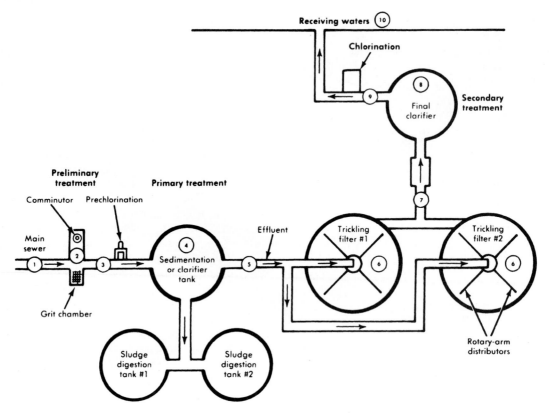

FIGURE 14-9
A flow diagram for a sewage treatment plant proceeds from preliminary treatment through primary (anaerobic) treatment, to secondary (aerobic) treatment, to final chlorination before returning the safe water back to a large body of water.

Intermittent sand filters are also used for secondary treatment. The underdrains are similar to those in the trickling filters. Surface distributing channels flood the effluent over the surface of the sand bed. Sand grains become coated with a gelatinous film, as do the stones in the trickling filters. In many respects, this is like the slow sand filtration method used in water treatment; it is highly effective but rather slow-acting. The surface of the sand bed must be cleaned and thus requires constant attention. The dry sludge is an effective fertilizer.

A new process that expands on the trickling filter system uses a deeper aeration tank and gently stirs the wastewater to further separate out the solids. At that point, air is bubbled through the wastewater, which is piped back through the clarifying tanks one more time, resulting in a cleaner end product. Known as a trickling filter solids contact process, the modified system cuts energy requirements.

Tertiary treatment. Most community sewage treatment plants now use a third process to remove or reduce certain chemicals such as phosphates, nitrogen, and carbon. Removal of these chemicals is desirable and even necessary because they can lead to eutrophication, a process that occurs naturally in bodies of water but normally takes thousands of years. The process is accelerated dramatically when excessive nutrients (such as nitrates and phosphates) stimulate marked growth of algae and other aquatic plants. The flourishing plants consume elements essential to marine life and to the natural purification of wastes. This essentially was the condition in Lake Erie for several years.

Phosphorus compounds that contaminate streams, lakes, and other bodies of water derive from synthetic detergents, domestic wastes, and runoff from farms and other land. Detergents are not the major source of phosphorus in the effluent of sewage treatment plants, and this phosphorus is no more difficult to remove than that from other sources. In community sewage more than 50% of the total phosphorus comes from domestic wastes, detergents account for about 35%, and the remainder comes from fertilizers used in farming and lawn care.

Removal of phosphorus involves conversion of soluble phosphorus into insoluble forms and then precipitation of the insoluble forms, which is usually done by adding metal salts—for example, aluminum sulfate or ferrous chloride. When settled out, the phosphorus compounds are removed with the sludge, which is disposed of where it will not enter a body of water.

Nitrogen removal is not so simple. One method for removing nitrogen uses a stripping tower from 25 to 50 feet high. The inside of the tower is laced with wooden slats. Effluent is pumped to the top of the tower and is distributed uniformly from a horizontal tray across the top of the latticework. As the falling water strikes the slats, droplets are formed. Droplet surface films are of minimum thinness, which favors the escape of ammonia gas from the droplets. Air in the tower enters through side louvers and, by completely surrounding the droplets, promotes a maximum transfer of ammonia from the water to the air. The process of water falling and forming new droplets is repeated at least 200 times.

This tertiary treatment vastly improves the efficiency of chlorination.

Tertiary treatment of most community sewage is imperative if the United States is to save its streams, lakes, and ponds. Ecology makes clear that all life on earth (human life included) depends on good-quality water. Complete sewage treatment will be expensive, but compared with the alternative, it will be essential.

Chlorination. Primary treatment of sewage may be all that is necessary when the effluent from community sewage is emptied into receiving waters (such as lakes or rivers) that provide extreme dilution. In some instances, dilution is sufficiently great that after secondary treatment it is safe to empty the effluent into the final disposal lake, river, or sea. When the population concentration is great and available bodies of water are not adequate, however, a good safety measure is to chlorinate the effluent coming from the primary or secondary treatment unit. In some instances chlorination is necessary only during the summer months when available stream flow is low. Two-stage chlorination, in which chlorine is added to the grit chamber at the beginning of treatment and again to the final effluent, provides added safety.

Besides destroying organisms, chlorine reduces the BOD and odor of effluents. The chlorine injection mechanism is similar to that used in water treatment plants.

Final disposal. The receiving waters into which the final effluent is emptied are usually public waters and, as such, are under the jurisdiction and supervision of a state agency. Other communities and citizens have a claim to the use of the waters. The larger the body of receiving water, the greater the safety factor. Although the supervising state agency recognizes practical considerations, no community has the right to jeopardize the public health. If a community is to be granted the privilege of disposing of its wastes, it must take reasonable precautions to ensure that its sewage effluent is not a threat to human life and welfare.

Lagoon Treatment

Cost of a typical sewage treatment plant can be beyond the financial means of a small community. Fortunately, raw sewage lagoons can provide economical and satisfactory treatment of community sewage. A lagoon is a shallow pond in which natural processes produce an acceptable purification.

A lagoon is usually located at least a quarter of a mile from residential areas, where seepage will not pollute groundwater that may be used for domestic purposes. A lagoon is a rectangular excavation, at least half an acre in area and from 3 to 5 feet in depth (Figure 14-10). The soil at the bottom of the lagoon should be relatively impervious to prevent excess loss of effluent by seepage. Embankments prevent outside surface drainage from entering the lagoon. The inlet from the community's sewerage system should be near the center of the lagoon.

Organic material that settles to the bottom of the lagoon is decomposed by bacteria and is converted into ammonia, carbon dioxide, and water. Algae feed on these soluble nutrients and, in the presence of sunlight, produce oxygen and thus maintain aerobic conditions and help prevent odor. If the lagoon freezes over, the ice shuts out sunlight and interferes with the treatment process.

Decontamination of sewage effluents may be necessary if they are being discharged into public waters, especially during the summer months. Raw sewage lagoon effluents are generally not discharged into public waters in quantities that would result in greater than 1 part effluent per 20 parts dilution.

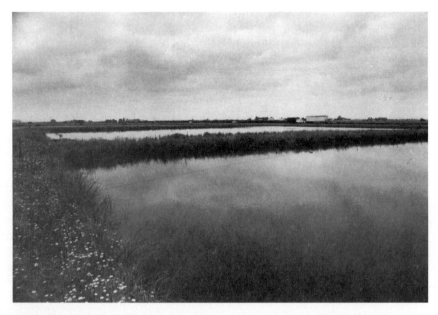

FIGURE 14-10
Lagoons serve as an alternative for sewage treatment in small communities that cannot afford a full-scale sewage treatment plant.

Lagoon treatment is not the equivalent of the standard methods of treatment, but it can be acceptable. It serves when the community concerned is not able to finance the more costly, more elaborate primary and secondary treatment plants.

Financing Sewage Treatment

Sewage treatment plants are costly but are a necessary community investment in protecting health, in maintaining an esthetic environment, and in disposing of community wastes. No fully equitable method has been developed for paying the costs of treatment plant construction and maintenance. Virtually all payment methods are based on the volume of water citizens use from the community's water supply.

Most communities in the United States find it necessary to issue bonds for the construction of a treatment plant. The security for the bonds is the community's ability to collect fees and levy taxes to redeem the bonds when due. All establishments connected to the public sewerage system are charged a monthly sewer fee that is based on the amount of water the establishment used during the month. The practice is based on the assumption that the amount of water a household uses is a reasonable index of the extent to which the household uses the sewer service. The sewer fee is usually higher during winter months than during summer, when the sewer rate is lowered to compensate for the fact that much of the water going through the meter is used for lawn sprinkling and does not go into the sewer lines.

Regulation of Sewage Disposal

In the United States construction and operation of sewage treatment facilities and disposal of the final effluent are the responsibility of the community, but the regulation of the sewage treatment plants and disposal of final effluents are the province of the state. This authority may be vested in the sanitary engineering division of the state department of health or in a special state sanitation authority. There are advantages in having a special authority to regulate sewage disposal, largely because water pollution is an increasing problem. In addition, a separate authority can deal with air pollution and other problems in the total environment.

The state can order a community to treat its sewage before emptying the final effluent into public waters. Courts have held this to be a proper function of the state and have ordered communities to raise the necessary funds to provide for proper sewage disposal. Plans for a community sewage treatment plant must be approved by state engineers, who also work with communities in an advisory role. Sewage disposal plant operators should pass state certification examinations, and the operation of the sewage plant must meet state sanitation requirements.

Septic Tanks

A serious community health problem may exist when a residential area is not served by sewers. A septic tank for each domicile is the means used for sewage disposal in such areas, which are usually the fringes of a city or the outlying districts just beyond the city limits.

A septic tank can be satisfactory for the disposal of household liquid wastes if the tank, drain tile, and seepage pit are properly constructed. When improperly installed, however, a septic tank can constitute a hazard to health and, esthetically, can be a severe nuisance. Sewage sporadically coming to the surface or, during flooding, washing over a neighborhood can constitute a hazard to the well-being of everyone in the vicinity. Such situations generally produce a certain pattern of citizen response: first, a long-time toleration of the situation; then, protests to the health officials or others; then, perhaps, court action. The final solution is usually the installation of sewers as a part of the community sewerage system. When at all feasible, even at considerable cost, sewer lines rather than septic tanks should be the choice.

Pit Latrines

The outhouse or pit latrine still does service in industrialized countries as a temporary facility on construction sites or at outside concerts, tent fairs, and picnic or park areas. In developing countries it is the primary means of shifting rural populations from unsanitary conditions of waste disposal to safe disposal. Pit latrine technology is simple, but the acceptability of designs is highly dependent on local toilet customs, cultural taboos, and environmental and economic conditions.

Cities without Sewage Systems

Cities with inadequate sewage systems pose possible danger to health and life. As a consequence, pressures are exerted on officials and on voters to provide the necessary finances and planning for an adequate sewage system for their community. Federal and state funding adds to the incentive to provide the community with an approved, safe means for water disposal.

Throughout the world one can find cities of more than 1 million inhabitants without a sewage system. Tokyo, with more than 10 million people, has one of the largest population of any city in the world, yet it depends on collection tanks and tanker trucks to collect and dispose of sewage.

Hiroshima was leveled by a nuclear bomb, which necessitated a complete rebuilding of the city. Environmentalists assumed that Hiroshima would begin by putting in a complete sewage system before erecting structures above the ground. The situation was ideal for this sequence. But no such system was built. The tank system apparently is preferred in Japan. This choice could cause Western countries to ask themselves whether they have overemphasized the necessity for all of the sewage systems they have built.

STREAM POLLUTION

Although stream pollution is generally thought of only in terms of a threat to human health, it actually affects many factors of economic and other significance. For example, it can render water unsuitable for industrial use. It affects agriculture by altering the taste of milk from cows drinking polluted water. Polluted irrigation water represents possible dangers. Waterfowl and other animals are exposed to botulism and cyanide poisoning. Turbidity and thermal pollution can destroy fish and other marine life. Decomposition of nitrogen wastes forms nitrates and, because all of the oxygen is consumed, green plants die and anaerobic bacteria (for example, botulism) survive. Farther down the stream where little pollution exists, green plant life may be profuse and give off oxygen. Pollution with acids may cause dock deterioration, and pollution from such industries as mining and quarrying may interfere with navigation and thus necessitate dredging.

Criteria of Stream Pollution

Organic criteria. In the final analysis, the most reliable single index of stream pollution can be the BOD, expressed as the quantity of oxygen required for oxidation of organic matter (expressed in pounds). The capacity of any body of water to oxidize organic wastes depends on its oxygen content, including oxygen resulting from photosynthesis in algae and other green plants. If oxygen use exceeds oxygen production, a negative oxygen balance occurs and an anaerobic condition results that produces undesirable bacterial action. A stream need not be in a state of negative oxygen balance to be badly polluted, however.

Chemical criteria. Trace metals polluting many rivers and streams include iron, manganese, copper, zinc, lead, chromium, nickel, tin, cobalt, cadmium, and mercury. These metals settle in the river sediment and can be transported to man, along with organic pollutants, by any of the routes shown in Figure 14-11.

Acid rain. Sunlight triggers the photochemical conversion of pollutants in the air to acidic substances. These combine with water vapor and return to the earth's surface as acid rain or snow. Sulfur dioxide emissions from coal-fired power plants are the main cause of acid rain, which contaminates surface waters and damages manmade structures in eastern North America and Europe. The most acidic rain ever recorded fell on Wheeling, West Virginia; it was 5000 times as acidic as unpolluted rain. Although not a direct health threat for man, acid rain is believed to account for a decline in fish populations in high-altitude lakes in the northeastern United States and Canada. The two countries are negotiating for a solution to the problem of acid rain. The acid rain falling on Canada is largely caused by

pollution produced in the United States. Much of the damage to forests and crops once blamed on acid rain is now attributed to ozone.

Like the EPA ''Superfund'' for cleanup of toxic dumps and the regulation of water pollution by industry, created by the Clean Water Act, the regulation of air pollution by industry has become a political and economic issue of greater proportion because of the problems of international trade balances. Some Western industries say the trade balances are tilted in favor of the countries with less costly controls on pollution. More on acid rain and ozone will be addressed in Chapter 17.

Standards. In the United States classification of streams was established by the first state stream regulating agency, the Pennsylvania Sanitary Water Board, created in 1923. This board established standards for three classes of streams. Class A streams

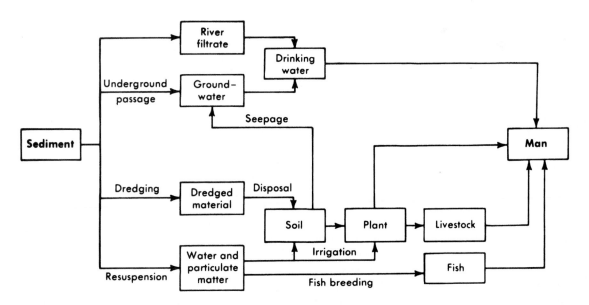

FIGURE 14-11
Several pathways are shown by which pollutants can work their way from the sediment at the bottom of a stream or river to human hosts.
Source: Courtesy Regional Office for Europe, World Health Organization.

are those in their natural state, probably subject to chance contamination by human beings but unpolluted or uncontaminated from any artificial source. They are generally fit for domestic water supply after chlorination, will support fish life, and may be safely used for recreational purposes. Class B streams are those that are more or less polluted. The extent of regulation, control, or elimination of pollution from these streams will be determined by a consideration of (1) the present and probable future use and condition of the stream, (2) the practicability of remedial measures for abatement, and (3) the general interest of the public through the protection of the public health, the health of animals, fish, and other aquatic life, and the use of the stream for recreational purposes. Class C streams are so polluted that they cannot be used as sources of public water supplies, will not support fish life, and are not used for recreational purposes. From the standpoint of the public interest and practicability, it is not necessary, economical, or advisable to attempt to restore them to a clean condition.

Other standards have been established by other stream pollution control boards. Some boards also zone rivers. The 1985 amendments for reauthorization of the Clean Water Act set the new timetables and standards for controlling the discharge of hazardous chemicals into lakes and streams and for industry to comply with the standards.

Control of Stream Pollution

The long-established principle of riparian rights holds that landowners have the right to have a stream come down to their property with its quality unimpaired and its quantity undiminished. Most people agree that there should be an equitable distribution of water, particularly between states and between communities. Obtaining some degree of equitable distribution while protecting natural waters is a formidable assignment.

The Federal Water Pollution Control Law went into effect in 1948. This legislation declared the pollution of *interstate* waters to be a public nuisance that must be abated. It protected the rights of the states in controlling water pollution. It also provided funds for surveys, investigations, and research. The essence of the law was the cooperation and coordination of all federal, state, and community agencies engaged in efforts to reduce or eliminate pollution of interstate waters and tributaries. Funds were made available for the construction of community sewage treatment facilities.

The 1965 Water Pollution Act passed by Congress provided that each state determine the uses of its lakes and rivers. This water quality approach has much to recommend it, but it proved to be difficult to administer. After 10 years, many states had not established water quality standards, and other states were unable to reconcile the relationship between pollutants and water use.

In 1971 the Federal Water Pollution Control Act went into effect. It shifted the emphasis from water quality standards to direct effluent limits, with the theoretical goal to be zero discharge. This act requires polluters to apply for a discharge permit from the EPA. The first phase of this program ended in 1976, by which time all firms and agencies were obligated to use the best available means to control water pollution. The goal of the second phase, which ended in 1981, was to achieve water clean enough for swimming and fish propagation. The goal for 1985 was the elimination of all effluents. That target date was deferred and will be debated in 1994.

Progress on reduction of stream pollution appears to have been steady from 1975 through 1981, but deregulation in the federal administrative policies of the early 1980s resulted in some reversals and slowing of the improvements. Both communities and industries have found the costs of effluent elimination to be the main hurdle. The National Council on Environmental Quality acknowledges that costs rise exponentially with the degree of cleanliness sought, so that the last 1% of treatment could cost as much as the previous 99%. Because costs may be prohibitive even with federal subsidies, zero discharge may be an unattainable and perhaps unnecessary goal. Something less may be satisfactory.

Some communities have developed land disposal systems in which wastes are routed through a simple treatment, then stored in lagoons, and finally sprayed over a wide acreage of land. Ecologists favor such an approach, because it returns invaluable nutrients to the soil. This type of simple technology may provide an acceptable, if not completely satisfactory, answer to the problem of effluent discharge.

Two or more states set up compacts when a stream adjoins more than one state. Some of these agreements are formal, others are informal. Usually, an interstate commission or water control council is created. Cooperation is the purpose for and the key to these joint programs for pollution control.

Within a state, responsibility for pollution control may be vested in the state department of health; or some other agency will be responsible for general environmental health problems, including water pollution. The state agency may set up districts or drainage areas to provide control measures best suited to particular problems in specific sections of the state. The state sanitation authority may establish standards of pollution, conduct surveys, and take action to abate a pollution nuisance. Only after all cooperative measures have failed will the state agency resort to legal measures. There is a need for waste disposal and a need for water protection. To reconcile the two is the task that faces every community and every country.

SOLID WASTES

Community solid wastes consist of garbage, ashes, rubbish (boxes, papers, other scraps), street sweepings, trade wastes, and occasionally such things as dead animals. Leaves, grass, and shrub cuttings will often be considered wastes that must be disposed of. Industrial wastes are normally not a community problem, because industries are expected to dispose of their own wastes.

Of the solid wastes of a community, garbage poses the most significant health menace, because it provides feed for stray dogs, rats, and insects. In some regions this may be a minor factor in health, but in other geographical areas dogs, rats, and mosquitoes are hosts of serious diseases and thus constitute a significant threat to health. Rubbish can also harbor rats and insects, but the removal of rubbish usually is more a matter of esthetics and convenience than of health.

Collection

Both the collection and the disposal of garbage and refuse are accepted government functions in most countries. Some communities collect household and commercial garbage and rubbish without charge, the cost being met through general tax funds; others charge for garbage and rubbish collections. The responsibility for collection usually rests with the department of public works or some other comparable department, and responsibility for proper sanitation relating to garbage and rubbish usually rests with the health authorities of the community.

Some communities contract with private firms to collect garbage and rubbish. Specifications for collections are set up by the city council, and bids are called for. The successful bidder is then granted a franchise for a period of about 5 years, when bids are again called for. The city council specifies what the charges will be and stipulates the frequency of collections. Each householder pays the disposal company for hauling garbage and refuse. Garbage is usually collected at regular intervals, whereas rubbish is hauled away only on the special request of the householder. Some cities have a can-exchange arrangement, in which the city provides a can, picks up the filled can, and leaves a clean, empty one at each collection location. The frequency of garbage collections in residential areas varies from weekly to every other day. When ashes are kept separate, a weekly collection of ashes is frequently the pattern. Collections from commercial districts are usually made six times a week.

A 30-gallon container for garbage or three large plastic bags per week is usually adequate for a typical family. Community regulations specify that the containers must be of plastic, metal, rubber, or other special composition. The containers must be watertight, fly-tight, and easily cleaned or disposable. A tightly fitting lid is required. The householder is responsible for cleaning out the container and occasionally decontaminating it with some strong germicide such as Lysol. Some communities require that garbage and ashes be separated when incineration is the method of disposal. This may also be required when reduction (garbage disposals in sinks or compactors) or hog feeding is the method of disposal.

Some communities require that garbage cans be lined with paper. Others require that garbage be wrapped either in ordinary paper or in wet-strength plastic bags. Again, wrapped garbage is not desirable when hog feeding or reduction is the method of disposal.

Enclosed trucks with hydraulic hoists for loading, compressing, and unloading are both sanitary and economical (Figure 14-12). At least once a week the trucks are steamed and cleaned with detergents.

Disposal

Open dumps, sanitary landfills, incineration, hog feeding, reduction, and grinding are the recognized methods of garbage disposal. Most communities use dumps for the disposal of garbage and refuse, but this choice is less than desirable. Burning at the dump creates a fire hazard and obnoxious smoke and odor. In addition, dumps are breeding grounds for rats and vermin. Only when the dump is in an isolated area and properly supervised can it be an acceptable method of disposal.

Sanitary landfills require a land depression or excavated trench into which garbage and refuse is dumped and then covered with dirt. This method serves to reclaim wastelands, does not require separation of ashes and garbage, can be virtually odorless, and can be free of rats and vermin. Availability of an acceptable area may be a problem, however.

Incineration is an expensive and controversial disposal method but is regarded as the most acceptable, especially in combination with a recycling program for plastic, glass and aluminum cans and bottles, and paper. Garbage and rubbish need not be separated. Ashes are excluded and usually magnetic separators are used to remove cans and other metal objects. Incinerators are composed of a receiving bin from which refuse is carried by conveyor to a hopper that feeds the refuse into a furnace. Oil, coal, or gas may be used as supplementary fuel for maximum combustion in the furnace. The final ash is removed from the bottom of the furnace and hauled to a dump or a landfill. When air pollution laws were enacted in the 1970s, they made incinerators less economical. Many facilities had to be closed. Recent shortages of landfill space have reversed this trend. Combined with energy generation from incinerators for some communities, incinerators have made a comeback.

Hog feeding is an old method of garbage disposal still in use but not approved by health authorities. It requires both a separation of garbage from other wastes and a sorting of the garbage. An area of 2 acres and a ton of garbage per day for 100 hogs is the usual standard. Even if the hog farm is well operated and is far removed from the community, feeding garbage to hogs is objectionable. Spreading garbage, raw and cooked, creates an unsanitary and malodorous environment where flies and rats proliferate. As a source of human trichinosis, garbage-fed hogs must always be regarded as a primary threat, even when an informed public cooks pork adequately before serving it.

Grinding of garbage and disposal of it in the community sewage is both effective and practical. A large grinding plant receives garbage from the collection trucks and empties the ground garbage into the trunk sewer. This task has been made easier with the widespread installation of home garbage disposals. Experience indicates that ground garbage causes no serious interference with sewage treatment. Oxygen demand of the sewage is increased, but not to a degree that would have an adverse effect on the

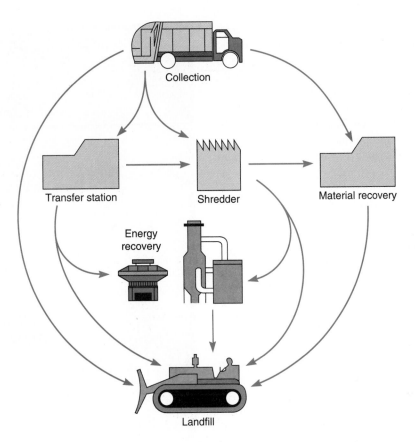

Collection

Transfer station

Shredder

Material recovery

Energy
recovery

Landfill

FIGURE 14-12
Raw refuse is collected by truck, shredded, and put thorugh a series of procedures to recover reusable material
and energy. The residual refuse then can be buried more safely in landfills, and the community benefits from
the salvage of materials and energy.
Source: Texas Department of Health.

treatment of the effluent or on the terminal waters into which the sewage effluent is emptied.

Domestic garbage grinders attached to kitchen sinks are highly satisfactory, although some objects must be separated out. The individual householder can purchase his or her own grinder from a commercial firm, the city may install home grinder units on a citywide basis and resell to the householder on an installment plan, or the city may retain ownership and charge a monthly rental fee. The municipal sewage treatment plant can handle the ground garbage if the biochemical oxygen demand is within a controllable range. To take care of household garbage in this manner, the community rightfully makes a regular monthly sewage charge.

Recycling

Recycling certain combustible and noncombustible solid wastes is receiving increased attention by research agencies and community officials. Over 75% of municipal solid waste in the United States is recyclable. Only 30% of these materials are being recycled because of deficiencies in technology, public cooperation, and markets. Community programs to increase this rate of recycling have included educational campaigns, incentives such as cash prizes, refundable deposits, and surcharges on garbage bags for nonrecyclable wastes. Mandatory programs obtain greater participation but also result sometimes in public antagonism and illegal private dumping on roadsides.

Successful community programs have emphasized colored containers in which residents can sort their recyclable materials and set them out with their trash cans. Garbage trucks are equipped with separate bins for the color-coded bags for glass, aluminum, plastic, and paper. The high visibility of the colored bags makes the recycling act a more public act that builds a neighborhood norm. Some communities have achieved 80% participation rates with such voluntary programs (Figure 14-13).

Wilton, New Hampshire, collects glass, metals, paper, and hazardous household wastes in separate containers with a mandatory program. This program has saved the town about $50,000 in waste-disposal costs per year and has brought in about $25,000 per year in revenue from the sale of recycled materials. Such programs do not necessarily pay for themselves, but for communities with dwindling landfill space and with air quality problems prohibiting incineration, recycling becomes increasingly attractive. Some states and communities are giving tax incentives to businesses that incorporate recycled materials into their manufacturing process. Recycled plastic is relatively inexpensive at $0.40 per pound compared with $0.60 per pound for pure plastic. Recycling appears to be a winning strategy for waste management on both the supply side and the demand side.

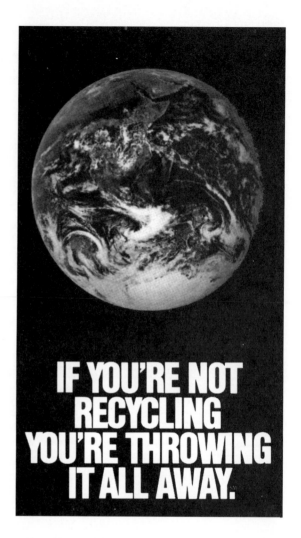

IF YOU'RE NOT RECYCLING YOU'RE THROWING IT ALL AWAY.

A little reminder from the Environmental Defense Fund that if you're not recycling, you're throwing away a lot more than just your trash.

You and your community can recycle. Write the Environmental Defense Fund at: EDF-Recycling, 257 Park Avenue South, New York, NY 10010, for a free brochure that will tell you virtually everything you need to know about recycling.

© 1988 EDF

EDF ™ Ad Council

FIGURE 14-13
Community recycling programs have been supported by national media campaigns to educate and encourage the public to sort and recycle its household wastes.
Source: Environmental Defense Fund and Advertising Council.

Reducing Litter

Litter serves as a signal of a blight on the community that disregards the common good. It would be difficult to establish a relationship between litter and physical health, but the effect of litter on mental health certainly could be appraised.

Litter reduction, to be effective, must be based on organization of resources and voluntary leadership. In the United States principal voluntary organizations for the prevention of litter are Keep America Beautiful, Inc. and the Sierra Club.

Some states and provinces have passed "bottle bill" legislation making mandatory a deposit for the return of certain containers and responsibility for preventing and controlling litter. Total litter in Oregon and Vermont was reduced by more than 10%.

SUMMARY

This chapter began with an examination of how water can be protected, derived, and treated for safe consumption. It ended with a discussion of ways in which that same water can be recycled back into the environment after domestic and other uses by treating wastewater and by handling other toxic wastes so that they do not contaminate the water supply beyond recovery.

The entire process of consumption and disposal of water is analogous to digestion on a community scale. The water must be protected, like other parts of the environment, if it is to remain usable without health risks. Protection includes treatment and testing of water supplies, disposal and treatment of wastes, control of pollution, and the maintenance of standards for these several processes.

Organic pollution of water has been controlled primarily with the use of chlorine. Inorganic pollution by trace metals and other toxic chemicals cannot be so easily neutralized with a single substance. The only hope for control of the thousands of possibly toxic chemicals polluting water is control of the disposal of toxic wastes. In addition to efforts to prevent the continuing pollution by industry and restrictions on agricultural use of pesticides, a "Superfund" had to be created for cleanup of the major sites where large quantities of toxic substances had been dumped in the past.

Disposal of human and industrial wastes has become a spiraling problem demanding greater investments and control. There is no other choice, for safe water and soil are essential to survival.

QUESTIONS FOR REVIEW

1. How does treating water for consumption differ from treating wastewater for release back into the environment?
2. If water is more important to a human being's health than any drug, why does water cost less than any drug?
3. If the total water supply in the world remains the same, why is water management important?
4. Who has the safer water, urban dwellers or rural dwellers?
5. What is the source of your community's water supply, and what are its merits and hazards?
6. How is it possible for water to be contaminated and still be safe?
7. Why is the bacteriological examination not directed at finding the typhoid bacillus?
8. Why are chemical wastes in water more difficult to test for and to neutralize than organic wastes?
9. What problems of waste disposal have been created by the development of suburban areas?
10. How would you initiate a program to make your community more conscious of its water protection needs?
11. What is the most equitable and efficient method of charging for sewage services?
12. If communities are responsible for the construction and operation of their own sewage treatment plants, why should the state be the regulating agency?
13. Industrial stream pollution has existed for more than 90 years; why is there so much concern about it now?
14. Why are toxic waste dumps in dry fields a threat to the water supply?
15. How can chemical or trace-metal sediment at the bottom of a stream reach people to do any harm?

READINGS

Buckley R: *Perspectives on environmental management,* Berlin, 1991, Springer-Verlag.

A collection of 15 essays examining environmental accounting, economics and taxation, environmental audit and insurance, institutional and administrative frameworks, regional environmental planning, and the growth of ecotourism. Concludes with trends for the 1990s.

Herwaldt BL, Craun GF, Stokes SL et al: Waterborne-disease outbreaks, 1989-1990, *MMWR* 40:SS-3, 1991.

Reviews the 26 outbreaks reported by 16 states where 4288 people became ill as a result of contaminated water intended for drinking. *Giardia lamblia* was implicated as the etiologic agent for a majority of the outbreaks.

Office of Technology Assessment, U.S. Congress: *Facing America's trash: what next for municipal solid waste?* New York, 1992, Van Nostrand Reinhold.

With 80% of existing landfill sites expected to close soon and new sites difficult to open, this guide to innovative waste management strategies offers technologies for solid waste reduction and management in environmentally sound and cost-effective long-term strategies. These include waste prevention, recycling, incineration, and landfills that can help ward off the impending waste crisis.

Sloan WM: *Site selection for new hazardous waste management facilities,* Geneva, 1992, World Health Organization, WHO Regional Publications, European Series, No. 46.

This guide to the selection of new sites where hazardous wastes can be collected, treated, stored, and disposed of in a safe manner acceptable to the general public gives particular attention to the measures to protect health, preserve environmental quality, and respect the social values and economic well-being of the host community.

BIBLIOGRAPHY

Aldrich T, Griffith J, editors: *Environmental epidemiology and risk assessment,* New York, 1992, Van Nostrand Reinhold.

Anderson B, editor: *Ecologue: the environmental catalogue and consumer's guide for a safe earth,* Englewood Cliffs, NJ, 1990, Prentice-Hall.

Benenson AS, editor: *Control of communicable diseases in man,* ed 15, Washington, DC, 1990, American Public Health Association.

British Medical Association: *Hazardous waste and human health,* Oxford, 1991, Oxford University Press.

Brown P, Mikkelsen EJ: *No safe place: toxic waste, leukemia, and community action,* Berkeley, 1991, University of California Press.

Bryant T, Fulton G, Budd G: *Disinfection alternatives for safe drinking water,* New York, 1992, Van Nostrand Reinhold.

Committee on Environmental Epidemiology, Board on Environmental Studies and Toxicology, Commission on Life Sciences: *Environmental epidemiology: public health and hazardous wastes,* Washington, DC, 1991, National Academy Press.

Committee on the Human Dimensions of Global Change, Commission on Behavioral and Social Sciences and Education: *Global environmental change: understanding the human dimensions,* Washington, DC, 1991, National Academy Press.

Committee on Restoration of Aquatic Ecosystems: *Restoration of aquatic ecosystems: science, technology, and public policy,* Washington, DC, 1992, National Academy Press.

DeLong JV: Public policy toward municipal solid waste, *Annu Rev Public Health* 14:137, 1993.

Elkington J, Hailes J, Makower J: *The green consumer,* Washington, DC, 1990, Tilden Press.

Environmental Resource Center: *Hazardous waste management compliance handbook,* New York, 1992, Van Nostrand Reinhold.

Fagliano J, Berry M, Bove F et al: Drinking water contamination and the incidence of leukemia: an ecological study, *Am J Public Health* 80:1209, 1990.

Federal-Provincial Working Group on Recreational Water Quality: *Guidelines for Canadian recreational water quality,* Ottawa, 1992, Canada Communications Group, for the Federal-Provincial Advisory Committee on Environmental and Occupational Health.

Fischhoff B, Bostrom A, Quadrel MJ: Risk perception and communication, *Annu Rev Public Health* 14:183, 1993.

Franceys R, Pickford J, Reed R: *A guide to the development of on-site sanitation,* Geneva, 1992, World Health Organization.

General Accounting Office: *Superfund: public health assessments incomplete and of questionable value,* Gaithersburg, Md, 1991, General Accounting Office.

Goldberg SJ, Lebowitz MD, Graver EJ et al: An association of human congenital cardiac malformations and drinking water contaminants, *J Am Coll Cardiol* 16: 155, 1990.

Greenberg AE, Clesceri LS, Eaton AD, editors: *Standard methods for the examination of water and wastewater,* ed 18, Washington, DC, 1992, American Public Health Association.

Hamlin C: *A science of impurity: water analysis in nineteenth century Britain,* Berkeley, 1991, University of California Press.

Hayes D: Harnessing market forces to protect the earth, *Issues in Science and Technology* 46:Winter 1990-91.

Health and Welfare Canada: *Guidelines for Canadian drinking water quality,* ed 4, Ottawa, 1990, Canada Communication Group.

Hosty JW, Foster P: *A practical guide to chemical spill response,* New York, 1992, Van Nostrand Reinhold.

Kerr C, editor: *Community health and sanitation,* London, 1990, Intermediate Technology Publications.

MacEachern D: *Save our planet,* New York, 1990, Dell.

Mihindu-Ngoma P: Clean water at low cost, *World Health:* 27, July-April 1992.

Monto A, Higashi G, Marrs C: Infectious agents. In Holland WW, Detels R, Knox G, editors: *Oxford textbook of public health,* ed 2, New York, 1991, Oxford University Press.

Reiff FM: Cholera in Peru, *World Health:* 18, July-August 1992.

Tarcher AB, editor: *Principles and practice of environmental medicine,* New York, 1992, Plenum.

Tonglet R, Isu K, Mpese M et al: Can improvements in water supply reduce childhood diarrhoea? *Health Policy Planning* 7:260, 1992.

Wagner TP: *The hazardous waste Q & A: an in-depth guide to the Resource Conservation and Recovery Act and the Hazardous Materials Transportation Act,* rev ed, New York, 1992, Van Nostrand Reinhold.

Warner DB, Laugeri L: The legacy of the Water Decade, *World Health:* 7, July-August 1992.

●●

Chapter 15

Residential, Occupational, and Other Environments

❖

*The rich are moving out of your cities two yards
a day, including weekends.*
CONSTANTINOS DOXIADIS

OBJECTIVES

When you finish this chapter, you should be able to:

- Describe the major health hazards in residential, occupational, and other environments
- Identify the agencies, standards, and laws regulating these environments
- Recognize strategies to improve or maintain the quality of housing, worksites, and other environments

The environments in which people live, work, and play obviously affect their quality of life. How much these environments influence health remains a matter of conjecture because it is nearly impossible to separate the environmental effects from other aspects of home, work, or recreation. When you consider the flight from cities referred to above by Doxiadis, a city planner from Greece, you can think immediately of ways in which housing, worksites, and recreational environments affect and are affected by the demographic, behavioral, economic, organizational, and genetic factors influencing community health. As discussed in Chapter 3, human ecology, demography, and epidemiology interact to produce community health problems and influence community health strategies. With the retreat of the more affluent people from the cities to the suburbs, for example, has gone much of the economic and organizational support for urban renewal, park and recreation construction, and even headquarter offices and commercial establishments. In short, these demographic shifts have simultaneously influenced housing, jobs, health, and life-style.

As Chapter 3 noted, the farm population declined

⅃5% of the North American population ⅃ʊ to less than 3% in 1990. The amount of land ⅃ea classified as urban doubled between 1960 and 1990, most of it in suburban development. These trends have been seen around the world, most dramatically in the developing countries. Migration from rural to urban areas has put new strains on cities to accommodate population growth with safe housing and jobs.

HOUSING: RESIDENTIAL ENVIRONMENTS

Housing is a private concern in most countries, and in some countries citizens are constitutionally protected against search and seizure of their homes and other property. Yet housing is also a public health responsibility, a matter of economics, and a measure of personal and family status. No wonder it arouses such emotion and controversy when threatened by neighborhood change, new zoning ordinances, or highway construction. Citizens have gone to court to bar waste disposal sites, mental health clinics, drug abuse and HIV treatment centers, and family planning clinics from being constructed in their neighborhoods. Nothing has felt more threatening to neighborhoods in recent years than toxic waste dumps and the construction of nuclear facilities.

Chapter 13 touched on the safety and injury prevention aspects of housing, occupations, and recreation. This chapter will concentrate on the ways in which these environments affect health and the ways in which communities respond.

Epidemiology of Housing and Health

To isolate the impact of housing on health would require an experiment in which people are randomly assigned to levels and types of housing. Of course, such an experiment could be carried out only under the most totalitarian yet totally egalitarian system of government. Random allocation of housing would deny personal preferences and tastes, personal

needs, and merit or status. In every society, these factors come into play in the selection of housing. In most societies income plays a large part in narrowing the range of available housing options. Higher income levels correlate with higher levels of education, and these together produce neighborhoods with greater access to medical care facilities, good nutrition, and social standards for child care and personal health practices, all of which influence health. The prospect of separating the contribution of housing from these other factors is remote. At best, those factors in housing related to human health can only be inferred.

Crowding. Crowding increases the transmission of communicable diseases, as studies on the incidence and spread of these diseases have revealed. Incidence rates of the common communicable diseases are higher for residents in densely populated areas than for the general population. The incidence of tuberculosis, for example, rises with increased crowding and substandard living conditions (see Chapter 11).

Indoor air. Insufficient **ventilation,** inadequate artificial lighting, and lack of sunshine can have adverse effects on air quality and health (Figure 15-1). In particular, the problems of indoor pollution resulting from inadequate ventilation have come to recent public attention as a consequence of improved insulation of housing (see the box on p. 456).

Structural factors. Defective heating units can cause carbon monoxide poisoning and fires. Defective or deteriorated floors, stairs, railings, and other structures account for high rates of injuries. Inadequate plumbing and toilet facilities can be a constant threat to health. These hazards were addressed in previous chapters.

Lead exposure. Lead in paint has long been recognized as the major source of high-dose lead exposure and asymptomatic lead poisoning for chil-

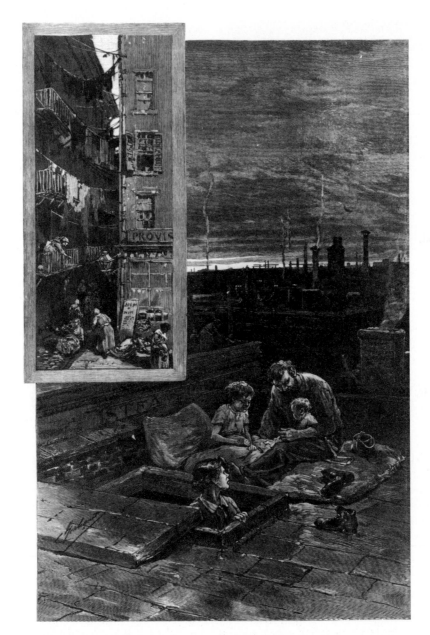

FIGURE 15-1
On the roof of a nineteenth-century New York tenement house in the summer. Crowding and poor ventilation drove people outdoors for sleep. Such conditions continue to exist.

Source: *Harper's Weekly* 29:497, Aug. 1, 1885. Courtesy, National Library of Medicine.

Indoor Pollution

An irony of the times is the price we are paying for the energy consciousness of the 1970s. All the caulking and weather-stripping has sealed out atmospheric air but has sealed in household pollutants. Cigarette smoke, paint odors, mildew, insecticide spray, **asbestos,** animal hairs, oven fumes, and **radon** (a radioactive by-product of the stones and soil under houses) all accumulate in unventilated household air. These indoor pollutants have been linked to increased respiratory distress (coughs, asthma, bronchitis, and flu-like symptoms), allergies, and increased risk of lung cancer and emphysema.

The attention given over the past 20 years to pollution in offices and public buildings has turned recently to air pollution in homes. A study sponsored by the Consumer Product Safety Commission of 40 homes in Oak Ridge, Tennessee, found hazardous chemicals numbering from 20 to 150 in each house. The indoor atmospheric concentrations of these chemicals were generally about 10 times (in one house, 45 times) higher than outdoor concentrations. In the early 1970s, the stagnant air inside an average home would have exchanged with outside air once every hour. Now, with improved insulation, the **air exchange rate** in many homes is only once in 10 hours.

If improved ventilation and controlled use of selected substances in the home are sufficient remedies for the indoor pollution threat, how would you mount a community program to address this problem? Considering the present consequences of measures taken to control energy expenditures, what community health problems might you expect in the year 2000 as a consequence of today's life-style and environmental modifications?

---

dren in the United States. Since 1977, paint produced for household use must, by regulation, contain no more than 0.06% lead. In contrast, some paints manufactured in the 1940s for indoor use contained more than 50% lead, and an estimated 27 million households in the United States remain contaminated by **lead paint.** Lead poisoning typically

occurs in children under 6 years old living in deteriorated, pre-World War II housing. It has been found also in children whose parents moved to older housing as "urban homesteaders," exposing the children to paint chips, dust, or fumes as the old lead-based paint was removed during remodeling or renovation. Other sources of lead exposure and the federal agencies responsible for dealing with them are shown in the box on p. 457.

Mental health. Poor housing conditions can be depressing and can lead to a decline in pride and motivation, both of which are essential to optimum mental health. There frequently follows a carelessness in living practices, in personal grooming, and in self-growth. Social and esthetic decline results from the uncleanliness and disorder often associated with substandard housing. Confusion, noise, and a lack of privacy are not conducive to a feeling of self-esteem. A person living in substandard housing conditions very easily acquires a feeling of being oppressed, powerless, and alienated.

Criteria of Substandard Housing

The American Public Health Association Committee on the Hygiene of Housing declared in 1952 that if *any four* of the following criteria existed, the term **slum** applied.

1. Contaminated water
2. Water supply outside (Figure 15-2)
3. Shared toilet or outside toilet
4. Shared bath or outside bath
5. More than 1.5 persons per room
6. Overcrowding of sleeping quarters
7. Less than 40 square feet of sleeping room per person
8. Lack of dual egress
9. Installed heating lacking in three fourths of the rooms
10. Lack of electricity
11. Lack of windows
12. Deterioration

The federal agencies—and their areas of responsibility—involved with regulating lead exposure or researching the effects of lead:

FDA has responsibility for regulating lead in:

- bottled water
- calcium supplements
- ceramic and other foodware
- commercial coffee urns
- decorated glassware
- food, including ingredients and packaging
- lead crystal
- lead-soldered food cans.

EPA (Environmental Protection Agency) researches and/or monitors lead content in air, water, and soil, and has some involvement monitoring lead-based paints.

NIOSH (National Institute for Occupational Safety and Health) conducts research and surveillance on occupational lead exposure and offers health hazard evaluation programs on worksites when requested and industrial hygiene training.

OSHA (Occupational Safety and Health Administration) regulates lead exposure at the worksite.

NIEHS (National Institute of Environmental Health Sciences) conducts basic biomedical research on human health effects of lead.

HUD (U.S. Department of Housing and Urban Development) funds public housing authorities to contain or remove lead-based paint in public housing units.

CPSC (Consumer Product Safety Commission) requires warning labels on lead solder for drinking water pipes; monitors lead paint on children's toys to ensure compliance with the federal standard limiting lead in paint to no more than 0.06 percent; regulates the labeling of artists' materials; and has issued safety warnings about hazards of use of lead-based paint in the home.

ATSDR (Agency for Toxic Substances and Disease Registry) is responsible for health assessment for areas near Superfund sites (toxic waste sites that pose an environmental threat); wrote case study on lead for health professionals; and authored 1988 congressional document about the nature and extent of lead poisoning of American children.

Source: FDA Consumer July-Aug. 1991, Food and Drug Administration.

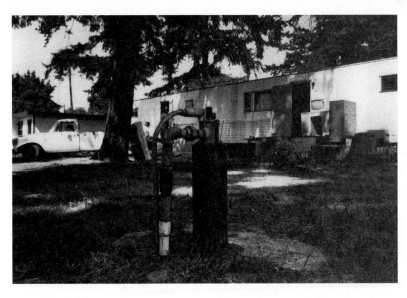

FIGURE 15-2
Remote and rural housing usually depends on ground water, which often lacks the purity controls that accompany community water supplies.

Substandard housing is to be found particularly in the blighted areas of cities, which is usually a deteriorating section between the business center and the principal residential sections of the community. This is the area on the fringes of the business section, where people live in retail store buildings that are no longer acceptable for commercial purposes. Many owners put nothing back into the buildings in the way of maintenance. As a consequence, deterioration, rubbish, garbage, flies, vermin, rats, and fire hazards prevail.

Principles of Healthful Housing

The American Public Health Association set minimum standards of housing based on fundamental human needs and necessary protection against hazards to health and life.

Fundamental psychological needs. Healthful housing provides adequate privacy for the individual, opportunities for normal family and community life, facilities that make possible the performance of household tasks without undue physical and mental fatigue and for maintenance of cleanliness of the dwelling and of the individual, possibilities for aesthetic satisfaction in the home and its surroundings, and concordance with prevailing social standards of the local community.

Protection against communicable disease. Healthful housing provides for a water supply of safe, sanitary quality, available to the dwelling, protected against pollution within the dwelling. It also provides toilet facilities of such character as to minimize the danger of transmitting disease, protection against sewage contamination of the interior surfaces of the dwelling, avoidance of unsanitary conditions in the vicinity of the dwelling, exclusion from the dwelling of vermin, which may play a part in the transmission of disease, facilities for keeping milk and food from decomposing, and sufficient space in sleeping rooms to minimize the danger of contact infection.

Protection against injury. Healthful housing is built with such materials and methods of construction as to minimize danger of injury due to collapse of any part of the structure. It provides for control of conditions likely to cause fires or to promote their spread; adequate facilities for escape in case of fire; protection against danger of electric shocks and burns, gas poisoning, falls and other mechanical injuries in the home, and protection of the neighborhood against the hazards of automobile traffic.

These basic housing needs may vary from one community to another, and even from one section of a community to another. Housing needs in the center of a metropolitan area may best be served by high-rise apartments; in the periphery by single-unit dwellings. The housing requirements set forth by the American Public Health Association can serve as a guide wherever needed, regardless of the circumstances.

Building Regulations and Codes

Regulation of housing construction has long been a recognized governmental function in most countries. In the community this authority is exercised through ordinances providing for building zones and for codes governing construction.

Zoning. Zoning is designed to control the type of building erected in a given section of a community. One zone may provide only for single-family structures. Another zone may provide for single- or two-family dwellings. In another zone the construction of multiple-dwelling structures may be permitted as well. Some areas may be zoned commercial, and others may be zoned industrial. Zoning protects the interests of those owning houses or other structures in an area against having their mode of life jeopardized and the value of their property reduced. It also provides a degree of uniformity in planning. In some communities a special planning commission considers matters of zoning and makes recommendations to the city council, which alone has the legal authority to enact local zoning ordinances.

Building codes. Community **building codes** have their roots in ancient history. As far back as 3500 BC, regulations applied to the making of bricks and hinges used in the construction of public buildings. Significant events that led to the evolution of the modern building code are shown in the box. Codes specify the type and quality of materials that may be used, standards of construction, the quality and proper installation of plumbing fixtures, wiring specifications. These and other provisions will give the prospective dweller, the neighborhood, and the community assurance that the building will meet the needs of the inhabitants in terms of safe and secure living. Communities can enforce building codes by requiring a permit to build. The fee for the permit may be nominal, but in granting the permit the issuing community authority specifies that the permit is issued on the provisions of the building code. Plans for the building must meet zoning and code standards and must be followed in the construction.

Model codes. The American Public Health Association developed a model housing ordinance regulating construction, maintenance, and occupancy of dwellings and dwelling units. The International Conference of Building Officials also developed a Uniform Housing Code. Both of these instruments can serve as excellent guides for health personnel and community authorities in developing local ordinances or codes.

A building erected before a building code was in effect will be bound by the requirements of the code if remodeling is to be done. Requiring a permit to remodel provides community officials with a means for requiring that the completed structure conform to code standards.

Deterioration. The housing problem of greatest general concern to the community—and of particular concern to the health department—is the building that was constructed years before a code existed

Milestones in the History of Building Codes

- 1700 BC—Babylonia's Code of Hammurabi stated that "if a builder has built a house for a man, and his work is not strong, and if the house he has built falls in and kills the householder, that builder should be slain."
- 1st Century—Roman Law regulated building heights, light, ventilation, sanitation, party walls (divisions separating properties) and setbacks.
- 1189 AD—England's "Henry Fitz-Elwyne's Assize of Buildings" addressed problems due to dense populations in cities, specifically party wall provisions and criteria for roof materials to decrease risk of fire spreading from building to building.
- 1625—In New Amsterdam, the first building law on record in America governed the types and locations of roof coverings to prevent fire transmission from sparks emitted from chimneys.
- 1666—After the "Great Fire of London," the first document resembling a building code was written and led to the passage of the Metropolitan Building Act which recognized the need for building officials to enforce codes.
- 1791—At the suggestion of George Washington, the Commissioners of Washington, DC, adopted the first official building regulations which limited the height of wood frame structures to 12 feet.
- 1850s—The first city building codes in North America were established by New York City.
- 1896—National Fire Protection Association was established in response to the need to create a standard for the uniform installation of sprinklers.
- 1915—Building Officials and Code Administrators (BOCA) was established.
- By 1920—The first mandatory statewide codes were developed and adopted by Wisconsin.
- 1922—International Conference of Building Officials (ICBO) was established.
- 1940—Southern Building Code Congress International (SBCCI) was established.
- 1972—Council of American Building Officials (CABO) was established.

Source: Trauma Foundation of San Francisco.

but that now has deteriorated to a substandard condition and will continue to decline. All of the objectionable aspects of deterioration will become progressively more apparent. In such cases it is doubtful that provisions of the building code can be enforced; thus the avenue for relief may be closed. In this type of situation health departments can play a vital role.

Sanction. When health officials judge a particular dwelling to be a threat to the health of the public, they can take necessary steps to abate the condition by consultation and negotiation with the owner or, as a last resort, court action to declare the condition a **public nuisance** (see Chapter 19). Inspections are made, hazards and other unsatisfactory conditions are reported, and a notice is issued to correct the unsatisfactory condition. Diplomacy and reasonable restraint are usually exercised by health officials. Legal measures are taken only as a last resort. Public support, always essential to the health department, is developed by a continuing program of public education and by the health staff's exemplary professional service to the community.

Community Responsibility

People living in substandard housing sometimes become so discouraged that they do not recognize the deterioration going on about them. Tragically, children growing up under these circumstances can become so conditioned that they expect nothing else. Many people in substandard housing would like to find something better, but their economic situation has them enslaved (Figure 15-3).

Government role. For centuries housing was left to the individual or to private enterprise, but country after country recognized that this was inadequate. The entry of governmental agencies was a logical development if government was to serve the public in fulfilling its needs, and one of the primary human needs is adequate housing.

In 1937 the U.S. federal government instituted a slum clearance and low-rent housing program by creating local housing authorities committed to slum clearance and to the construction of low-rent housing. Community agencies constructed and operated the housing. Federal funds made up 90% of the financing, with the remainder from municipal or private sources. Loans of federal funds at low interest rates were available. Communities receiving funds were required to eliminate a slum dwelling unit for each new low-cost dwelling unit constructed.

The Housing Act of 1949 further extended federal aid to housing by authorizing financial assistance to communities for the clearing of blighted

---

EPA Puts Federal Government Focus on Radon in New Homes

If the Environmental Protection Agency has its way, new homes built in high-risk radon areas would be automatically equipped with passive radon control systems that it says could save 200 lives over 5 years.

The EPA proposed in 1993 that state and local organizations charged with developing and enforcing building codes adopt model standards to render new homes radon resistant. The EPA estimates that 7,000 to 30,000 U.S. lung cancer deaths per year can be attributed to lethal indoor radon levels.

Because of the threat, Florida, Washington, New Jersey, and Montgomery County, Md., have already adopted radon reduction building codes.

Installing a radon control system during construction is not only good preventive medicine but also can save homeowners significant amounts of money, the EPA says. For example, a passive system costs about $350 to $500 per house when installed during construction, but retrofitting existing homes may run from $800 to $2,500 for the same system.

The proposed model standards recommend that passive radon control techniques be routinely installed in all new homes built in high-risk radon areas and that new homes be tested to confirm that the systems keep indoor radon levels below 4 picocuries per liter of air (See Figure 15-4).

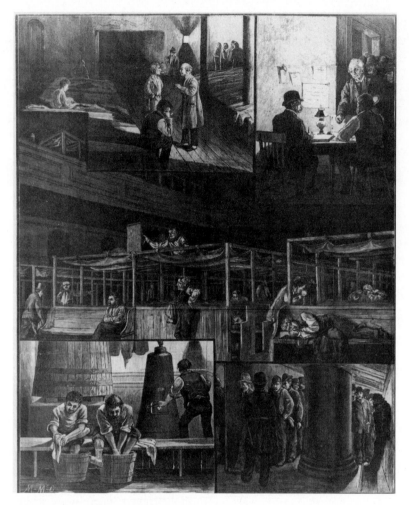

FIGURE 15-3
Wood-engraved vignettes of a "tramp's lodging house" in New York City around 1875. Housing improvements in the nineteenth century have been credited with a large proportion of the reduction in communicable diseases in that century, but poor people in cities depended on charity and shared sleeping areas.
Source: National Library of Medicine.

areas and slums and for redevelopment sites. Federal financial assistance for housing was also given to private enterprise through local agencies. Communities, in turn, could build on the cleared sites or could interest private capital in purchasing the sites from the city and in building approved dwellings or other structures. Certain tax benefits were granted to private purchasers and developers.

Urban renewal. Urban renewal was established by the Housing Act of 1954 as a combination of federal, community, and private resources to replace

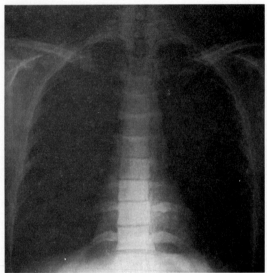

WARNING: RADON IS DEADLY IN THIS AREA.

You can't see it, smell it or even feel it. It just quietly attacks your lungs, until one day you find you have lung cancer.

It's called Radon. A naturally occurring, radioactive gas that seeps into your home. In fact, it is the second leading cause of lung cancer in America.

If your home has high levels of Radon, you're being exposed to as much radiation as having literally hundreds of chest x-rays in one year.

But there is something you can do about it. Testing for Radon is simple and inexpensive. And homes with high levels can be fixed. Call 1-800-SOS-RADON to get your test information.

RADON, THE HEALTH HAZARD IN YOUR HOME THAT HAS A SIMPLE SOLUTION.   &EPA   Ad Council

FIGURE 15-4

Testing for radon levels in homes has been promoted by the U.S. Environmental Protection Agency (EPA) in the early 1990s with public service advertisements such as this one.

Source: Advertising Council.

slum and blighted areas with adequate residential and business facilities. To qualify for federal aid, the community had to agree to certain requisites, such as a comprehensive plan of development including administrative organization, financial adequacy, citizen participation, and responsibility for adequately relocating persons displaced by urban renewal. Not all urban renewal leads to better housing, but the business and other structures that were constructed during this period were in harmony with the concept of urban renewal and contributed to the aesthetic improvement of communities.

Urban decline. In the 1960s there was a breakdown of the environment within the semipublic domain—that which falls between the responsibility of the individual household family on one hand (for example, indoor cleanliness, safety) and municipal government on the other (public water supply, public sanitation, sewage disposal, etc.). Most of the problems in this domain are with low-rent apartment or tenement housing.

Poor maintenance was the primary problem. Buildings often were structurally sound but poorly maintained. Building superintendents were poorly paid.

Shelter poverty of the 1970s. Soaring interest rates, inflation, and the dramatic appreciation of housing costs in the 1970s and early 1980s put rents and mortgage rates out of reach for many young couples and individuals. In addition, the changing family structure put relatively more single individuals in search of housing. For many people, the consequence was "shelter poverty"—the inability to meet the need for other necessities after paying the cost of housing. During the 1970s, the number of shelter-poor households increased by 34%, or 6.4 million. The rate of increase was greater for renters than for homeowners, who had tax advantages in owning even though their mortgage payments were usually as high as the rent paid by renters. By 1980, over 25 million households—32% of all households in the United States—were shelter-poor.

Homelessness. The shock of the 1980s was the realization that many of the people who were shelter-poor in the 1970s were now without homes. The most widely quoted estimate was that over the course of a year 3 million Americans were **homeless.** At any time, from 250,000 to 400,000 people in the United States had no home. About 41% of the homeless had chronic physical disorders, 33% had psychiatric problems, and 38% of the homeless were alcohol or drug abusers. Slightly more than half were minorities, 25% women, 10% children aged

15 or less. The homeless are defined as those who routinely sleep in bus, train, airport, or subway terminals, in abandoned buildings, or outside on steam heating grates and in parks. Mortality is high. Dozens of the homeless froze to death during the winter of 1984-85. Twenty died in New York City alone. Many more suffered pneumonia or tuberculosis.

The 1987 homeless assistance act. The growing national embarrassment of homelessness spurred the U.S. Congress to enact the Stuart B. McKinney Homeless Assistance Act, which was signed into law in July 1987. The Act provides for a range of services for the homeless, including primary health care services. The hope was that the "seed money" provided by the federal government under this act would get local health care for the homeless programs going and that state and local communities would eventually assume the costs of the programs. Today the total numbers have changed little, and the percentage of homeless who are mentally ill or have alcohol or drug problems remains around 70%.

Economic strategies. Other strategies to ease the housing problem in the United States focus primar-

---

Homeless Mental Patients

An especially disturbing dimension of the problem of the homeless is the growing number of the mentally ill in this population. Rescue mission workers estimate that a third of those who seek help are former mental patients with nowhere else to turn. In the United States, the number of patients in psychiatric wards has been halved since 1970. In some states, two thirds of the beds have been emptied by court orders allowing mental hospitals to keep only those patients judged a threat to themselves or others. Mayor Edward Koch of New York City, which had at least 40,000 homeless people, complained in 1985 that many neighborhoods had been turned into "outdoor psychiatric wards."

Los Angeles estimates that, because of the city's warm climate, the number of homeless people in the downtown district doubles in winter to more than 15,000. The county mental health department claims that other communities give one way bus tickets to Los Angeles to many of their chronically mentally ill homeless as part of a "Greyhound therapy" plan to clear their own communities of the housing burden.

Like toxic agents, the homeless are seen by many communities as something to be dumped in other communities. How can communities be supported in taking greater responsibility for the housing of homeless people? How can homelessness be prevented?

A Case Study

The East Harlem Environmental Extension Service, Inc. (a nonprofit corporation representing housing groups, owners, tenants, and job training organizations working with the Department of Community Medicine of the Mount Sinai School of Medicine and New York City's Board of Education), initiated a training, stipend and field service program for east Harlem residents. The extension service began its training programs with three training cycles of 15 participants. During training each participant received $80 per week rising to $100. Subjects taught were boiler maintenance, plastering, painting, electrical work, simple plumbing, carpentry, fire prevention, and rodent and pest control. Red Cross first aid training was a key part of the program, and a field manual on health and safety was put to use. The program was linked with family health workers, public health workers, public health nurses, and community health guides.

The program improved the housing in east Harlem and gave the trainees vocational skills that afforded them better opportunities for employment. It showed the way and encouraged other communities to assess their situation and to develop programs that provided improved housing for their citizens. A similar concept demonstrated in Baltimore, Maryland, activated inner city youth enrolled in a community pediatric center to repair broken windows in their neighborhoods. Community leaders have the opportunity to initiate and develop projects for housing betterment.

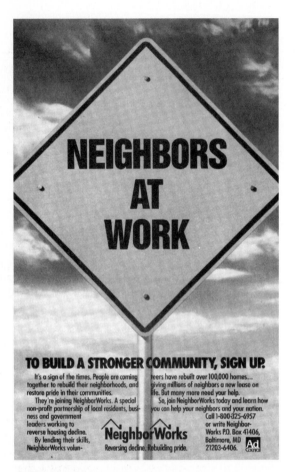

NEIGHBORS AT WORK

TO BUILD A STRONGER COMMUNITY, SIGN UP.

It's a sign of the times. People are coming together to rebuild their neighborhoods, and restore pride in their communities.

They're joining NeighborWorks. A special non-profit partnership of local residents, business and government leaders working to reverse housing decline. By lending their skills, NeighborWorks volun-

teers have rebuilt over 100,000 homes... giving millions of neighbors a new lease on life. But many more need your help.

So, join NeighborWorks today and learn how you can help your neighbors and your nation.

Call 1-800-325-6957 or write Neighbor-Works P.O. Box 41406, Baltimore, MD 21203-6406.

NeighborWorks
Reversing decline. Rebuilding pride.

FIGURE 15-5
Community cooperation between volunteers, businesses, and public agencies has been stimulated in the face of declining housing quality in neighborhoods.
Source: Advertising Council.

ily on taxation policies. One such approach would increase the personal income-tax exemption to give low-income taxpayers more discretionary income. Another would eliminate home-owners tax deductions, especially on second homes used for vacation purposes, on the grounds that these deductions primarily subsidize interest rates for high-income tax-

payers. A third would put a heavier tax on short-term capital gains from the sale of housing. This would discourage speculative buying and selling of real estate for short-term profits, which artificially inflates the cost of housing. A federal housing bank is needed to finance low-income housing at minimal or zero interest rates. One strategy that has had the most publicity because of former President Jimmy Carter's active participation is the mobilization of volunteers and local businesses to redevelop neighborhood housing (see Figure 15-5).

It is likely that Medicaid cuts in the United States, combined with reductions in subsidized low-cost housing and more stringent criteria for Social Security payments, and continuing deinstitutionalization of mental patients will result in continuing homelessness in the years ahead, especially for the mentally ill.

OCCUPATIONAL HEALTH ENVIRONMENTS

Occupational environments must be organized to protect the personal health of the worker. Modern occupational health has been extended to include nonoccupational as well as occupational factors that affect the health of workers.

Management usually has a legal responsibility for factors affecting the health of workers. In some instances management goes beyond legal requirements. Management occasionally concerns itself not only with the well-being of workers but also with the welfare of their families. This policy may be regarded as benevolence by some people and is criticized as paternalism by others. Yet, at times, it is necessary to extend the health program beyond the work environment to the home environment.

Attempts to promote the health of workers should be encouraged as a product of collective bargaining if not as the self-initiating action of management. The protection of workers by preventing occupational hazards, however, is of such public concern

Health Status and Risk Reduction Objectives for Occupational Health and Safety for the Year 2000

- Reduce deaths from work-related injuries to no more than 4 per 100,000 full-time workers. (Baseline: Average of 6 per 100,000 during 1983-87)

Special Population Targets

Work-Related Death Rate (per 100,000)	1983-87 Average	2000 Target	Percent Change
Mine workers	30.3	21	
Construction workers	25.0	17	
Transportation workers	15.2	10	
Farm workers	14.0	9.5	

Annual Survey of Occupational Injuries and Illnesses. The Bureau of Labor Statistics collects these data for businesses with 11 or more workers.

- Reduce work-related injuries resulting in medical treatment, lost time from work, or restricted work activity to no more than 6 cases per 100 full-time workers. (Baseline: 7.7 per 100 in 1987)

Special Population Targets

Work-Related Injuries (per 100)	1983-87 Average	2000 Target	Percent Change
Construction workers	14.9	10	
Nursing and personal care workers	12.7	9	
Farm workers	12.4	8	
Transportation workers	8.3	6	
Mining workers	8.3	6	

Annual Survey of Occupational Injuries and Illnesses.

- Reduce occupational skin disorders or diseases to an incidence of no more than 55 per 100,000 full-time workers. (Baseline: Average of 64 per 100,000 during 1983-87*)
- Increase to at least 75% the proportion of worksites with 50 or more employees that mandate employee use of occupant protection systems, such as seatbelts, during all work-related motor vehicle travel. (Baseline data available in 1991*)
- Reduce to no more than 15% the proportion of workers exposed to average daily noise levels that exceed 85 dBA in 1992*)
- Eliminate exposures which result in workers having blood lead concentrations greater than 25 μg/dL of whole blood. (Baseline: 4505 workers with blood lead levels above 25 μg/dL in 6 states in 1988*)
- Increase hepatitis B immunization levels to 90% among occupationally exposed workers. (Baseline data available in 1991†)

*National Institute for Occupational Safety and Health.
† Center for Prevention Services.

that it must be translated into legal codes recognizing minimum responsibility for reducing such hazards. Most managements accept this responsibility willingly and go beyond legal stipulations, but some are governed entirely by the requirements of the law in dealing with occupational health and safety, and some violate the law in their negligence.

Because many workers are overlooked in the promotion of industrial health, the community must be concerned. This concern should extend beyond mere legal requirements to the sphere of whatever measures are essential for protection and promotion of the health of every worker.

Epidemiology of Occupational Illness

In the United States the National Institute for Occupational Safety and Health (NIOSH) estimates that each year 100,000 Americans die from occupational illnesses. Nearly 400,000 new cases of occupational diseases occur annually. (These estimates are controversial, but no better ones are available.) When multiple etiological factors are considered, between 10% and 20% of all cancer cases may be related to carcinogens in the workplace.

An occupational health program properly goes beyond the prevention of hazards to physical and mental health and extends into the positive promotion of the health of workers. Health education, rest, recreation, treatment of sudden illness, optical services, and even diagnosis of ailments are aspects of modern occupational health. A competent, trained worker is a valuable asset in industry. The same worker possessing a high level of health is an even more valuable asset. Management is interested in its employees' quality of health for economic reasons, which include concerns with absenteeism, productivity, and morale which relates to satisfaction with working conditions. Some hazards to health are always present in any occupation, operation, plant, or industry. What is important is the degree of danger facing workers. Some hazards are so extreme that

they must be eliminated or markedly reduced, while others are of less concern.

Injuries. Injuries pose an immediate threat in virtually all occupations, as Chapter 13 indicated. Industries alert to their responsibilities in injury control are concerned almost entirely with the safety of their own employees. In some industries such as transportation, however, safety concerns include possible injuries to others as well as to employees.

Dusts, gases, and fumes. Dusts, gases, and fumes can be a hazard to the general public as well as to employees. Fortunately, means are available to reduce these hazards to tolerable levels. Maximum allowable concentration values adopted for various industrial poisons refer to average concentrations that can be tolerated continuously 8 hours per day without impairment to health immediately or in the future (Figure 15-6).

Dusts are generally classed as inert, irritating, and toxic. Inert vegetable and animal dusts are present in papermaking, weaving, spinning, and other manufacturing processes that use wool and similar raw materials, but the dangers are not great. Mineral and metallic dusts are more dangerous. Stonecutters, drillers, miners, grinders, and polishers encounter respiratory damage resulting from inert dusts. Granite and quartz dust cause damage to the lungs resulting in *silicosis,* a lung disease that is fatal unless the condition is recognized early and exposure to dust is prevented.

Dusts pose two problems. The first is that of concentration. The second is the important matter of particle size. Both concentration and size of dust particles can be measured.

Inert and irritating dusts usually can be kept to a minimum level. Wet processing reduces the production of dust. Enclosing work that creates dusts, combined with the use of exhaust systems, can reduce dust to a level below the danger point.

Toxic dusts, gases, and fumes such as asbestos,

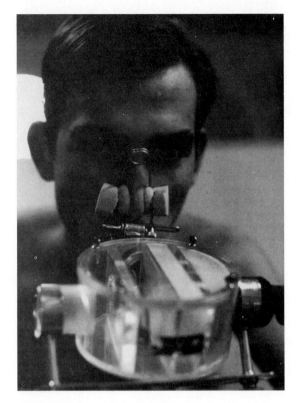

FIGURE 15-6
A worker undergoing a breathing test to assess effects of exposure to occupational gas emissions.
Source: World Health Organization, photo by P. Larsen.

arsenic, mercury, lead, iron oxide, sulfuric acid, carbon monoxide, and manganese pose specific problems of control (Table 15-1). Management is usually alert to hazards of this type and is constantly devising procedures to reduce or eliminate these dangers. Research, often with an assist from governmental agencies, is developing measures for the prevention of these industrial hazards. Although the immediate concern is for the worker within the plant, management also has a concern for possible effects on the general public. It is generally conceded that no industrial process hazardous to human health is so in-

dispensable to the economy that it could not be eliminated if it cannot be altered sufficiently to protect the health of workers.

Excessive temperature or humidity. Blast furnaces, smelters, kilns, tanneries, textile mills, laundries, and breweries are examples of industrial processes that make temperature or humidity control difficult. Dermatitis, gastrointestinal disturbances, eye inflammations, and even exhaustion result from atmosphere extremes. Air conditioning can bring atmospheric conditions to tolerable levels. Some workers are physiologically not equipped to tolerate even moderate atmospheric change.

Excessive noise. Industry recognizes that noise is more than a health hazard, as it affects production. Noise is an arbitrary descriptor that includes frequency, quality, and loudness of sounds. Loudness is measured in **decibels.** The lowest sound the human ear can detect is 1 decibel. Loudness is expressed as multiples on a logarithmic scale of the smallest distinguishable difference in sound. Thus a sound of 10 decibels is 10 times louder than 1 decibel; a sound of 20 decibels is 100 times louder than 1 decibel. This logarithmic expression is used as a convenience in avoiding the use of numbers in four or more figures. Long doses of 90 decibels can cause hearing loss. Higher levels can be injurious to hearing, and lesser levels can be disturbing. The annoyance threshold for intermittent sounds is 50 decibels to 90 decibels, discomfort occurs at 110 decibels, and the pain threshold is in the vicinity of 120 decibels. A short exposure to a noise of 150 decibels can cause permanent hearing loss.

Decibel levels correspond to the following: whisper, 10 decibels; quiet street, 50 decibels; normal conversation, 50 to 60 decibels; truck or sports car, 90 decibels; pneumatic jackhammer 95 decibels; loud outdoor motor, 100 decibels; loud power mower, 105 decibels; siren, 125 decibels; riveting, 130 decibels; jet takeoff, 150 decibels. Rock music

TABLE 15-1
Major occupational hazards and the estimated numbers of workers exposed in the United States

Potential dangers	Diseases that may result	Workers exposed (U.S.)
Asbestos	White-lung disease (asbestosis); cancer of lungs and lining of lungs; cancer of other organs	Miners; millers; textile, insulation and shipyard workers—estimated 1.6 million exposed
Lead	Kidney disease, anemia; central nervous system damage; sterility; birth defects	Metal grinders; lead-smelter workers; lead storage-battery workers—estimated 835,000 exposed
Arsenic	Lung cancer, skin cancer, liver cancer	Smelter, chemical, oil-refinery workers; pesticide makers and sprayers—estimated 660,000 exposed
Benzene	Leukemia; aplastic anemia	Petrochemical and oil-refinery workers; dye users; distillers; chemists; painters; shoemakers—estimated 600,000 exposed
Cotton dust	Brown-lung disease (byssinosis); chronic bronchitis; emphysema	Textile workers—estimated 600,000 exposed
Coal dust	Black-lung disease	Coal miners—estimated 208,000 exposed
Coke-oven emissions	Cancer of lungs, kidneys	Coke-oven workers—estimated 30,000 exposed
Radiation (x-rays)	Cancer of thyroid, skin, breast, lungs and bone; leukemia; reproductive effects (spontaneous abortion, genetic damage)	Medical technicians, uranium miners; nuclear power and atomic workers
Vinyl chloride	Cancer of liver, brain, lung	Plastic-industry workers—estimated 10,000 directly exposed

Source: Occupational Safety and Health Administration; Nuclear Regulatory Commission, U.S. Depts. of Energy, Interior, and Health and Human Services; Health and Welfare Canada.

bands have adversely affected the hearing of their members, indicating a hazard of that occupation.

Infections. Infections are a latent hazard in all occupations and are a particularly serious hazard in some industries. Slaughterhouse employees, dairy workers, and others who handle livestock or hides are exposed to such diseases as brucellosis and anthrax. Health care workers may be exposed to the HIV virus through unsafe handling and disposal of used needles. Other workers handle substances that serve as media for pathogens of humans. The use of disinfectants and sterilizing methods should prevent most infections in these categories. Medical atten-

tion to all suspected cases of infection is necessary in industry as well as elsewhere.

Toxic chemicals. Harmful substances other than gases and fumes can be present in industry (see Table 15-1). Chemicals used in plant operations can cause harm to the skin. Chronic poisoning can occur in workers improperly handling materials in routine operations. Knowledge of the presence of these hazards and proper regulations governing their handling reduce or virtually eliminate the danger. Legal regulations and management alertness combine to make poisoning rather rare in modern industry.

Radiation. Health hazards of radiation are not a new concern. Luminous paints containing radioactive compounds were recognized as a hazard more than 70 years ago, during World War I; a number of women died after ingesting considerable amounts of radium through the habit of licking the points of their brushes while painting the luminous dials on watches.

Today, the use of radioactive products requires special precautions of shielding and the use of personal safety measures such as protective clothing. A necessary safeguard is the use of meters for monitoring the amount of exposure to radiation. Standards for maximum permissible concentration (**MPC**) of radiation have been established for various circumstances.

Disposal of radioactive wastes in the United States is in accordance with standards set by the U.S. Atomic Energy Commission. Sufficient knowledge about radiation hazards is now available, and industry is applying this knowledge to prevent any radiation danger to employees or to the general public.

The current opposition to nuclear reactors is partially the usual backlash when new developments are introduced, according to those who work with radioactive materials. But the concerns about environmental effects as well as health effects are justifiable in the wake of Chernobyl.

Sanitation. Proper sanitation measures have long been a concern and accepted responsibility of industry. Industrial sanitation programs are designed to provide conditions that will safeguard the health of employees as well as provide for maximum production.

A safe and adequate water supply is a first requisite. Industries usually obtain their water from an approved municipal supply. If a private source is used, the water should be free from turbidity and contamination and should be tested regularly. A daily test would be called for when threat of contamination is present; once a week can be ample at other times. About 20 gallons per worker per day is necessary for all purposes, although the amount varies with the kind of industry involved. Approved drinking fountains should be placed in convenient locations in the plant, the number depending on the number of workers and the nature of their work.

When an auxiliary water supply is used for fire protection, flushing, and other such purposes, this second supply should be safe for human consumption or so controlled that there will be no possibility that workers will use the unsafe water for drinking or handwashing purposes. Using red or some other color for such faucets or fixtures is a common safeguard.

An approved type of sewage system for liquid wastes is an indispensable sanitation measure. If the plant sewage system cannot be connected to a community system, then provisions must be made for plant sewage disposal.

Washrooms must be of good construction with adequate toilets and washbasins. The number of toilet units varies from 1 per 10 workers to 1 per 30 workers. When urinals are installed, only two thirds as many units are needed.

Washing faucets may be preferred over washbasins because they are less likely to be a means of infection spread. Automatic control of temperatures at 125° F (52° C) is possible with the mixture of hot and cold water running from the same faucet. Liquid soap is preferred because bar soap too easily finds its way to the floor. Shower heads are attached to the wall usually just below average worker chin level.

Illumination. Lighting that meets recommended standards reduces accidents and eyestrain and improves efficiency and productive output. Where highly detailed work is involved, as much as 100 footcandles of illumination is recommended. Illumination of at least 50 footcandles is required in such areas. Along hallways, or where no great visual discrimination is called for, from 10 to 20 footcandles can be adequate. It is always important to avoid great contrasts in degree of illumination from one area to another. A ratio of 5 to 1 is preferred, with 10 to 1 the outside limit.

Ventilation. Proper ventilation of industrial plants is designed to provide physical comfort by controlling the temperature, humidity, and movement of air. Either natural or artificial means are employed. Removing body heat and moisture in the summer and providing circulation and moderate temperature in the winter are the customary goals. Temperature between 66° and 72° F (19° and 22° C) with a relative humidity of 50%, combined with movement of air, provides for physical comfort.

Some industries have the problem of removing dusts, gases, vapors, and fumes, for which exhaust systems are employed. If air is recirculated, the ventilation system must be operating efficiently at all times. This requires competent maintenance.

Responsibility for Occupational Health

Management, workers, unions, local government, and the national government all have responsibilities in occupational health. Local health departments are rarely equipped to provide the highly technical professional services that occupational health problems demand. Whether the local health department can provide extensive or decidedly limited service, the overall approach must be that of cooperation between all persons and organizations concerned with a particular occupational health problem. Health departments do not enter these situations as a police force but as public servants ready to help remedy existing health problems. Only when industrial management fails to live up to established and accepted standards will the force of legal authority be exercised.

Setting standards. The identification of occupational hazards and illnesses calls for the development of standards for major common health hazards for injury and toxic exposures. Setting and main-

---

> ### Services and Protection Objectives for Occupational Health and Safety for the Year 2000
>
> - Implement occupational safety and health plans in 50 states for the identification, management, and prevention of leading work-related diseases and injuries within the state. (Baseline: 10 states in 1989: 32 states in 1992.*)
> - Establish in 50 states exposure standards adequate to prevent the major occupational lung diseases to which their worker populations are exposed (byssinosis, asbestosis, coal workers' pneumoconiosis, and silicosis).
> - Increase to at least 70% the proportion of worksites with 50 or more employees that have implemented programs on worker health and safety.
> - Establish in 50 states either public health or labor department programs that provide consultation and assistance to small businesses to implement safety and health programs for their employees.
> - Increase to 75% the proportion of primary care providers who routinely elicit occupational health and safety exposures as a part of patient history and provide relevant counseling.
>
> *Public Health Foundation.

---

taining standards require increased numbers of health hazard evaluations, and routine questioning about occupational health risks by physicians and other health care providers as part of their patients' medical history. National objectives also relate to increasing workers' knowledge of hazards at their worksite. Educational objectives to increase workers' knowledge of occupational risks include informing workers routinely of their personal exposure measurements, of the results of their health examinations, and about life-style behaviors that interact with factors in the work environment to increase risks.

A state or provincial occupational health division

may be in the department of health or the department of labor. In either arrangement, the purpose of the occupational health staff is to assist all industry with health problems unique to the industry, to conduct surveys, and to enforce regulations relating to occupational health. Teamwork between industry, workers, and official occupational health personnel is the key to effective programs for the promotion of occupational health.

Priorities. Allocation of resources for occupational health must be based on considerations of frequency of occurrence, severity of effect, and the likelihood of effective prevention. These three criteria have led to the following list of priorities:

Ten leading work-related diseases and injuries

---

1. Occupational lung diseases
2. Musculoskeletal injuries
3. Occupational cancers
4. Severe occupational traumatic injuries
5. Occupational cardiovascular diseases
6. Disorders of reproduction
7. Neurotoxic disorders
8. Noise-induced hearing loss
9. Dermatological conditions
10. Psychological disorders

OSHA. On the national level in the United States the National Institute for Occupational Safety and Health (NIOSH) was created by the Occupational Safety and Health Act of 1970 (PL 91-596). The Occupational Safety and Health Administration (**OSHA**) was created to implement most of the regulatory provisions of the act. Congress declared as its purpose and policy in this act ''to assure as far as possible every working man and woman in the Nation safe and healthful working conditions and to preserve our human resources'' by encouraging employers and employees in their efforts to reduce the number of occupational safety and health hazards at their places of employment, and to institute new ... to perfect existing programs for providing safe and healthful working conditions.

Hazard Prevention and Occupational Health Promotion

Components of a comprehensive workplace health program include the implementation of regulatory policies promulgated by federal and state agencies, but also the other channels of influence suggested by Figure 15-7. Specific interventions follow:

Educational and informational measures. Measures that communities and employers or unions can take to support behavior and to increase awareness include the following:

- Reviewing, recommending, initiating, and publicizing occupational health and safety standards and practices necessary for monitoring and surveillance of on-the-job health and safety standards, including environmental health requirements
- Initiating by management, in concert with workers and their representatives, experimental and innovative educational programs relevant to workers' occupational health and safety needs
- Initiating and expanding methods designed to motivate labor and management responsibility for the development and maintenance of a safe and healthful work and community environment
- Developing awareness of the potential interactions between occupational health hazards and life-style habits and their effects on health
- Developing worker awareness through electronic and print media, vocational training programs, information from health care providers, campaigns aimed at high-risk worker groups (for example, asbestos workers, newly em-

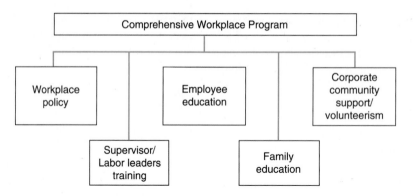

FIGURE 15-7
Channels for implementing a comprehensive occupational health program include more than just the regulatory mechanisms implied by policies. They also include involvement of workers, supervisors, community organizations and volunteers, families of workers, and labor leaders.
Source: Centers for Disease Control and Prevention.

ployed workers, and elderly workers), and organized labor programs

- Training professional occupational health and safety personnel, including occupational health physicians and nurses, industrial hygienists, toxicologists, and epidemiologists, and including occupational health education in the curricula of medical and nursing schools and in continuing education for health professionals
- Developing awareness in other groups involved with workers or the workplace, including engineers, managers, teachers, social workers, and health care workers
- Developing public awareness of occupational disease and injuries and their high cost to the nation
- Using labeling in simple language to inform workers, employers, health professionals, and the public of occupational hazards, associated risks, and symptoms as appropriate
- Including occupational health as part of the comprehensive health education curricula in high schools

Service measures. Organizational supports for behavior conducive to worker health include the following:

- Implementing well-designed corporate occupational health programs that include preventive and treatment services directed at nonoccupational as well as occupational health
- Promoting consultation services of governmental agencies to assist small businesses to identify problems and to establish suitable programs for eliminating or controlling these problems (Figure 15-8)
- Encouraging small businesses to form cooperative groups to seek occupational health expertise
- Developing a personal health service delivery system in which the diagnosis and treatment of occupational illnesses and injuries will be coordinated and integrated with all other health services that are provided the worker and his or her family
- Upgrading capabilities of state or provincial and local health departments to participate in occupational health and safety services, in-

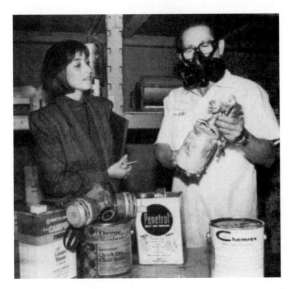

FIGURE 15-8
Paints produce fumes from their solvents, some of which pose respiratory hazards, especially when combined with cigarette smoking. Surveillance of equipment, precautionary practices, and protective clothing are difficult with construction workers because of their transient rather than stationary work patterns.
Source: University of Texas Health Science Center at Houston.

cluding monitoring, surveillance, and consultation to small businesses

Technological measures. Ways to improve the physical environment of the workplace to make it more conducive to health include

- Improved architectural and engineering design of worksites to prevent injuries
- Control technology to protect workers, including development of safe substitutes for toxic substances, design of process units to eliminate worker exposure, implementation of safe maintenance procedures, and modification of jobs to eliminate harmful physical and mental stress
- Measurement technology to enable quick, accurate, and economical assessment of hazard

levels in the workplace by workers, employers, or health professionals

Legislative and regulatory measures. Some of the political and legal strategies possible include

- Fully implementing laws related to workers' health and provisions for product control
- Recommending, initiating, and evaluating measures designed to improve and expand occupational health and safety legislation, paying particular attention to the possibility of standardizing benefits through a national system of worker's compensation
- Developing criteria and documents recommending standards
- Promulgating new health standards for hazardous substances
- Requiring annual inspections by industrial hygiene compliance officers
- Conducting mandated industry-wide studies and health hazard evaluations for carcinogenicity and reproductive effects that could lead to temporary emergency standards
- Changing worker's compensation laws to put stronger economic pressures on employers to reduce hazardous conditions at the worksite

Economic measures. Government agencies can further support improvements through fines and negative publicity for companies with poor health and safety conditions and through tax deduction measures for capital investment in control technology or occupational health programs.

Relative strength of the measures. Given the broad nature and scope of occupational safety and health problems, the relative strength of the measures varies with the problem at hand, with the nature and adequacy of enforcement efforts and with research capacity. Most occupational health problems require the simultaneous or consecutive application of several types of measures as a comprehensive strategy for hazard eradication. For example, eradication of the asbestos hazard might be achieved by

- Banning all nonessential uses of asbestos
- Substitution of other materials found to be nonhazardous
- Research to determine all human exposure during the "life cycle" of the fiber
- Worker education to minimize exposure that may still occur during demolition and repair work
- Rigid enforcement of control standards wherever use of asbestos remains necessary
- Professional education for physicians to assure proper medical help for exposed individuals

This type of eradication program focuses public attention on the problem and goes beyond merely establishing a standard for permissible exposure levels.

Finally, better data and better surveillance systems are required if occupational safety and health are to be measurably improved.

OTHER ENVIRONMENTS

This section will concentrate on a few remaining health concerns arising out of environmental aspects of recreation. These concerns tend to be overrated by the public. Given that 65% of the average North American's time is spent inside his or her home, and 22% is spent at work, this chapter has already addressed the environments in which people spend 87% of their time. Future predictions suggests that North Americans will spend increased time at home "cocooning." Of the remaining time, another 6% is spent in transit between home and work, leaving a total of only 7% at other locations, such as shops, banks, and recreational settings. If exposure time is a criterion of health risk, recreational and other environments pose a limited threat. The fact that recreation is an optional, discretionary use of one's

time makes the public more avid in seeking information about and assurances of safety and health protection in these settings.

Smoking in Public Places

Some studies indicate that ambient smoke can adversely affect the health of nonsmokers. Thus, regulating smoking in public places is desirable. Bars and other drinking establishments are notorious for their reputation as smokefilled places, but restaurants in many parts of the world now offer nonsmoking areas. City and state ordinances require nonsmoking sections in many establishments and ban smoking in some, such as theaters, elevators, public buildings and—increasingly—transport vehicles.

Swimming Areas

Recent developments in swimming pool construction and natural bathing areas have caused health officials to expand their programs for regulating public swimming facilities. This regulatory authority of state, provincial, and community health departments extends to pools and natural bathing areas of motels, hotels, resorts, parks, and other enterprises serving the public.

Health aspects of swimming facilities. On the positive side, swimming can promote both physical and mental well-being. On the negative side, accidents associated with swimming represent a great threat to health and life. In recent years, unsupervised motel pools have taken a frightful toll of lives by drowning. Slipping on slick walkways and in shower and locker rooms has been a source of serious injuries. Diving also has resulted in numerous injuries and deaths. Long hair trapped in Jacuzzi jets has resulted in drowning in relatively shallow water.

Disease spread via swimming facilities is always a possibility, but the general public harbors many misconceptions about the role of such facilities in disease spread. It is extremely doubtful that respiratory diseases are ever spread by water in a pool or other swimming facility. No tangible evidence exists that such diseases as the common cold, influenza, tuberculosis, or poliomyelitis are spread via pool water. The close social contact of swimmers may be a factor in the transfer of respiratory diseases, but the pool itself is not a vehicle of spread. Pinkeye (conjunctivitis) is not spread by pool water, but swimmers using the same towel may thus communicate it.

Diseases most likely to be transmitted via water in swimming facilities are those of the intestinal tract. Typhoid fever and bacillary dysentery may be conveyed by water, but it is doubtful that salmonellosis is ever transmitted in this way. If water in a swimming pool is chlorinated properly, however, the danger of typhoid fever and dysentery spread is zero.

Certain skin infections are transmitted from swimmer to swimmer by physical contact associated with activities at the pool, the locker room, or the shower room, or by handling common objects. Athlete's foot (tinea pedis), boils (furunculosis), and impetigo contagiosa can be transmitted through contact associated with swimming activities. Swimmers' itch and schistosomiasis can be contracted from natural swimming waters. However, the simple measure of dragging a bag of copper sulfate around a lake behind a boat will rid the waters of schistosomes.

Swimming pools. Many types of swimming pools are constructed: competitive pools, diving tanks, instructional pools, recreational pools, and pools for other purposes. Yet, as specified by the American Public Health Association, there are certain common construction needs—impervious, permanent materials for walls, bottom, vertical ends and sides; inlets submerged in a safe place; outlets synchronized with inlets; overflow gutters all around to allow slight overflow; and nonslip walkways at least

5 feet wide all around the pool. Showers and locker rooms should be well lighted, well ventilated, and clean.

Artificial pools are classified on the basis of water-fill methods, which affect the quality of the water.

1. *Fill-draw* means the pool is filled and emptied at regular intervals. Timing is determined by the physical appearance of the water and the bathing load. This type of pool can be acceptable when properly operated. However, whether this type is used depends on the cost of water and the nature of pool use. Fill-draw pools are acceptable where use by swimmers is limited, but they are seldom constructed today.

2. *Flow-through* means there is a continuous passage of water in and out of the pool and the chlorine content is controlled. This type of pool is highly acceptable, but the cost of water makes it highly uneconomical.

3. *Recirculating* means that the water from one part of the pool is removed by pumps and, after being filtered and decontaminated by chlorination, is returned to the pool. Using the water over and over again is economical. In addition, the water quality is excellent. For these two reasons, this type of pool is most frequently constructed.

Water in swimming pools is usually decontaminated by chlorination, although bromine and ozone are also used. Bromine is more stable and tenacious than chlorine, but bromine fumes are highly irritating to the eyes and respiratory tract. Ozone is extremely expensive and little used, except for pools on ships, on estates, or at clubs.

When chlorine is used, a chlorine residual from 0.4 to 0.6 ppm should be maintained. This chlorine level may be irritating to the eyes of some swimmers. Alkalinity of the water should be maintained at pH between 7.2 and 8.2. Not more than 15% of water samples should contain more than 200 bacteria per milliliter, as determined by the standard agar plate count, or contain more than 1 coliform organism per 50 milliliters of sample.

Wading pools. Much less sanitary than swimming pools, wading pools are frequently little more than cesspools. The usual practice is to add water constantly, using a standard of 0.5 ppm chlorine residual for decontamination purposes. Under moderate or heavy use, a wading pool should be drained and refilled at least twice a day.

Spas and hot-tubs. Like wading pools, spas and hot-tubs can become a medium for pollutants, especially if used by small children. Because of their heat and small size, spas and hot-tubs can give rise to great concentrations and rapid growth of organisms. Another danger is that of overheating, which can cause burns and cardiovascular problems; people are especially susceptible to overheating when they are drinking alcoholic beverages. New guidelines have been promulgated by the Centers for Disease Control for special maintenance of spas and hot-tubs.

Natural bathing areas. Lakes, rivers, and ponds used for swimming purposes are frequently dangerously polluted. Sewage, cesspool drainage, and other effluents may contaminate such water. Many public swimming areas are unsupervised, but even those that are supervised are not always safe.

Supervision of natural bathing areas consists of identifying and preventing all possible sources of pollution and then keeping a close check on the degree of contamination. A permissible maximum coliform count of 1000 per 100 milliliters is standard. Areas are also classified by the following average coliform index:

Class	Coliforms per 100 Milliliters
A	0-49
B	50-499
C	500-999
D	Over 1000 (unacceptable)

Because of the danger of typhoid, dysentery, and staphylococcus infections, even a relatively low coliform index does not make a swimming area safe. For this reason, health officials, using other data, sometimes close down swimming areas that may have been used for many years without any apparent mishaps.

Regulations. All public swimming pools are subject to official regulation. A pool is classed as a **public pool** if it is used by people other than the owners or their families. Whether a charge is made for the use of the pool is not a consideration in classifying a pool as public. In the United States authority to regulate public swimming facilities rests with the state. However, if the state legislature has granted home rule to a county or city, the county or city has authority to regulate public swimming pools within its territorial jurisdiction.

State regulation of public swimming facilities is usually vested in the state department of health. Permits to operate a public swimming facility are issued annually to those individuals or organizations having pools that meet all state specifications relating to construction and maintenance. A nominal fee is charged for the permit. Annual renewal is contingent on safe operation and the maintenance of conditions acceptable to the state inspectors, who make periodic inspections.

Community regulation of public swimming pools is based on an ordinance and related regulations. Many communities use as a guide the *Suggested Ordinance and Regulations Covering Public Swimming Pools,* a model developed by the Joint Committee on Swimming Pools of the American Public Health Association in cooperation with the U.S. Public Health Service. This model ordinance is a guide to be used in the design, construction, operation, and maintenance of public swimming pools. Provisions are reasonable and are not restrictive or punitive. The ordinance begins by requiring submission of plans and specifications and outlining acceptable materials and construction. This includes specifications for dressing rooms, showers, and toilet facilities. Guidelines for pool operation, pool maintenance, and supervision of swimmers are given, including safety requirements and lifesaving equipment. In all respects, this model ordinance can be adapted to all situations and can serve admirably for communities accepting their responsibilities in regulating public swimming pools.

The county or city health department is customarily charged with responsibility for enforcement of the swimming pool ordinance. Health department sanitarians include this function in their regular responsibilities. In addition, sanitarians provide a consulting service for citizens requesting information or advice relating to private residential pools. Sanitarians also make regular inspections of conditions in natural bathing areas and take such action as is necessary to protect the public against hazards. Much of the work in swimming facilities regulation goes unnoticed, yet it is becoming a progressively more significant public health function as the population and its recreational activities expand.

SUMMARY

People spend over four fifths of their time in home and work environments. These environments therefore deserve special attention from community health agencies to assure their safety and freedom from serious health risks. Where risks cannot be eliminated, people need to be informed of the risks, of ways to avoid or minimize them, and of tests they can obtain to determine the safety of their environment or to assess their health status in relation to the risks.

Major hazards in residential environments include substandard facilities, crowding, lead paint, and indoor pollution. Building regulations and codes protect the public against some of these hazards, and informed residents can prevent or minimize others through proper ventilation, cleaning, storage, and repainting practices. Population and economic trends have led to increased numbers of people who are homeless, even in Europe and the

United States. Deinstitutionalization of the mentally ill has added a particularly vulnerable population to the homeless.

Occupational risks other than injuries, which are discussed in Chapter 13, include dusts, gases, fumes, chemicals, excessive noise, poor ventilation, inadequate lighting, temperature and humidity extremes, infections, and radiation. Employers and workers share the responsibility for reducing occupational hazards, with government setting standards, regulations, and enforcement procedures through laws such as the Occupational Safety and Health Act in the United States.

People spend only a small proportion of their time in recreational and other nonresidential, nonoccupational environments, but it can be a high-risk proportion. Public places are increasingly regulated to reduce potential exposure to health risks. Smok-

---

To Improve Occupational Safety and Health, by the year 2000 . . .

Objectives target reducing deaths from work-related injuries; reducing work-related injuries, cumulative trauma disorders, occupational skin disorders, and hepatitis B infections; increasing the proportion of worksites that mandate employee use of occupant protection systems; reducing worker exposure to high daily noise levels; eliminating exposures that result in workers having high blood lead concentrations; increasing hepatitis B immunization levels among occupationally exposed workers; implementing State occupational safety and health plans for the identification, management, and prevention of work-related injuries and diseases; establishing exposure standards to prevent major occupational lung diseases, and public health/labor department programs that provide assistance to small businesses to implement employee safety and health programs; increasing worksite programs on worker health and safety and back injury prevention and rehabilitation; and increasing the primary care providers who routinely elicit occupational health exposures as a part of patient history and provide relevant counseling.

ing in public places has been banned or restricted in many communities and on some public transportation. Swimming facilities present minimal risks, other than injuries, if properly managed, but wading pools and spas or hot-tubs require extra precautions.

QUESTIONS FOR REVIEW

1. Why is it so difficult to determine scientifically the effect of housing on health?

2. How has improved insulation produced a problem of increased indoor pollution?

3. How do building regulations and zoning codes protect the public's health and safety?

4. What were the major factors leading to the shelter poverty of the 1970s and the homelessness of the 1980s and 1990s?

5. Why should employers want to invest in the health of workers?

6. What factors might account for the improving record of occupational illness and injury over the past decade?

7. Thinking of the college or university as a workplace, how would you organize efforts to improve the health conditions for workers or students?

8. Why should recreational environments be of any less concern for health purposes than home and work environments?

9. Why has smoking in public places become such an issue?

10. With all the people sharing public swimming pools, why are such facilities not a great health hazard?

11. Why are spas and hot tubs at greater risk of causing disease than swimming pools?

READINGS

American Public Health Association and American Academy of Pediatrics: *Caring for our children—national health and safety performance standards: guidelines for out-of-home child care programs,* Washington, DC, 1993, American Public Health Association.

Guidelines for the development and evaluation of the health and safety aspects of family/group day care homes and child care centers, beginning with the environmental quality of the care and recreational facilities.

Panel on Dosimetric Assumption Affecting the Applications of Radon Risk Estimates: *Comparative dosimetry of radon in mines and homes,* Washington, DC, 1991, National Academy Press.

Household radon risk may be overestimated, this panel concluded from its study of evidence for the Environmental Protection Agency. After several years of warning the public about the risk of lung cancer from exposure to radon in the home, based on estimates derived from radon exposure in mines, the conclusion is that the exposure rate is 30% less in a home than the occupational risk in a mine with the same level of radon gas, mainly because a miner is breathing harder under working conditions.

Shinn M: Homelessness: what is a psychologist to do? *Am J Community Psychol* 20:1, 1992.

Comparing person-centered and structural explanations for homelessness from data on the distribution of poverty, inadequate and unaffordable housing and 700 families requesting shelter in New York City, this article draws implications for research and action by psychologists.

Sprague JF: *More than housing: lifeboats and children,* Stoneham Mass, 1991, Butterworth Architecture.

New environments responding to the critical social needs of homeless mothers and children are described in this book. Building plans and environmental requirements include descriptions of new zoning laws, childcare services, and shared spaces. Examples range from emergency housing to transitional and permanent dwellings for single-mother families.

Weeks JL, Levy BS, Wagner GR: *Preventing occupational disease and injury,* Washington, DC, 1991, American Public Health Association.

The up-to-date handbook has a public health orientation to occupational disease with strategies for prevention, legal and regulatory resources, worker education and training and an alphabetical listing of disease entities with methods of identification, occurrence, causes, pathophysiology, prevention, and further readings on each.

BIBLIOGRAPHY

American Institute of Architects: *An architect's guide to building codes and standards,* ed 2, Washington, DC, 1991, American Institute of Architects.

Baser ME: The development of registries for surveillance of adult lead exposure, 1981 to 1992, *Am J Public Health* 82:1113, 1992.

Burrell R, Glaherty D, Sauers LJ: *Toxicology of the immune system: a human approach,* New York, 1992, Van Nostrand Reinhold.

Consumer Product Safety Commission and American Lung Association: *Biological pollutants in your home,* Washington, DC, 1990, Consumer Product Safety Commission.

Corn JK: *Response to occupational health hazards: An historical perspective,* New York, 1992, Van Nostrand Reinhold.

Fawcett T, Moon RE, Philip JF et al: Warehouse workers' headache; carbon monoxide poisoning from propane-fuelled forklifts, *J Occup Med* 34:12, 1992.

Fischer DB, Boyer A: State activities for prevention of lead poisoning among children—United States, 1992, *MMWR* 42:165, 1993.

Greeley A: Getting the lead out . . . of just about everything, FDA Consumer Mag reprint (revised from July-Aug 1991 issue), DHHS Publ. No. (FDA) 92-2249, Washington DC, 1992, U.S. Government Printing Office.

Guidotti TL, Clough VM: Occupational health concerns of firefighting, *Annu Rev Public Health* 13:151, 1992.

Hall JR: *U.S. experience with smoke detectors,* Quincy, Mass, 1992, National Fire Protection Association.

Lewis RJ Sr: *Sax's dangerous properties of industrial materials,* ed 8, New York, 1992, Van Nostrand Reinhold.

Lovato CY, Green LW: Maintaining employee participation in workplace health promotion programs, *Health Educ Q* 17:73, 1990.

Mood EW, editor: *Housing and health: APHA-CDC recommended minimum housing standards,* Washington, DC, 1986, American Public Health Association.

National Institute for Occupational Safety and Health: NIOSH health hazard evaluation program, Pub No 648-004/40829, Atlanta, 1992, Centers for Disease Control, Public Health Service, U.S. Government Printing Office.

New South Wales Cancer Council and New South Wales Health Department: *Developing policies for schools,* Sydney, 1991, NSW Cancer Council.

Office of Technology Assessment, U.S. Congress: *Neurotoxicity: Identifying and controlling poisons of the nervous system,* New York, 1992, Van Nostrand Reinhold.

Pauls J: Safety standards, requirements, and litigation in relation to building use and safety, especially safety from falls involving stairs, *Safety Sci* 14:125, 1991.

Sciarillo WG, Alexander G, Farrell KP: Lead exposure and child behavior, *Am J Public Health* 82:1356, 1992.

Tarter SK, Robins TG: Chronic noise exposure, high-frequency hearing loss, and hypertension among automotive assembly workers, *J Occup Med* 32:685, 1990.

Tenforde TS: Biological interactions and potential health effects of extremely-low-frequency magnetic fields from power lines and other common sources, *Annu Rev Public Health* 13:173, 1992.

Toro PA, McDonnell DM: Beliefs, attitudes, and knowledge about homelessness: a survey of the general public, *Am J Community Psychol* 20:53, 1992.

Trauma Foundation: Special issue on housing codes, *Injury Prev Network Newsletter* 9:1, 1992.

Upton AC, Shore RE, Harley NH: The health effects of low-level ionizing radiation, *Annu Rev Public Health* 13:127, 1992.

Wallerstein N, Rubenstein H: *Teaching about job hazards: a guide for workers and their health providers,* Washington, DC, 1993, American Public Health Association.

Webb GR, Redman S, Sanson-Fisher RW: Work injury experience at an industrial worksite, *J Occup Health Safety Austral NZ* 8:143, 1992.

Winkleby MA, Rockhill B, Jatulis D et al: The medical origins of homelessness, *Am J Public Health* 82:1394, 1992.

Wintemute GJ: Drowning in early childhood, *Ped Annals* 22:417, 1992.

Yoon PW: *Guidelines for baseline surveys and impact assessments: training papers in population and family welfare education in the worksetting,* No 1, Albany, NY, 1992, International Labor Office, United Nations, ILO Publications Center.

Zaebst D, Stern F, Heitbrink W et al: Evaluation of techniques for reducing diesel forklift emissions, *Appl Occup Environ Hyg* 7:17, 1992.

Chapter 16

Community Food and Vector Control

❖

I aimed for the public's heart and hit it in the stomach.

UPTON SINCLAIR

OBJECTIVES

When you finish this chapter, you should be able to:

- Describe the modes of transmission of disease by food and other vehicles and vectors
- Identify the major food protection and vector control strategies for communities and sources of their authority
- Develop objectives for a community food and vector control program

---

Sinclair's novel *The Jungle* (1906) exposed filthy conditions in the Chicago stockyards and meatpacking plants, which aroused public indignation to a level that enabled passage of the U.S. Pure Food and Drug Act and the Federal Meat Inspection Act. To put these landmark legislative acts in perspective, you might review some of the milestones of public health listed in Chapter 1 and note in particular the landmarks listed on the next page. These reflect people's centuries-old search for safe food (Figure 16-1).

The first Pure Food and Drug Act, passed by Congress in 1906, was directed primarily at food adulteration. Even when supplemented by the Copeland-Tugwell Act of 1938, which was directed at proper sanitation in processing and handling of foods, the act was considerably watered down from the original proposal as the result of lobbying by manufacturers with vested interests. The Food and Drug Administration (FDA) has the main responsibility to protect the safety and quality of foods.

Most countries hold the food producer, processor, or manufacturer legally responsible for sanitary and safe food, which means food that is clean and

Milestones in Food Protection		
1203	England's King John promulgates the first Assize of Bread, the foundation of all food regulation in the English-speaking world.	
1785	Massachusetts passes the first comprehensive food adulteration law in the United States.	
1820	Friedrich Accum publishes *Treatise on Adulteration of Food and Culinary Poisons.*	
1850	Lemuel Shattuck's report for Massachusetts recommends control of adulterated food as part of a comprehensive public health system.	
1862	Congress establishes the U.S. Department of Agriculture and authorizes scientific experiments relating to agricultural chemistry.	
1880	The National Board of Trade conducts a competition for a draft of a national food law, which ultimately leads to the Pure Food and Drug Act of 1906.	
1884	The Bureau of Animal Industry is created within the Department of Agriculture to prevent interstate shipment or export of diseased cattle.	
1890	Congress passes a law to prohibit the importation of adulterated food.	
1906	The Pure Food and Drug (Wiley) Act prohibits interstate commerce in misbranded and adulterated foods, drinks, and drugs. Federal Meat Inspection Act passed.	

1916	USDA publishes *Food for Young Children,* first dietary guidance pamphlet.
1917	U.S. Food Administration established to supervise World War I food supply. USDA's first dietary recommendations—*Five Food Groups.*
1924	Addition of iodine to salt to prevent goiter, first U.S. food fortification program.
1927	Food, Drug, and Insecticide Administration established. Name is changed to Food and Drug Administration (FDA) in 1932.
1933	Agricultural Act amendments permit purchase of surplus commodities for donation to child nutrition and school lunch program.
1938	The Food, Drug and Cosmetic (FD&C) Act includes provisions for food standards, FDA nutrition research program established. Social Security Act supports role of nutrition in health.
1941	President Roosevelt's National Nutrition Conference and first Recommended Dietary Allowances by the Food and Nutrition Board. FDA promulgates standards for enrichment of flour and bread with B-complex vitamins and iron.
1946	National School Lunch Program established.

continued

safe for human consumption. This has long been referred to in common law as the implied warranty or guarantee that the product is safe. Those selling food cannot claim ignorance of the fact that food is contaminated or otherwise objectionable as a valid defense. Regulatory control of foods sold to the public is still necessary. The closer the implementation of this control is to the consumer, the more effective the control. On the state or provincial level, the departments or ministries of agriculture and of health have responsibility for controlling foods. On the community level, the county, district, or city health department usually has this responsibility.

EPIDEMIOLOGY OF FOOD-BORNE DISEASE

Unsavory as it may be to consume dirty or decomposed food, the epidemiology of food control is concerned only with threats to health. Food must be sanitary and safe if it is not to be a **vehicle** for the transmission of disease-causing toxins or organisms or intolerable levels of carcinogens.

Modes of Transmission

Food can transfer disease by five different means: inherently harmful characteristics, allergy, ptomaine poisoning, toxin transfer, and infection transfer.

Milestones in Food Protection—cont'd	
1958 Food Additives Amendment for FD&C Act Prohibits use of a food additive until safety established by manufacturer. Delaney Clause prohibits carcinogenic additives. GRAS (Generally Recognized as Safe) list established.	1988 DHHS publishes *The Surgeon General's Report on Nutrition and Health.*
1965 Food Stamp Act passed by Congress. Nationwide Food Consumption Survey collects first data on dietary intake of individuals.	1989 The National Academy of Sciences releases reports on *Diet and Health* and the role of pesticides in agriculture and food safety.
1967 U.S. Congress passes first major meat inspection law since 1906, requiring states to have inspection requirements at least equal to federal requirements.	1990 The U.S. *Healthy People 2000* objective for the nation includes four objectives for reduction of foodborne illnesses (see later box).
1972 USDA establishes Special Supplementary Food Program for Women, Infants, and Children (WIC). Agriculture and Consumer Protection Act provides price support to farmers Amendments to Older Americans Act of 1965 establish a congregate and home delivered meals program.	1991 FDA completes the Total Diet Study on Americans' dietary intake of pesticide residues, concluding that the levels on domestic and imported foods were ''quite low and represent no appreciable public health risk.''
	1992 USDA publishes the Food Guide Pyramid (Figure 16-2) and, together with the U.S. Public Health Service, endorses the use of irradiation as an adjunct to other food safety technologies and procedures.
1980 USDA and USDHHS jointly issue *Nutrition and Your Health Dietary Guidelines for Americans.* DHHS issued *Promoting Health/Preventing Disease: Objectives for the Nation,* with 17 nutrition objectives for the year 1990.	1993 Federal policy on pesticides reversed by FDA, EPA, and USDA, now endorsing the use of ''integrated pest management'' with beneficial insects and crop rotation for some pesticides.
1984 The U.S. Surgeon General's Workshop on Breastfeeding and Human Lactation develops strategies for promoting breastfeeding.	1994 New food labels required on all U.S. canned and packaged foods to enable consumers to make informed nutritional choices.

Other harmful effects of food consumption behavior have been addressed in the chapter on health promotion in terms of excess consumption of dietary fats, cholesterol and alcohol, and insufficient consumption of nutrients and fiber. The focus in this chapter is on the environmental aspects of food protection and the related behavioral aspects of gathering, processing, transporting, storing and preparing food.

Inherently harmful foods. Food poisoning is a term used so generally that it encompasses a spectrum of digestive disorders, but distinction should

be made between a food that is itself poisonous and a food that merely serves as a vehicle for the transmission of pathogens to humans. Some 70 to 80 species of mushrooms are inherently poisonous to all people. Yet these poisonous plants are not a serious community health problem because the general public is well informed in this regard. Commercial producers of such foods as mushrooms have both the knowledge and the legal responsibility to provide the market with safe foods.

Food allergies. A food may also be classed as poisonous for a person who is allergic to it. By ''al-

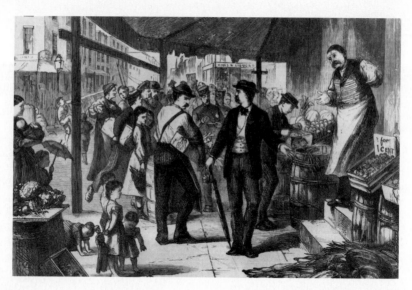

FIGURE 16-1

Inspection of fruit in New York markets by order of the Board of Health, circa 1873. Today the public's concern with fruits, vegetables, and grains, as well as meat, fish, and poultry, is the residual pesticides or chemical fertilizers that might make them hazardous to health, just when public health and nutrition advocates are recommending increased (for most people) consumption of high-fiber grains, fruits, and vegetables (see Figure 16-2).

Source: After R. Lewis, *Harper's Weekly* 17:796, 1873. Courtesy National Library of Medicine.

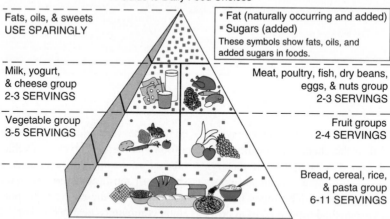

Food Guide Pyramid
A Guide to Daily Food Choices

Fats, oils, & sweets
USE SPARINGLY

- Fat (naturally occurring and added)
- Sugars (added)
These symbols show fats, oils, and
added sugars in foods.

Milk, yogurt,
& cheese group
2-3 SERVINGS

Meat, poultry, fish, dry beans,
eggs, & nuts group
2-3 SERVINGS

Vegetable group
3-5 SERVINGS

Fruit groups
2-4 SERVINGS

Bread, cereal, rice,
& pasta group
6-11 SERVINGS

FIGURE 16-2

After several years of field testing with diverse populations, USDA issued this graphic, "The Food Guide Pyramid," in 1992 to communicate three key dietary guidance concepts—variety, moderation, and proportionality. Food safety was not addressed, either in the dietary guidelines of the United States and Canada, or in the Food Guide Pyramid. In fact, however, the relative safety of foods is somewhat proportional to the relative frequency with which they are recommended.

Source: U.S. Department of Agriculture.

lergy'' is meant a condition of altered tissue reaction, in which reexposure to a substance produces disturbing effects. About 30% of Americans have food allergies. Rarely does a person have an allergy to a single food. Community health strives through public health education to assure that the public knows that food allergy may cause **rhinitis,** asthma, gastrointestinal disturbances, cardiovascular disturbances, and various skin disorders. Informed citizens can then seek medical services to determine whether they have allergies that would account for having one or more of these symptoms.

Ptomaine poisoning. A ptomaine is a toxin formed in the decomposition of protein through bacterial action. Meat that is sufficiently decomposed to possess ptomaines would be totally unpalatable. Even if meat is this badly decomposed, there would be no harmful results if it were well cooked before being eaten because the heat would break up the protein chains that compose the ptomaines. It is doubtful that anyone in the United States dies of ptomaine poisoning.

Toxin transfer by food. Food occasionally serves as the vehicle for transferring toxins to the digestive system of humans. Normal cooking processes usually disintegrate toxins, but because of a lack of understanding people may fail to take precautions necessary to protect themselves against poisoning by foodborne toxins.

Botulism is caused by a neurotoxin produced by the spore-forming organism *Clostridium botulinum,* which is found in alkaline and neutral soils. Raw vegetables have vast numbers of the organism on them but are not a threat to health because the organism is **anaerobic,** meaning that it does not produce toxin in free air. A person eating raw beans, peas, beets, or other vegetables would not be affected. However, if these vegetables are subjected in the canning process to an ordinary boiling temperature of 212° F (100° C), the spores withstand

Botulism Case Studies

Case 1

A 22-year-old California man awoke at 2 AM with vomiting, blurred vision, and a ''thick tongue.'' Symptoms progressed to total quadriplegia, then respiratory failure requiring mechanical ventilation. Two days earlier the patient had eaten stew prepared by his roommate from fresh ingredients (including meat and unpeeled potatoes and carrots) then left overnight at room temperature. The roommate ate it hot on the first night with no subsequent illness. The patient tasted it without reheating 16 hours later and complained of a bad taste. The roommate confirmed a sour taste, immediately spit it out, rinsed his mouth and remained well. The patient was treated with antitoxin and recovered after extended hospitalization.

Case 2

A man of Egyptian descent, age 32 years, was admitted to the hospital after a series of emergency visits because of rapidly progressive problems including dizziness, facial drooping, dry mouth, weakness, and respiratory failure requiring mechanical ventilation. Three family members developed similar symptoms the next day. The New Jersey Department of Health traced the source of botulism to an ethnic preparation of fish known as moloha, an uneviscerated, salt-cured fish product. The family consumed the moloha without cooking or heating it the day before the man appeared with symptoms. The fish market from which the family bought the fish denied selling moloha or similar fish products, and none could be found on the premises. The public was alerted through the news media to avoid eating moloha. No additional cases were reported.

Why did these incidents occur even though the food was not home canned and had been cooked in one case?

Cases summarized from reports in *MMWR* 34:146, 1985; and 41:521, 1992.

that temperature and the organism survives. Placed in the anaerobic conditions of a can or jar, the organism produces toxin. If the vegetables are well cooked before they are eaten, the toxin is destroyed. If the vegetables are eaten without being brought to a boil, however, the toxin can be fatal, as it is one of the most potent of known poisons.

About 24 hours after the toxin has been ingested, gastrointestinal symptoms may appear. An acute poisoning of the nervous system becomes apparent, and paralysis of the respiratory system or the muscles of swallowing occurs. Treatment of botulism is by antitoxin, given intravenously. The antitoxin should be administered as soon as possible to be effective.

Commercial canners eliminate the possibility of botulism poisoning by using pressure cooking at 248° F (120° C). The community health problem is that of educating the public about the need either to use pressure cookers for canning or to use tyndallization, which means bringing the food to a boil (212° F) on 3 consecutive days before canning. The public should know that, in any case, the best preventive measure is always to bring previously cooked vegetables or meat to a boil before serving.

Infection transfer by food. A food cannot transfer pathogens unless the following favorable conditions exist:

1. The organism must be virile and exist in large numbers.
2. The time interval from reservoir to a new host must be short.
3. The temperature must be favorable (in the neighborhood of 100° F [38° C], which is optimum for pathogens of humans).
4. Moisture must be available.
5. Very little light can be present.

Many pathogens of humans are not transferred by food. Except for a few respiratory diseases transferred via milk, virtually all infectious diseases transferred by food are those of the digestive system—amebic dysentery, salmonellosis, tapeworm, trichinosis, typhoid fever, and viral hepatitis. Because cow's milk can be an excellent medium for pathogens affecting the respiratory and other human systems, a few other diseases also transferred by milk must be mentioned—bovine tuberculosis, brucellosis, diphtheria, human tuberculosis, Q fever, and streptococcal infections (Figure 16-3). Protection of food primarily seeks to prevent food becoming a vehicle of pathogen transmission, a task that can be accomplished by preventing pathogens from reaching food and by destroying the organisms that have reached food.

Control of Milk and Dairy Products

Pathogens can enter milk from many sources, but there will likely be only two reservoirs: the cow, and human beings who handle the milk. Accordingly, all cows should be tested for tuberculosis, brucellosis, and mastitis, and all reactors should be culled from the dairy herd. Even though pasteurization would destroy the organisms causing these diseases, it would be foolhardy not to take the extra precaution of preventing pathogens from entering milk to be consumed by humans. Clinical examination of dairy personnel is of questionable value except where there is a history of tuberculosis or typhoid fever.

Milk processing. With the use of modern equipment, milk can go from the cow's udder to the bottle without ever being exposed to light. Yet even with the finest equipment, milk protein still requires training of the operating personnel, well-constructed stables with cement gutters, ample light, well-maintained ventilation, and fly control. A separate milking room has merit from the standpoint of sanitation. Whether hand milking or machine milking isused, all objects that might contaminate the milk should be decontaminated or removed from the milkhouse.

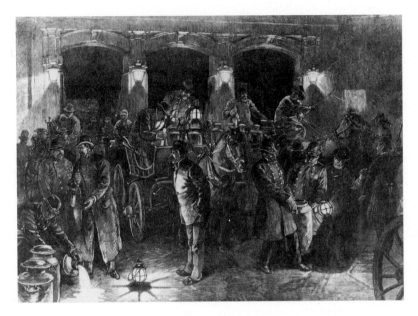

FIGURE 16-3
Concerns in the nineteenth century with food adulteration and inspection were expressed in dramatic novels such as Upton Sinclair's *The Jungle,* and in drawings such as this depiction of an early morning inspection and throwing out of adulterated milk by New York Board of Health inspectors.
Source: After W.A. Rogers, *Harper's Weekly* 26:185, March 25, 1882. Courtesy National Library of Medicine.

Producing farms should filter, or strain, all milk and cool it to 50° F (10° C) immediately after milking.

Pasteurization. As the best available safeguard against transmission of disease via milk, pasteurization consists of heating to a temperature for a period of time that will destroy pathogens but will not appreciably affect the quality of the product. The ''holding'' method of pasteurization heats the milk to 143° F (62° C) and holds it at this level for 30 minutes. This method destroys pathogens but does not affect taste, proteins, fats, sugars, or salts. It does reduce the level of vitamin C, but milk is not relied on as a source of this nutrient anyway, since the vitamin C content of milk is normally low. The ''flash'' method of pasteurization does the same job by heating the milk to 161° F (72° C) for 15 seconds.

Cooling and bottling should be done immediately after the pasteurizing. A temperature of 50° F (10° C) should be maintained. Paper containers have some advantages over bottles.

Salmonellosis outbreaks. The largest outbreak ever recorded of **salmonella** poisoning in the United States occurred in 1985 in Illinois. The Illinois Department of Public Health confirmed 5770 cases of salmonellosis. The pathogen was isolated from unopened containers of two lots of 2% milk processed at the same dairy plant in Illinois. The milk must have been inadequately pasteurized or contaminated after pasteurization. The contaminated milk was sold in three supermarket chains in Illinois, Indiana, Iowa, and Michigan. After the source of the outbreak had been identified, the dairy plant was closed immediately and all milk produced by the plant was removed from store shelves. In addition to the Illinois cases of salmonellosis, 289 cases were reported in Indiana, 43 in Michigan, and 28 in Iowa. Three other states reported 19 cases among persons returning from one of those states.

The rate of salmonellosis cases, excluding typhoid fever, increased in the United States from 1955 when the rate was only 3 per 100,000 population to 1987 when the rate was 22 per 100,000 population. A slight downward trend has occurred since then. The cause (or causes) of the increase is unknown, but the rate increases since 1977 have occurred primarily among the older age groups. The continuing increase in the number of outbreaks can be seen clearly in the trend shown in Figure 16-4.

Regulation of milk supplies. In some countries, state or provincial agricultural departments regulate milk supplies. In others the agricultural department

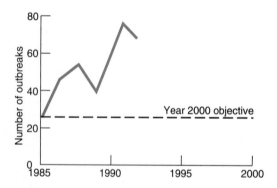

FIGURE 16-4
The year 2000 objective to reduce outbreaks of infections due to *Salmonella enteritidis* to fewer than 25 reported outbreaks per year will be difficult to achieve if recent trends in new outbreaks continue.
Source: U.S. Department of Agriculture, Centers for Disease Control and Prevention, and the Food and Drug Administration.

regulates economic factors and the health department regulates sanitation of milk supplies. Some states have a milk control board. State regulations set standards, but the most effective control exists on the local level. Accordingly, on the recommendation of the city health department, cities pass ordinances regulating the sale of milk in the community. A county, through its health department, also can regulate the sale of milk within its jurisdiction. These regulations can exceed state standards but cannot be lower than state standards.

The U.S. Public Health Service has developed a model ordinance governing the marketing of milk. Communities adopt ordinances adapted from this model. The model ordinance recognizes two grades of milk to be sold to the public. In addition to specifications dealing with farm facilities, processing methods, and other essentials, the ordinance sets up laboratory examination criteria of grades of milk.

Regulations are enforced by the issuance of a permit to sell milk following approval of the farm, the processing facilities, and other factors. Periodic inspections by sanitarians will apprise the dairy farmer of the sanitary quality of his or her operation. A health department, after reasonable warnings, may order a dairy farmer or milk plant to discontinue the sale of milk or refuse to renew the permit when it expires. The seller has the right to appeal to the governing health board or to the courts.

Milk Products. Manufacture of milk products has become big business, with processes controlled through state or provincial regulation, supplemented by local supervision, protecting the community against epidemics.

Ice cream mixes are pasteurized and stored at 10° F ($-12°$ C). Contamination would come from containers, dippers, and dispensers. Processing of frozen desserts generally comes under the same official scrutiny as does processing of other dairy products.

Butter requires pasteurization at higher levels than market milk. The fat is promptly cooled and then held in vats for churning. Cheese, because its curing process kills most pathogens, is relatively safe. "Green" cheese (not time-cured) can transmit pathogens such as the typhoid bacillus. Some cheese manufacturers take the precaution of pasteurizing the milk they use, but most do not deem this necessary. Cottage cheese, unless pasteurized and stored at 40° F (4° C), could easily transmit pathogens of humans.

The managers of most processing plants take pride in their business and can be relied on to produce a safe product. The relationship between processors and inspectors is usually harmonious. Inspectors serve in an advisory capacity on sanitation as well as in a regulating role. Legal measures to enforce sanitary standards for dairy products are usually employed only after all other means have failed.

Control of Meat, Fish, and Poultry

The public rebels against eating the meat from diseased animals. Even though cooking or curing kills pathogens, biochemical changes in the animal can give the meat a foul taste and even produce human illness. In addition, how meat is processed after slaughter affects its palatability and nutritional qualities. Improper canning can also be a danger to humans in that pathogens conveyed to the meat can survive and cause disease. The public also expects to be protected against the adding of cornmeal or other grains to ground meat or processed meats.

Control measures. Training of personnel, health education, demonstrations, and conferences have supported proper meat processing. Nevertheless, there remains a need for governmental inspection of meat on the national, state or provincial, and local levels.

The Meat Inspection Act of 1906 created the Meat Inspection Division of the U.S. Department of Agriculture. The act sought to safeguard the public by eliminating diseased or other bad meat from distribution, to supervise the sanitary preparation of meat and meat products, and to prevent the use of false or misleading names or statements on labels. Technically, the authority of the federal agency extends only over meats and meat products shipped in interstate or international commerce. In recent years, however, courts have interpreted "interstate" so broadly that virtually all transported meat is being so classed. This has caused some conflict between federal and state inspection functions, particularly in those states with decidedly inadequate meat inspection programs. In general, the large meat plants have fallen under federal regulation and the small local plants have been left to state or community inspection.

In 1967 Congress passed the first substantive legislation on meat inspection since the original act of 1906. The new act provided that the states had to have inspection requirements at least equal to those of the federal government. The act authorized the U.S. Secretary of Agriculture to take over interstate meat inspection in states falling below the federal standards. Title I of the act greatly broadened the scope of inspection, so that more than 500 additional plants were subject to federal regulation.

In 1992 the U.S. Public Health Service and the U.S. Department of Agriculture endorsed the use of **irradiation** as a safe and effective means to control *Salmonella* and other foodborne bacteria in raw chicken, turkey, and other poultry. Up to 60% of poultry sold in North America is contaminated with *Salmonella,* and studies suggest that all chicken may be contaminated with the *Campylobacter* organism. Consumer apprehension of irradiation has been a drawback to implementing the procedure, even though irradiation does not make food radioactive or increase human exposure to radiation. Some states either banned or issued a moratorium on the sale of irradiated foods in response to public fears. The World Health Organization concluded that irradiation can substantially reduce food poisoning, although it should not be used as a substitute for careful handling, storage, and cooking of food. Irradiated poultry can become recontaminated.

In January 1993 one the worst food-poisoning outbreaks ever to occur in the United States left 450 people sick, 230 with culture-confirmed infection with *Escherichia coli* 0157:H7, resulting in bloody diarrhea and hemolytic uremic syndrome affecting kidneys, sometimes acute renal failure. At least one toddler died. Investigations linked cases to consumption of hamburgers from one fast-food restaurant chain. *E. coli* 0157:H7 was isolated from epidemiologically implicated lots of ground beef. The company initiated an interstate recall to its Jack-in-the-Box outlets in three Pacific Northwest states in addition to Washington.

How could this outbreak have been prevented? The U.S. Department of Agriculture has undertaken a review of the national meat inspection system and processing phases, from slaughterhouse handling to meat grinding, transport, storage, sufficient cooking, and hygienic practices of restaurant personnel. Ground meats are most dangerous because grinding equipment may be a source of contaminants. Ground meat also has more surfaces on which microorganisms can multiply. The ultimate protection against these sources of contamination and reproduction of the organism would have been more thorough cooking, which would kill the *E. coli* organisms. The federal government and many states now recommend that all ground meats be cooked well past the pink stage at 155°F. and that the public avoid eating raw or pink hamburger.

Based on Centers for Disease Control and Prevention: *MMWR* 42:85, 1993; and Griffin PM, Tauxe, RV: The epidemiology of infections caused by *Escherichia coli* 0157:H7, other enterohemorrhagic *E. coli*, and the associated hemolytic uremic syndrome, *Epidemiol Rev* 13:60, 1991.

One other control measure not yet adopted in North America, but developed recently in Japan and widely used there and gradually in Europe, is **high-pressure food processing.** Not to be confused with home pressure cooking, this commercial process uses water pressure instead of heat. In conventional pasteurizing of packaged liquid products, food mak-

ers typically boil the food in batches to kill bacteria, but this destroys some taste and up to 30% of vitamins and minerals. High-pressure food processing preserves the fresh taste and nutritional quality of the food. It is most widely used with jams and other fruit products but is increasingly applied to meat, fish, and poultry processing.

Fresh meats. Some slaughterhouses limit their activities to slaughtering and the necessary cold storage, but many meatpacking plants combine slaughtering, cold storage, freezing, smoking, and pickling operations. In the United States most states supplement the federal meat inspection program by having their own inspection services for most slaughterhouses and all packing plants not under federal inspection.

Inspection of animals before slaughter serves to detect any disease or other adverse conditions. Killing, bleeding, and postmortem inspections of the hides, carcasses, and organs will detect gross pathology, and tissue examination will further detect disease conditions. Questionable carcasses are condemned, although the meat may be used for some purposes. A ''grade'' stamp on meat designates the grade quality of the meat, while the ''inspection'' stamp indicates that the meat has been passed as being safe.

Beef is placed immediately after slaughter in a cooler at 34° F (1° C), where it will be stored from 4 to 6 weeks. This storage improves flavor and texture because of the autolysis that occurs. Beef frozen at −15° F (−26° C) can be stored for more than a year. Pork, veal, and mutton are usually held for 3 days before being cut (see Table 16-1).

Cured and processed meats. Curing of such products as bacon, ham, and frankfurters calls for chilled meat that is moderately moist, pickling solution and brine, and a covered vat to prevent contamination. Cured meats are not necessarily completely protected against spoilage or deterioration. Proper storage is always necessary.

TABLE 16-1

Guidelines for market and home storage of fresh meats and dairy products underscore the importance of "use by" dating of products to indicate how long a product will retain optimum quality before consumption

Product	Storage period in . . .	
	Refrigerator	*Freezer*
Fresh meat		
Beef		
Ground	1-2 days	3-4 mo
Steaks and roasts	3-5 days	6-12 mo
Pork		
Chops	3-5 days	3-4 mo
Ground	1-2 days	1-2 mo
Roasts	3-5 days	4-8 mo
Cured meats		
Lunch meat	3-5 days	1-2 mo
Sausage	1-2 days	1-2 mo
Gravy	1-2 days	3 mo
Fish		
Lean (such as cod)	1-2 days	up to 6 mo
Fatty (such as blue, perch, salmon)	1-2 days	2-3 mo
Chicken		
Whole	1-2 days	12 mo
Parts	1-2 days	9 mo
Giblets	1-2 days	3-4 mo
Dairy products		
Cheese—Swiss, brick, processed	3-4 wk	*
Milk	5 days	1 mo
Eggs		
Fresh in shell	3-5 wk	—
Hard-boiled	1 wk	—

*Cheese can be frozen, but freezing will affect the texture and taste.
Sources: Food Marketing Institute for fish and dairy products; USDA for all other foods.

Processed meats pose the greatest danger of all meats and meat products. The usual processing of luncheon meats does not assure the destruction of all pathogens. Packaging and storage under inadequate refrigeration can provide a medium in which pathogens of humans can readily multiply; once the package is opened and the food handled, the remaining meat is often left at room temperature for some time, and then, in many instances, placed in refrigerators with temperatures considerably above 50° F (10° C).

Canned meats. Canned meats are first cooked. High temperatures and pressures are used without seriously affecting the quality of the product. Bacterial contamination can occur, with *C. botulinum* being one of the pathogens that might survive. Modern methods of meat canning minimize this risk.

Fish and shellfish. Fish is processed much like beef products. Fish can be held at a temperature of 40° F (4° C) for 2 weeks and be in excellent condition. Quick-freezing of fish, followed by a dip into clean water, produces an airtight coat of ice around each fish. All equipment used in processing fish should be decontaminated daily.

Other seafood, especially raw shellfish and fish harvested in unfavorable environments, pose a greater risk of foodborne illness. Ranking highest in risk of transmitting seafood-borne illness are raw or undercooked molluscan shellfish (oysters, clams, and mussels). The human risk is 1 illness per 250 servings of raw shellfish, whereas the risk from other seafood is 1 illness per 5 million servings. The comparative risk for poultry is 10 times less—1 in 25,000 servings. Raw shellfish account for 85% of all the illnesses caused by eating seafood.

Waters polluted with human sewage produce most of the problems. The most effective ways of protecting the safety of this food supply is preventing human wastes from getting into the waters and improving the monitoring of estuaries to prevent illegal harvesting of shellfish from polluted waters.

Proper cooking, once again, is the best self-protective measure individuals, families, and other food preparers can take. On-site inspection methods (sight and smell) between these two ends of the food protection chain cannot detect the viruses that cause hepatitis and the several types of bacteria that cause gastroenteritis from contaminated shellfish (Figure 16-5). Unlike meat and poultry, seafood is not sub-

ject to comprehensive mandatory inspections in North America. The FDA inspects only a tiny fraction of the 2.9 billion pounds of seafood imported each year, despite the fact that 50% of all seafood consumed in the United States is imported.

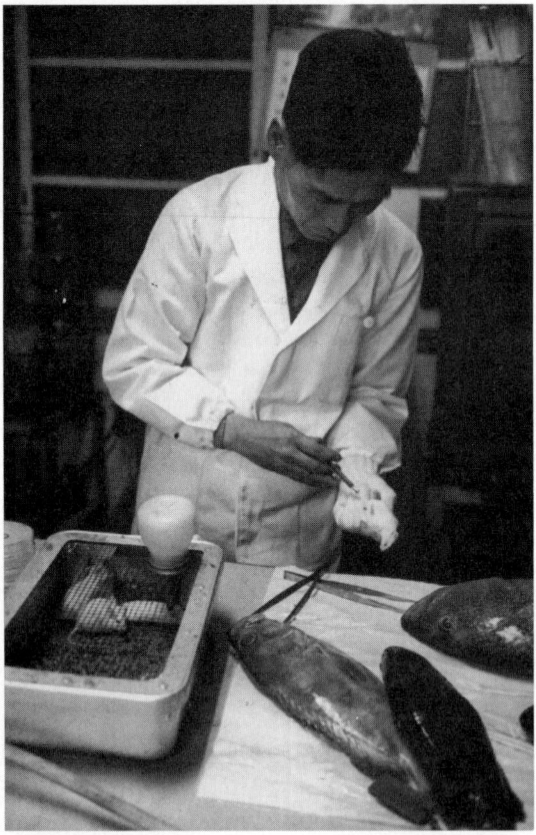

Canada has become increasingly concerned with the growing presence of toxins found in its fish. This is becoming a greater problem in Canada than the problems of bacteria or virus in seafood, especially for Native Indian and Inuit populations that depend heavily on fish for sustenance and for the regions in which heavy runoff of pesticides in agricultural areas are finding their way up the food chain to fish. The Great Lakes produce fish with high levels of industrial chemicals, and these are harvested as game fish.

Poultry. Poultry should be observed for a few days before killing. Poultry is quick-frozen at $-30°$ F ($-34°$ C) and stored at $-10°$ F ($-23°$ C). Canned poultry is processed under steam pressure of about 15 pounds per square inch, which should kill the *Salmonella* organism that fowl may harbor. If cold turkey or chicken is eaten without having been refrigerated since being served hot, salmonellosis transmission might occur.

Modern refrigeration and cooking facilities leave no excuse to transmit disease via meat. Unfortunately, handling of cold meats by a person who has an active case of or is a carrier of one of the foodborne diseases remains a likely mode of disease transmission via meat (Figure 16-6).

FIGURE 16-5
As North Americans become more concerned with high-fat foods, they are turning more to fish and experiencing more seafood-borne illnesses. Japan has long depended more on fish and has developed a wider range of inspection and testing methods, especially with those varieties used in sushi and other raw fish preparations.
Source: World Health Organization.

EATING ESTABLISHMENT REGULATIONS

No overwhelming evidence exists that dust or other dirt or a person coughing on food will transfer disease to the person who eats the food. Yet the public is entitled to sanitary and safe food when it eats in a public eating establishment. Cases of salmonellosis and viral hepatitis acquired in public eating places are more common than is generally realized.

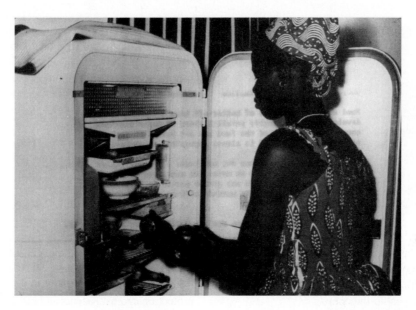

FIGURE 16-6
Food storage, preparation, and eating patterns of better-off town residents in the developing world roughly parallel those of industrialized countries, but much of their food has not passed through the food protection chain of the Western marketplace and is almost impossible to control. Thorough cooking is the best protection in these and other questionable circumstances.
Source: African Regional Office, World Health Organization and Food and Agriculture Organization. Photo by P. Pittet.

Amebic dysentery and typhoid fever can also result from eating in restaurants, schools, company cafeterias, and other institutions.

Citizens patronizing a public eating establishment may be neither qualified nor in a position to judge its sanitation. They must depend on the expertise and vigilance of the community health staff. Yet a better informed public could be a positive aid to the health staff by looking for restaurant ratings and by insisting that all public eating places practice sanitation standards set forth by the health department. Children and the elderly deserve special protection because they are more vulnerable.

Control Measures

Licensing of public eating places provides the instrument of control. To qualify for a license, the establishment must satisfy the equipment and operating requirements of the health department. Once the license has been issued, health department sanitarians make periodic inspections. Frequency and timing of inspections will depend on the known conditions of the restaurant and the number of available sanitarians.

Inspections

Rating of the restaurant usually follows the first inspection. Sanitarians find precise numerical rating to be difficult. Some health departments give A, B, or C ratings. Other departments give a rating of ''approved.'' A restaurant disapproved following an inspection will be given a probationary period in which to correct the deficiencies shown on the inspection form. Renewal of the operating permit will be denied if the establishment has failed to correct its faults. The owner may appeal to the community board of health and, in the event of an adverse decision, may appeal to the courts.

Personnel. Clinical examinations of new employees, even if accompanied by laboratory tests, are of limited value as a means for preventing disease spread via the restaurant. A more effective measure is to have employees well informed on the nature of disease spread and to enlist their active support in control. Above all, they should not come to work when they may have a communicable disease. Workshops for food handlers are held periodically by health departments to protect the patrons of eating establishments against infectious disease.

Facilities. A second key factor in the protection of the public is a safe water supply in the eating establishment. A third factor is proper toilet and lavatory facilities, with approved methods of waste disposal. Proper refrigeration and storage of food is highly important. Corrosion-proof utensils and equipment should be properly sanitized with detergents, decontaminants, and hot rinse water. All other safety factors are significant but perhaps not as vital as those enumerated above. Many sanitarians contend that rodent control is particularly important.

A meaningful overview of a full inspection can be garnered from the items in eating and drinking establishments that most local departments of health require their sanitarians to inspect. These items are listed not by order of importance, but for inspection convenience (see box on p. 495 and Figure 16-7).

The integrity of the management and the training and supervision of the employees produce restaurant personnel who are aware of their responsibility to the public and who know how to prepare and serve food properly.

Bakeries and confectionaries. Safeguards in producing bakery and confectionary products are similar to those essential to restaurant operations but are somewhat less demanding. Employee exclusion when necessary as a communicable disease control measure, safe water supply, proper waste disposal, protection against rodents and insects, proper refrigeration, and sanitizing of utensils are all important. The use of sanitary ingredients and the exercise of sanitary precautions during manufacture are also significant. Wrapping and other sanitary provisions are essential in handling and storing the finished product. Fortunately, cleanliness is the very nature of the bakery and the confectionary and, although sanitary inspections should be made at intervals, these establishments are rarely a cause of disease transmission.

Retail food stores. In retail food stores, safety of food is a first consideration in protecting the public. Refrigeration and storage are of primary importance. Elimination of all spoiled foods should be prompt and complete. Employees convalescing from an infection of the digestive tract should not handle uncovered foods. It would be difficult for organisms they might transfer to lettuce, tomatoes, or other produce to survive the customer's journey home, but the risk should not be ignored.

Cleanliness is a second consideration. Because of modern packaging, the customer is usually assured of clean food. Self-service gives customers an opportunity to do some inspecting themselves. Yet the

A Food Inspector's Checklist

Floors

Cleanable, good repair; smooth, nonabsorbent; cleaned properly.

Walls and Ceilings

Clean, good repair; finished, light color; washable to level of splash.

Lighting

Adequate light; working surfaces; storage rooms, preparation areas; fixtures clean.

Ventilation

Adequate ventilation; free from odors, condensate; stove hoods and ventilators, adequate design.

Toilet Facilities

Clean, ventilated; convenient, ample number; proper construction, good repair.

Water Supply

Adequate supply and pressure; approved construction; safe, complies with state standards.

Lavatory Facilities

Adequate, convenient to kitchen; hot and cold water; soap, sanitary towels, or air dryer; clean; good repair.

Construction of Utensils, Equipment

Cleanable construction; self-draining, no corrosion; free from cracks, chips; no open seams; no toxic utensils.

Cleaning of Equipment

Clean cases, counters, shelves, tables, meat blocks, refrigerators, stoves, hoods, can openers, freezers, and so on; clean cloths used.

Cleaning of Utensils

Single service used only once; dishwasher, sinks, drainboards, approved and maintained; kitchenware, tableware clean; dishwashing procedures approved.

Bacterial Treatment of Utensils

Approved sanitization, time, temperature, chemical concentration; machine properly operated; kitchenware adequately treated; dishtowels not being used.

Storage and Handling of Utensils

Protected from contamination; no handling of contact surfaces; single serviceware properly handled; dippers kept in running water.

Disposal of Wastes

Approved liquid waste disposal; plumbing complies with state code; approved garbage cans; covered, pending removal; clean and in good repair; garbage storage and removal approved.

Food Temperatures

Cold perishable food below 45° F (7° C); hot perishable food above 140° F (60° C); ice storing, handling approved; thermometer in each refrigerator; refrigerators maintained.

Wholesomeness of Food

Clean, no spoilage, safe; approved sources.

Wholesomeness of Milk Products

Milk, milk products approved; milk dispensed properly.

Wholesomeness of Shellfish

Approved sources; stored in original containers.

Preparation and Storage of Food

No contamination by immersion, leaking, or condensation; neat storage, off floor.

Display and Serving of Food, Drink

Minimum manual contact; food wrapped or covered; cafeteria front protected.

Vector Control

Fly control approved; roaches, insects controlled; rodents under control; structure rat-proof; no animals or fowls; all poisonous compounds stored away from food, proper use.

Cleanliness of Employees

Clean outer garments; clean hands and nails; no spitting, no tobacco used in rooms where food is prepared.

Housekeeping

Site, premises neat and clean; no operations in private quarters; adequate clothing lockers and dressing rooms kept clean; storage of soiled clothing, linens, mops, and so on.

Control

No person at work with any communicable disease, sores, or infected wounds; washing sign posted in all toilet facilities.

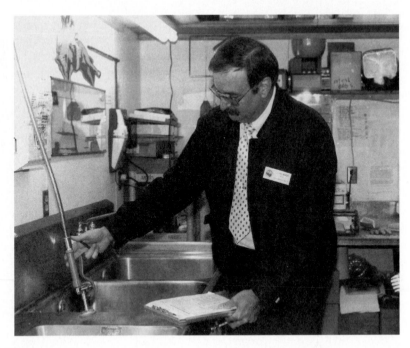

FIGURE 16-7
A sanitary inspector for a local health department examines the water supply and dishwashing facilities of a restaurant, with his checklist on a clipboard.
Source: Photo courtesy Lincoln-Lancaster County Health Department.

cleanliness of the whole store is desirable, and store managers know they will not be in business long if their store is not clean. Safe water should be used for all store purposes.

Community health departments do not find retail food stores a great problem. Occasionally the health department will have complaints against a market. For example, failure to dispose of discarded produce does pose a problem when employees are lax. A written warning by the health department sanitarian usually produces the necessary remedy.

Appraisal of Food Control Measures

Constant vigilance by health officials is essential to protect the public against foodborne diseases. Citi-zens cannot make their own inspections of restau-rants, dairies, slaughterhouses, or canneries and they cannot see what goes on in the back room of retail stores and bakeries. They must depend on the tech-nical expertise of officials paid from taxes. Yet cit-izens can aid their own cause by being knowledge-able and by cooperating with public officials who are protecting the public.

Many technical fields have provided communi-ties with methods and procedures for protection against the transmission of disease and poisons. Freezing as an alternative to canning is both con-venient and safe. Chemical additives lend protection as well as danger. Legislation protects consumers against the indiscriminate use of ingredients such as soybeans in hamburgers. Legislation also protects

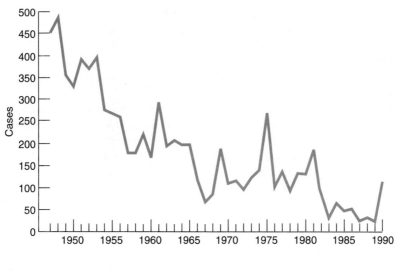

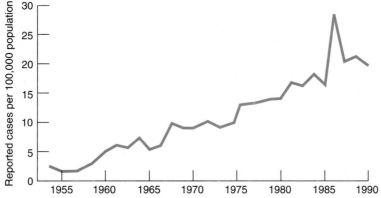

FIGURE 16-8

A, Declining numbers of reported trichinosis cases, 1947-1990. **B**, Increasing numbers of salmonellosis (excluding typhoid fever), 1955-1989, United States.

Source: **A**, McAuley JB, Michelson MK, Schantz PM: Trichinosis surveillance, United States, 1987-1990, *MMWR* 40:SS35, 1990. **B**, U.S. Public Health Service: Food safety: preventing foodborne disease, *Prev Rep*, Jan 1991.

the public by requiring sanitation and proper food handling in the retail business. This has become increasingly important with the growth of food chains and franchise marketing. The ''natural food'' fads have required some degree of official supervision, though largely in the area of fair trade rather than as vehicles of disease spread.

Despite the many technical advances in safeguarding the food the public eats, the need for individual citizens to contribute to their own protection is ever present. Such self-supervision requires public health education to be fully effective.

New foodborne diseases, such as *Campylobacter,* are emerging and previously common but usually benign organisms, such as *E. coli* and *Salmonella,* are increasingly sources of outbreaks, even as scourges of the past, such as botulism and trichinosis, are declining (Figure 16-8). Actual numbers of cases and deaths for the new illnesses caused by known organisms are difficult to pin down because mild cases often go undiagnosed. Several factors account for the rise in foodborne illnesses, including, ironically, the health interests of large numbers of people seeking lower-fat alternatives in poultry and fish. Per capita consumption of chicken in the United States rose from 40 pounds in 1970 to 70 pounds in 1990. Other causes lie in new food processing technologies introducing new risks, the aging of the population, and growing numbers of immunosuppressed people with HIV infections who are more susceptible to foodborne illness and more vulnerable to severe outcomes. Food control measures become more important as new technologies allow transport and prolonged storage of foods produced in large, centralized plants. This means that a single contaminated product can infect more people in a larger geographic area. Similarly, the global marketplace makes the variations in regulations between countries more problematic.

Community control mechanisms provide a critical link in the food safety chain, but individuals must still exercise caution and hygienic practices to protect themselves. Consumers today cook less, use more rapid cooking methods such as microwaves, rely on prepared foods, and often have less training and experience in food handling than in times past. The federal governments of the United States and Canada encourage communities to develop tailored educational materials to increase consumer and food handler awareness of methods to prevent foodborne diseases. Farm management strategies and fishery practices to reduce pathogens in poultry, fish and shellfish, and to reduce pesticide residues

in fruits, vegetables, and fish are of growing importance.

FOOD PROTECTION OBJECTIVES

The overall goal regarding community food sources is to protect the community from foodborne illness. Specific objectives for a given community should be adapted from the Model Standards (APHA, 1991) and from the national objectives shown in the box on p. 499.

VECTOR AND ZOONOSES CONTROL

In community health practice the term **vector** is not limited strictly to forms of the class Insecta but includes allied arthropods such as ticks and mites. The health interest in these forms is in their role as vectors of pathogenic organisms. Virtually all of these are biological vectors in that the pathogen passes through part of its life cycle inside the intermediate invertebrate host. The common housefly, however, is strictly a mechanical vector. Some biological vectors, under certain circumstances, can be mechanical vectors by transferring pathogens on their wings, feet, or body.

Zoonoses are the infections or infectious diseases transmissible under natural conditions from vertebrate animals to human beings.

Epidemiology of Vectors

The tick and the common housefly may transfer pathogens even in the northern climates. Communities everywhere have to contend with the nuisance of mosquitoes, flies, lice, and other arthropods, but the significant health problem is their role as vectors of disease.

Transmission of disease by vectors can be described by three patterns or routes over which a disease is transmitted.

Health Status Objectives

Reduce infections caused by key foodborne pathogens to incidences of no more than:

Disease (per 100,000)	1987 Baseline*	2000 Target
Salmonella species	18	16
Campylobacter jejuni	50	25
Escherichia coli 0157:H7	8	4
Listeria monocytogenes	0.7	0.5

Reduce outbreaks of infections due to *Salmonella enteritidis* to fewer than 25 outbreaks yearly. (Baseline: 77 outbreaks in 1989.)*

Risk Reduction Objectives

Increase to at least 75% the proportion of households in which principal food preparers routinely refrain from leaving perishable food out of the refrigerator for over 2 hours and wash cutting boards and utensils with soap after contact with raw meat and poultry. (Baseline: For refrigeration of perishable foods, 70%; for washing cutting boards with soap, 66%; and for washing utensils with soap, 55%, in 1988.)†

Services and Protection Objectives

Extend to at least 70% the proportion of states and territories that have implemented model food codes for institutional food operations and to at least 70% the proportion that have adopted the new uniform food protection code ("Unicode") that sets recommended standards for regulation of all food operations. (Baseline: For institutional food operations currently using FDA's recommended model codes, 20%; for the new Unicode to be released in 1991, 0%, in 1990.)‡

*Baseline data source: Center for Infectious Diseases.
†Baseline data source: FDA Food Safety Survey, USDA Diet-Health Knowledge Survey.
‡Baseline data source: Center for Food Safety and Applied Nutrition.

Humans—vector—humans
Humans—vector—lower vertebrate—vector—humans (zoonoses)
Lower vertebrate—vector—humans (zoonoses)

Vector–disease relationships. Known vector–disease relationships indicate that a specific pathogen is transmitted via a specific vector. To say that the mosquito transmits yellow fever is not a complete statement. Only the specific *Aedes aegypti* mosquito serves as the intermediate host for the pathogen causing yellow fever. For present purposes, however, a list will serve that identifies the general type of vector with the disease or diseases it transmits to humans.

From Food to Vectors in History

In 1668 near Florence, Italy, Francesco Redi laid to rest the theory of **spontaneous generation,** which held that food and other organic matter rotted because maggots "spontaneously" grew out of it. Redi noted that when he covered meat in a jar with a gauze screen, flies could not land on it and the meat did not develop the usual maggots. He transferred this knowledge to show how insects also contaminated plants. In 1687 Bunomo, a student of Redi, took Redi's theory of insect as **vector** and Leeuwenhoek's Dutch microscopic methods to study scabies, a common skin disease of the time. Bunomo took a magnifying glass and an artist into a prison to examine the skin of prisoners with scabies. He found mites on the skin and set his artist to work drawing them. As the artist peered intently and patiently through the crude microscope, he saw the mites laying eggs. This confirmed Redi's experiment with flies and maggots and established the vector theory of disease transmission.

How does this account reflect the convergence of knowledge and technology and their diffusion from one generation to another and from one country to another? How does Redi's discovery differ in its relevance for community health from more basic biomedical discoveries?

Mosquitoes: yellow fever, malaria, encephalitis, filariasis

Fleas: bubonic plague, murine typhus

Ticks and mites: Rocky Mountain spotted fever, tularemia, Lyme disease

Biting flies: tularemia

Lice: epidemic typhus, relapsing fever

House flies: salmonellosis

In addition, roaches are suspected of transmitting enteric diseases, and bedbugs are suspected of conveying relapsing fever. AIDS cannot be transferred by food or animal vectors.

Food Safety and Vector Control Agencies, Federal Level

United States

Three U.S. federal agencies share responsibility for animal agriculture and food protection.

- **Food and Drug Administration.** *The Center for Veterinary Medicine* oversees the development of animal drugs and feed additives and monitors animal health products to ensure they are safe and effective. *The Center for Food Safety and Applied Nutrition* monitors drug residues in milk through its Milk Safety Branch.
- **U.S. Department of Agriculture.** *The Food Safety and Inspection Service* randomly tests for drug residues in animals at the time of slaughter. *The Animal and Plant Health Inspection Service* regulates the approval of vaccines, diagnostic test kits and biologicals, which are used to detect or enhance an animal's immunity to infection.
- **Environmental Protection Agency.** *The Office of Pesticide Programs* oversees the approval of chemicals used topically on animals to control pests.

In Canada

Salmonella and Food-borne Disease Unit, Health of Animals Directorate, Food Production and Inspection Branch, Agriculture Canada.

Control measures. The first principle of vector control is to identify the specific vector and to plan control measures accordingly. When the tick is the known vector, for example, control measures will differ from measures taken when a mosquito is the intermediate host. Yet three factors must always be considered: elimination of breeding places, destruction of the insect or its larva, and protection of possible human hosts by preventing the vector from reaching humans.

Mosquito control is representative of the classic techniques of insect control, whether the particular species is a vector or simply a general annoyance (Figure 16-9). Control measures cover all three of the previously mentioned factors and apply with minor variations for ticks, flies, lice and mites.

- Eliminating breeding places
  —Destroying or emptying containers holding water
  —Filling water holes
  —Draining ponds, marshes, and swamps
  —Rendering bodies of water unsuitable for breeding by using larvicides, releasing water at high velocities, and fluctuating the water level
  —Diverting stream flow
  —Trimming the banks of ponds, lakes, and streams to prevent swamps
  —Introducing natural antagonists of mosquito larvae, such as fish *(Gambusia)*
- Destroying adult insects
  —Spraying insecticide in areas populated by mosquitoes
  —Spreading insecticide-impregnated sawdust on surface of flowing streams
  —Putting oil-solution insecticide over rain barrels and other water containers
- Protecting humans against contact by mosquito
  —Screening
  —Clothing
  —Nets
  —Repellents

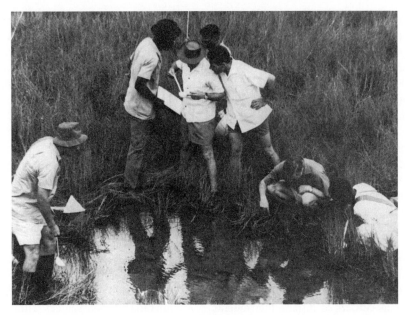

FIGURE 16-9
Reconnaissance is the first step in mosquito control and malaria eradication. Here a team of entomologists investigate the density of mosquito larvae in streams and marshy land in Togo.
Source: World Health Organization, photo distributed by United Nations Environmental Programme.

Insecticides

Like most technologies, insecticides can have harmful as well as beneficial effects. People, lower vertebrates (wildlife especially), and vegetation (including crops) can be harmed if the insecticide solution is too highly concentrated. Controlling the use of insecticides is imperative. Overuse of insecticides is destroying wildlife. Air and water pollution can be created by insecticides. Unfortunately, because the effects of insecticides on vector populations are only temporary, it is necessary to spray or otherwise apply the insecticide weekly.

The community has a responsibility to reduce vector populations in its area. In North America this is usually a function of the community health department and is carried out in cooperation with state or provincial agencies. Community authorities also have a responsibility in regulating the use of insecticides by private citizens. This is primarily a problem of public education directed to specific groups or individuals. Research on insecticides is being carried on by governmental agencies and by scientists in universities and colleges. Identifying permissible concentrations of insecticides is the immediate problem, but the long-range objective is that of developing insecticides that destroy insect vectors but are harmless to people, other animals, and vegetation.

Rodent and Zoonoses Control

The term *rodent* encompasses all animals belonging to the order Rodentia and includes squirrels and other animals as well as rats and mice. The ground squirrel can harbor the pathogens that cause Rocky

Mountain spotted fever and tularemia in humans and can transmit rabies directly. A vector must transmit most pathogens from rodent to human—for example, the tick for Rocky Mountain spotted fever and the horsefly for tularemia. In the United States control of squirrels is essentially a state and federal problem, and both the federal and state governments have extensive programs to eliminate ground squirrels. Field teams using guns, traps, and poisons carry on a constant campaign to eliminate ground squirrels in regions with endemic Rocky Mountain spotted fever and tularemia.

In communities the rodent problem is essentially confined to rats and mice. These rodents cause economic loss, create aesthetic problems, and transmit disease. Rats and mice destroy and eat poultry and eggs, grains and sprouts, and corn. They also destroy merchandise. Despite the enormity of this economic loss, it is as carriers of disease that rodents pose the greatest threat to communities.

Rat-borne diseases. Rats harbor several pathogens. In many instances the rat dies of the disease. In other instances it remains a carrier of the disease over a considerable period of time. Although many misconceptions exist regarding the relationship of rats to human disease, at least six diseases of humans are definitely known in which the rat (or house mouse) serves as a reservoir of infection.

Murine typhus: rat—rat fleas—humans
Bubonic plague: rat—rat fleas—humans
Weil's disease (infectious jaundice): urine of rat
Salmonellosis: feces of rat and house mouse
Rat-bite fever: bacteria via bite
Rickettsialpox: house mouse—mite—humans

Obviously, not all rats harbor pathogens of humans, but the greater the rat population, the greater the potential reservoir.

Varieties of rats. Three types of rats are of health concern. The black rat lives in walls and between floors. It has a pointed muzzle, slender body, long

tail, and a sooty color. The roof rat is more brown but otherwise resembles the black rat and usually lives off the ground. The brown rat is also called the sewer rat, wharf rat, and Norway rat. It is a large rodent with a blunt head, short ears, and short tail. It burrows and nests in the ground. Also of concern is the house mouse, which lives in walls, furniture, and other protective places.

Control measures. A community rodent control program must begin with a well-thought-out plan based on surveys and participation by residents. Education of the public is essential to ensure the type of cooperation on which a successful program must be based. When all residents make their premises rat-free, the task of community officials is not a difficult one.

A community program has five aspects: surveys, elimination of food sources, elimination of nesting and breeding places, rat-proofing, and killing of rats. Each aspect involves certain measures.

1. Surveys
   a. Poor sanitation areas
   b. Substandard housing
   c. Tenements
   d. Railroad areas
   e. Areas near dumps
2. Elimination of food sources
   a. Placing all food in rat-proof containers
   b. Covering garbage cans
   c. Prohibiting dumping of food wastes in open areas
3. Elimination of nesting and breeding places
   a. Disposing of debris
   b. Burning trash and rubbish
   c. Prohibiting piles of building materials
4. Rat-proofing
   a. Closing external openings
   b. Placing screens and metal over cracks and openings
   c. Eliminating all possible passages
5. Killing of rats
   a. Trapping

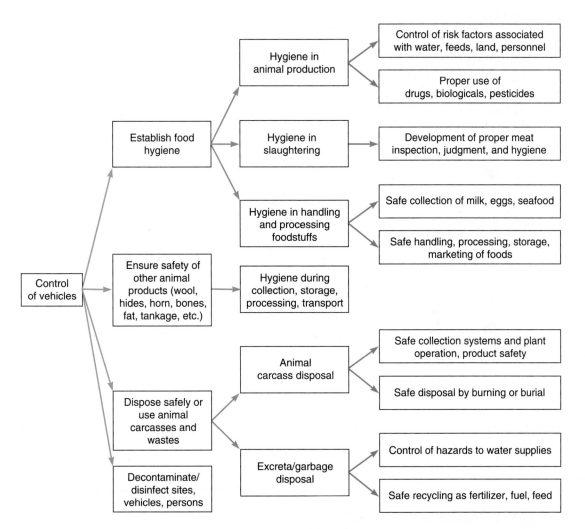

FIGURE 16-10
Summary of methods of control of food and other vehicles of disease transfer.
Source: Extracted and modified from various Expert Committees on Bacterial and Viral Zoonoses of the World Health Organization.

b. Use of approved rodenticides with all possible safeguards

c. Fumigation with warning signs and other safeguards

Droppings of infected rats and mice on food consumed by humans transmit disease. Keeping all food where rats and mice cannot reach it is of primary importance. Of secondary importance is the practice of all possible safety measures when using rodenticides and fumigation to kill rats. Eliminating mice by trapping is relatively simple.

SUMMARY

Food is essential to life and health, yet it can transmit disease and can be a poison itself. Much of our food supply comes from animals. Insects facilitate the pollination of food-producing plants. Much of the grain grown as food is shared with animals. Yet these animals can become vehicles of disease transmission to man, and food can become contaminated by animals, including rodents and insects acting as vectors. The food chains and cycles inherent in the relations between people and other animals are countless in their variety, their potential benefits, and their potential hazards. This chapter has emphasized only those relationships controlled by health agencies in the interests of community food protection and community health.

The essential features of these relationships can be summarized in the flow chart in Figure 16-10. This figure ties this chapter's content with the con-

cepts introduced in earlier chapters on communicable disease control and epidemiology. In Figure 16-10, the control of disease-transmitting vehicles, including animals and food itself, is divided into four broad strategies. Among these, food hygiene is divided into the phases of food production and distribution. Each of these phases has specific objectives and activities associated with it, as seen on the right side of Figure 16-10.

QUESTIONS FOR REVIEW

1. Why do manufacturers of food, tobacco, and alcohol products lobby against proposed legislation that is designed in the public interest?

2. In terms of health protection, what is the value of home freezers?

3. Why are most cases of foodborne infections to be found in the lowest economic, social, and educational groups?

4. In your community and state or province, is there overregulation of the food industry?

5. To what extent is the prevention of foodborne disease a matter of community health education?

6. In home canning, botulism occurs from improper procedures in preparation. How can this be corrected?

7. Why are respiratory diseases not transmitted via solid foods such as vegetables, fruits, and baked goods?

8. If pathogens are destroyed by pasteurization, why are cows with brucellosis, tuberculosis, or mastitis culled out as producers?

9. A dairy inspector once remarked that a certain dairyman could not produce satisfactory milk if he had the best equipment in the world. What was meant and what is the significance of the remark?

10. Why is more attention given to underpasteurization than to overpasteurization of milk?

11. When some cases of disease, such as salmonellosis, are traced to pasteurized milk, what are some possible breakdowns in the milk processing operation that could account for the disease transmission?

Objectives to Insure Food Safety by the Year 2000
Objectives target reductions in the incidences of foodborne diseases; reduction in salmonella infection outbreaks; improving food handling techniques on the part of consumers; and increasing the number of states that adopt model food codes.

12. Should governmental officials prohibit adding ingredients to meats or permit adding ingredients under governmental inspection and control?

13. Which is more important in restaurant sanitation: what is done in the dining area or what is done in the food preparation area—and why?

14. In restaurant rating, which system do you prefer, an A, B, or C rating or an ''approved'' or ''not approved'' rating—and why?

15. How does the control of vectors such as flies and rodents protect the community food supply?

READINGS

Abdussalam M, Kaferstein FK: Safety of street foods, *World Health Forum* 14:191, 1993.

Street vendors supply large amounts of food at affordable prices, particularly in developing countries. The need to regulate this trade for safety and quality must be weighed against diminishing the availability and accessibility of produce to poor people.

American Public Health Association and Model Standards Work Group: *Healthy communities 2000 model standards: guidelines for community attainment of the year 2000 national health objectives,* ed 3, Washington, DC, 1991, American Public Health Association.

As for each of the other sets of national objectives shown in previous chapters, this volume provides community-level elaborations of the year 2000 objectives for the nation in food safety and vector control.

Miller RW: *Get hooked on seafood safety,* DHHS Publ No (FDA) 91-2246, Washington, DC, 1991, Food and Drug Administration. (Reprinted from *FDA Consumer Mag*)

Reviews the results of the Centers for Disease Control risk assessment study for various types of seafood compared with poultry in producing foodborne illnesses.

Vanderzant C, Splittstoesser D, editors: *Compendium of methods for the microbiological examination of foods,* ed 2, Washington, DC, 1992, American Public Health Association.

Presents a comprehensive selection of proven methods for processing and testing the safety and quality of foods. Chapters on microorganisms involved in processing and spoilage of foods, pathogenic organisms, foodborne illnesses, and rapid and automated methods of food processing.

World Health Organization: *WHO Expert Committee on Rabies, eighth report,* Tech Rep Ser No 824, Geneva, 1992, World Health Organization.

Reviews new knowledge from basic and applied research on rabies and the prevention of this zoonotic disease. Prospects for controlling the spread of rabies in wild animal populations with new oral vaccines are discussed.

BIBLIOGRAPHY

Ahmed FE, editor: *Seafood safety,* Washington, DC, 1991, Committee on Evaluation of the Safety of Fishery Products, Food and Nutrition Board, Institute of Medicine, National Academy Press.

Auld ME, Weinreich DA: Foundations of American food safety, *Top Clin Nutr* 6:32, 1990.

Barkan ID: Industry invites regulation: the passage of the Pure Food and Drug Act of 1906, *Am J Public Health* 75:18, 1985.

Bello M: Lower lead limits eyed for food additives, *NRC News Rep* 41:14, 1991.

Blumenthal D: *Food irradiation: toxic to bacteria, safe for humans,* DHHS Publ No (FDA) 91-2241, Washington, DC, 1991, Food and Drug Administration. (Reprinted from *FDA Consumer Mag* Nov 1990.)

Centers for Disease Control: Update—milk-borne salmonellosis, Illinois, *MMWR* 34:215, 1985.

Centers for Disease Control and Prevention: Preliminary report: foodborne outbreak of *Escherichia coli* 0157: H7 infections from hamburgers—Western United States, 1993, *MMWR* 42:85, 1993.

Committee on Assessment of Technology and Opportunities for Marine Aquaculture in the United States: *Marine aquaculture: opportunities for growth,* Washington, DC, 1992, National Academy Press.

Committee on Evaluation of USDA Streamlined Inspection System for Cattle, Food and Nutrition Board, Institute of Medicine: *Cattle inspection,* Washington, DC, 1990, National Academy Press.

FAO Panel of Experts on Pesticide Residues in Food and the Environment and the WHO Expert Group on Pesticide Residues: *Pesticide residues in food—1991,* Geneva, 1992, World Health Organization.

Food Safety and Inspection Service: *A quick consumer guide to safe food handling,* Home and Garden Bull No 248, Washington, DC, 1990, U.S. Department of Agriculture.

French G, Pavlick A, Felsen A et al: Outbreak of type E botulism associated with an uneviscerated, salt-cured fish product—New Jersey, 1992, *MMWR* 41:521, 1992.

Griffin PM, Tauxe RV: The epidemiology of infections caused by *Escherichia coli* 0157:H7, other enterohemorrhagic *E. coli,* and the associated hemolytic uremic syndrome, *Epidemiol Rev* 13:60, 1991.

Isaacson RL, Jensen KF, editors: *The vulnerable brain and environmental risks,* vol 2, *Toxins in food,* New York, 1992, Plenum.

Jaret P: The disease detectives: stalking the world's epidemics, *National Geographic* 114(Jan): 19, 1991.

McAuley JB, Michelson MK, Schantz PM: Trichinosis surveillance, United States, 1987-1990, *MMWR* 40: SS35, 1990.

Management and Analysis Branch: *Residue monitoring—1991,* Washington, DC, 1991, Food and Drug Administration.

National Association of State Public Health Veterinarians, Inc: Compendium of animal rabies control, 1992, *MMWR* 41:1, 1992.

Office of Communications, National Institute of Allergy and Infectious Disease: *Lyme disease: the facts, the challenge,* NIH Publ No 92-3193, Bethesda, 1992, U.S. Department of Health and Human Services.

Palmer S, Bakshi KS: Chemical contaminants in food. In Tarcher AB, editor: *Principles and practice of environmental medicine,* New York, 1992, Plenum.

Parmer D, Murray E, Pannarella K et al: Update: *Salmonella enteritidis* infections and shell eggs—United States, 1990, *MMWR* 39:909, 1990.

Patlak M: Looking ahead to the promises of food science in the future, *NRC News Rep* 41:13, 1991.

Richardson GH, editor: *Standard methods for the examination of dairy products,* 15 ed, Washington, DC, 1985, American Public Health Association.

Sabetta JR, Hyman S, Smardin J et al: Foodborne nosocomial outbreak of *Salmonella reading*—Connecticut, *MMWR* 40:804, 1991.

Scale M, Collier C, Hinkle CJ et al: Foodborne hepatitis A—Missouri, Wisconsin, and Alaska, 1990-1992, *MMWR* 42:526, 1993.

Shaffer N, Wainwright RB, Middaugh JP et al: Botulism among Alaska Natives: the role of changing food preparation and consumption practices, *West J Med* 153: 390, 1990.

Tarcher AB, editor: *Principles and practice of environmental medicine,* New York, 1992, Plenum.

Telzak EE, Bell EP, Kautter DA et al: An international outbreak of type E botulism due to uneviscerated fish, *J Infect Dis* 161:340, 1990.

U.S. Public Health Service: Food safety: preventing foodborne disease, *Prevention Rep* (Office of Disease Prevention and Health Promotion), Jan 1991.

Williams T, Moon A, Williams M: *Food, environment and health: a guide for primary school teachers,* Geneva, 1990, World Health Organization.

World Health Organization and United Nations Environment Programme: *Insect and rodent control through environmental management: a community action programme,* Geneva, 1992, World Health Organization.

Chapter 17

Control of Air, Radiation, and Noise Pollution

The atmosphere is a blanket for the Earth. Too much blanket or too little, and we're in trouble
CARL SAGAN

OBJECTIVES

When you finish this chapter, you should be able to:

- Describe the major sources and the health effects of atmospheric pollution
- Identify the major methods of atmospheric pollution control
- Identify objectives and strategies for environmental protection pertaining to the control of air pollution, radioactivity, and noise in your community

---

Carl Sagan's statement quoted above reflects an ecological concern: Each individual adds to and takes away from the atmospheric blanket covering you and the entire earth. Community actions can affect the health and quality of life of every human being. The burning of coal in China contributes to a parched American sunbelt. The fossil fuels used in North America can contribute decades later to more starvation in sub-Saharan Africa. Like water, air is a limited and shared resource that knows no national boundaries. It accumulates chemicals, carbon dioxide, and other gases in one geographical region and dumps them as **acid rain** in another or adds to the warming ''greenhouse effect'' of the atmosphere for everyone.

This chapter offers you further analyses of the delicate balance of the environment and how social organization and human behavior, especially since the Industrial Revolution, have upset this balance. The natural history of most life forms, including human beings, evolved over millions of years before humankind had the capacity to affect the environment so vastly. In just the last century or so the human population has imposed a social history so destructive to the environment that people now must seek ways to control or compensate for the resultant

507

health effects. In relation to the atmosphere this means controlling air pollution, use of radioactive materials, and production of noise.

AIR POLLUTION

Air pollution can be defined as the presence in the **ambient** (surrounding) atmosphere of substances in concentrations sufficient to interfere directly or indirectly with one's comfort, safety, or health, or with the full use of one's property. From the earliest of times man-made pollution has been the main concern, though naturally occurring pollution can be a threat to health and livelihood as well.

Epidemiology of Air Pollution

Air pollution comes from industrial exhausts, home heating, incineration, open fires, open dumps, road dust, engine exhaust, crop spraying, construction debris, chemicals including radon and other sources. Everyday tools have also come under criticism for their contribution to pollution, including gasoline-powered lawn mowers, leaf blowers, hedge trimmers, snow blowers, and chain saws. These machines produce up to 50 times more air pollution per horsepower than trucks.

Pollutants may be in the form of solids, liquids (vapors), and gases. The atmosphere of a representative industrial area will have about 22% of its pollutants from industrial sources, about 10% from commercial sources, and the remaining 68% from public sources. Pollution becomes a problem when a receptor—essentially plants or animals, including human beings, are adversely affected by the pollution.

Smog. Smog resulting from ozone pollution is a persistent problem not only in cities but also in suburbs and rural areas. **Ozone** in the upper atmosphere protects the earth from harmful solar radiation. In contrast, ozone near the earth's surface is a primary ingredient of smog. Vapors from gasoline, and other organic products mix with atmospheric chemicals in sunlight and are "cooked" to form photochemical smog.

Two basic ingredients in this recipe for pollution are nitrogen oxides and volatile organic compounds (VOCs). Nitrogen oxides come primarily from the incomplete combustion of fossil fuels by motor vehicles and electric power plants. VOCs are produced by motor vehicles, evaporating solvents, chemical and petroleum industries, natural vegetation, and natural events such as volcanic eruptions and forest fires (Figure 17-1).

Health aspects. Smog has both an irritating and a direct toxic effect on human beings. Smog containing ozone causes respiratory problems when air pollution is high. The ingredients of smog also cause environmental problems. Chlorofluorocarbons (CFGs), a type of VOCs, are a family of organic compounds that are nontoxic, long-lived and nonflammable. While ideal for some uses such as refrigerators and fire extinguishers, their longevity al-

---

Global Deforestation

Since preagricultural times, the world has lost about one fifth of all its forests, from more than 12 billion acres to under 10 billion acres. Each year a tropical forest about the size of Washington State is cleared from the planet for agricultural or developmental purposes. In the past, much of this loss has been from the developed countries in Europe, Asia, and North America. Now the tropical forests are disappearing most rapidly in Latin America, Asia, and Africa. This loss is considered one of the most serious global problems to some environmental experts because of the role these forests play in regulating the global climate. Through photosynthesis, the forests absorb huge quantities of carbon dioxide. Many scientists believe that if carbon dioxide is not kept in check it will cause significant warming of the earth in a process known as the greenhouse effect.

How life begins in the forest.

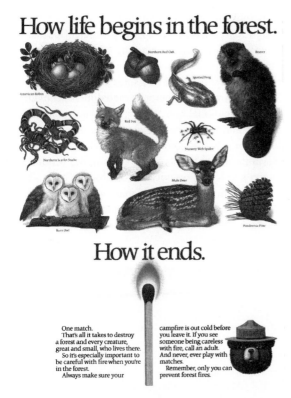

How it ends.

One match.
That's all it takes to destroy a forest and every creature, great and small, who lives there. So it's especially important to be careful with fire when you're in the forest.
Always make sure your

campfire is out cold before you leave it. If you see someone being careless with fire, call an adult. And never, ever play with matches.
Remember, only you can prevent forest fires.

FIGURE 17-1
Besides the direct destruction of life caused by forest fires, the indirect effects by way of atmospheric pollution are more subtle but potentially far-reaching. The purposeful destruction of rain forests have even broader effects. The "Smokey the Bear" campaigns over the past several decades have been the most successful, at least in terms of public recognition, of the American public service advertising field.
Source: Advertising Council for Forest Service, U.S. Department of Agriculture, and State Foresters.

lows them to remain in the atmosphere long enough to rise to the stratosphere. There they break down under intense solar radiation and they destroy the ozone. Reduced ozone in the upper atmosphere allows increased ultraviolet radiation to reach the earth, with possible harm to humans, animals, and vegetation. In the lower atmospheres the CFGs contribute to global warming. Together with water vapor, carbon dioxide, methane, and nitrous

oxide, they absorb infrared radiation, warming the earth.

As a threat to human well-being, the most devastating effect of air pollution results when a **temperature inversion** occurs. The Denver and Los Angeles areas in the United States are particularly plagued by this problem because of their topography. Surface air normally rises, but during an inversion a layer of warm air resting on top of relatively cool air pins the cool air down much like a lid on a kettle. Smog results when pollution cannot escape.

More research is necessary before precise statements can be made on the specific effects of pollution on human health. Sufficient empirical evidence does exist to alert communities to the possible dangers of air pollution. Some effects are acute and can be fatal, while other effects are delayed and may be apparent as chronic diseases only after years of exposure.

Several cities have experienced acute air pollution disasters in this century. In 1930 in the Meuse Valley, Belgium, 60 people died as the result of heavy air pollution. In Donora, Pennsylvania, in 1940, a reported 20 people died from pollution. In London in 1952, during a 2-week period of air pollution, about 4000 more people died than normally would have. And on December 3, 1984, a chemical plant in Bhopal, India, accidentally leaked a cloud of methyl isocyanate that killed about 2000 residents of that city. Leaks from railroad cars and trucks carrying chemicals have led to local community evacuations in many North American communities. In the first three incidents most of those who died had had chronic respiratory or circulatory diseases, and a large proportion were the elderly. The Bhopal tragedy and transportation accidents illustrates the increasing vulnerability of whole communities to the possibility of industrial or nuclear accidents that could unleash massive doses of air pollutants. Regulating the construction and safety procedures of such plants has become an onerous responsibility of governmental agencies.

Chernobyl in the former U.S.S.R. and Three Mile Island in the United States both experienced meltdowns at nuclear power plants. These resulted in the release of nuclear radiation into the atmosphere. In Chernobyl hundreds of people died immediately. Concern with long-term effects of radiation continue as the radioactive cloud from Chernobyl drifted across northern Europe polluting food chains as far away as Sweden.

People with asthma and other respiratory diseases have their condition aggravated by air pollutants. Eye, nose, and throat irritation caused by air pollution may be mild, moderate, or severe, depending on the individual's sensitivity and the pollutants involved. Irritation of the lungs may make individuals more susceptible to lung infections. Carbon monoxide poisoning may affect heart action adversely and have delayed ill effects on a person. Gastrointestinal disturbances, especially in children, appear to be more prevalent during periods of heavy air pollution.

Economic and aesthetic aspects. Air pollution can damage trees, shrubs, and flowers and ruin crops. Cattle become ill from air pollutants. Air pollution causes damage to residences and other structures. It can interfere with the enjoyment of an otherwise attractive environment. Air pollution properly can be declared a nuisance on esthetic as well as health grounds.

Persons who believe that they have been harmed or inconvenienced or have suffered monetary loss from single-source pollution can obtain redress in court. A suit against the firm or persons creating the objectionable air pollution can result in a judgment of monetary compensation for the damage to the plaintiff's person or property. Courts have awarded compensation for harm to cattle resulting from air pollution caused by industrial plants producing aluminum products.

Volcanic ash. Volcanic ash presents a threat to health in some areas. Not ''ash'' at all, but pulverized rock, it often contains small pieces of lightweight, expanded lava called **pumice.** Because a volcano gives advance warning of an eruption, officials usually have time to move persons in the immediate neighborhood to a safer area perhaps 20 or 30 miles away. Long before evacuation is necessary, local and national personnel should have conducted classes and used other means to inform nearby residents of what actions should be taken at the first warning of a volcanic eruption, as in the Mount St. Helen's volcanic activity in the United States. The 1991 eruption of the Mt. Pinatubo volcano in the Philippines forced the evacuation of 16,000 U.S. military personnel, dependents, and civilians from

---

A Volcanic Winter

In the summer of 1816, New England and New York experienced freezing temperatures and 10 inches of snow, killing much of the green growth in large areas of North America. In Virginia, Thomas Jefferson applied for an emergency bank loan because of his crop failures. England referred to 1816 as ''the year without a summer.'' A typhus epidemic that killed 65,000 people in the British Isles in 1816 was blamed on famine induced by the cold and by crop failures. All of these phenomena were brought about by the eruption in 1815 of Mt. Tambora, a volcano in the Dutch East Indies (now Indonesia). Spewing 25 cubic miles of ash into the upper atmosphere, the Tambora eruption was probably the worst in 10,000 years. Mount Vesuvius in Italy is more famous for its sudden burial of an entire city in molten lava during the time of the Roman Empire, but the Tambora eruption put a massive cloud of debris into the atmosphere that stayed aloft for months, circled the globe, and blanketed the Northern Hemisphere.

What lessons can you draw from this account of the eruption of Mt. Tambora? Could the great American floods of the midwest in 1993 be attributed to the Mt. Pinatubo eruption in the Philippines in 1991? Is air pollution confined in its effects to the place of origin?

Clark Air Force Base and 20,000 Filipinos living near the volcano. Only two people were killed.

After a volcanic eruption, intermittent ashfalls may continue over several years. They may cause people to move away from the area, but some residents apparently accept that pattern of life as a challenge. When residents of a threatened volcanic area refuse to leave, officials may order residents to move. If some families need assistance, help is provided by officials. All in all, this is a localized problem with relatively low loss of life and few serious injuries. It is an area in which governmental agencies assume a major responsibility, but in which citizen cooperation is important.

Air Pollution Control

To control and regulate air pollution by solid particles is least difficult. Various smoke-inspection devices are available for measuring the density of smoke and other particles in the air (Figure 17-2). With established means for measuring smoke pollution, cities have passed ordinances limiting the emission of smoke to periods of 6 minutes in 1 hour for industrial plants. Proper firing and design of coal furnaces eliminates 90% of smoke from industrial plants.

Control of pollution by smoke is relatively easy. Unfortunately, the most serious air pollutants are sulfur oxide, nitrogen oxide, and motor vehicle emissions, and these are more difficult to measure.

Sulfur oxides. Pollution arises principally from the combustion of sulfur-containing coal and fuel oil and is highly injurious to human health, to property, and to vegetation. Using low-sulfur fuels or removing sulfur from fuels before they are burned reduces pollution. Natural gas, which is relatively free of sulfur, is preferable to other fuels in terms of reduction of air pollution. Coal is the nemesis, because only a fraction of its sulfur content can be removed before burning. Efforts are now directed toward re-

moving the sulfur oxides from the combustion gases before they escape into the air.

Nitrogen oxides are a by-product of all combustion processes, including those from automobiles. At present, nitrogen oxide pollution is not as serious a problem as sulfur oxide pollution, but as fuel combustion increases, the nitrogen oxide pollution problem will increase proportionately unless control methods are discovered and implemented.

Motor vehicle air pollution is more extensive than sulfur oxide and nitrogen oxide pollution, but motor vehicle air pollution is partially yielding to newly developed control techniques. Among the methods effective in reducing tailpipe emissions are the modification of motors to achieve more complete combustion, the injection of air into the exhaust system to oxidize the gases before they reach the tailpipe, and the passage of exhaust gases through afterburners before they are released into the air. Some of these methods are applied by U.S. automobile manufacturers in the form of catalytic converters and exhaust gas recirculation to comply with the standards established by the Clean Air Act.

U.S. legislation. In the era when air pollution meant smoke pollution, community ordinances could be enacted to control the problem because the smoke constituted an obvious nuisance. In addition, the degree of smoke pollution could be measured with some precision. Today, air pollution is more subtle and can no longer be regarded as a strictly localized concern. It has become a national and international problem that recognizes no geographical or political boundaries.

U.S. federal air pollution control was first established in 1955 as a consequence of the action of Congress, which passed PL 84-159 ''to provide research and technical assistance relating to air pollution control.'' With the adoption of the **Clean Air Act** in 1965, Congress acknowledged that federal financial assistance is essential for the development of programs to control air pollution. Matching funds encouraged state and local governments to initiate

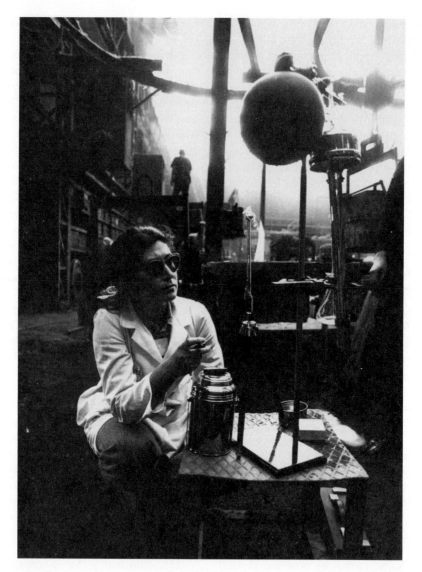

FIGURE 17-2

In situ evaluation of chemical and particulate matter in the air of a factory assists industry in the design of necessary control installations on furnaces, incinerators, and dust-producing equipment and procedures. This inspection is in Ankara, Turkey.

Source: International Labour Organization photo by Jean Mohr, courtesy United Nations Environmental Programme and World Health Organization.

The Double Edge of Public Policy

Automobiles continue to be a major source of air pollution. The highways that carry these vehicles were expanded greatly under the Highway Act of 1956. Over $50 billion was committed to building more than 40,000 miles of highways. It was the largest public works project in history. This highway construction was in part inspired by fear of nuclear attack during the "red" paranoia of the 50s. In lobbying Congress for funding, President Eisenhower, a World War II army hero, pointed out that American cities needed broad avenues of escape if threatened by nuclear weapons. By addressing one problem, public escape routes, highways created other problems with congestion, pollution, and scarring of the landscape. Today, many lobby for abandoning automobiles in favor of mass public transportation or bicycles. If such transportation solutions are supported, what problems will they solve? What problems are they likely to create?

air pollution control programs. The act encouraged area-wide, interjurisdictional or regional control of air pollution.

The Air Quality Act of 1967 authorized the federal government to step in to control air pollution when the state fails to act. No national emission standards for specific pollutants were set up, but provisions were made to study the problem of standards.

The Clean Air Act of 1970, the most ambitious and costly environmental legislation in history, led to a vast national cleanup. The most deadly emissions—sulfur oxides and toxic particles from industry—declined sharply enough to increase the life of the average American by a full year, although the less dangerous smog caused by car emissions remains a problem.

The Clean Air Act was an aggressive piece of legislation that grew out of an era when polls showed that Americans were rating pollution above crime as a serious problem. It was the year of Earth Day 1970, a time when Girl Scouts wearing gas masks crowded into congressional air quality hearing rooms in support of irate citizens demanding cleaner air. Declaring air "our most vital resource" and seizing the political initiative to the dismay of Democrats, President Richard Nixon asked Congress in 1970 for sweeping and stringent new clean-air legislation.

The resulting Clean Air Act was in the form of amendments to earlier laws. It ordered the automobile industry to cut emissions 90% by 1975—a deadline that was pushed back repeatedly. Specific emission allowances were set for various industries. National standards were set for allowable levels for seven air pollutants—sulfur dioxide, particles, hydrocarbons, nitrogen oxide, carbon monoxide, ozone, and lead—and states were ordered to meet these standards or to forfeit federal highway and sewer money (Table 17-1).

After further amendments in 1977, however, the initiative began to lose momentum. By 1978 the Carter administration was singling out federal clean-air rules as a chief cause of inflation. Today, polls show North Americans, especially Canadians, are about twice as concerned about air pollution as they were in 1985 (Figure 17-3). The Reagan administration eased the standards and control measures in its efforts toward **deregulation** of industry. The Clinton administration appears to be committed to restoring and furthering the environmental agenda.

The 1990 amendments. In 1990 major new amendments were made to the Clean Air Act designed to control virtually every important source of air pollution and substantially reduce health and environmental damage caused by acid rain, smog, urban ozone pollution, toxic chemicals and destruction of the earth's atmospheric ozone shield. Congressional debate over the bill considered the economic and health trade-offs in the Act. These trade-offs were debated in the 1990 election. The then-future vice president, Al Gore, argued that environmental protection would create jobs; the then-sitting vice president, Dan Quayle, working through the Com-

TABLE 17-1

The seven air pollutants for which U.S. standards exist, their main sources, and their health effects

Pollutant	Description	Main sources	Health effects
Ozone	Main component of smog, formed in air when sunlight "cooks" hydrocarbons (like gasoline vapors) and nitrogen oxides from automobiles	Not directly emitted but formed from emissions of automobiles, etc.	Irritation of eyes, nose, throat; impairment of normal lung function
Carbon monoxide	By-product of combustion	Cars and trucks	Weakens heart contractions; reduces oxygen available to body; affects mental function, visual acuity and alertness
Particles	Soot, dust, smoke, fumes, ash, mists, sprays, aerosols, etc.	Power plants, factories, incinerators, open burning, construction, road dust	Respiratory and lung damage, in some cases cancer; hastens death
Sulfur dioxide	By-product of burning coal and oil, and of some industrial processes; reacts in air to form sulfuric acid which can return to earth as "acid rain"	Power plants, factories, space heating boilers	Increases acute and chronic respiratory disease; hastens death
Nitrogen dioxide	By-product of combustion; is "cooked" in the air with hydrocarbons to form ozone (smog); on its own, gives smog its yellow-brown color	Cars, trucks, power plants, factories	Pulmonary swelling; may aggravate chronic bronchitis and emphysema
Hydrocarbons	Incompletely burned and evaporated petroleum products; are "cooked" with nitrogen dioxide to form ozone (smog)	Cars, truck, power plants, space heating boilers, vapors from gasoline stations	Negligible
Lead	A chemical element	Leaded gasoline	Brain and kidney damage; emotional disorders; death

Source: Adapted from U.S. Environmental Protection Agency.

petitiveness Council, argued that new requirements would result in job losses.

Current issues. Other difficulties plague the Clean Air Act in the political and economic climate of the 1990s. Some cities—for instance, Los Angeles—will never meet today's air pollution standards unless people there are kept out of their cars by force. Relatively clean areas of the nation must meet even tougher standards designed to prevent them from developing air pollution, causing manufacturers to

complain that industrial growth is being hindered in the "sunbelt" West and South, and communities in the "rust belt" North to complain of lost jobs. Different standards for different industries and tougher standards for newer plants tend to encourage the retention of old, inefficient factories. The slow-down in capital investment and the lagging efficiency of American industry are major culprits blamed for recession and balance-of-trade deficits.

Air pollution has rebounded as a major public issue and a high-priority item on the national agen-

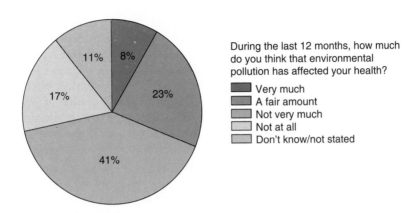

During the last 12 months, how much
do you think that environmental
pollution has affected your health?

■ Very much
■ A fair amount
■ Not very much
□ Not at all
▨ Don't know/not stated

FIGURE 17-3

Impact of environmental pollution on one's own health as perceived by Canadians age 15 and over, 1990. The Canadian Health Promotion Survey found that the perception of a health effect was not particularly related to people's own environmental health practices, but public perceptions do appear to influence support for legislative reforms.

Source: Geran L: Environmental practices of Canadian households, *Can Soc Trends* 28117, 1993; Peters L: Environmental health practices. In Stephens T, Fowler Graham D, editors: *Canada's health promotion survey 1990: technical report*, O'Hawa, 1993, minister of supply and services, Canada (Cat no H39-2632-1990E).

das of Canada, Mexico, and the U.S. with the North American Free Trade Agreement (NAFTA). After two decades of experience, researchers can estimate the number of lives saved by the control of the most dangerous air pollutants—sulfur oxides and particles. Emission restrictions and requirements to burn low-sulfur coal that were imposed on power plants and factories cut the U.S. mortality rate 7%, increasing the average life of Americans by a year.

Cost-benefit analysis. The problem in determining the effects of pollution on health is that pollutants do their damage over long periods of time. The U.S. Congress dealt with such uncertainties by ordering national standards set low enough to protect the most sensitive people with ''an adequate margin of safety'' and without regard for what this might cost industry and consumers. That principle was supported by the National Commission on Air Quality, an independent group that studied the act in preparation for the congressional debate. It was supported in 1980 by the Supreme Court in its rejection of an

Environmental Protection Agency (EPA) proposal to use **cost-benefit analysis** in setting new (less restrictive) standards. Both the commission and the Supreme Court concluded that government must act to control potentially harmful pollutants despite scientific uncertainty about the precise harm they cause, the levels of exposure that cause harm, and the cost. This was the congressional mandate in its ''adequate margin of safety'' principle.

The principle was challenged by U.S. industry and the Reagan and Bush administrations, who sought to replace it with a less demanding one that would define a health hazard in terms of ''significant risk of adverse effects.'' The argument is that the air has already been cleaned enough to save most of the lives that could be saved by pollution-control measures, so further expenditures should be limited, with cost to industry and consumers as a consideration. Yet, asthma deaths have continued to rise.

Scientists now believe that for certain dangerous pollutants there is no threshold below which nobody is affected. If this is true, then to meet the congressional mandate could require the closing of many industries. The law will be amended again before that happens. The unions obviously oppose closing of industries, which means that the traditional coalition of Democrats and conservationists has come apart on this issue. Industry, in the meantime, must continue to seek alternative production methods and pollution control devices, because even where there is no direct harm to human life, pollution causes indirect damage to health and the quality of life. **Acid rain,** for example, results from sulfur oxide pollutants carried in rain clouds and can affect marine and plant life, thereby interfering with food chains (see Chapter 14).

State programs. States were slow to initiate pollution control programs. The stimulation of federal legislation and funding is needed to change this picture. The recognized minimum per capita expenditure for an adequate state program is set at $0.25, and few states have reached this level, indicating that most state programs are not yet in that stage where effective control measures can be taken.

An effective state or provincial air pollution control program requires the following factors:

1. A sanitary authority with status, funds, and research including field studies
2. Regional approach to air pollution control
3. Calculated program to reduce pollution each year
4. Licensing of new industries and new operations based on realistic appraisal of all factors involved
5. Industrial zoning based on an intensive study of all factors involved, including the economic benefits to be gained for each proposed industrial installation
6. Impartial application of regulations, but with a policy permitting changes in regulations, as dictated by experience

Community Programs. Few local and regional air pollution control programs in U.S. cities and coun-

ties spend enough on air pollution control. On all levels—federal, state and local—successful programs are being developed, but some communities have a more serious pollution problem today than they had 5 or 10 years ago. National standards of pollution await enforcement of pollution control by communities. Emission standards for pollution control should be applied more rigorously and alternative sources of energy should be developed (Figure 17-4).

Standards. Table 17-1 identifies the seven widespread pollutants for which the EPA has set standards. Levels of all pollutants measured for the United States and Canada have been reduced in recent years. The standard for particles is inadequate because there is now evidence that only the tiniest ones, those that penetrate deep into the lungs, are dangerous. The standard as now written measures particles of all sizes, including large ones that are trapped in the nose and cause no damage.

Table 17-2 shows that most metropolitan communities that had serious problems in their control of automobile carbon monoxide pollution have made progress. Ozone pollution, however, worsened between 1988 and 1990 for Atlanta, Atlantic City, Baton Rouge, Birmingham, Dallas-Fort Worth, Houston, Kansas City, the Portland-Vancouver corridor, San Diego, Santa Barbara, and Washington, D.C.

In addition to the seven widespread pollutants for which it has standards, the EPA has identified a group of cancer-causing pollutants that it labels hazardous: asbestos, mercury, beryllium, vinyl chloride, benzene, radionuclides, and arsenic. Of 700 atmospheric contaminants, 47 have been identified as recognized carcinogens (adequate evidence), 42 as suspected carcinogens (limited evidence), 22 as cancer promoters, and 128 as mutagens. These pollutants are emitted in small quantities, but there potential adverse effects on health are more severe than those of the widespread pollutants. The EPA is studying them and has set emission limits for some.

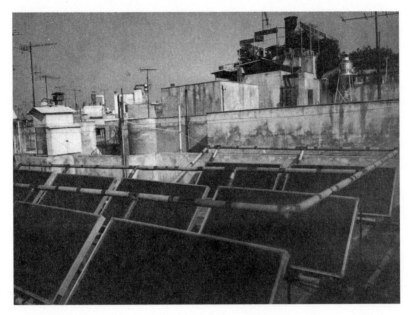

FIGURE 17-4
Equipping apartment houses and even single-family houses with solar captors on their roofs provides enough energy to supply hot water and at least minimal electricity needs of residents in lieu of some of the energy required from highly polluting electricity-generating plants. These work best, of course, in sunny regions such as Athens, Greece, shown here, and the U.S. southwest.
Source: UNEP Photo by T. Farkas, courtesy World Health Organization.

Concern about carcinogenic pollutants also is beginning to focus on the growing popularity of diesel automobile engines because, while they emit lower levels of carbon monoxide and hydrocarbons, they emit more nitrogen oxides and 30 to 100 times more particles, which contain some carcinogenic compounds. Nevertheless, the U.S. National Academy of Sciences has found no conclusive evidence that breathing diesel exhaust causes cancer, birth defects, or lung disease in humans, although diesel materials painted on or fed to rats may cause cancer in them. Studies of workers regularly breathing diesel exhaust found no higher rate of cancer among these employees.

Indoor air pollution. As buildings are being sealed more tightly to conserve energy, they seal in dangerous pollutants. As is often the case, solving one problem, energy loss, creates another problem, indoor air pollution. Tighter insulation prevents the infiltration of outdoor pollutants, but most ventilation systems for smaller and older buildings results in indoor concentrations of inert gases and smaller particles that are as high as outside levels (Figure 17-5).

In addition to particles from the outside that can become trapped in sealed buildings, including radon, there are many indoor sources of air pollution including gas ranges, smoking cigarettes, building materials, furnishings, paints, solvents, cleaning agents, and cosmetics. Germs can grow in air conditioning units. Indoor air pollution also occurs in airplanes and other sealed spaces.

Common household products emit smog-form-

TABLE 17-2
Metropolitan areas failing to meet national ambient air quality standards for carbon monoxide—
number of days exceeding standards; 1989 and 1990. Note progress in all but Anchorage
and Reno.

Metropolitan area	1989	1990	Metropolitan area	1989	1990	Metropolitan area	1989	1990
Albuquerque, NM	6	3	Hartford, CT	1	—	Phoenix, AZ	9	4
Anchorage, AK	3	12	Klamath County, OR[1]	2	—	Portland, OR-WA	2	2
Baltimore, MD	—	1	Lake Tahoe S. Shore, CA	(NA)	5	Provo-Orem, UT	12	11
Boston, MA-NH	—	—	Las Vegas, NV	26	17	Raleigh-Durham, NC	2	2
Chico, CA	1	1	Longmont, CO	(NA)	—	Reno, NV	2	7
Cleveland, OH	1	—	Los Angeles, CA	72	47	Sacramento, CA	18	11
Colorado Springs, CO	1	—	Medford, OR	15	—	San Diego, CA	4	—
Denver-Boulder, CO	6	3	Memphis, TN-AR-MS	2	1	San Francisco, CA	6	2
Duluth, MN	2	—	Minneapolis-St. Paul, MN-WI	2	1	Seattle-Tacoma, WA	2	2
El Paso, TX	5	4	Missoula County, MT[1]	2	1	Spokane, WA	11	6
Fairbanks, AK[1]	3	2	Modesto, CA	8	2	Stockton, CA	4	2
Fort Collins, CO	1	—	New York, NY-NJ-CT	16	4	Syracuse, NY	2	1
Fresno, CA	13	1	Ogden, UT	(NA)	3	Washington, DC-MD-VA	1	—
			Philadelphia, PA-NJ-DE-MD	2	—			

—Represents zero.
NA Not available.
[1]Not a metropolitan area.
Source: U.S. Environmental Protection Agency, press release, November 1991, and Statistical Abstract of the United States, 1992.

ing chemicals. The 16 products that account for half of all hydrocarbons (one of two principal ingredients of ozone) from the consumer, include air fresheners, automotive windshield washer fluids, bathroom and tile cleaners, engine degreasers, floor polishers, furniture maintenance products, general-purpose cleaners, hair sprays, hair mousses, hair-styling gels, glass cleaners, aerosol insect repellents, laundry prewash products, oven cleaners, nail polish removers, and aerosol shaving cream. By far the biggest smog contributor among the 16 products is hair spray.

One of ironies of indoor air pollution is that staying indoors is often the recommended solution for outside air pollution (Figure 17-5). Furthermore, the average American adult spends about 80% of his or her time indoors. Fresh air is a good general solution for most indoor air problems. Reduction, or elimination of sources is most desirable.

Asbestos. Widely used for its resistance to heat and chemical corrosion, asbestos has over 3000 uses. Many of these uses are in building products, including insulation, fireproofing, and floor tiles. In the early 1970s the EPA listed asbestos as a hazardous air pollutant and established safety standards for it. New regulations will ban most uses of asbestos by the mid-1990s.

When properly maintained, asbestos does not appear to be a health hazard. When it is damaged or deteriorated, however, mineral fibers may become airborne and become a health hazard. Once released into the air, the fibers can remain suspended for days or weeks. If not removed, fibers can pollute the building for a lifetime and become airborne whenever dust is stirred up. Asbestos is known to cause asbestosis, a lung disease that is usually fatal, as well as cancer of the lung, stomach, and chest lining.

Removal of asbestos is not always the answer.

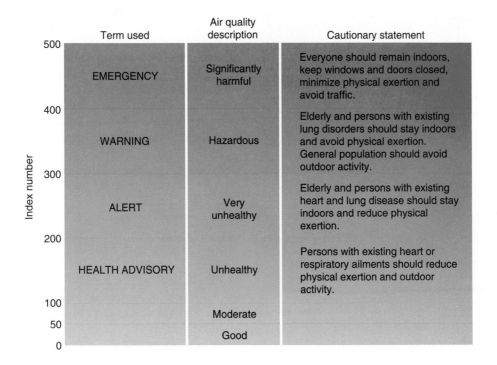

FIGURE 17-5

The Pollution Standard Index numbers correspond to the warnings issued to the U.S. and Canadian publics. The United States uses the terms on the left to describe the air quality in media announcements, along with the cautionary statements. The Canadian "Haze Watch" for air quality is now published along with the sun intensity indicators to warn people to cover their skin.

Sources: U.S. Environmental Protection Agency and Ministry of Environment Canada.

Material in good condition and inaccessible may be left until the building is demolished. Some materials may be covered, treated with an encapsulating agent, or repaired. If damaged, deteriorated, or located in areas where it is readily accessible and susceptible to disturbance, it may need to be removed. Removal, however, should only be done by qualified personnel. The removal process itself can be hazardous to the health of workers and that of building occupants if the asbestos is not handled properly.

Second-hand smoke. After reviewing the cumulative evidence, the U.S. Environmental Protection Agency declared in 1992 that second-hand tobacco smoke is a human carcinogen and a cause of serious respiratory problems in infants and young children (Figure 17-6). The strongly worded government report concluded that environmental tobacco smoke (ETS) should be added to a select list of the most toxic substances known to cause cancer in humans. The report estimated that 3000 lung cancer deaths each year and as many as 300,000 lower respiratory tract infections (including bronchitis and pneumonia) among children each year could be attributed to ETS. It also linked ETS to new cases of asthma and to the aggravation of symptoms in some 20% of the 2 to 5 million asthmatic children in the United States (Figure 17-7).

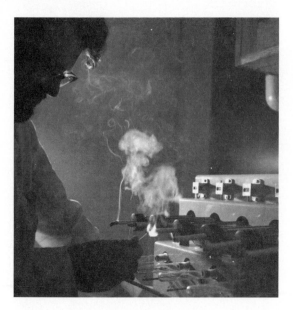

FIGURE 17-6
After years of growing research evidence, passive smoking or environmental tobacco smoke was declared a human carcinogen by the U.S. Environmental Protection Agency in 1992.
Source: Environmental Protection Agency.

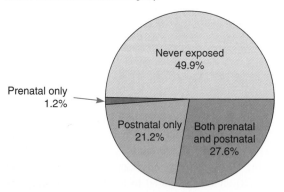

Prenatal only 1.2%

Never exposed 49.9%

Postnatal only 21.2%

Both prenatal and postnatal 27.6%

FIGURE 17-7
Over half of children 5 years of age and under have been exposed to smoke before or after birth in the United States. These exposures are estimated to account for higher rates of children born with abnormal lung functions and others developing early pulmonary morbidity, including bronchitis, pneumonia, and asthma after birth.
Source: National Center for Health Statistics. Overpeck MD, Moss AJ: *Children's exposure to environmental cigarette smoke before and after birth: health of our nation's children, United States, 1988. Advance data from vital and health statistics*, no 202, Hyattsville, Md, 1991, National Center for Health Statistics.

RADIATION POLLUTION

Human populations have always been exposed to natural sources of radiochemical activity and cosmic radiation. This type of radioactivity is referred to as background radiation, and all people are exposed to a harmless amount of about 0.1 R (roentgens) per year. Not until the splitting of the atom did radioactive atmospheric pollution become a problem.

Radioactivity is a natural physical process. Although atoms of most substances are stable, some complex radioactive atoms—known as radioisotopes—are unstable because they have too much energy. They become more stable by releasing extra radiation energy in a process known as radioactive decay. The particles released from this process cannot be seen, smelled, tasted, or heard, but radioactivity is hazardous. Radiation can penetrate human tissue. Depending on the level of exposure the effects on human organs can range from nausea, to localized skin burns, to death.

Epidemiology of Exposure to Radioactivity

Medical sources. The use of radioactive materials for treatment, research, and other purposes must always be regarded as a potential hazard, but these possible sources of radioactivity are usually well controlled and are not a danger to the general public. The immediate danger is to those people working with radioactive materials, and they have the necessary knowledge to use proper shielding and to take other precautions for protecting themselves.

Nuclear weapons. The prevention of nuclear war has been described by some as the ultimate public health problem. The atomic bomb has been used twice as a weapon of war. The United States dropped the bombs on August 6, 1945, in Hiroshima, Japan and on August 9, 1945, in Nagasaki, Japan. At each site 75,000 people died immediately; many more suffered the effects of radiation-related illnesses, even until today.

When nuclear weapons were tested in the atmo-

Nuclear Winter

Based on studies of the Mount Tambora effects of 1816 and on other volcanic and climatological analyses, a group of scientists postulated in 1983 the concept of a disastrous man-made winter caused by nuclear war. The fires and explosions that would follow the detonation of only half of the world's nuclear arsenals would propel at least 180 million tons of smoke and 15 million tons of dust into the atmosphere. These clouds would blanket the earth for at least 6 to 20 weeks, dropping temperatures 18° to 55° F in Europe, North America, and China if the war occurred during spring or summer, or in the Southern Hemisphere if it happened in their spring or summer. The pall of smoke and dust would block out 99% of the sunlight, destroying agriculture for at least a year. Famine would be unavoidable for survivors of the war in all parts of the world.

How long a nuclear winter would last is incalculable. The rainfall that might flush the skies could be disrupted by the accumulation of the sun's heat in the upper atmosphere. Even sunlight that did penetrate the blanket of dust would present the additional danger of lethal ultraviolet radiation because much of the protective ozone layer in the upper atmosphere would have been burned away. Given the effects of freezing temperatures, radiation exposure, general air pollution, famine, and the resulting inadequately treated diseases, wounds, and burns (since little medical care would be left available), nuclear winter presents the possibility of human extinction.

sphere, explosions sprayed the atmosphere with long-lived radioactive particles. These particles, such as strontium-90 and cesium-137, settled to the earth. Such fallout represents a threat to human life because penetration of body cells by radioactive particles causes ionization of the atoms of cells, particularly cells undergoing division. The extent of damage depends on the dose received and whether it is received externally or internally. For doses received or applied externally, the unit of measurement is the **roentgen**—the amount of radiation that causes two ionizations per cubic micron. An adult exposed to 1 R would receive about 10 to 17 ionizations over the whole body. A dose of less than 100 R produces no symptoms in a person, but 500 R in one dose is fatal. The U.S. Atomic Energy Commission reports that the average external dose from nuclear weapons test fallout was from 0.001 to 0.005 R per year, less than 5% of the annual dose from background radiation.

Internal dosage is expressed by the strontium unit (SU), which is equivalent to 0.003 R per year exposure of bone tissue. Internal doses result from ingesting radioactive water, milk, and other foods (Figure 17-8). This type of exposure to radioactivity poses a greater health threat than does external exposure. Strontium-90 is chemically similar to calcium and thus is deposited in bone. In young children strontium-90 is distributed throughout the bones, where localized high doses may cause malignancies. In adults the cancellous (spongy) bone is usually affected, causing acute poisoning.

Maximum permissible concentration (**MPC**) has not been established to the satisfaction of scientists in the field of radiation. The U.S. National Academy of Sciences has proposed 50 SU as the MPC, but the U.S. National Committee on Radiation sets the standard 25% higher. It should be noted that the level of radioactive fallout from nuclear tests was greater in the United States than in any other country.

Nuclear arms proliferation is a great threat and could become a by-product of nuclear energy technology if the technology is converted to arms by terrorists. The Europeans and New Zealanders have been the most vociferous in objecting to nuclear arms on their territory, but health professionals elsewhere have become increasingly concerned with the health implications of a world faced with the possibility of "the ultimate epidemic." Nuclear disarmament initiatives of Russia, the North Atlantic Treaty Organization, and the United States are hopeful signs.

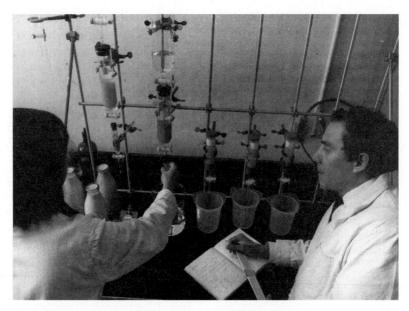

FIGURE 17-8
Radiochemical analysis of milk, testing for the presence of strontium 90, has been necessary in regions affected by fallout from nuclear reactor accidents or by nuclear weapon testing.
Source: Photo by P. Larsen, courtesy World Health Organization.

Nuclear reactors. Nations' energy needs are increasing at a rate faster than the rate of population growth, and it is apparent that fossil fuel sources are inadequate to meet rising energy needs. The next most readily available source is nuclear energy, which can be converted to electrical energy. To obtain this additional electrical power, governments and public utility companies have developed nuclear reactors. Protesters have raised objections to the proposed plant sites and even to the construction of such plants. They are concerned about the possibility of constant emissions from the reactors, thermo-pollution from heated water emptied into streams, unsafe disposal of radioactive wastes, and—foremost of all—accidents that would saturate the atmosphere with lethal radioactive ions. The 1979 incident at the Three Mile Island reactor in Penn-sylvania and the more recent Chernobyl incident confirmed the validity of some of these concerns.

Emissions of nuclear reactors are controlled by shielding and the use of other proven methods. Water is cooled before being discharged into streams. Wastes are buried 2500 feet underground or otherwise rendered distant or relatively harmless to human beings. Accidents that would threaten communities have probabilities close to the order of zero, but Chernobyl demonstrated that "close" is not good enough. Those who work at nuclear plants are the most exposed to any possible danger and the most knowledgeable. These experts who understand the situation tend to minimize any reason for fear. When tapping solar energy becomes more feasible, reducing the need for nuclear reactors, the public will be more reassured.

Surveillance. The U.S. Public Health Service, with monitoring stations distributed across the nation, keeps a close surveillance of nuclear plants and atmospheric radiation and takes all possible action to control sources of radiation. Similar agencies in other countries serve this purpose. On the state or provincial and community level, detection and correction of radiation ''leaks'' from x-ray machines, fluoroscopic equipment, and other sources of radiation is a continuous effort by health officials and special agencies set up to safeguard the public. At present, the general public is relatively safe from radiation hazards, but constant vigilance is imperative.

PRESSURIZED GASES

Gases held under pressure in containers pose direct threats to health and long-term threats to the atmospheric environment.

Fluorocarbon Gases

For some time health scientists have recognized that **fluorocarbon propellants** can produce atmospheric effects harmful to human health. Some American investigators have done research in this field, but Russian and German scientists have been doing a major share of the ongoing studies.

Fluorocarbon propellants from aerosol spray containers (Figure 17-9) do not decompose chemically in the lower atmosphere because they do not react with any other gases. Rainwater does not remove these propellants from the air. Fluorocarbons drift slowly into the upper regions of the stratosphere and release chlorine after being subjected to ultraviolet rays. The released chlorine atoms react with ozone molecules to produce chlorine oxide and oxygen. This reaction in turn decreases the amount of ozone, eventually reducing the ozone concentration by as much as 4%. Recovery to normal levels

Electric and Magnetic Fields: A New Health Issue?

Over 300,000 miles of power lines stretch across the U.S. Both electric and magnetic fields exit between the overhead conductors and the ground whenever current flows. Both electric and magnetic fields transfer electrical energy to conductive objects, including humans. There is a debate in current research about whether these fields independently or in combination cause health problems. A small body of epidemiologic research reports an association between low-level background residential alternating-current magnetic fields and childhood cancer. Regulatory, judicial, and media involvement have raised public awareness and fear on the issue. The challenge now is to determine the risk better through solid research and implement ways to avoid it. Until then, we can expect opposition to new transmission facilities, reluctance to buy homes near power lines, labor concerns, and personal damage litigation. Keeping the public informed will be an important public health education responsibility.

of ozone may take more than 100 years. When the ozone level is lowered, more ultraviolet rays reach the earth, which could result in such effects as cancer, particularly of the skin.

The cooling fluid used in most refrigerators and some radiators has a similar effect on the ozone. These are being phased out by treaties signed in 1990 among most Western countries, but large, Third World countries are just beginning to enjoy the benefits of widespread home refrigeration. The human respiratory tract can be directly affected by fluorocarbons. In the nonciliated part of the nasal junction, fluorocarbon particles move slowly, but particles deposited in the ciliated tissue move more rapidly. Thus there can be an immediate threat to the lungs of exposed users as well as possible long-term effects from atmospheric changes created by fluorocarbons.

Few products remain on the market in North

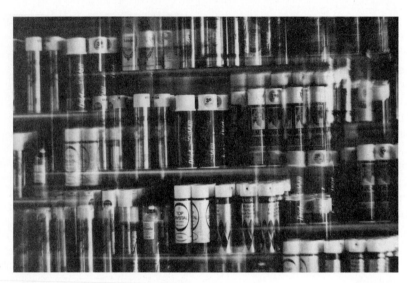

FIGURE 17-9
Fluorocarbon propellant spray cans as a source of indoor pollution and ozone depletion have been gradually replaced by other forms of spray cans without fluorocarbons. The indoor pollution problem remains, while attention on the ozone depletion issue has shifted to refrigerants containing similar ozone-depleting chemicals.
Source: Photo by T. Farcas, courtesy World Health Organization.

America that use fluorocarbon-driven propellants in spray cans. These containers have been replaced by different types of spray cans such as pump or water-driven sprays. The U.S. government either could require that industry label containers using fluorocarbon propellants as being dangerous to human health or could completely ban these propellants.

Some states have taken action through legislation that bans the sale of containers using fluorocarbon propellants. An Oregon law provides that violation of the state's ban on propellants is a class "A" misdemeanor, a criminal violation punishable by fines up to $1000 and 1 year in prison.

Other Pressurized Gases

Pressurized gases other than fluorocarbons also present dangers. Oxygen in containers can be a fire hazard if released near a flame. Stored in hallways or near vehicles, compressed gas cylinders can be knocked over and explode with devastating results. Rusty cans of ether can be volatile fireballs when kicked. Teenagers sniff aerosol chemicals for a dangerous high. Small children can incur lung damage or poisoning from breathing aerosol fumes. Finally, much of the problem of indoor pollution addressed in Chapter 15 is attributable to pressurized gases sprayed or leaked into the contained air spaces of unventilated houses or buildings.

NOISE AND HEAT POLLUTION

Noise and heat are increasing in significance as public concerns. The growing magnitude and complexity of society have brought increases in noise levels to a degree that calls for programs to relieve people of distress. Not all sound is objectionable, nor is all sound classed as noise. Technically, noise is any disturbing sound that interferes with work, comfort, or rest. It is doubtful that death has ever been caused by noise, yet noise can have an adverse effect on health, particularly mental health. Sounds are measured in decibels. Noise over 90 decibels can cause stress, even hearing loss. Prolonged exposure to noise of 85 to 115 decibels have been linked to a variety of mental and social problems.

Epidemiology of Noise

The urgency of the problem created by noise depends on the frequency of the occurrence, the absolute as well as the relative loudness, and whether the noise is necessary or unnecessary. The honking of an automobile horn may be objectionable, but the siren of a fire truck may not be. Some sounds that may be objectionable nevertheless must be accepted. For example, as much as the public objects to the boom when jet planes break the sound barrier, citizens in certain locations have had to learn to live with this noise. Airports change flight schedules and paths to accommodate some citizen complaints.

Industry noise control. In many industries noise represents a problem of some significance. Exposure to high noise levels can cause deafness. Noises of lower levels can affect workers' efficiency and be otherwise objectionable. Industry usually makes surveys of noise intensities and takes necessary corrective measures, as described in Chapter 15. Segregating noisy operations, insulating for sound control, redesigning machinery, and changing operations are among the possible corrective measures. Where noise intensity cannot be avoided, providing workers with ear protectors will safeguard their hearing.

Community noise control. Certain noises in the modern community, such as from traffic, street work, construction work, locomotives and certain industries, may be ever present. The public generally accepts a certain noise intensity from these sources, but will lodge complaints when the noise rises above a certain level of intensity.

City planning, including restricting industrial or commercial operations to particular zones, is a first measure. Cooperation resulting from communication between all parties concerned is the key to dealing with noise problems that arise and that are not covered by existing ordinances. Community organization efforts should precede court action, but if all other efforts fail, a court injunction will prohibit the offender from continuing the noise nuisance or will order the offender to reduce the noise to a defined, tolerable level.

Noise-control laws have been enacted in various cities. New York enacted the first noise-pollution law in the 1970s. Laws dealing with contemporary noise sources include banning rolling "boom-boxes" and cars with mega-watt stereos. Limits have been set on car and home alarms in some areas.

From July 1 to 13, 1993, the eastern part of the United States suffered a heat wave implicated in 84 deaths in the Philadelphia area alone, especially among elderly and infirm people (Figure 17-10). Three cases occurring in other parts of the country follow:

Case 1. A one-year-old infant left sleeping for approximately 75 minutes in the back seat of an automobile with the windows closed was found dead from hyperthermia.

Case 2. On July 7, a 48-year-old woman was found unconscious at her kitchen table in her mobile home. She was pronounced dead on arrival at a local emergency department. Rectal temperature measured at the emergency department after the 20-minute air-conditioned ambulance ride was 108° F (42° C). All the windows in the decedent's mobile home were closed and fans turned off when she was discovered. She had been dehydrated the day before when she arrived for her appointment at a local health department clinic.

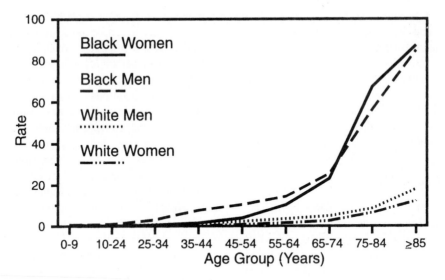

FIGURE 17-10
Rate per 100,000 population of heat-related deaths, by age and race—United States, 1979-1988.
Source: Merchandani et al: Heat-related deaths—United States, 1993, *MMWR* 42:559, 1993.

Case 3. On July 8, a 68-year-old man, last seen alive on July 5, was found in a slightly decomposed state in his apartment. Room temperature exceeded 100° F (38° C). Direct cause of death was atherosclerotic heart disease, but hyperthermia was recorded as a contributing factor.

How might these deaths have been prevented at a community level of action?

AIR QUALITY OBJECTIVES

The overall goal of community air quality control programs is to achieve and maintain adequate air quality to avoid adverse effects on human health and welfare and to minimize damage to structures and vegetation, visibility reduction, odor, and other nuisance effects or esthetic insults to the population. Specific objectives for a given community should be developed by inserting realistic target dates and levels of results anticipated using the national objectives from the box on p. 527.

ENVIRONMENTAL PROTECTION AGENCIES

With the growing concern about environmental health problems it was logical that special agencies should be created to safeguard the interests of the general public in the protection and promotion of environmental quality. These agencies are found at all levels of government and basically are regulating agencies. At the national level in most countries is an agency such as the EPA in the United States. State or provincial agencies are variously named, but a common designation is Department of Environmental Quality. Some metropolitan areas have environmental control departments, but the nature of environmental quality, being geographically broad rather than localized, dictates that the state agency serve all state needs in matters of environmental control.

State or Provincial Agencies

A state or provincial department of environmental quality is usually governed by an unpaid lay commission appointed by the governor or premier. The

U.S. National Health Objectives for Air Pollution in the Year 2000

Health status objectives

- Reduce asthma morbidity as measured by a reduction in asthma hospitalizations to no more than 160 per 100,000 people. (Baseline: 188 per 100,000 in 1987)

Special Population Targets

Asthma hospitalizations (per 100,000)	1987 baseline	2000 target
Blacks and other nonwhites	334	265
Children	284*	225

*Children aged 14 and younger

Risk reduction objectives

- Reduce human exposure to criteria air pollutants, as measured by an increase to at least 85% in the proportion of people who live in counties that have not exceeded any Environmental Protection Agency standard for air quality in the previous 12 months. (Baseline: 49.7 in 1988)

Proportion Living in Counties That Have Not Exceeded Criteria Air Pollutant Standards in 1988 for:

Ozone	53.6%
Carbon monoxide	87.8%
Nitrogen dioxide	96.6%
Sulfur dioxide	99.3%
Particulates	89.4%
Lead	99.3%
Total (any of above pollutants)	49.7%

Note: An individual living in a county that exceeds an air quality standard may not actually be exposed to unhealthy air. Of all criteria air pollutants, ozone is the most likely to have fairly uniform concentrations throughout an area. Exposure is to criteria air pollutants in ambient air. Due to weather fluctuations, multi-year averages may be the most appropriate way to monitor progress toward this objective.

Baseline data source: Office of Air and Radiation, Environmental Protection Agency.

- Increase to at least 40% the proportion of homes in which homeowners/occupants have tested for radon concentrations and that have either been found to pose minimal risk or have been modified to reduce risk to health. (Baseline: Less than 5% of homes had been tested in 1989)

Special Population Targets

Testing and modification as necessary in:	Baseline	2000 target
11.6a Homes with smokers and former smokers	—	50%
11.6b Homes with children	—	50%

Baseline data sources: Office of Radiation Programs, Environmental Protection Agency; Center for Environmental Health and Injury Control.

- Reduce human exposure to toxic agents by confining total pounds of toxic agents released into the air, water, and soil each year to no more than:

  0.24 billion pounds of those toxic agents included on the Department of Health and Human Services list of carcinogens. (Baseline: 0.32 billion pounds in 1988)

  2.6 billion pounds of those toxic agents included on the Agency for Toxic Substances and Disease Registry list of the most toxic chemicals. (Baseline: Approximately 2.62 billion pounds released in 1988)

Baseline data source: Toxic Chemical Release Inventory.

- Reduce human exposure to solid waste-related water, air, and soil contamination, as measured by a reduction in average pounds of municipal solid waste produced per person each day to no more than 3.6 pounds. (Baseline: 4.0 pounds per person each day in 1988)

Baseline data source: Characterization of Municipal Solid Waste in the United States: 1990 Update.

commission appoints a full-time professional director, who in turn appoints the professional staff, subject to approval by the commission. Usually the state or province is divided into districts, and members of the professional staff are assigned to the different districts. Responsibilities of the staff in each district usually are as follows:

1. *Air quality:* investigating complaints of air pollution and obtaining necessary corrections; monitoring air quality problems in the district; conducting surveys and collecting samples of air; reviewing and preparing permits for emissions

2. *Water quality:* investigating complaints of water pollution and developing necessary controls and enforcement procedures to protect state or provincial water standards; investigating and reviewing proposed waste treatment plant locations; conducting inspections and surveillance of existing sewage treatment plants and sewage collection systems; conducting inspections and surveillance of existing industrial treatment facilities and waste discharges; preparing waste discharge permits for treatment facilities; conducting water quality basin surveys

3. *Solid wastes:* investigating solid waste disposal sites; evaluating proposed sites; preparing permits for solid waste disposal facilities

4. *Community and interagency responsibilities:* providing technical assistance and advice to local health departments and officials on such matters as sewage disposal, solid waste disposal, industrial waste disposal, and water quality surveys; consulting with the public, industry representatives, engineers, and city, county, state or provincial, and federal officials regarding plans, programs, and permits related to the design, construction, and operation of sewage treatment facilities, industrial waste treatment facilities, air treatment systems, and solid waste disposal systems; providing public information to local groups on all aspects of environmental quality.

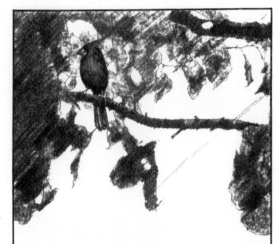
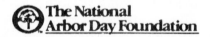
FIGURE 17-11
Tree planting in urban areas has helped control temperature levels, which reduces the evaporation of water and the production of greenhouse gases.
Source: The National Arbor Day Foundation.

While these state or provincial environmental quality agencies are often separate from the state or provincial health departments, cooperation and a close relationship are important. The magnitude of environmental health problems in modern society makes imperative the existence of a self-contained agency to be responsible for environmental quality. Health departments still carry on their traditional functions, perhaps more effectively after being relieved of the many tasks inherent in environmental health programs. Voluntary organizations concerned with the environment also contribute (Figure 17-11).

SUMMARY

As Carl Sagan warned, the atmosphere is a sensitive, protective shield for the earth. Because it extends across community and national boundaries, cooperation between governmental jurisdictions to control air pollution is essential. The potential for community-wide and world-wide drift of pollutants and clouds of chemicals, dust, or smoke makes the responsibility of each industry, each community, and each nation greater. This has been illustrated most poignantly by the experience of the 1816 "year without a summer," the Bhopal disaster in India in 1984, and the Chernobyl nuclear disaster in 1987.

Problems with radioactivity are attributable to industry, medical care (x-rays), government (nuclear power plants and weapons), and radon gas. Fifty percent of the current U.S. population dose comes from naturally occurring background radiation, such as cosmic radiation and radioactive materials in the water, soil, and air; 45% results from diagnostic and therapeutic medical applications; and the remaining 5% is accounted for by fallout, industrial use, production of nuclear power, and consumer products. Thus roughly half the exposure of the population at large comes from human sources. Low levels of ionizing radiation can produce delayed effects, such as cancer and genetic anomalies, after a latent period of many years.

As society becomes increasingly complex, the need to control adverse environmental factors becomes more urgent. No one has the right to jeopardize others' welfare by making the environment threatening to health or unpleasant (as in the case of air and noise pollution). The community must impose requirements on its residents for the protection of all. Besides the authority of the community represented in legislative requirements, community officials must provide services that will assist citizens in maintaining the best possible environment from the standpoint of health. Equally important, each citizen should understand his or her responsibility for a healthful environment and be motivated to assume responsibility for the quality of the community's environment. A "blitz" program or cleanup campaign may be justified on occasion but should not be the regular mode of community effort. Constant promotion of environmental health is the effective prescription.

QUESTIONS FOR REVIEW

1. Why does air pollution control require cooperation between governmental jurisdictions?
2. How do chemicals, smoke, and ash produce too much "blanket" in the earth's atmosphere?
3. How do chemicals produce too little "blanket"?
4. Why does smog accumulate?
5. What role do volcanic eruptions play in the theory of nuclear winter?
6. Why has there been an increased interest in environmental health despite the great advances in the understanding and overall control of environmental pollutants?
7. If an industrial firm that will employ 3000 people wishes to set up in your community a plant that will cause a great deal of air pollution, what would be your stand and your rationale for it?
8. In the past year, to what radiation dangers have you been exposed?
9. What safeguards and assurances do you get from the burial method of nuclear waste disposal?
10. What questions would you ask if the Department of

Energy proposed to put one of the nuclear waste disposal sites in your community?

11. Why is nuclear war referred to as the ultimate epidemic?

12. What are the characteristics of fluorocarbon propellants from aerosol spray cans that enable them to drift to the upper atmosphere and decrease the protective ozone layer?

13. In what ways will the environment of the future be more or less hazardous to human health than the environment of today?

14. How can noise be considered a form of air pollution?

15. Which agencies have jurisdiction over environmental controls in your community?

under have been exposed to environmental cigarette smoke either from prenatal maternal smoking or from sidestream smoke from household members after their birth, or both, according to this analysis of data from the latest National Health Interview Survey.

Waller RE: Field investigations of air. In Holland WW, Detels R, Knox G, editors: *Oxford textbook of public health,* vol 2, ed 2, Oxford, 1991, Oxford Medical.

This review of field investigation methods for air pollution covers the characteristics of air pollutants including smoke, other suspended particulate matter, sulphur dioxide, and others, human exposures, studies of acute affects, and associations of air pollution with chronic respiratory disease and lung cancer.

READINGS

Committee on Tropospheric Ozone Formation and Measurement, Board on Environmental Studies and Toxicology, Commission on Geosciences, Environment, and Resources: *Rethinking the ozone problem in urban and regional air pollution,* Washington, DC, 1992, National Academy Press.

This National Research Council study, mandated by the Clean Air Act of 1990, reviews ozone pollution, one of America's most stubborn environmental problems. The report suggests city, state, and federal (FDA) roles in controlling nitrogen oxides and volatile organic compounds producing ozone.

O'Riordan MC, Brown AP: Ionizing radiation. In Holland WW, Detels R, Knox G, editors: *Oxford textbook of public health,* vol 2, ed 2, Oxford, 1991, Oxford Medical.

This review of the public health aspects of radiation covers quantities and units of measurement, sources of ionizing radiation, exposure to radon, biological action of ionizing radiation, carcinogenic and genetic effects of radiation, principles of radiological protection, and radiation accidents.

Overpeck MD, Moss AJ: Children's exposure to environmental cigarette smoke before and after birth: health of our nation's children, United States, 1988, Advance data from vital and health satistics; no 202, Hyattsville, Md, 1991, National Center for Health Statistics.

About one half of all U.S. children 5 years of age and

BIBLIOGRAPHY

Adair RK: Constraints on biological effects of weak extremely-low-frequency electromagnetic fields, *Phys Rev A* 43:1039, 1991.

Becker SW: Air pollution information activities at state and local agencies—United States, 1992, *MMWR* 41: 967, 1993.

Beral V: Leukaemia and nuclear installations, *Br Med J* 300:411, 1990.

Bromet EJ, Parkinson DK, Dunn LD: Long-term mental health consequences of the accident at Three Mile Island, *Int J Mental Health* 19:48, 1990.

Cassano PA, Koepsell TD, Farwell JR: Risk of febrile seizures in childhood in relation to prenatal maternal cigarette smoking and alcohol intake, *Am J Epidemiol* 132:462, 1990.

Environmental Defense Fund: *Investing in prevention: opportunities to reduce disease and health care costs through identifying and reducing environmental contributions to preventable disease,* Washington, DC, 1993, Environmental Defense Fund.

Fox NL, Sexton M, Hebel JR: Prenatal exposure to tobacco. I. Effects on physical growth at age three, *Int J Epidemiol* 19:66, 1990.

Geran L: Environmental practices of Canadian households, *Can Soc Trends* 28:17, 1993.

Gregor MA, Van Amburg G, Thrush JC et al: Unintentional deaths from carbon monoxide poisoning—Michigan, 1987-1989, *MMWR* 41:881, 1992.

Hatch MC, Wallenstein S, Beyla J et al: Cancer rates after the Three Mile Island nuclear accident and proximity to the plant, *Am J Public Health* 81:719, 1991.

International Agency for Research on Cancer: Extremely low-frequency electric and magnetic fields and risk of human cancer, *Bioelectromagnetics* 11:91, 1990.

International Commission on Radiological Protection (ICRP): Recommendations of the International Commission on Radiological Protection, ICRP Publ No 60, *Ann ICRP* 21:1, 1991.

Jablon S, Hrubec Z, Boice J: Cancer in populations living near nuclear facilities. A survey of mortality nationwide and incidence in two states, *JAMA* 265:1403, 1991.

Leaf A: Potential health effects of global climatic and environmental changes, *N Engl J Med* 321:1577, 1989.

Lednev VV: Possible mechanism for the influence of weak magnetic fields on biological systems, *Bioelectromagnetics* 12:71, 1991.

Merchandani H, Pace P, Hameli AZ et al: Heat-related deaths—United States, 1993, *MMWR* 42:558, 1993.

Murdock BS: Global warming: will it affect health? *Health Env Digest* 4:1, 1990.

Neel JV, Schull W, Awa A et al: The children of parents exposed to atomic bombs: estimates of the genetic doubling dose of radiation for humans, *Am J Hum Genet* 46:1053, 1990.

Office of Disease Prevention and Health Promotion: It's official: passive smoking poses health risk, *Prev Rep,* June/July 1993.

Paris P, Rappaport S, Lieber K et al: Populations at risk from air pollution, *MMWR* 42:301, 1993.

Peters L: Environmental health practices. In Stephens T, Fowler Graham D, editors: *Canada's health promotion survey 1990: technical report,* Ottawa, 1993, Minister of Supply and Services Canada.

Pettersson B, Tillgren P, Finer D et al, editors: Playing for time ... creating supportive environments for health: report from the 3rd International Conference on Health Promotion, Sundsvall, Sweden, 1992, The Sundsvall Conference on Suportive Environments, Peoples' Health Vastermorrland.

Read PP: *Ablaze: the story of Chernobyl,* Toronto, 1993, Secker and Warburg.

Savitz DA, John EM, Kleckner RC: Magnetic field exposure from electric appliances and childhood cancer, *Am J Epidemiol* 131:763, 1990.

Schnorr TM, Grajewski BA, Hornung RW et al: Video display terminals and the risk of spontaneous abortion, *N Engl J Med* 324:727, 1991.

Seager J, editor: *State of the earth atlas,* New York, 1990, Simon and Schuster.

Shope RE: Vector-borne diseases: will warmer climates move them? *Health Env Digest* 4:3, 1990.

Smilkstein MJ, Burton BT, Keene W et al: Acute respiratory illness linked to use of aerosol leather conditioner—Oregon, December 1992, *MMWR* 41:965, 1993.

Stevens W, Thomas DC, Lyon JL et al: Leukemia in Utah and radioactive fallout from the Nevada test site, *JAMA* 264:585, 1990.

Tenforde TS: Biological interactions and potential health effects of extremely-low-frequency magnetic fields from power lines and other common sources, *Annu Rev Public Health* 13:173, 1992.

Thomas D, Stram D, Dwyer J: Exposure measurement error: influence on exposure-disease relationships and methods of correction, *Annu Rev Public Health* 14:69, 1993.

Upton AC, Shore RE, Harley NH: The health effects of low-level ionizing radiation, *Annu Rev Public Health* 13:127, 1992.

Wang JX, Inskip P, Boice J Jr et al: Cancer incidence among medical diagnostic X-ray workers in China, *J Natl Cancer Inst* 82:478, 1990.

Weiss KB, Gergen PJ, Wagener DK: Breathing better or wheezing worse? the changing epidemiology of asthma morbidity and mortality, *Annu Rev Public Health* 14:491, 1993.

Weitzman M, Gortmaker S, Sabol A: Racial, social and environmental risks for childhood asthma, *Am J Dis Child* 144:1189, 1990.

Wilson BW, Stevens RG, Anderson LE, editors: *Extremely low frequency electromagnetic fields: the question of cancer,* Columbus, Oh, 1990, Battelle.

PART FIVE

• •

Health Resources and Services

The targets of community health action are life-style, environment, and organized health services. These are the three modifiable components of the health field concept introduced in Part 1. Part 2 showed how these applied at various stages of the life span, from infancy to old age. Part 3 presented health promotion strategies directed primarily at the life-style or behavioral determinants of health, and Part 4 discussed environmental strategies to protect health. In this concluding part the resources and services necessary to organize the planning, implementation, and evaluation of community health strategies are identified. Resources and services are described first in the broader global and national context, then in the state or provincial context. Finally, the community and personal health services themselves are described.

Chapter 18

World and National Context of Community Health Services

Think globally; act locally.
Anonymous

OBJECTIVES

When you finish this chapter, you should be able to:

• Identify the sources of authority in national and international health agencies and actions

• Describe the placement of typical governmental functions at the national level and how they support community health and national health objectives

• Identify major agencies, foundations, and associations supporting community health at national and international levels

---

The roots of community health services are historical, philosophical, scientific, political, and economic. The historical conditions affecting a community's health services reflect not just the history of that community, but the history of the nation and the world that have shaped the community. The philosophies guiding the provision of community health services stem from the national and global philosophies defining health services as a right, and community self-determination and self-sufficiency as an ideal. Health science is universal by definition.

National and international politics and economics determine the resources available to communities. They set the foundation for the authority and capability of communities to provide services to meet their own health needs.

GLOBAL STRATEGY OF HEALTH FOR ALL

The clearest and most widely accepted articulation of a basic set of values for health, as these relate to world development, is contained in the Declaration of Alma-Ata (see box). The principles were articulated in a 1978 conference sponsored by the World Health Organization and the United Nations Children's Fund (WHO/UNICEF). The Declaration has been endorsed by most countries, including the United States and Canada. The Declaration acknowledges health as a human right, not a privilege, and ties health status to economic and social status. It establishes health as a common concern of all countries.

SOURCES OF AUTHORITY IN HEALTH

The **authority** of national governments in matters of health varies from country to country, depending on whether the country is under constitutional, imperial, or martial law. At one extreme, constitutions that create a republic, federation, or commonwealth of disparate states tend to reserve most powers for the states and grant only essential powers for the *common* good to the central government. This is the case, for example, in Australia, Canada, the United Kingdom, and the United States. At the other ex-

---

Declaration of Alma-Ata, Summary

Article I: "Health . . . is a fundamental human right and . . . the attainment of the highest possible level of health is a most important worldwide social goal whose realization requires the action of many other social and economic sectors in addition to the health sector."

Article II: "The existing gross inequality in the health status of the people, particularly between developed and developing countries as well as within countries, is politically, socially, and economically unacceptable and is, therefore, of common concern to all countries."

Article III: "Economic and social development, based on a New International Economic Order, is of basic importance to the fullest attainment of health for all and to the reduction of the gap between the health status of the developing and the developed countries. The promotion and protection of the health of the people is essential to sustained economic and social development and contributes to a better quality of life and to world peace."

Article IV: "The people have the right and the duty to participate individually and collectively in the planning and implementation of their health care."

Article V: "Governments have a responsibility for the health of their people which can be fulfilled only by the provision of adequate health and social measures. A main social target of governments, international orga-

nizations, and the whole world community in the coming decades should be the attainment by all peoples of the world by the year 2000 of a level of health that will permit them to lead a socially and economically productive life. Primary health care is the key to attaining this target as part of the development in the spirit of social justice."

The basic philosophy of Primary Health Care (PHC) is described under the Declaration of Alma-Ata as follows:

Article VI: "Primary health care is essential health care based on practical, scientifically sound, and socially acceptable methods and technology made universally accessible to individuals and families through their full participation and at a cost that the community and country can afford to maintain at every stage of their development in the spirit of self-reliance and self-determination. . . ."

The development of PHC is clearly identified not only as a national priority for developing countries, but as an international mission in Article IX of the Declaration:

"All countries should cooperate in a spirit of partnership and service to ensure primary health care for all people since the attainment of health by people in any one country directly concerns and benefits every other country."

treme, small countries, some monarchies, many socialist countries, and countries under martial law tend to centralize power at the national level and depend on state or local governmental bodies merely to carry out central plans and directives. Most countries swing between these extremes during their history.

Centralized Functions and Powers

The U.S. federal government provides many indispensable health services, as outlined in this chapter. Although the U.S. Constitution grants the federal government no *direct* authority to engage in public health activities, authority to promote health is conferred by general clauses concerning federal responsibilities. The British North America Act of 1867 similarly established Canada with a clear division of responsibility between federal and provincial governments, leaving jurisdiction over most health matters to the provinces. The many health functions carried on by the U.S. and Canadian federal governments derive their authority from the few specific centralized powers of the federal government. These powers are typical of those generally reserved by nations at the federal or central level.

Regulation of interstate commerce. Most national charters reserve the right to regulate interstate commerce. In the U.S., Australia, and Canada, this provision gives Congress and Parliament the right to pass legislation controlling shipment and quality of foods and drugs and governing movement of people and livestock on interstate carriers. Control of insects, air pollution, stream pollution, and other health threats becomes a federal function under the authority to regulate interstate commerce.

Taxing power. Most countries tax health-related products. In the case of the United States, Congress controls narcotics, alcohol, and tobacco by requiring a tax for a permit to possess and sell narcotics and

a tax on each transaction for the sale of cigarettes and alcohol. Oddly, the courts have held that these particular measures are primarily for revenue rather than for regulatory purposes.

Postal power. The U.S. and some other national governments prohibit the use of the mails in any frauds, including health frauds. Misbranded or fraudulent drugs, patent medicines, and foods cannot legally be shipped through the mails, nor can any promotional material relating to fraudulent drugs or foods.

Patent authority. Many national governments require that any newly developed drug or medicine to be distributed to the public must be registered or patented. International copyright and patent codes have ensured some uniformity among nations on patents, but the procedures for approval of drugs for marketing vary widely among countries.

Treaty-making power. National governments enter into agreements with other nations for control of communicable diseases, regulation of sanitary conditions, exchange of health information, and other health matters that are international in nature.

National war power. National governments have the authority to protect and maintain the health of all personnel in their armed forces.

Local authority. National governments have the responsibility to govern and to provide health services for local populations in federal trust territories, such as Canberra in Australia and the District of Columbia in the United States. For example, the authority to govern the District of Columbia carries an implied responsibility for the health of residents of the District.

Power to appropriate money. Responsibility for the general welfare, together with the right to create agencies, forms the great umbrella under which most federal health activities operate. Appropriating money for health agencies of the national, state or provincial, and local governments, for the construction of hospitals, for research, for health personnel training, for stream pollution control, and for other health projects has been the major contribution of national governments to health.

Power to create agencies. Responsibility for the general welfare has enabled national governments to set up agencies to deal with each health problem that arises. For example, within each of the U.S. federal executive departments there exist bureaus, divisions, or branches directly or indirectly concerned with some aspect of health.

OFFICIAL FEDERAL HEALTH AGENCIES

In countries as large as Australia, Canada, and the United States, various federal ministries, departments, bureaus, and other agencies are engaged in some sphere of health work. In most cases health is a partial or subordinate function of the agency. For example, the U.S. Department of Health and Human Services (DHHS) is concerned not only with health, but with welfare, housing, and a host of other human services. Arguments can be made about the relationship of health to such services, but no particular overall organizational relationship exists between these agencies. When cooperation does occur, it is the result of the judgment and action of the administrators involved or occasionally by legislative requirement for joint action.

Sometimes the assignment of health functions to government agencies does not appear connected to agency purposes. For example, health departments in many states were assigned responsibilities for administering Medicaid services. This responsibility pulled them away from traditional community health and prevention services toward health care services. In other cases, government agencies appear

to be a composite of special interests. This can occur when groups succeed in having a certain health program assigned to a particular agency. Once the program has been lodged with a certain agency, the special interest group will guard the agency's prerogative.

Most of the federal agencies with health functions are concerned with special problems or serve special groups. In the United States the Public Health Service is the only federal agency that truly deals with general health protection and health promotion. All others contribute one or more of the health services of the jigsaw puzzle referred to as the federal health program.

U.S. Executive Departments with Health Services*

In most national governments, every executive department or ministry has one or more branches directly or indirectly involved in health work. In almost every instance, health is not a sole or principal concern of the department or ministry. For the purpose of the present discussion, only a limited number of agencies in each executive department of the U.S. federal government will be identified and their health activity indicated. These U.S. agencies provide direct health services, regulatory services, advisory services, and grants-in-aid, and they loan personnel, conduct special studies, disseminate information, and conduct research, as well as provide other services related to their primary mission. Similar departments exist in most other countries as ministries.

Department of Health and Human Services (DHHS). The DHHS is continually restructuring its operating divisions, all of which are involved in matters of health in one form or another. Table

*At the time this edition went to press, Canada had just reorganized Health and Welfare Canada into a Ministry of Health and a Ministry of Human Resources. Further major changes may be expected following the election of a prime minister in late 1993.

18-1 shows DHHS expenditures toward achievement of the year 2000 health objectives. As of 1993, there were four major divisions within DHHS (Figure18-1), two devoted primarily to health and two devoted primarily to other human services.

For administration closer to the grass roots,

TABLE 18-1
U.S. health promotion and prevention priority areas

	(Dollars in thousands)	
	Fy 1990	*Fy 1991*
1. Physical activity and fitness	$21,789	$23,528
2. Nutrition	600,730	627,967
3. Tobacco	14,128	15,170
4. Alcohol and other drugs	667,025	750,475
5. Family planning	334,463	365,438
6. Mental health and mental disorders	1,002,136	1,294,088
7. Violent and abusive behavior	32,951	42,248
8. Educational and community-based programs	811,307	1,053,723
9. Unintentional injuries	40,499	48,806
10. Occupational safety and health	111,612	124,662
11. Environmental health	236,111	253,795
12. Food and drug safety	489,353	566,852
13. Oral health	89,612	102,040
14. Maternal and infant health	3,730,315	4,275,359
15. Heart disease and stroke	124,500	130,410
16. Cancer	591,535	845,571
17. Diabetes and chronic disabling conditions	686,980	768,291
18. HIV infection	1,637,623	2,098,378
19. Sexually transmitted diseases	97,174	102,555
20. Immunization and infectious diseases	380,284	432,629
21. Clinical preventive services	445,291	580,096
22. Surveillance and data systems	198,966	205,663
23. Cross-cutting and other	28,794	46,189
Total Resources	$12,373,178	$14,753,933

DHHS has 10 regional offices (see box). Most divisions of the DHHS have offices and personnel in these regional headquarters. The organization and functions of this Department and its four constituent units will be presented in more detail following a brief account of the health-related activities of the remaining departments of the executive branch of the federal government.

Department of Agriculture (USDA). This department administers a variety of programs with prevention components, including food and nutrition programs. In 1990 the USDA and DHHS jointly updated and published the *Dietary Guidelines for Americans.* The guidelines set standards for nutrition programs offered by the department. Other pre-

DHHS Regional Offices		
Region	*Area*	*Office Location*
1	Connecticut, Maine, Massachusetts, New Hampshire, Rhode Island, Vermont	Boston, MA
2	New Jersey, New York, Puerto Rico, Virgin Islands	New York, NY
3	Delaware, Maryland, Pennsylvania, Virginia, West Virginia, District of Columbia	Philadelphia, PA
4	Alabama, Florida, Georgia, Kentucky, Mississippi, North Carolina, South Carolina, Tennessee	Atlanta, GA
5	Illinois, Indiana, Michigan, Minnesota, Ohio, Wisconsin	Chicago, IL
6	Arkansas, Louisiana, New Mexico, Oklahoma, Texas	Dallas, TX
7	Iowa, Kansas, Missouri, Nebraska	Kansas City, MO
8	Colorado, Montana, North Dakota, South Dakota, Utah, Wyoming	Denver, CO
9	Arizona, California, Hawaii, Nevada, American Samoa, Guam, Trust Territory of the Pacific	San Francisco, CA
10	Alaska, Idaho, Oregon, Washington	Seattle, WA

DEPARTMENT OF HEALTH AND HUMAN SERVICES

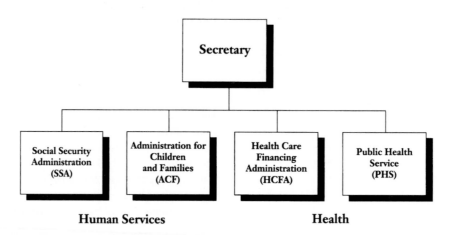

FIGURE 18-1

The four major administrative units, each with an assistant secretary, reporting to the Secretary of the Department of Health and Human Services, who reports in turn to the president. Of the two dealing primarily with health, HCFA administers Medicare and Medicaid, the other is the Public Health Service, which includes most of the agencies relating to community health (see Figure 18-5).

vention activities include food safety, family health, and nutrition education.

Food assistance programs—including the Food Stamp Program, the National School Lunch and School Breakfast programs, and the Child and Adult Care Food Program. The Special Supplemental Food Program for Women, Infants, and Children (WIC) provides supplemental foods and nutrition education to low-income pregnant, breastfeeding, and postpartum women, as well as to infants and children up to age 5 who are at nutritional risk.

Cooperative Extension Service—is USDA's direct educational network for food and nutrition information, reaching adults and children in 3150 counties in the U.S. Educational programs address all aspects of agricultural safety and health, including prevention of traumatic injury and reduction of exposure to infectious agents.

Food Safety and Inspection Service—provides food safety information to consumers and the food service industry. Targeted information is provided to those who are at risk for developing foodborne illness.

Agricultural Research Service—conducts research to define the nutrient requirements of humans at all stages of life.

Department of Commerce. Research is conducted by this department on fishery resources and the safety, quality, and identity of fishery products through the National Oceanic and Atmospheric Administration (NOAA). This agency and the Food and Drug Administration jointly developed a Voluntary Seafood Inspection Program to ensure the safety, wholesomeness, and proper labeling of seafood products.

Department of Defense. The initial health promotion program launched by this department in 1986 focuses on the improvement and maintenance of military readiness and enhancement of the quality of life for the department's personnel and other beneficiaries. Programs are focused on key risk reduction areas, including smoking prevention, exercise, nutrition, stress management, alcohol and drug abuse, and early identification of hypertension. Each of the armed services has implemented physical fitness programs. A strong policy against drug abuse has been established. A long history of efforts to control sexually transmitted diseases has met with varied success.

Department of Education. The Drug-Free Schools and Communities Act supports school-based and community-based drug, alcohol, and tobacco prevention programs. Other health-related activities include spinal cord injury prevention, services to infants and toddlers with disabilities, dropout prevention programs, and comprehensive school health education programs.

Department of Housing and Urban Development. This department contributes to community health through the provision of decent, safe, and sanitary housing to program participants.

Lead-based paint hazard removal—involves research, testing, and abatement of lead-based paint in both public and private housing.

Radon contamination in housing—includes cooperative efforts with DHHS to conduct radon contamination research and testing initiatives primarily with department-owned and subsidized housing.

Housing and community development assistance programs—set minimum property standards for housing design and construction to reduce the potential risk to public health from both man-made and natural hazards and irritations such as toxic dumps, power lines, and drainage canals.

Other health-related programs include the Public Housing Drug Elimination Grant Program, child care demonstration projects in public housing developments, and, under the McKinney Act, funding to enable homeless persons to find housing and supportive services.

Department of the Interior. Through the management of nationally owned public lands and natural resources, this department offers a variety of programs supporting health. The National Park Service administers more than 340 public areas that offer a wide variety of scenery, recreation, and enjoyment. Interpretation and educational programs provide opportunities that are educational, as well as directed at preventing injuries in parks.

Department of Justice. Funding, technical assistance, and training are provided in areas such as crime prevention and control, drug abuse prevention, family violence, child physical and sexual abuse, and AIDS as it relates to the criminal justice system.

"Weed and seed"—begun in 1991 as a comprehensive law enforcement and community revitalization strategy, this program seeks to drive crime out of neighborhoods and reclaim them for law-abiding citizens.

Preventing and controlling gang violence—involves a study to examine the nature and scope of the gang problem nationally, strategies to address these problems, and a National Clearing House to collect, analyze, and disseminate information on anti-gang programs.

Drug demand reduction activities—drug prevention programs for high-risk youth; multiservice, neighborhood-based programs for youth and their families; and the widely recognized National Citizens' Crime Prevention Program, featuring McGruff the Crime Dog, who urges youth not to experiment with drugs, are all designed to complement the supply-side strategies of interdiction and law enforcement to reduce drug smuggling and drug selling.

Other Justice Department health-related programs include those for missing and exploited children and assistance to victims of crime.

Department of Labor. A number of preventive and rehabilitative health programs of this department involve the development of health and safety standards to protect workers exposed to work-related hazards, provision of information to employers and employees to gain compliance with these standards, enforcement of standards, and compensation programs for those injured or made ill at work.

Occupational Safety and Health Administration—OSHA develops, enforces, and educates about safety and health standards intended to provide workers with job environments as free as feasible from health and safety hazards. Worksite inspections are accompanied by citations and penalties for violations. Health standards are set to protect workers against a wide variety of chemicals.

Mine Safety and Health Administration—develops and enforces safety and health rules for all mining and mineral processing operations from two-person sand and gravel pits to large underground coal mines.

Department of Transportation (DOT). Safe transportation and the environmental impact of transportation are found in the multiple agencies of this department.

National Highway Traffic Safety Administration—sets safety standards for motor vehicles, conducts public information programs (Figure 18-2), and implements other programs to reduce deaths, injuries, and economic losses resulting from traffic accidents. Programs in this administration include the use of seat belts and child safety seats, reduction of alcohol-related fatalities, pedestrian safety, motorcycle safety, and prevention of trauma and injury.

Federal Highway Administration—has a mission to prevent injuries on the roadways. In the last few years it has broadened its regulation of com-

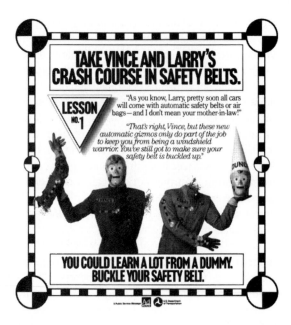

FIGURE 18-2
The National Highway Traffic Safety Administration, like most federal agencies, conducts public information programs to increase awareness of laws, regulations, and ways in which people can protect themselves in the absence of laws and regulations.

Source: National Highway and Traffic Safety Administration, U.S. Department of Transportation.

mercial motor vehicle safety through such actions as removing unsafe and unqualified drivers from the highways. Commercial motor vehicles operating in interstate commerce must pass, at least annually, a thorough inspection to comply with federal standards.

Federal Aviation Administration—The FAA contributes to reduction of aviation injuries through a comprehensive regulatory program that includes the design, manufacture, operation, and maintenance of aircraft, their component systems, and spare parts. This administration also operates the nation's air traffic control system.

Other prevention-related programs of DOT include protection of the marine environment and boating safety by the Coast Guard, railroad standards and safety, and the Urban Mass Transportation Administration, which enables the elderly and handicapped to use public transportation through specially equipped vehicles.

Department of the Treasury. Certain regulatory and law enforcement agencies of the Treasury Department, such as the Bureau of Alcohol, Tobacco, and Firearms (ATF), provide health-related prevention activities. DHHS and the ATF work together on the labeling of ingredients and substances that may pose a public health problem (Figure 18-3). Other programs include the health-warning labeling of alcoholic beverages and testing for the contamination or alteration of alcoholic beverages. Through testing, the ATF has found problems such as the presence of pesticides and methanol in alcoholic beverages, leading to product recall.

Department of Veteran Affairs. The former Veterans Administration was elevated to department status in 1989. It has a preventive medicine program that focuses on 11 risk factors representing diseases that have high mortality and morbidity for the VA patient population. Each VA medical center and independent outpatient clinic engages in prevention programs.

Independent U.S. Federal Agencies and Health Services

Environmental Protection Agency (EPA). The mission of this agency to abate and control pollution is accomplished through a variety of standard setting, monitoring, enforcement, education, and research activities. Major programs address air quality, water quality (including safe drinking water), pesticides, solid waste, toxic substances, the protection of groundwater and wetlands, climate change, and environmental hazards in homes, such as radon (Figure 18-4).

The Toxic Release Inventory is conducted annually to determine the toxic chemical release from

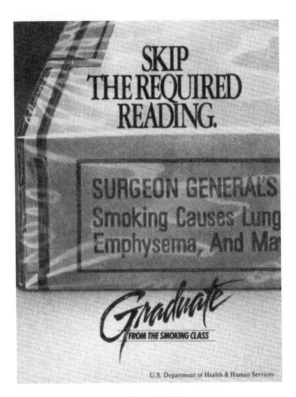

FIGURE 18-3

The Alcohol, Tobacco, and Firearms agency of the U.S. Treasury Department has responsibility for labeling substances that may pose a public health hazard, but the U.S. Department of Health and Human Services conducts health education campaigns to draw public attention to these labels and to use them as a springboard or theme for other educational messages.

Source: Office on Smoking and Health, Centers for Disease Control and Prevention, U.S. Department of Health and Human Services.

manufacturing facilities to air, water, land, and off-site transfers. Results of the survey are available to the public through the Emergency Planning and Community Right-to-Know program to contribute to the identification of releases of potential concern.

The EPA works with industry, the military, and other governmental organizations to ensure the lowest achievable levels of emission of chlorofluorocarbons (CFCs) and halons to prevent further destruction of the ozone layer. Nonessential uses of CFCs as aerosol propellants were banned in 1978.

RADON. THE HEALTH HAZARD IN YOUR HOME THAT HAS A SIMPLE SOLUTION.

Call 1-800-SOS-RADON to get your Radon test information.

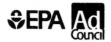

FIGURE 18-4

The Environmental Protection Agency is one of several outside the U.S. Department of Health with a broad range of health responsibilities. Some of these reach down to the community and link the federal government with the household level of environmental concerns.

Source: Environmental Protection Agency.

The Clean Air Act Amendments of 1990 endorsed the phaseout by the year 2000 of CFCs and halons and imposed more stringent intermittent targets and fines.

Consumer Product Safety Commission. The commission was created in 1973 to protect consumers from unreasonable risks of injury associated with consumer products. It identifies products that present the more serious safety problems and deals with them on a priority basis. Identification of such products is aided by the National Electronic Injury Surveillance System, which is a cooperative effort with selected hospitals that provide data about product-related injuries treated in emergency rooms across the country.

Products and issues highlighted in the commission's recent prevention activities include cigarette lighters, cigarette ignition, swimming pools and hot tubs, toys with choking hazards, playground equipment, riding lawn mowers, gas detection, poison prevention, chemical hazards, and heat tapes.

Other agencies. A considerable number of other somewhat independent federal agencies provide health services to a significant degree. From a long list, a few of these agencies are identified as examples.

Federal Trade Commission—control of deceptive advertising of foods, drugs, cosmetics, and devices shipped in interstate commerce

Interstate Commerce Commission—enforcement and promotion of health standards in the operation of interstate carriers

National Science Foundation—development of fundamental research in biological, physical, medical, and health sciences

Scores of federal agencies are thus engaged in health work. In each case the service is significant—in some, essential. Yet the principal health organization in the U.S. federal government, the one that carries on virtually all health service functions to an extended degree, is the Public Health Service (PHS).

U.S. DEPARTMENT OF HEALTH AND HUMAN SERVICES
Public Health Service

History. What began in 1798 as the Marine Hospital Service in the Treasury Department evolved into the Public Health and Marine Hospital Service in 1902. In 1912 the name was changed to the U.S. Public Health Service. The responsibilities of the agency have increased dramatically over the years. In 1917 it was charged with responsibility for the physical and mental examinations of all immigrants to the United States. In the same year a national leprosarium was opened in Carville, Louisiana, and the Public Health Service was designated as the operating agency. In 1929 the medical care of federal prisoners and narcotic addicts became a responsibility of the Public Health Service. In the same year a program in mental hygiene was launched. The Social Security Act of 1935 further extended the responsibilities of the Public Health Service. All grants-in-aid to states to strengthen local and state health departments were administered by the Public Health Service.

A series of congressional acts continued to increase the functions of the Public Health Service. In 1937 the National Cancer Act was passed, followed by the Venereal Disease Control Act a year later. In 1939 the U.S. Public Health Service was moved from the Treasury Department to the Federal Security Agencies.

The Public Health Law enacted in 1944 was a landmark in the development of the Public Health Service, because this act provided for an expansion, reorganization, and consolidation of the agency and a revision of laws relating to public health. When the Department of Health, Education, and Welfare (now the Department of Health and Human Services) was established in 1953, the Public Health Service became a part of the new department.

In 1980, the Department of Education was created, and the Department of Health, Education, and Welfare was renamed the Department of Health and Human Services (DHHS). Today, the Assistant Secretary for Health is the administrative head of the eight divisions of the Public Health Service. The head of the Commissioned Corps of Uniformed Public Health Service Offices is the Surgeon General.

Mission. The mission of the PHS, broadly stated, is to protect and advance the health of the American people by

- Conducting and supporting biomedical, behavioral, and health services research and communicating research results to health professionals and the public;
- Preventing and controlling disease, identifying health hazards, and promoting healthful behaviors for the nation's citizens;
- Monitoring the adequacy of health personnel and facilities available to serve the nation's needs;
- Improving the organization and delivery of health services and bringing good health care within the reach of all Americans;
- Ensuring that drugs and medical devices are safe and effective and protecting the public from unsafe foods and unnecessary exposure to radiation;
- Administering block grants to the states for preventive health and health services; alcohol, drug abuse, and mental health services; maternal and child health services; and
- Working with other nations and international agencies on global health problems and their solutions.

Organization. Eight units of the Public Health Service contain numerous offices, bureaus, centers, institutes, and divisions that change their names, locations, or functions to some degree with every major health bill passed by Congress. They grow, shrink, split, or disappear with each year's appropriations. Of the 62 units of DHHS that were listed in the 1973 edition of this book, only a few still exist under the same administrative division and with the same name in 1993, and it is expected that President Clinton will continue to make major bureaucratic changes as promised in his election campaigns. Table 18-2 outlines the current units by their bureaucratic names and budgetary commitments to prevention. The mission and activities of the office of the

TABLE 18-2
Prevention is an important part of the mission of each Public Health Service (PHS) agency. Noted below is the FY 1991 distribution by agency of investments in prevention. Also noted is the contribution from other Health and Human Services (HHS) agencies outside PHS

Public Health Service	
Agency for Health Care Policy and Research	$45,195,000
Alcohol, Drug Abuse, and Mental Health Administration*	$753,907,000
Centers for Disease Control	$1,134,116,000
Food and Drug Administration	$669,100,000
Health Resources and Services Administration	$1,113,211,000
Indian Health Service	$706,000,000
National Institutes of Health	$1,927,963,000
Office of the Assistant Secretary for Health	$46,148,000
Total PHS	**$6,395,640,000**
Administration for Children and Families	**$811,693,000**
Health Care Financing Administration	**$7,546,600,000**
Total Funds for Prevention (HHS)	**$14,753,933,000**

*Effective October 1, 1992, ADAMHA was reorganized as the Substance Abuse and Mental Health Services Administration.

Assistant Secretary for Health and each of the eight PHS units are highlighted below.

Office of the Assistant Secretary for Health (OASH). The Assistant Secretary for Health is responsible for overseeing the work of the eight units of the Public Health Service. This includes overseeing national programs and policies related to health services delivery, disease prevention and health promotion, and biomedical research.

Objectives. *Healthy People 2000: National Health Promotion and Disease Prevention Objectives* were developed in this office and released on September 6, 1990. The Office of Disease Prevention and Health Promotion (ODPHP) was instrumental in the

cooperative effort undertaken to develop the objectives. Over 375 national membership organizations, 56 states and territories, and many agencies of the federal government participated in the effort. Some of the over 300 objectives for improved health promotion, health protection, preventive services, and surveillance were included in the early chapters of the book to demonstrate national prevention intents. These 300 objectives distribute among the 23 prevention priority areas shown in Table 18-1 with budgetary expenditures for each.

Organization. Besides ODPHP, the President's Council on Physical Fitness, currently chaired by Arnold Schwarzenegger, is also located in this office. Numerous programs directed at improving the physical fitness of youth are run by the council, including the President's Challenge Physical Fitness Test, summer fun programs, and 4-H projects.

Other staff offices that advise the assistant secretary on prevention issues, policies, and programs in targeted areas include the Office of Women's Health (OWH), National AIDS Program Office (NAPO), National Vaccine Program Office (NVPO), Office of International Health (OIH), Office of Minority Health (OMH), and Office of Population Affairs (OPA). Also reporting directly to the Assistant Secretary for Health are the administrators of the eight agencies or administrations shown in Figure 18-5 and described below.

Substance Abuse and Mental Health Services Administration (SAMHSA). The administration was created in 1992 through reorganization of the former Alcohol, Drug Abuse, and Mental Health Administration (ADAMHA). The administration has lead responsibility for the federal government's support and conduct of research on mental illness, substance abuse, and addictive disorders.

The Center for Substance Abuse Prevention (CSAP) is SAMSHSA's chief prevention component. Its mission is to prevent alcohol and other drug

PUBLIC HEALTH SERVICE

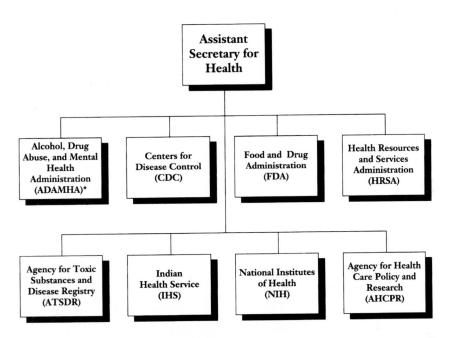

FIGURE 18-5

The Assistant Secretary for Health reports to the Secretary of the U.S. Department of Health and Human Services and has responsibility for the eight line agencies of the Public Health Service shown here, as well as staff units such as the Office of the Surgeon General and the Office of Disease Prevention and Health Promotion. Effective October 1, 1992, ADAMHA was reorganized as the Substance Abuse and Mental Health Services Administration. In 1993 the name of CDC changed to Centers for Disease Control and Prevention, but the initials CDC continue to be used.

abuse. Targeted programs include those aimed at pregnant and postpartum women, infants, college students, drinking drivers, and children of alcoholics. CSAP operates a National Clearinghouse on Alcohol and Drug Information and provides training through the National Training System to communities, professionals, and state agencies on substance abuse prevention. Multiple program evaluation efforts are being undertaken to assess the impact of training and other CSAP interventions.

The National Institute on Alcohol Abuse and Alcoholism (NIAAA) is the lead federal agency for basic and applied research on the causes, conse-quences, treatment, and prevention of alcohol-related problems. *The National Institute on Drug Abuse (NIDA)* is the agency with primary responsibility for research on the epidemiology, etiology, prevention, and treatment of drug use and abuse. The mission of the *National Institute of Mental Health (NIMH)* is to improve the understanding, treatment, and rehabilitation of the mentally ill, prevent mental illness, and foster the public's mental health. Examples of research conducted by these three agencies include the impact of alcoholic beverage control policies, such as server training, mass media programs to heighten public awareness about drug abuse, and training on coping skills for youth at risk of suicide.

Centers for Disease Control and Prevention. Based in Atlanta, the Centers for Disease Control and Prevention (CDC) is well known for its efforts to combat communicable diseases. Indeed, its original name was Office of Malaria Control in War Areas (1942). As of 1993 CDC had a $1.5 billion budget and over 7300 employees, including epidemiologists, microbiologists, entomologists, physicists, toxicologists, chemists, physicians, nurses, dentists, public health advisors, pharmacologists, veterinarians, health education specialists, writers, statisticians, social scientists, environmental engi-

neers, industrial hygienists, skilled technicians, and administrative and support personnel.

The major operating units of CDC are shown in Figure 18-6. In 1993 the name of the organization was expanded to emphasize its prevention focus. The mission of the CDC is to improve health by preventing disease, disability, and injury; monitoring health status; promoting healthful behaviors; and fostering healthful environments.

A major CDC activity is tracking disease incidence and trends and exchanging epidemiological information with health authorities throughout the United States and the world to enable them to take quick action in response to outbreaks, epidemics, and natural disasters. CDC is the lead PHS agency

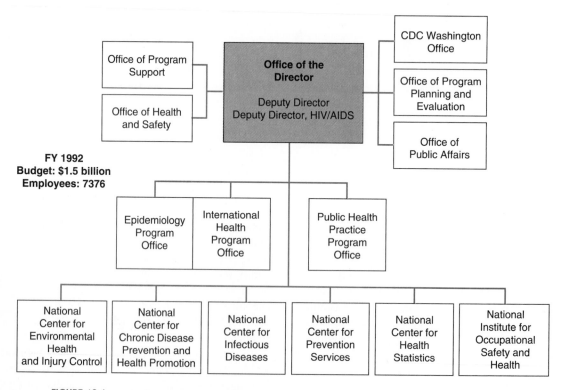

FIGURE 18-6

The organization of the Centers for Disease Control and Prevention as of June 1992.

Source: Centers for Disease Control: *CDC Fact Book,* FY 1992, U.S. Department of Health and Human Services.

for working with the states and communities to track and implement *Healthy People 2000* objectives. The distribution of the program budgets for CDC is shown in Figure 18-7.

CDC works closely with state and local health departments in developing and operating disease control programs, including programs for sexually transmitted disease control, childhood immunization, diabetes control, and community water fluoridation. Also provided are laboratory diagnostic services for unusual problems. CDC supplies rare vaccines, immunoglobulins, and therapeutic drugs that are not otherwise available for preventing and treating uncommon diseases. Annually, CDC personnel assist state health departments in investigating disease outbreaks. The investigation of fast-food hamburgers contaminated with *E. coli* in 1993 in Washington State is a good example of these cooperative efforts; other examples are the investigations of toxic shock syndrome, Reye's syndrome, Lyme disease, and acquired immunodeficiency syndrome (AIDS). CDC trains state and local health officials in epidemic control and in operating local disease prevention and health promotion programs.

On the international front, CDC works with governments of other nations and with the World Health Organization (WHO) to help control diseases before they can spread from one country to another. Programs focus on decreasing morbidity and mortality among infants and children, preventing the spread of HIV infection, improving conditions for refugees, and strengthening public health capacities overseas. For example, CDC administers a national quarantine program, which is carried out not only at U.S. ports of entry but also at strategic locations overseas, to protect the United States against the introduction of diseases from other countries. It also provides assistance and consultation when needed in the case of epidemics, as requested by health administrations of other nations.

CDC has been active in assessing special health-related problems, such as the impact on health of the volcanic eruption of Mount St. Helens, the health consequences of the nuclear accident at Three Mile Island, the potential risks associated with toxic waste disposal, and the effects of heat waves on communities. CDC cooperates with federal, state, and local officials in carrying out designated activ-

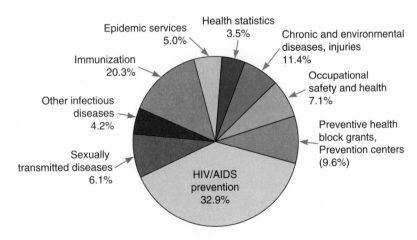

FIGURE 18-7
Percentage of CDC funding by program area, fiscal year 1992. Nearly one third of the program budgets are devoted to prevention and control of HIV/AIDS.
Source: Centers for Disease Control: *CDC Fact Book,* FY 1992. U.S. Department of Health and Human Services.

ities related to health effects of exposure to toxic substances. Scientists at CDC's National Institute for Occupational Safety and Health (NIOSH) conduct laboratory research and epidemiological studies to determine hazards in the working environment and steps that should be taken to eliminate them. NIOSH recommends acceptable exposure limits for toxic substances and harmful physical agents that workers may encounter; it also evaluates health conditions at specific work sites in response to requests from employers or employees.

An inaccurate laboratory diagnosis can be as great a threat to health as an untreated disease or an industrial hazard, which is why CDC monitors the licensing and certification of clinical laboratories and administers a comprehensive program to improve the nation's laboratory service.

CDC's health education activities seek to develop better ways of educating people about their health through school systems, health care providers, community organizations, and other channels. CDC also has educational programs in AIDS, family planning, smoking cessation, exercise, and violence prevention.

Food and Drug Administration (FDA). The FDA regulates products that run the gamut of modern life, including food, drugs, the nation's blood supply, vaccines, food and drugs for animals, cosmetics, heart pacemakers, x-ray machines, and microwave ovens. It is estimated that the FDA regulates products that account for 20 cents of every dollar spent by consumers. The work of the FDA's scientists— physicians, chemists, nutritionists, microbiologists, pharmacologists—forms the basis of its regulatory activities.

The FDA's 1991 budget of $681 billion represents recent increases in resources. Those funds, however, do not match all the activities required of the FDA by legislation. The mismatch of resources to mandated activities was publicly highlighted in the late 1980s when irregularities in generic drug enforcement were uncovered. A 1990 report to the

secretary of DHHS recommended that the FDA be removed from the Public Health Service and report directly to the secretary. The recommended reorganization would increase FDA autonomy, clarify its mission, and increase its enforcement authority.

Health Resources and Services Administration (HRSA). Leadership is provided by this Administration to promote access to health care services, primarily through programs that increase the availability and accessibility of community health resources. Priority programs are those that improve the availability of primary care for the medically underserved and for specific at-risk populations.

Among the health-related services provided is the Healthy Start Initiative, which involves collaboration of the administration with states and communities to reduce infant mortality. Other responsibilities include administration of the National Organ Transplant Program; support of states to plan and deliver health care to the underserved urban and rural area residents, migrant workers, and the homeless; assistance in ensuring health and workplace standards for federal employees; and provision of services for AIDS patients, including education and construction of non-acute care facilities.

The administration provides leadership in health resources through the education, distribution, and utilization of health professionals, including increasing the number of minorities in all health professions. The National Health Service Core provides primary care physicians, psychiatrists, dentists, and other health professionals to underserved areas in return for scholarship or loan repayment.

Agency for Toxic Substances and Disease Registry (ATSDR). The ATSDR was created in 1980 as a separate entity of the PHS by the Comprehensive Environmental Response, Compensation, and Liability Act, commonly known as the Superfund. The mission of this agency is to prevent or lessen the adverse effects of substances in the environment that are hazardous to both human health and quality of life. The work of the agency is carried out through research at potentially hazardous Superfund sites, development of databases linking exposure to substances and subsequent health and environmental effects, and dissemination of scientific information about the health effects of exposure to hazardous substances. To date, the toxicological profiles of 130 hazardous substances on the Superfund list have been identified.

Indian Health Service (IHS). The IHS assists Indian tribes in developing the capacity to staff and manage health programs for American Indians and Alaska Natives through activities that include health and management training, technical assistance, and human resource development. It also helps tribes to coordinate health planning, obtain and utilize health resources available through the government, design and operate comprehensive health care services, and develop community sanitation facilities.

The IHS provides health care for approximately 1.8 million American Indians and Alaska Natives through a network of 43 hospitals, 66 health centers, 4 school health centers, and more than 51 health stations. Among the prevention focuses of the IHS are maternal and child health, child abuse and neglect, community injury control, fluoridation, and substance abuse prevention. The IHS has a $1.8 billion budget to conduct its activities.

A new law will put the IHS on par with other public health agencies by requiring its director to be approved by the Senate for the first time. In addition, the new law sets 61 health goals for Native Americans to be met by the year 2000, including reduced rates of cancer, infant mortality, and alcoholism. The law authorizes $334 million for that effort in fiscal 1993.

National Institutes of Health. In 1887 the Marine Hospital Service founded a research laboratory at the Marine Hospital, Staten Island, New York. In 1891 the name was changed to Hygienic Laboratory, and the unit was moved to Washington, D.C.

In 1930 the Hygienic Laboratory became the National Institutes of Health (NIH) and moved to Bethesda, Maryland.

The mission of the NIH is the development of new knowledge for the prevention and control of disease. A broad, complex program is designed to meet the needs in biomedical science. The NIH includes 13 Institutes of Health, each with its own medical or health focus (see box). The focus of these institutes reflects not only physiological logic, but political pressure. The emphasis on the production of new knowledge through research has been balanced in recent years with the dissemination of knowledge through public education campaigns (Figure 18-8). Although scientists in the laboratories and clinical centers of the NIH carry on part of the

---

National Institutes of Health

The National Institutes of Health is a federation of organizations that includes 13 Institutes of Health, each with its own medical or health focus:

- National Cancer Institute (NCI)
- National Heart, Lung, and Blood Institute (NHLBI)
- National Institute of Diabetes and Digestive and Kidney Diseases (NDDK)
- National Institute of Arthritics and Musculoskeletal and Skin Diseases (NIAMS)
- National Institute of Allergy and Infectious Diseases (NIAID)
- National Institute of Child Health and Human Development (NICHD)
- National Institute of Aging (NIA)
- National Institute of Dental Research (NIDR)
- National Institute of Environmental Health Sciences (NIEHS)
- National Institute of General Medical Sciences (NIGMS)
- National Institute of Neurological Disorders and Stroke (NINDS)
- National Eye Institute (NEI)
- National Center for Research Resources (NCRR)

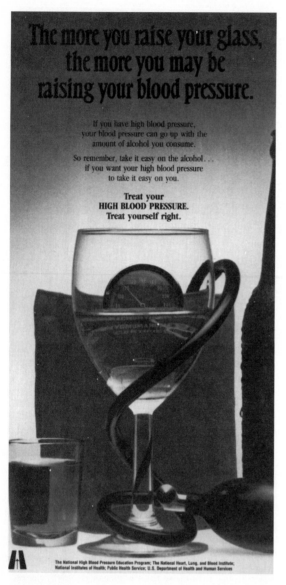

The more you raise your glass, the more you may be raising your blood pressure.

If you have high blood pressure,
your blood pressure can go up with the
amount of alcohol you consume.

So remember, take it easy on the alcohol . . .
if you want your high blood pressure
to take it easy on you.

**Treat your
HIGH BLOOD PRESSURE.
Treat yourself right.**

The National High Blood Pressure Education Program; The National Heart, Lung, and Blood Institute;
National Institutes of Health; Public Health Service; U.S. Department of Health and Human Services

FIGURE 18-8
The National High Blood Pressure Education Program of the National Heart, Lung, and Blood Institute is an early example of NIH taking on more public health education and knowledge dissemination to help close the gap between new knowledge generated through research and its application by health professionals and the public.

Source: National Institutes of Health.

program of research, most of the research is done by others through grants administered by the NIH. About 90% of the institute's **appropriation** of more than $8 billion yearly goes to the **extramural** program of grants to scientists and research institutions throughout the nation and the world.

The grants program is planned to provide a continuous supply of competent scientists in biomedical disciplines. In addition to the training grants, fellowships, and traineeships, the program also provides facilities, equipment, and other resources, including computers and primate centers. Basic research now cuts across several of the traditional biomedical areas. Special attention is given to national trends and to neglected areas of research.

The NIH has an international research program that seeks to make use of the abilities of qualified scientists the world over. Grants have been made to scientists in various health disciplines in many countries. The NIH has also provided opportunities for promising young American scientists to work abroad as members of established research groups. No foreign grants are made unless they are of a high value and are related to health objectives of value to the United States. Nobel Prize awards in medicine and physiology have been made to foreign investigators who were working under grants from the NIH.

The NIH makes contracts with foreign institutions to conduct research and provides fellowships to American scientists to study at foreign research centers of excellence. NIH also promotes a visiting program that brings distinguished scientists to the United States to work in the NIH laboratories or the John E. Fogarty International Center.

NIH finances research in hospitals, medical schools, and nonprofit research centers. Altogether, it underwrites about 40% of all the biomedical research done in the United States.

Agency for Health Care Policy and Research (AHCPR). Established in 1989, the agency serves as the federal focal point for health services research to enhance the quality of patient care services. The broad goals of the agency are to promote improvements in clinical practice and patient outcomes through more appropriate and effective health care services, to promote improvements in the financing, organization, and delivery of health care services, and to increase access to quality care. Among the Agency's activities are support for conferences on primary care research, support and dissemination of health policy research, and the provision of pre and postdoctoral support for academic training and for research concerning health services research methods and problems.

Other administrations in the Department of Health and Human Services. The U.S. Public Health Service and its eight major units play the major role in federal prevention efforts. Three other administrations within DHHS also have prevention efforts (Figure 18-1).

Social Security Administration (SSA). Through its Social Security Administration, DHHS operates the world's largest social insurance program. As of May 1991, a total of 40,119,000 people received a total of $236 billion annually in social security benefits. Most beneficiaries are retired workers. Some are disabled workers and their family members. Others are young children or eligible spouses of workers who have died (Figure 18-9). As of December 1992, the average monthly benefits payable to retired workers was $629; the average benefits for disabled workers was $609.

The Social Security System is financed through payroll taxes of working Americans. The employed worker and his or her employer share the tax equally. To qualify for benefits, the worker must have worked in covered employment long enough to become insured. Just how long depends on when the worker reaches age 62 or, if earlier, when he or she dies or becomes disabled. Spouses, including some aged-divorced spouses, and children under 18 of retired or disabled workers are eligible for benefits. Workers who become so severely disabled that they are unable to work may be eligible for benefits until they are no longer disabled.

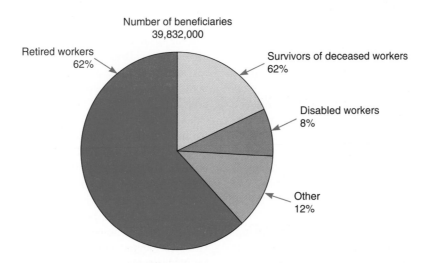

Number of beneficiaries
39,832,000

Retired workers
62%

Survivors of deceased workers
62%

Disabled workers
8%

Other
12%

FIGURE 18-9
Percentage of persons receiving monthly Social Security benefits, by type of beneficiary, 1990.
Source: U.S. Bureau of the Census and Social Security Administration, *Statistical Abstract of the United States,* 1992.

With the aging of the U.S. population, decreases in the number of young workers, and the huge federal deficit, the future of the Social Security Program has provoked intense discussion. By the year 2030, every fourth American will be 60 years of age or older. Organizations such as the American Association for Retired Persons (AARP) carefully watch actions of the government that may chip away at entitlements for the nation's seniors. The financial questions raised about the future of Social Security have sparked debates between the pre-World War II generation, who are now eligible for benefits, and "Generation X," who are just entering the work force, with the baby boomers caught in the middle between their own parents and children. Can we afford Social Security as it exists now? Who will pay?

Administration for Children and Families (ACF). Established in 1991, this Administration provides leadership in the administration of assistance and services programs designed to promote family stability, self-sufficiency, responsibility, and economic security. Programs focus on improving the health and well-being of low-income families, neglected and abused children and youth, Native Americans, and individuals with lifelong disabilities. These targeted populations are those at special risk in the *Year 2000 Objectives for the Nation's Health.*

The Head Start program intends to do as its name implies—provide a "head start" to low-income preschool children aged 3 to 5 and their families before they enter the public schools. The developmental services provided under this program include education, parental involvement, social services, and health services. Over 600,000 children are enrolled in over 31,000 Head Start classrooms.

Aid to Families with Dependent Children (AFDC) and Job Opportunities and Basic Skills Training (JOBS) are administered by the Office of Family Assistance to help low-income individuals and families meet immediate financial needs to become and remain economically self-sufficient. The Office of Child Support Enforcement helps locate absent parents, establishes paternity, and enforces regulations that require the so-called "deadbeat dads" to support their own children financially.

Title XX Social Services Block Grants, which totaled $2.8 billion in 1991, are intended to prevent or remedy the neglect, abuse, or exploitation of children and adults unable to protect their own interests. Other programs provide aid such as help with home heating and cooling bills for low-income households, the National Youth Sports Program, and emergency grants to help the homeless out of poverty.

The theme of economic independence that runs throughout these programs reflects the economic realities and political debates of our times. Changes in the executive and legislative branches of the government lead to renewed debate as to whether these types of social service programs, in the long run, promote independence or dependence in their recipients. The existence of multiple generations of a family on social services is used by some as an argument for the dependence fostered by such programs. The desperate plight of homeless children and the disabled who are unable to care for themselves are evidence to others of the need for such services. How these debates are resolved will shape both the structure and programs offered by the government.

Administration of Aging (AoA). The AoA is part of the ACF and was established to provide a focal point in government for the concerns and needs of older people and to coordinate federal policies that affect them. It supports community-based nutrition and companionship programs, transportation services, legal aid, homemaker and home health services, residential repair, and recreational activities for older people. A primary goal of all programs for the elderly is to provide supportive services in the community that will enable them to lead fully independent lives, avoid unnecessary institutionalization, and be a part of the community.

Health Care Financing Administration (HCFA).
Medicare and Medicaid, legislated in 1966, culminated a quarter century of legislative efforts to ensure that no elderly, disabled, or poor American need forego basic health care because of cost. Within DHHS, the Medicare and Medicaid bureaus are managed by the Health Care Financing Administration. These programs will be described in greater detail in Chapter 21.

Medicare provides low-cost health insurance for aged and disabled Social Security and railroad retirement beneficiaries.

Medicaid, jointly funded by federal and state governments, provides virtually free health coverage for those unable to afford any other kind of insurance or health care.

The Health Care Financing Administration also develops and enforces standards to ensure high-quality health care and to guarantee the safety and quality of all health services financed by federal funds.

Refugee health. Not since the early years of this century have Canada and the United States received such high numbers of immigrants as in the 1980s. The difference between the immigration waves then and now is that the early immigrants to the North American "melting pot" were primarily from Europe, especially the British Isles. Today the immigrants come predominantly from Latin America and Asia (Table 18-3). The language and cultural differences are greater and, for many of today's refugees such as the "boat people" from Vietnam, Cambodia, Haiti, and Cuba, the burden of prior disease, malnutrition, and physical and mental suffering is greater.

What lessons might be learned from North America's previous immigration waves in caring for the

TABLE 18-3
Estimated refugee arrivals in Canada and the United States by country of origin, 1990

Country of birth, citizenship, or last permanent residence	Canada	U.S.
Europe (mostly Eastern Europe)	15,831	33,111
Asia and Middle East	13,545	51,867
Central America, Haiti, and Cuba	5,393	9,910
South America	811	264
Africa	4,048	2,212
Total	39,628	97,364

Sources: Employment and Immigration Canada; U.S. Immigration and Naturalization Service.

new immigrants and protecting the health of the resident population? What do students preparing today for careers in the health professions need to learn about multicultural health services? What is the role of the federal government, as distinct from the role of communities, in refugee health?

PROFESSIONAL HEALTH ORGANIZATIONS

Professional societies or associations are formed by people who have completed a prescribed curriculum and training and have met standards of certification. These people of common purpose organize to uphold professional standards and to serve society better through their united efforts. The basic preparation of future practitioners as well as the continuing professional education of current practitioners is of concern to these organizations. While the primary purpose of a professional society is to promote the interests of the profession and its members, its image and prestige depend on its service to humankind, and members of these professional societies are fully aware of this fact. What best serves the public should be in the best interests of the profes-

sional organization. Examples of the more promi-
nant community health professional societies follow, but many more allied and specialty health
professional groups are active in each country and
many states.

American Medical Association

The American Medical Association (AMA) was
founded in 1847. Its constitution states that "the object of the Association is to promote the art of medicine and the betterment of public health." Primarily, the AMA serves the interests of private medical
practitioners, but its activities are planned to protect
and serve the interests of the public and particularly
to provide the best possible medical service.

The AMA is a federation of state societies, and
these in turn are made up of county societies, which
means that the national organization is an association of state societies rather than of individual practitioners. The AMA strives to improve the quality
of medical service by informing members of ad-
vancements in medicine and related fields. It has had
programs and committees investigating possible
fraud in drugs, foods, cosmetics, and related products that might jeopardize the health of the public.
The AMA also participates in the accreditation of
hospitals.

The *Journal of the American Medical Association* is a weekly publication and is generally regarded as a leading journal in its field. The AMA
also publishes health-related pamphlet material for
distribution.

In recent years the AMA has lent its considerable
political weight to numerous community health issues. It helped pass the legislation that eliminated
smoking on all domestic commercial airline flights
of 2 hours or less. It supported legislation that would
outlaw plastic handguns that could not be detected
in airport metal detectors and another bill that would
require a 7-day waiting period and background
check on all handgun purchasers. These and other

lobbying efforts are directed toward protection of
the public as well as of the interests of physicians.

American Dental Association

The American Dental Association was formed in
1860 to advance the dental profession by raising the
quality of dental education and dental practice. The
association is the profession's agency for keeping
practitioners informed of new developments in
equipment, procedures, and techniques.

In its early years the American Dental Association was an organization of individual dental practitioners; later it became an association of state
societies, which in turn are composed of representatives from county societies. The American Dental
Association publishes the *Journal of the American
Dental Association* and a yearly index of periodical
dental literature. The association also publishes
pamphlets for distribution to patients.

American Public Health Association

The American Public Health Association was established in September 1872 and rapidly expanded its
scope from a limited interest in sanitation to a broad
public health program encompassing all factors affecting the health of the people.

The American Public Health Association carries
on a wide variety of activities through 22 sections:
laboratory, alcohol, tobacco, and other drugs, health
administration, community health planning and policy development, statistics, environment, radiological health, food and nutrition, international health,
maternal and child health, public health education
and health promotion, gerontological health, social
work, population and family planning, public health
nursing, epidemiology, school health education and
services, oral health, mental health, occupational
safety and health, pediatric health, vision care, and
medical care. The association has developed standards and procedures that have been widely ac-

cepted and adopted, including methods for the inspection of water and sewage, guidelines for the operation of swimming pools, diagnostic reagents and procedures, the appraisal of local health work, a model health code for cities, and standards for the accreditation of public health training. The association conducts surveys and other studies, which it initiates and carries out at the request of organizations or of individuals. Its publication, the *American Journal of Public Health,* is issued each month. In addition, the association publishes *The Nation's Health,* a monthly newsletter, pamphlets, special reports, and other material.

American Nurses Association

In the years since 1896, when nurses first banded together to form their national professional organization, the American Nurses Association has represented registered nurses in setting standards of practice, standards of education, and standards for nursing services. An ethical conduct guide was adopted by the association in 1950 as the Code for Nurses. Standards of practice in specialized areas of nursing and advocacy for the baccalaureate degree as the appropriate entry level preparation for nurses have been reflected in the credentialing and licensure procedures for nurses, and accreditation procedures for nursing schools and nursing services. ANA publications number over 200 with about 20 new titles each year. The *American Journal of Nursing* is published monthly. *The American Nurse,* a monthly newspaper, keeps the 50 constituent state nurses' associations in communication with each other.

Canadian Public Health Association

The CPHA, incorporated in 1912 as a national nonprofit association, serves some 25 community health disciplines in conducting and supporting national and international health programs. CPHA works in partnership with federal and provincial government departments, international agencies, and nongovernmental organizations in conducting research and programs. Representing public health in Canada, the membership believes in universal and equitable access to the basic conditions necessary to achieve health for all Canadians. The mission of the association is "to constitute a special national resource in Canada that advocates for the improvement and maintenance of personal and community health according to the public health principles of disease prevention, health promotion and protection, and healthy public policy."

CPHA publishes the *Canadian Journal of Public Health,* the *CPHA Health Digest, Canadian AIDS News, A Miracle in the Making,* and *Partners Around the World.* The CPHA Health Resources Centre is the sole Canadian distributor of WHO publications and various books of interest to community health professionals. Affiliated with CPHA are the Canadian Society for International Health and the Canadian Association for Teachers of Community Health.

National League for Nursing

The National League for Nursing was formed in 1952 when three national nursing organizations and four national committees combined their resources and programs—the National League of Nursing Education (founded in 1893), the National Organization for Public Health Nursing (1912), the Association of Collegiate Schools of Nursing (1933), the Joint Committee on Practical Nurses and Auxiliary Workers in Nursing Services (1945), the Joint Committee on Careers in Nursing (1948), the National Committee for the Improvement of Nursing Services (1949), and the National Nursing Accrediting Service (1949).

The principal purpose of the National League for Nursing is simply stated, "That the nursing needs of the people may be met." The National League for Nursing continues the practices and objectives of the previous National Organization for Public Health Nursing, including the following:

1. To stimulate responsibility for the health of the community by establishing and extending public health nursing
2. To bring about cooperation among nurses, physicians, and all others interested in public health
3. To develop standards of public health nursing
4. To maintain a central bureau of information and assistance in such services
5. To publish periodicals and bulletins

The league has both professional and nonprofessional members, including both public health nurses and friends of public health nurses. The official periodical of the National League for Nursing is *Nursing Outlook.* The league also publishes *Nursing Research.*

Society for Public Health Education

The Society for Public Health Education was formed in 1958 as the Society of Public Health Educators. Its change in name reflects its commitment to promotion of health education of the public, which transcends the interests of its professional members. With a membership of less than 1500, the society has been remarkably effective in influencing national policy related to health education, including the Health Information and Promotion Act of 1976 (PL 94-317). The society publishes *Health Education Quarterly* and meets annually in conjunction with the American Public Health Association.

American Alliance for Health, Physical Education, Recreation and Dance

The American Alliance for Health, Physical Education. Recreation and Dance began in 1885 as the American Association for the Advancement of Physical Education. It became a department of the National Education Association in 1937. "Alliance" refers to its several constituent organizations, including the Association for the Advancement of Health Education. Several areas of alliance activity are related to health; these include school nursing, school medical service, health teaching, nutrition education, dental health, mental health, and recreation. The alliance recommends program standards for communities. It publishes the monthly *Journal of Physical Education, Recreation and Dance, Journal of Health Education,* and the *Research Quarterly for Exercise and Sport.* (For more information, write AAHPERD, 1900 Association Drive, Reston, VA 22091.)

HEALTH FOUNDATIONS

Many philanthropic foundations are engaged in community health programs. Some foundations are international in scope; others are national or even limited to a region or city. Some have broad programs and operate in a variety of fields; others are specific in their activities and tend to concentrate on relatively few projects. Six foundations will be described as examples of the different types that engage in health projects.

Milbank Memorial Fund

The Milbank Memorial Fund was established in 1905 with the objective "to improve the physical, mental, and moral condition of humanity and generally to advance charitable and benevolent objectives." Its activities for the most part have been in preventive medicine. Objectives of the organization have been attained through grants and fellowships. Contributions of the fund have been to the fields of public health, medicine, social welfare, research, and education. The fund has sponsored population studies, demonstrations, projects, a recent study of schools of public health, and the measurement of various aspects of public health services. The organization has extended its activities to mental hygiene, school lunches, food research, vision care, dental studies, prenatal and postnatal instruction, and public health demonstrations.

Rockefeller Foundation

The Rockefeller Foundation was chartered in 1913 under the laws of the state of New York for the purpose of "promoting the well-being of mankind throughout the world." In its organization the foundation carries out work in five areas: (1) international health, (2) medical sciences, (3) natural sciences, (4) social sciences, and (5) humanities.

The international health effort is an operating agency with its own laboratories and staff of scientists. Three phases of work have been pursued: (1) control of specific diseases such as yellow fever, tuberculosis, and influenza, (2) aid to health departments, and (3) health demonstrations, aid to selected schools, public health education, and grants of postgraduate fellowships in public health. Out of the research laboratories of the foundation have come many significant contributions in the treatment of yellow fever, typhus, influenza, and malaria.

The other divisions of the Rockefeller Foundation support university, laboratory, and other research groups. Fellowships for postdoctoral work are also granted. These divisions support a wide range of activities through various grants and appropriations.

Commonwealth Fund

The Commonwealth Fund was founded in 1918 with a simple but meaningful objective: "To do something for the welfare of mankind." Activities have included health, medical education and research, education, and mental hygiene. The fund has been instrumental in advancing public health practices and procedures through research, improved teaching in medical schools, extension of public health services to rural communities, provision and improvement of hospital facilities, and strengthen-

ing of mental health services in the United States and Great Britain.

W.K. Kellogg Foundation

The W.K. Kellogg Foundation was established in 1930 to "help people to help themselves" and for "the promotion of health, education, and the welfare of mankind, but principally of children and youth, directly or indirectly, without regard to sex, race, creed, or nationality." A functional problem-solving approach has been used rather than one of research or relief. For example, grants have been made to various counties to establish county health departments. Recognizing society's difficulty in putting available knowledge to use for human benefit, Mr. Kellogg gave the foundation its distinctive commitment to "the application of knowledge to the problems of people." The foundation remains true to this philosophical concept and addresses significant human issues with direct, pragmatic answers.

From modest beginnings, with programs relating to the health and educational needs of children in south-central Michigan, the foundation has grown to a position of national and international prominence for its contributions in meeting social goals. Managed independently by its own board of trustees and administration, it is one of the largest philanthropic organizations in the United States. Since its inception the foundation's total expenditures have exceeded $643 million. As a private grant-making foundation, it provides financial assistance to organizations and institutions that have identified and analyzed problems and have designed constructive action programs aimed at practical solutions.

For many years the W.K. Kellogg Foundation has funded projects in the United States, Canada, Latin America, selected European countries, Australia, and New Zealand. Revised programming priorities for the 1990s limit grants outside the United States and Latin America to the Kellogg International Fellowship Program and to international networks of activities related to the current programming interests. These include coordinated cost-effective health services, a wholesome food supply, and adult continuing education.

Ford Foundation

Founded in 1936 by automobile manufacturer Henry Ford and his son Edsel, the Ford Foundation devoted most of its resources prior to 1950 to charitable and educational institutions in Michigan. Since becoming a national and international foundation with headquarters in New York, it has distributed more than $5 billion to organizations and individuals in 100 countries.

In education and research the foundation makes grants to universities, colleges, and other institutions and supports higher education assistance for minority students. It also provides help for blacks and other minorities through community action, housing, and job training.

In communications the Ford Foundation has provided grants since 1952 to aid noncommercial broadcasting. The foundation helped establish the Public Broadcasting Service.

In international affairs, the foundation makes grants to developing countries to help build institutions needed for long-range growth. Some of its most notable contributions have been in family planning programs through the Population Council, based in New York. Until 1972, the Ford Foundation was the largest philanthropic foundation contributing to the health field.

Robert Wood Johnson Foundation

The Robert Wood Johnson Foundation began its work on the national scene in 1972, with offices just outside Princeton, New Jersey. Foundation grants put primary emphasis on improving access to general medical and dental care. The statistics on access have improved considerably, so two additional priorities have been added: (1) support for research programs to make health care more effective and more affordable and (2) support for research, development, and demonstration projects that show promise of helping large numbers of people avoid disabilities and maintain or regain maximum possible functioning in their everyday lives.

One of the new programs of the Robert Wood Johnson Foundation, initiated in 1989, is a $26 million grant program to support community-based substance abuse prevention programs.

COOPERATION AND COORDINATION

Foundations and voluntary health agencies have made a significant contribution to health in Western nations and the world. Each agency is free to choose its own course of action and is sufficiently flexible to adjust to changing conditions and needs. These agencies tend to specialize and demonstrate what can be done in a specific field of health. In theory, when this has been accomplished, the task or field is taken over by an official health agency and the need for the voluntary agency no longer exists. In practice, few voluntary agencies are ever dissolved, and overlapping of programs exists to some degree.

National Health Council

To meet the long-existing need for cooperation and coordination, in 1921 the National Health Council was organized with about 50 voluntary national groups represented. The U.S. Public Health Service served as an advisory member. At the outset the council was well financed and well staffed. Within 5 years of its inception, however, it had become ineffective and had abandoned many of its projects. Some revitalization has occurred in recent years through the organization of National Health Forums, the inauguration of Community Health Week, the creation of working committees, and various publications. The council assisted in the establishment of a National Center for Health Education now based in New York, and cosponsored a series of

Regional Health Promotion Forums with the U.S. Office of Disease Prevention and Health Promotion.

Voluntary Health Organizations

Voluntary health organizations perform a unique and important role in the promotion of health in every U.S. state and in most nations. No health program is complete in the sense that it serves every individual who could benefit from the program. Thus there is a need for these organizations to expand and intensify their services. Furthermore, there are areas of health needs that receive little attention and less service. Perhaps the National Foundation for Infantile Paralysis (now the March of Dimes Birth Defects Foundation) charted the course that all existing voluntary as well as official agencies might consider. When the agency's original goal of preventing poliomyelitis was virtually achieved, the agency directed its attention and energies to other health problems in need of solution, such as the prevention of birth defects. Voluntary health organizations will be described in the remaining chapters.

OFFICIAL INTERNATIONAL HEALTH ORGANIZATIONS

For more than a century, health scientists of the world have worked cooperatively and harmoniously in promoting the health of all people. National interests have given way to world interests. Exchange of health knowledge, loan of the services of experts, and united efforts in preventing the spread of disease have characterized the international activities of public health personnel the world over. In the early years of international health activities, virtually all attention was directed to the control of communicable diseases (see box on p. 562), but programs have expanded to encompass the entire spectrum of health promotion.

International congresses on hygiene and epidemiology have been held at irregular intervals since 1852, when the first congress met in Brussels. After a series of such meetings, the International Office of Public Health was created in 1907, by agreement among 40 nations. Until the formation of the Health Section in the Secretariat of the League of Nations, the International Office of Public Health served as the medium for the international exchange of health knowledge and for cooperation on health matters. In 1950 the International Office of Public Health was absorbed by the World Health Organization (WHO) under the United Nations.

World Health Organization

Origins. The International Health Conference that convened in New York City on June 19, 1946, ushered in a new era in health cooperation. The conference was attended by representatives from all of the member states of the United Nations and by observers from 13 countries that were not members. At the closing session on June 22, the final instruments for the creation of the World Health Organization were approved and signed by the conference. They included a protocol providing for the absorption by WHO of the International Office of Public Health and the League of Nations Health Section. The constitution of WHO came into force on April 7, 1948. That date is commemorated each year as World Health Day. Today WHO is an intergovernmental organization within the United Nations system.

Purpose. The founding principles of WHO, which include a widely quoted definition of health, are set forth in the preamble of its constitution:

> Health is a state of complete physical, mental, and social well-being and not merely the absence of disease or infirmity.
>
> The enjoyment of the highest attainable standard of health is one of the fundamental rights of every human being without distinction of race, religion, political belief, or economic or social conditions.

Milestones in World Health Cooperation

1830 Cholera pandemic spreads across Europe.

1851 First International Sanitary Conference fails in Paris to establish an international sanitary convention.

1892 Limiting focus on cholera, International Sanitary Convention passes.

1897 International conventions for prevention of plague adopted.

1902 Pan American Health Organization (PAHO) created as International Sanitary Bureau, later to become regional office of the World Health Organization.

1907 L'Office International d'Hygiene Publique created in Paris.

1919 League of Nations created with the Health Organization of the League of Nations set up in Geneva.

1926 International Sanitary Convention revised to encompass measures for prevention and control of smallpox and typhus.

1935 International Sanitary Convention for aerial navigation.

1938 Conseil Sanitaire, Maritime et Quarantinaire at Alexandria handed over to Egypt, later becomes WHO Regional Office for the Eastern Mediterranean.

1945 United Nations Conference on International Organization in San Francisco approves resolution to establish new, autonomous, international health organization.

1946 Constitution for World Health Organization (WHO) approved at International Health Conference in New York.

1947 WHO Interim Commission organizes first international health cooperation to assist Egypt in cholera epidemic.

1948 WHO Constitution ratified on April 7, now celebrated each year as World Health Day. First World Health Assembly held with 55 member governments.

1951 New International Sanitary Regulations replace earlier International Sanitary Conventions.

1973 Twenty-sixth World Health Assembly, noting widespread dissatisfaction with health services and the need for radical changes, decides that WHO should collaborate with, not "assist," its member states in developing national health care systems.

1974 Expanded Program on Immunization launched by WHO to protect the world's children from poliomyelitis, measles, diphtheria, whooping cough, tetanus, and tuberculosis.

1977 Health for All by the Year 2000 set as a target "to permit all people to lead a socially and economically productive life."

1978 Alma-Ata Declaration on Primary Health Care adopted as the key to attaining Health for All (see box on p. 536).

1979 United Nations General Assembly affirms that health is a powerful lever for socioeconomic development and peace. Worldwide eradication of smallpox certified by Global Commission.

1981 United Nations General Assembly endorses Global Strategy for Health for All by the Year 2000 and urges other international organizations to collaborate with WHO.

1986 WHO designated dracunculiasis (guinea worm disease) as the next disease scheduled to be eradicated (by 1995) after smallpox.

1987 Global Program on AIDS launched with WHO.

1988 On fortieth anniversary of WHO, resolution adopted to eradicate poliomyelitis by the year 2000.

1991 Pandemic of cholera spreads across South and Central America, requiring renewal of cooperation that led to first International Sanitary Conference in 1851.

The health of all peoples is fundamental to the attainment of peace and security and is dependent upon the fullest cooperation of individuals and states.

The achievement of any state in the promotion and protection of health is of value to all.

Unequal development in different countries in the promotion of health and control of disease, especially communicable disease is a common danger.

Healthy development of the child is of basic importance: the ability to live harmoniously in a changing total environment is essential to such development.

The extension to all peoples of the benefits of medical, psychological, and all related knowledge is essential to the fullest attainment of health.

Informed opinion and active cooperation on the part of the public are of the utmost importance in the improvement of the health of the people.

Governments have a responsibility for the health of their peoples that can be fulfilled only by the provision of adequate health and social measures.

Financing. The WHO budget is raised by assessment of member states according to a formula, with a limitation that no nation shall pay more than 25% of the total assessment. In addition, the organization receives funds from various other sources, such as the Pan American Health Organization, and voluntary contributions from governments, institutions, and individuals.

Organization. The democratic nature of WHO is reflected in its organization, where legislation, administration, and services are under the direction of the 166 member states. A great deal of the services of participants are contributed without any cost to the organization.

The World Health Assembly is the legislative branch of WHO. Delegates of the member states and nongovernmental associate members meet annually in Geneva, Switzerland. The World Health Assem-

bly establishes policy and decides on the program and budget for the next year.

The executive board is the board of directors of the organization. The board is composed of 31 persons qualified in health matters. It meets at least twice a year to advise and act for the assembly. Each year the assembly elects eight governments to designate members to serve for 3 years.

The secretariat designates the professional management of WHO at headquarters in Geneva and in 166 countries of the world. The director-general is the chief executive, and in organization the secretariat is composed of three departments: advisory services, central technical services, and administration and finance. Each department is composed of divisions that in turn are made up of sections.

Regions are used for effectiveness in decentralized organization and operation. For WHO pur-

---

Declaration of Global Eradication of Smallpox

The Thirty-third World Health Assembly, on this the eighth day of May 1980:

Having considered the development and results of the global programme on smallpox eradication initiated by WHO in 1956 and intensified since 1967;

Declares solemnly that the world and all its peoples have won freedom from smallpox, which was a most devastating disease sweeping in epidemic form through many countries since earliest times, leaving death, blindness and disfigurement in its wake and which only a decade ago was rampant in Africa, Asia and South America:

Expresses its deep gratitude to all nations and individuals who contributed to the success of this noble and historic endeavour:

Calls this unprecedented achievement in the history of public health to the attention of all nations, which by their collective action have freed mankind of this ancient scourge and, in so doing, have demonstrated how nations working together in a common cause may further human progress.

poses, the world is divided into six regions, each with its own organization consisting of a regional committee composed of delegates from governments in the region, and a regional office that administers WHO-aided projects and supervises the staff in the various projects. Regional offices of WHO are logically distributed as shown in Figure 18-10.

Each regional office has its own staff and method of operation. In addition, there are now more than 1000 health-related institutions around the world designated officially as WHO collaborating centers.

Advisory panels consist of more than 12,000 scientists, health administrators, and educators from many nations. These panels provide expert advice in their respective fields. Committees of experts are chosen from these panels to provide the necessary expertise to deal with particular health problems.

Functions of WHO. To meet the objectives of its charter, WHO recognizes specific functions as its responsibilities.

1. International health—to act as the directing and coordinating authority on world health
2. International conventions—to propose conventions, agreements, and regulations and make recommendations concerning international health matters
3. International standards—to develop, establish, and promote international standards for food, biological, pharmaceutical, and similar products
4. Nongovernmental organizations—to promote cooperation among scientific and professional groups that contribute to the advancement of science
5. Research—to promote and conduct research in health

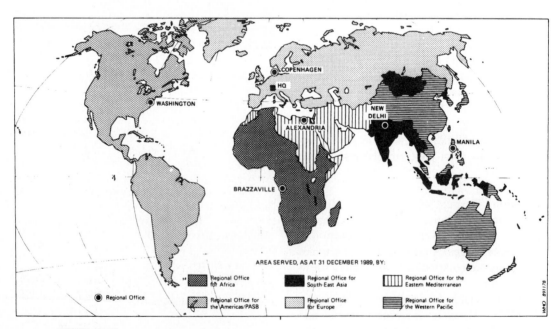

FIGURE 18-10
The distribution of regional offices of WHO, the regions they serve, and the headquarters in Geneva.
Source: World Health Organization.

6. Public health—to study and report on public health and medical care from preventive and curative points of view, including hospital services and social security

7. Primary health services—to assist governments, upon request, in strengthening primary health care services

8. Maternal and child health—to promote maternal and child health and welfare and to foster the ability to live harmoniously in a changing environment (Figure 18-11)

9. Diseases—to stimulate and advance work to eradicate epidemic, endemic, and other disease

10. Diagnosis—to standardize diagnostic procedures as necessary

11. Living conditions—to promote the improvement of nutrition, housing, sanitation, recreation, economic, or working conditions, and other aspects of environmental hygiene

12. Accidents—to promote the prevention of accidental injuries

13. Mental health—to foster activities in mental health, especially those affecting human relations

14. Education—to promote improved standards of teaching and training in health, medical, and related professions

WHO is helping many nations to solve many health problems. In helping a nation, it is always the objective of WHO to build up the nation's potential and train its personnel so that eventually outside help will not be needed. In some cases the services of WHO are merely advisory, but in many instances the organization's personnel are on the scene to do the job that is necessary. WHO also operates closely

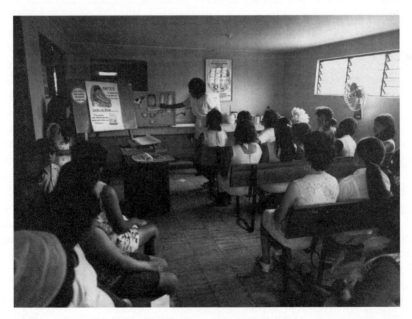

FIGURE 18-11
At the Puerto Malarino Health Centre of Cali, Colombia, a nurse educator explains to a group of pregnant women the best uses of powdered milk and eggs and the rules of good nutrition.
Source: World Health Organization, photo by Almasy.

with the United Nations Children's Fund (UNICEF), the United Nations Specialized Agencies, especially the Food and Agriculture Organization (FAO), and the United Nations Educational, Scientific and Cultural Organization (UNESCO), the United Nations Development Program (UNDP), and the International Labor Organization (ILO).

Health for All by the Year 2000. In 1978 WHO joined with UNICEF in a declaration of principles of primary health care for all people by the year 2000. This declaration, which grew out of a jointly sponsored conference in Alma-Ata, then U.S.S.R., has come to be known as the Alma-Ata declaration and has since shaped WHO policy for the 1980s and 1990s. The main features of the Alma-Ata declaration were highlighted at the beginning of this chapter. The principle of participation in the declaration is what makes national and international health resources today more relevant to and supportive of community health.

Pan American Health Organization

Origins. Creation of the Pan American Sanitary Bureau was authorized by the Second International Conference of the American Republics, which met in Mexico City in 1902. It was formally organized as the International Sanitary Office at the First Inter-American Sanitary Conference, held in Washington, D.C. The fifth such conference, which met in Santiago, Chile, in 1911, changed the name to Pan American Sanitary Bureau.

Accomplishments. From its inception the Pan American Sanitary Bureau devoted its attention primarily to the control of communicable diseases. The participating nations cooperated with each other by exchanging vital statistics reports, exchanging health information on travelers, reporting new advances in disease control, exchanging knowledge on advances in sanitation procedures, training health personnel, and making technical experts available to

other nations on a consulting basis. The Pan American Sanitary Bureau is now known as the Pan American Health Organization (**PAHO**). Although an independent health organization, it is integrated with the World Health Organization (**WHO**) as one of its regional offices.

Of the many accomplishments in health since PAHO was founded at the turn of the century, one of the most spectacular was the eradication of smallpox from the Western Hemisphere in 1973. The Americas were the first region to succeed in the global campaign against the disease, which was eradicated worldwide in 1979. Other significant accomplishments include reducing the incidence of other communicable diseases, cutting the infant mortality rate in half between 1960 and 1980, reducing the incidence of major childhood diseases as a prime cause of death through a hemisphere-wide immunization campaign, increasing life expectancy, providing safe water and basic sanitation, and improving nutrition.

Yet for a majority of the people living in the Americas, disease and health risks still cast dark shadows over the future. More than one third of the people in Latin America and the Caribbean have no access to clean water. More than two thirds have no access to basic sanitation. And 40% of this population has no access to health care.

Much work remains to be done to extend health services to those millions now lacking them; to provide clean water, basic sanitation, adequate immunization, and good nutrition; and to achieve prevention, early detection, and cure of disease. PAHO and its member governments are committed to meeting that challenge and making the universal right to health a reality in the Americas.

Priorities and objectives. To provide all citizens access to primary health care, PAHO's member countries have identified priority health areas and specific strategies for developing their infrastructures. Elements of national strategies that various countries have in common have been incorporated into hemisphere-wide strategies and a basic plan of action. The plan is a framework for the design of specific programs at regional and national levels. The hemisphere-wide strategies contain several specific goals, including

- Life expectancy at birth of 70 years or more
- An infant mortality rate of less than 30 per 1000 live births
- Mortality in children aged 1 to 4 years of less than 2.4 deaths per 1000
- Immunization of all infants less than 1 year old against diphtheria, whooping cough, tetanus, tuberculosis, measles, and poliomyelitis
- Tetanus vaccination for all pregnant women in areas of risk
- Provision of safe drinking water for 100 million rural residents and 155 million urban inhabitants
- Provision of sewage disposal services for 140 million rural residents and 250 million urban inhabitants by 1990, and for 130 million more people by the year 2000
- Extension of health services to ensure that everyone has access to them

The plan for meeting these goals emphasizes health promotion and disease prevention, combined with health restoration, rehabilitation, and improvements in the environment.

SUMMARY

This chapter has cast the subject of community health services in the broader context of the global and national structures that provide resources for them. These structures include the national or federal authority that allocates responsibilities to various agencies and levels of government. In most republics, this authority comes from a constitution reserving certain generic powers for the central or federal government. Many federal governments, such as those of Australia, Canada, and the United States, leave the majority of specific health respon-

sibilities to the states or provinces. Numerous federal agencies in the United States carry health authority and health-related responsibilities. Chief among these is the Department of Health and Human Services (DHHS), comparable to Health Canada in that country and to the ministries of health in most countries. Within DHHS, the chief responsibility for health lies with the Public Health Service. Programs throughout multiple organizations of the PHS are directed toward achievement of the *Year 2000 Health Objectives* discussed in the early chapters of this book. Within the Public Health Service, the major agency having direct relationships with states and communities is the Centers for Disease Control and Prevention.

At the global level, the structures supporting community health services include various philanthropic foundations and international agencies representing multigovernmental concerns. Major health-related foundations include the Rockefeller, W.K. Kellogg, Ford, and Robert Wood Johnson foundations. Several of the United Nations' agencies carry health responsibilities, but chief among these is the World Health Organization. Of its six regional offices, the Pan American Health Organization represents the governments of North, Central, and South America and the Caribbean. The most significant recent development in international health-related agencies has been renewed commitment to community health services, epitomized by the Alma-Ata Declaration on Primary Health Care and the WHO global policy goal of "Health for All by the Year 2000."

QUESTIONS FOR REVIEW

1. In your judgment, which of the eight broad general clauses of the Constitution of the United States provides the federal government with the best means for the promotion of health, and what is your reasoning?
2. How has the government used the taxing power in matters of health?

3. Why is it difficult to recall any time that you or any member of your family received a direct health service from a federal agency?

4. What reasons can you give for and against lodging the function of stream pollution prevention and control in the U.S. Department of the Interior?

5. What are your reasons for or against establishing the U.S. Public Health Service as an independent agency?

6. What is the significance of the fact that 95% of the professional public health people in the United States are nonmedical people?

7. Why should appropriations for health represent investments rather than expenditures?

8. What justification is there for the NIH subsidizing the research of scientists in other countries?

9. Why should the federal government concern itself with research in the health sciences?

10. In your judgment, what specific health problem is most in need of more extensive and intensive research?

11. What voice does a local medical practitioner have in the policies of the AMA?

12. Which of the professional health organizations do you regard as most public-spirited and least self-interested? Why?

13. Why do most Western nations give far more to WHO than they receive? What is your comment?

14. Why does WHO place so much emphasis on communicable disease control in view of all the recent technological advances in this field?

15. Why is it so important that WHO place primary emphasis on helping nations to help themselves?

READINGS

El Bindari-Hamad A, Smith DL: *Primary health care reviews: guidelines and methods,* Ottawa, 1992, Canadian Public Health Association Health Resources Centre.

Using a variety of approaches developed by the World Health Organization, this book provides detailed guidelines on monitoring the implementation of the global strategy of Health for All by the Year 2000 through country-level strengthening of primary health care organization.

Office of Disease Prevention and Health Promotion: *Prevention '91/'92: federal programs and progress,* Washington, DC, 1992, U.S. Department of Health and Human Services, Public Health Service, U.S. Government Printing Office 332-838.

This annual compilation shows the budgetary and programmatic contribution of each department and agency of the federal government toward achieving the year 2000 objectives for the nation in disease prevention and health promotion.

Pan American Health Organization: *The crisis of public health: reflections for the debate,* Ottawa, 1992, Canadian Public Health Association Resources Centre.

The programmatic priorities established by PAHO's governing bodies for the Western Hemisphere set the agenda for future debate at the country level concerning critical issues in public health.

World Health Organization: *Facts about WHO,* Geneva, 1990, World Health Organization.

This monograph covers the history of WHO and international cooperation in public health, and the objectives, functions, targets, strategies, organization, achievements, and challenges of WHO. Details of the Health for All by the Year 2000 global initiative for primary health care and decentralization.

BIBLIOGRAPHY

Aday LA: *At risk in America: the health and health care needs of vulnerable populations in the United States,* San Francisco, 1993, Jossey-Bass.

Andrus JK, de Quadros CA, Olive J-M: The surveillance challenge: final stages of eradication of poliomyelitis in the Americas. In CDC surveillance summaries, *MMWR* 41:21, 1992.

Bennett A, Adams O, editors: *Looking north for health: what we can learn from Canada's health care system,* San Francisco, 1993, Jossey-Bass.

Basch PF: *Understanding health care in the context of world medicine,* New York, 1989, Oxford University Press.

Brown LD, editor: *Health policy and the disadvantaged,* Durham, NC, 1991, Duke University Press.

Canadian Public Health Association: *Position paper sustainability and equity: primary health care in developing countries,* Ottawa, 1990, Canadian Public Health Association.

Coyte PC: Comparative health systems, Canada, *Adv Health Econ Health Serv Res* 1(suppl):103, 1990.

Crichton A, Hsu D, Tsang S: *Canada's health care system: its funding and organization,* Ottawa, 1990, Canadian Hospital Association Press.

Grant JP, editor: *The state of the world's children 1990,* New York, 1990, Oxford University Press.

Hancock T: The evolution, impact and significance of the Healthy Cities/Healthy Communities movement, *J Public Health Policy* 14:5, 1993.

Harmon RG: *Health Resources and Services Administration 1992 annual report: progress on year 2000 goals and objectives,* Rockville, Md, 1993, Public Health Service, U.S. Department of Health and Human Services.

Healthy people 2000: national health promotion and disease prevention objectives, Washington, DC, 1991, U.S. Department of Health and Human Services, Government Printing Office.

Hopkins DR, Ruiz-Tiben E: Surveillance for dracunculiasis, 1981-1991. In CDC surveillance summaries, *MMWR* 41:1, 1992.

Jelliffe DB: *Community nutritional assessment,* New York, 1990, Oxford University Press.

Jonas S: *An introduction to the U.S. health care system,* ed 3, New York, 1992, Springer.

Lawson J: *Public health in Australia: an introduction,* Roseville, NSW, 1991, McGraw-Hill Book Co. of Australia.

Litman TJ, Robins LS: *Health politics and policy,* ed 2, Albany, NY, 1991, Delmar.

McGinnis JM: *ODPHP Director's report,* Washington, DC, 1993, Office of Disease Prevention and Health Promotion, Public Health Service, U.S. Department of Health and Human Services.

Monekosso GL: African universities as partners in community health development, *J Community Health* 18:127, 1993.

National Highway Traffic Safety Administration: *Protecting our own: community child passenger safety programs,* ed 2, Washington, DC, 1990, U.S. Department of Transportation.

National Highway Traffic Safety Administration: *Idea sampler: Buckle up America,* Washington, DC, 1991, U.S. Department of Transportation.

National Highway Traffic Safety Administration: *Fatal accident reporting system 1989: a decade of progress,* Washington, DC, 1991, U.S. Department of Transportation.

National Institute on Drug Abuse: *Drug abuse technology transfer,* DHHS Publ No (ADM) 91-1764, Rockville, Md, 1991, Alcohol, Drug Abuse, Mental Health Administration.

PHS action plan for women's health, Washington, DC, 1991, Office of Disease Prevention and Health Promotion, U.S. Department of Health and Human Services.

Public Health Service Task Force: A plan to strengthen public health in the United States, *Public Health Rep* 106(Suppl 1):1, 1991.

Roemer MI: *National health systems of the world,* New York and Oxford, 1991, Oxford University Press.

Roper WL, Baker EL, Dyal WW et al: Strengthening the public health system, *Public Health Rep* 107:609, 1992.

Schneider D, Greenberg MR, Choi D: Black leaders' perceptions of the year 2000 public health goals for Black Americans, *Am J Public Health* 83:1171, 1993.

Stephen WJ: *Primary health care in the Arab world,* Wells, England, 1992, Somerset House.

U.S. Bureau of the Census: *Statistical abstract of the United States,* ed 112, Washington, DC, 1992, U.S. Department of Commerce.

Vugia DJ, Koehler JE, Ries AA: Surveillance for epidemic cholera in the Americas: an assessment. In CDC surveillance summaries, *MMWR* 41:27, 1992.

Williams SJ: *Contemporary issues in health services,* Albany, NY, 1993, Delmar.

World Health Organization: *The work of WHO 1988-1989. Biennial report of the Director-General to the World Health Assembly and to the United Nations,* Geneva, 1990, World Health Organization.

World Health Organization: *WHO global programme on AIDS: 1991 progress report,* Geneva, 1992, World Health Organization.

World Health Organization: *Implementation of the global strategy for Health for All by the Year 2000: second evaluation,* Geneva, 1993, World Health Organization.

Wunderlich GS, editor: *Toward a national health care survey: a data system for the 21st century,* Washington, DC, 1992, National Academy Press.

Chapter 19

State or Provincial Health Resources and Services

❖

The powers reserved to the several states will extend to all the objects which . . . concern the lives, liberties and properties of the people, and the internal order, improvement and prosperity of the state.

JAMES MADISON, *The Federalist Papers*

If public health is to maintain the reputation it now enjoys, it will be because in everything we do, behind everything we say as the basis for every program decision—we are willing to see faces.

WILLIAM H. FOEGE, M.D., former director, Centers for Disease Control

OBJECTIVES

When you finish this chapter, you should be able to:

- Identify the source and extent of state or provincial authority for health-related functions
- Describe the organization, resources, and services typical of state or provincial health agencies
- Describe ways in which states or provinces plan and promote health legislation

This chapter takes you a step closer to home, from the global and national context of community health to the state or provincial context. You should become increasingly aware of the broader constitutional and legal frameworks within which community health operates and the resources available to your community from higher levels of organization. The most effective community health programs are those that take full advantage of such resources and support while developing their own local resources and self-sufficiency.

Federalism pertains to the recognition of the vast differences between the states in their needs and their traditions. Likewise, communities must understand their own local needs and demand their share of state and national resources.

The "New Federalism" of the 1980s sought to return many of the rights to states or provinces that seemed to have been taken over by federal agencies. Unfortunately, the transfer of resources to states did not accompany the transfer of responsibility. The U.S. federal contribution to the states declined during this period from approximately 25% of state and local budgets in the late 1970s to 17% by 1990. With this decrease in contribution, tax revolts at home, rising health costs, and increasing demands from entitlement programs, state, provincial, and local governments across North America face challenges to provide health care and prevention programs in the 1990s. In a variety of approaches states have been at the forefront pushing the United States toward health care reform. In the 1992 presidential election health care reform was a key issue, and it is a commitment of the Clinton administration. Prevention services are a key component of reform efforts.

CLOSER TO HOME

The most compelling argument for decentralization from federal to state or provincial and local levels is to make services and the allocation of resources more sensitive to the needs of the people intended to be served—the "faces" referred to by Dr. Foege in the quotation at the beginning of this chapter. Program requirements for public health agencies differ depending on the characteristics of the population served. For example, state populations range from a low of a half million in Alaska to 28 million in California. Rural populations vary from 9% in California to 66% in Vermont. Public health agencies often care for the most needy of the population, who range from a low of 6% below the poverty line in New Hampshire to a high of 25% in Mississippi. These different population characteristics place different demands on the nature, location, and administration of public health programs.

In most countries health planning and resources are coordinated at some level between the local community and the national agencies responsible for public health. In the United States this intermediate level is the state health agency (SHA), usually named the state Department of Health.* The state constitution provides the SHA with broad functions. The state constitution also permits or directs the state legislature to pass supplemental statutory provisions. In Australia and Canada state ministers of health also sit as elected legislators of parliament. Canada and most European countries have provincial or district health agencies, called ministries of health, which have varying degrees of autonomy and independence from their national ministries of health. In small countries, such as Ireland, the county functions as the equivalent of a state or province.

The function of state and provincial health agencies is to develop a long-range, equitable, comprehensive, and balanced approach to the diverse needs of many communities. If states allow each com-

*We will use the abbreviation SHA to refer broadly to health agencies at the state (United States or Australia) and provincial (most other countries) level.

munity to have complete autonomy in addressing short-range health concerns of local interest groups, the programs will tend to serve only the most affluent or the most politically powerful.

State and provincial agencies support the community health department. They provide the services of experts when requested or needed for an important local health problem. The SHAs also provide local health departments with laboratory services and with equipment and facilities for special surveys and other purposes. Devices for measuring air pollution, and other types of equipment are made available by the state to local authorities for the protection or promotion of community health.

The SHA acts as the link between national health agencies and local health departments. Federal health funds are allocated by the SHA to the local health agencies. Through the SHA, community health departments are able to obtain the services of national or federal health experts to solve unique or difficult health problems or to deal with an emergency when summary action is required.

HEALTH AUTHORITY AND RESPONSIBILITY

Sovereignty, or ultimate authority, in matters of health rests with the people. This authority is vested in local and state or provincial governments to pass such legislation and take such action as may be necessary to promote the health and general welfare of the people. As stated by James Madison, who more than anyone set the tone of the U.S. Constitution, the state in the United States has virtually unlimited authority to do what is necessary to promote the greatest good for the greatest number of people. There is but one limitation on the state's power to pass legislation regarding health matters—a statute may not violate or be inconsistent with the provisions of the U.S. Constitution. In the exercise of the state's police power in matters of health, the action taken must be *reasonable* and *constitutional*.

Delegation of Authority

The people of a state or province approve a constitution, which in some cases mentions health only in providing that the legislature set up health agencies and pass laws to protect and promote the public's health. In some states in the United States the constitution delineates in some detail what the state health organization and services shall be. Most public health authorities agree that the state constitution should contain broad, general provisions granting to the state legislature authority to establish the necessary health agencies, their responsibilities, and their authority. This type of general constitutional provision would provide for changes through legislation as new needs arise.

In some states, notably California in recent years, the people's impatience with the legislative process has led to numerous health initiatives by referendum on the state ballot. These have included an increase in cigarette taxes to pay for more health education and smoking prevention programs, as well as health care to help pay for the medical costs incurred by tobacco use (see Figure 19-1).

Most legislatures choose to delegate their health authority to a state or provincial board of health to pass health regulations, standards, and requirements, with the provision that the health boards must restrict themselves to health matters. In effect the state or provincial board of health acts as a quasilegislative body. The legislature also charges the health board with the responsibility for the enforcement of these regulations, which have the force of law.

Health Agencies in the State or Province

Each state or province has both official health agencies and voluntary health agencies. An **official health agency** or service is one supported by tax funds and recognized as a governmental agency or service. Examples of such agencies are the Minnesota Department of Public Health, the Maryland Department of Health and Mental Hygiene, and the Brit-

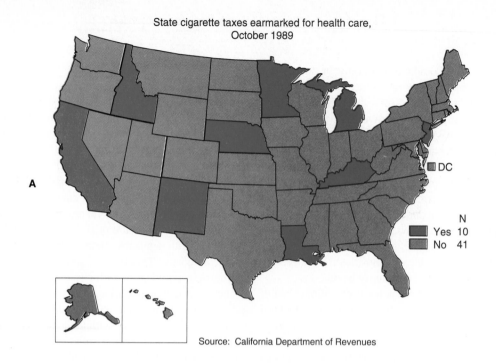

State cigarette taxes earmarked for health care,
October 1989

A

N
Yes 10
No 41

Source: California Department of Revenues

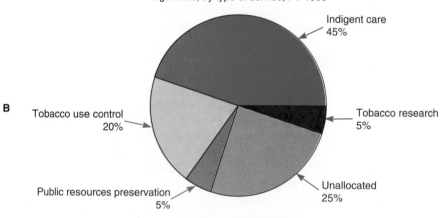

Distribution of revenues from California's tax on
cigarettes, by type of service, FY 1990

B

Indigent care
45%

Tobacco research
5%

Tobacco use control
20%

Unallocated
25%

Public resources preservation
5%

TOTAL: $603 MILLION

FIGURE 19-1

A, Tobacco sales taxes have been dedicated to health care expenditures in 10 states to recover some of the costs imposed on the state by the health effects of tobacco. **B,** California has dedicated its more substantial cigarette tax revenues to several additional purposes related to health.

Source: California Department of Health Services.

ish Columbia Ministry of Health. Official health agencies have staffs appointed by some official governmental body; the staff members are government employees and may be classified as officials.

A **voluntary health agency** is one supported entirely or primarily by financial contributions from citizens and private organizations. These agencies may bid on and accept government contracts to perform health services. Examples of such agencies are the American Lung Association, the American Cancer Society, and the Canadian Heart and Stroke Foundation. Services of voluntary health agencies are carried on at the state level by full-time, salaried, professional personnel. Most of the recognized voluntary health agencies in the United States have a national organization with state divisions and local chapters or affiliates. The effective, principal sphere of operation of most voluntary agencies is at the state level where funds are raised, programs are planned, and services are developed. Some of the funds raised in the state are contributed to the national office, and some may be channeled to the local chapters or affiliates.

Official Agencies Serving Health

All states, the District of Columbia, eight U.S. territories, and the provinces of Canada have a government agency responsible for the administration of public health services. Depending on how activities in a state are organized, public health responsibilities and authority may not be located in the SHA. For example, four SHAs are the state mental health authority and only 15 SHAs are the lead environmental agency (Table 19-1).

Many other official agencies also engage in health promotion and environmental health protection. Most of these agencies provide health as a secondary service or even an incidental activity. Often health benefits are a by-product of the primary activities of the agency. Nevertheless the composite activities of these agencies amount to a significant contribution to health.

TABLE 19-1

Responsibilities of state health agencies (SHAs) in 50 states and the District of Columbia, 1990

Responsibilities	SHAs (N = 51)	
	n	*%*
State public health authority	51	100
Institutional licensing agency	41	80
Institutional certifying authority for federal reimbursement	40	78
State agency for children with special health care needs	39	77
State health planning and development agency	22	43
State institutions/hospitals	16	31
Lead environmental agency in the state	15	29
State professions licensing agency	10	20
Medicaid single state agency	5	10
State mental health authority	4	8

More than one agency may carry on the same health function. This duplication usually results from empire building, long-established custom or priority, and political patronage or protectionism. On the state or provincial level as well as the local and national levels, agencies multiply and often outgrow their original purpose, so they create new activities to justify their continuing existence.

SHAs are usually organized in one of two ways: as a freestanding independent agency responsible directly to the governor or the board of health, or as a component of a superagency. Thirty-two states are organized according to the first model; 18 states and the District of Columbia are organized by either the superagency or state board model. Figure 19-2 shows an example of a state, Massachusetts, with a freestanding independent state health agency. The Massachusetts Commissioner of Health reports directly to the Governor of Massachusetts. Figure 19-3 shows a superagency structure in Delaware where the Commissioner of Public Health heads one of many subagencies reporting through two bureaucratic layers to the governor. In a state larger than Delaware

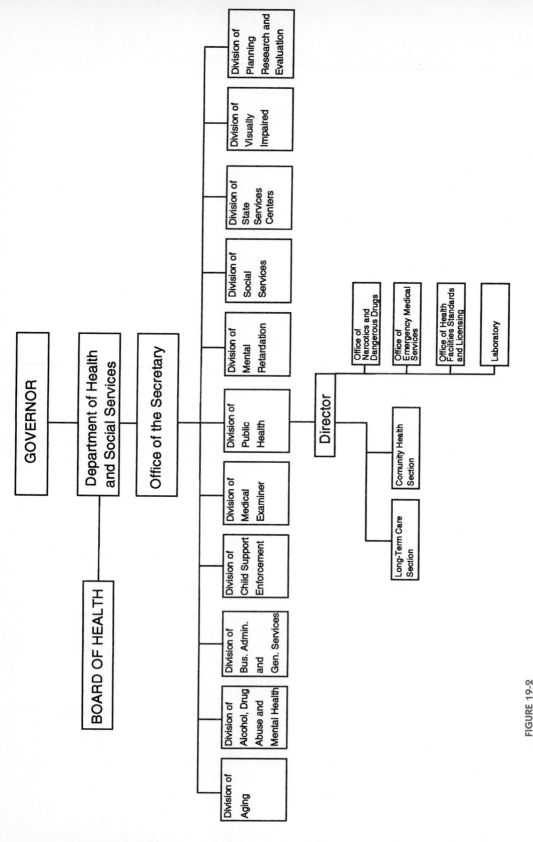

FIGURE 19-2

Massachusetts Department of Health's organization chart for 1990 illustrates the typical structure of a state health agency with a free-standing, independent relationship to the governor of the state. Issues with high priority such as Narcotics and Dangerous Drugs often have a staff office to give them freer access to several of the line agencies below the director or commissioner.

Source: Centers for Disease Control: *Profile of state and territorial public health systems: United States, 1990,* Atlanta, 1991, U.S. Department of Health and Human Services.

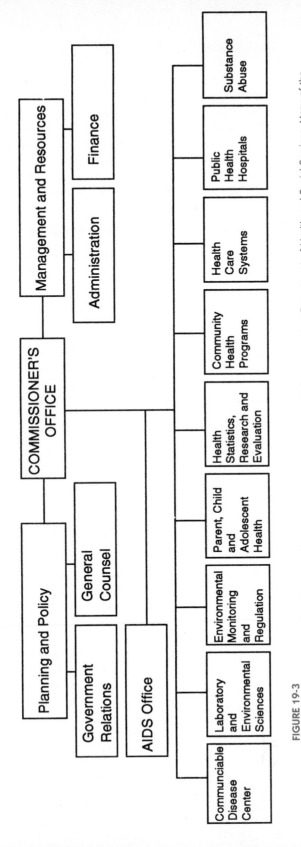

FIGURE 19-3

The Delaware Division of Public Health in 1990 was located two layers deep in the superagency Department of Health and Social Services. Many of the usual functions of a state health agency, such as aging, alcohol and drug abuse, reside in other agencies at the same level.

Source: Centers for Disease Control: *Profile of state and territorial public health systems: United States, 1990,* Atlanta, 1991, U.S. Department of Health and Human Services.

this would put the public health program at some disadvantage in competing for state resources.

To note all the other state or provincial agencies that perform health services to some degree would produce an almost interminable list. The agencies and organizations found in most states will indicate the spectrum. In many cases the title of the agency gives some indication of the nature of its health function.

Department of Agriculture
Department of Education
Department of Labor and Industry
Department of Welfare
Department of Conservation
Department of Mental Health
Department of Motor Vehicles
Department of Public Safety
Department of Civil Service and Registration
Department of State Institutions
Department of Parks and Recreation
Drug and Alcohol Agency
Universities
Colleges
Experiment Stations
Commissions
   Blood pressure
   Cancer
   Children's abuse
   Blind
   Governor's Council on Physical Fitness
   Mental health
   Dairy and food
   Hotel
   Workers' compensation
   Hospital
Boards
   Industrial inquiry
   Water resources
   Examining and licensing
      Medicine
      Dentistry
      Nursing
      Medical laboratory
      Podiatry

Important as the health services given by these agencies are, the administrative need for combining agencies and for coordinating services is apparent. Such reorganization can result in a reduction in costs and in an improvement in services. In large states, however, consolidation sometimes creates overly complex and confusing bureaucracies.

Cooperation with Other Sectors

The U.S. objectives for the nation for 1990 and 2000 in disease prevention and health promotion captured the imagination of many health professionals and the commitment of some health organizations. As of January 1993, 27 states had completed their own year 2000 objectives in health promotion and disease prevention based on national objectives; another 20 states are pursuing development of objectives (Figure 19-4). Most of these objectives could not be accomplished by health professionals and official health agencies alone. Attaining them will require the active participation of other sectors, other professionals, and other institutions than those primarily identified with health.

It is remarkable that health objectives draw any attention at all, considering their remote and sober character. They hardly have the siren call raised by the devastating epidemics of the past. They scarcely compete even with economic concerns, much less with threats of war and nuclear holocaust. It is little wonder, then, that other sectors and the public at large often respond with indifference when called on to help achieve the national or state objectives in disease prevention and health promotion.

Building on mutual interests. Two reasons seem to explain the little interest in health promotion that has been shown by other sectors. One is the perceived demand of the public; the second is the possibility that support could contribute to other goals that they seek.

Perceiving a public demand for health promotion, many organizations outside the health field have taken up health-related programs. Business and

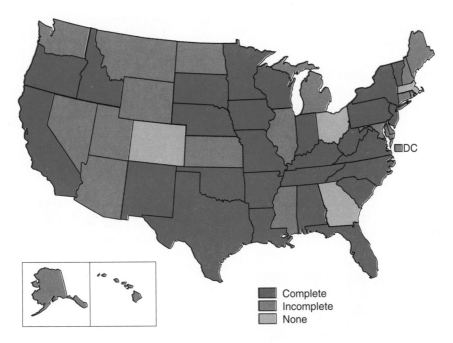

Complete
Incomplete
None

FIGURE 19-4
The 27 states that had completed by early 1993 their year 2000 objectives and plans for disease prevention and health promotion programs in line with the *Healthy People 2000* document of the U.S. Department of Health and Human Services are shown in dark color.
Source: U.S. Department of Health and Human Services: PHS Update, February & March 1993.

industry, in particular, have risen to the challenge of consumer demand, providing health and fitness products and services. Many companies have begun to offer health promotion programs or facilities for their employees. Some have justified these expenditures on the grounds that such programs provide the organization a competitive edge in attracting and holding the best employees.

How did this consumer demand come about? Can it be sustained or even nurtured to gain further support from other sectors? At least part of the answer to these questions lies in an enlightened public. Continuing health information and education programs produce increased consumer discretion in matters of health. Increased interest and discretion in turn stimulate commercial and news media to provide yet more information, some of which inevitably is inaccurate and misleading. Conflicting information

stirs debate and controversy, further whetting the public's appetite for more health information and education.

The downside to this growing market for health ideas is the consequent glutting of information. Some of the innocent bystanders in the withering crossfire of health information despair at ever avoiding all the risks to health that are reported by the media. The public pleads for relief from this tumult. Nowhere does the cooperation of health organizations in various sectors promise greater relief for the public than in the development of consensus on selected health messages and the dissemination of joint communications such as the dietary guidelines for Americans, which were formulated jointly by the U.S. Department of Agriculture and the U.S. Department of Health and Human Services. The objectives for individual states in disease prevention and health promotion offer greater potential for consensus than do national objectives.

Linking health to other objectives. The second motive accounting for interest shown by other sectors in health promotion is the possibility that such promotion might contribute to their own mission, which is something other than health. In the business sector the hope of many executives—and the conviction of some—is that their employee health promotion programs will contribute to improved morale, greater productivity, and reduced health insurance claims (see Figure 19-5). Some even support these programs with no conviction that they

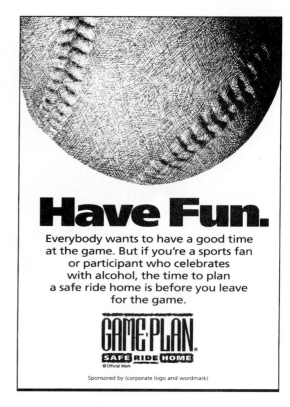

Have Fun.

Everybody wants to have a good time at the game. But if you're a sports fan or participant who celebrates with alcohol, the time to plan a safe ride home is before you leave for the game.

GAME·PLAN
SAFE RIDE HOME
ⓡ Official Mark

Sponsored by (corporate logo and wordmark)

FIGURE 19-5
Other sectors besides health agencies at the state or provincial level sometimes see ways in which they can support or promote health objectives relevant to their own objectives. This ad was sponsored by the Insurance Corporation of British Columbia, which insures automobiles and crash liability. Any company or vendor such as a sports stadium owner can put their own logo at the bottom of the ad.

Source: Courtesy Insurance Corporation of British Columbia.

The Coordination Paradox of Health Promotion Today

Not since the seventeenth century has the medical establishment—or, for that matter, the public health establishment—been more irrelevant to the task of improving the public's health. The health professions know what must be done to improve health—hence they have the ability to state achievable objectives for the year 2000. But they are helpless by themselves to achieve most of these objectives. Success depends on reaching people where their daily decisions about environment and life-style are influenced and made. This means reaching them in schools, at worksites, and in other nonmedical settings in the community.

Some health professionals assume that a wave of the coordinating wand will bring disparate interests into line if only the wand is waved at a high bureaucratic level. Such wishful thinking has given the health care sector the mistaken impression that other sectors of human services are all too willing to set their own priorities aside if presented with a health problem requiring attention. Perhaps there was once a time when coordination was easier, when epidemics were threatening enough to galvanize concerted community action, but this is very seldom the case today.

What must be done to gain the cooperation of other sectors and to build statewide coalitions for health promotion?

---

will influence health, so strong is their belief that the programs will improve morale and productivity. These alternative "bottom lines" should remind health professionals that the cooperation and the support of other sectors depend in part on an ability to translate the objectives into terms that relate to these sectors' goals.

Health professionals sometimes lose sight of the fact that for most people health is not a terminal value. Rather, people seek health as an instrumental means in order to gain other ends. Similarly for organizations whose mission is not health, health promotion can nevertheless serve as a means to achieve their ends. The education sector provides a poignant example of the need to shift the ''health-for-its-own-sake'' orientation of the objectives for disease prevention and health promotion. Schools today are leaping to the task of raising the cognitive learning scores of children in basic subjects. This has resulted in abandoning certain courses, often including health education. But health promotion in the schools and in other community settings that reach children can contribute to children's greater alertness and improved cognitive performance in basic subjects. Presenting this thesis to the education sector should make it possible to regain the schools' cooperation in health promotion for productivity motives not unlike those of industry in supporting employee health promotion programs.

ORGANIZATION AND FUNCTIONS

In four states in the United States the state constitution names the department responsible for the activities necessary to protect and promote health and specifies its functions. In the remaining states the state constitution delegates this authority to the state legislature. Massachusetts established the first state health board in the United States in 1869. (Local official health agencies had been in operation for more than a century prior to the creation of the Massachusetts State Board of Health.) No two states have precisely the same structure for their health programs. The head of the SHA is appointed by the governor to a cabinet-level position in 32 states; the head of the SHA resides in the superagency in 14 and in the state board of health in 4 (Mississippi, Oklahoma, South Carolina, and Texas).

State Board of Health

State boards or councils of health are used for citizen input into the operation of the SHA in 40 states.

These boards or councils function in a policy-making capacity in 21 states, in an advisory capacity in 17, and in both capacities in 2 states. The usual practice is to appoint a board of about nine members. Board members are appointed by the governor—subject to approval by the legislature—and serve without pay but are reimbursed for personal expenses in connection with their duties, such as attending meetings and participating in special functions. Board members usually are appointed for terms of 6 years, with terms staggered to provide for changes in board membership yet still ensure desirable continuity. The board is not generally composed of health specialists but ideally is made up of a cross-section of the population of the state or province and is representative of various interests, geographical areas, and backgrounds. The board's role is to reflect the viewpoints, interpretations, desires, and needs of the public. There could be no objection to having a physician on the board, but to have the membership dominated by health professionals would defeat the very purpose for which the board is created. Just as education policies are left to nonexperts in education rather than to professional academicians, general health policies are decided by lay citizens with the viewpoint and judgment of the general public. Services of experts are provided to the board by the professional staff of the health department and other consultants as needed.

Powers of the board of health. The state or provincial board of health has such powers and functions as have been granted to it by the state or provincial constitution and the legislature. Seven acknowledged powers of any board of health include: code making, quasijudicial powers, administration, investigation, supervision and consultation, education, and coordination with other health agencies.

Code making is a quasilegislative function, giving the board the authority to make necessary rules and regulations to carry out the functions granted to it by the legislature. The professional health staff recommends these rules and regulations and assembles them into a sanitary code. This code has the effect of law when approved by the board of health. Courts have upheld the power of the board to enact binding rules and regulations, providing these rules and regulations do not go beyond the bounds of health matters.

Quasijudicial powers are exercised by the board in its authority to summon before it anyone alleged to have violated state or provincial health regulations. The board has the further recognized authority to summon witnesses. Hearings may be held by the board before granting or revoking a license. In all cases the citizen concerned has the right to contest any adverse action of the board by filing an appeal in court.

State or provincial director of health. Administrative functions of the state or provincial board of health are delegated to the full-time staff of health specialists. In Australia, Canada, and many Asian, African, South American, and European countries, the chief provincial health officer is called the minister of health. In most states of the United States the chief administrator is called the health commissioner, although ''health officer,'' ''health director,'' ''secretary of health,'' and other titles are used. In some states of the United States the board elects the commissioner; in others the governor appoints the commissioner. Twenty-three states require that the head of the SHA have an M.D. degree. Top leadership positions tend to be filled by non-physicians, although SHAs usually have physicians on staff or access to input from physicians with preparation and experience in public health. The commissioner has certain recognized responsibilities: (1) general administration, (2) recommendation of health legislation, rules, and regulations for consideration by the board, (3) appointment of personnel, (4) preparation of the budget, (5) supervision of divisions or bureaus, (6) enforcement of health rules and regulations, and (7) coordination of relationships with official agencies, organizations, and the public.

Departmental Organization

The structure of the health department or organization varies (see Figures 19-2 and 19-3). At the top of the administrative pyramid is the health commissioner, officer, or minister of health. At the next level are the primary administrative units, usually called *divisions,* which in turn are divided into *bureaus* or *sections.* There may be further subdivisions, but this would be necessary only in departments in heavily populated states or provinces. A large state or provincial health department may have 10 divisions, whereas a small one may have only half that number. Each division, bureau, or section has a director or chief. In most instances, the title of the division or bureau, as shown in Figure 19-2, indicates the function or areas of health service.

The distribution of program effort can be illustrated by reviewing the functions of the units of a typical state health department in the United States.

Functions of a Department of Health

Emergency medical services. Recent federal and state legislation has made the SHA responsible for many aspects of an **emergency medical services system.** Responsibilities of the SHA include ambulance vehicle licensing and inspection, ambulance consultation, emergency medical communications, ambulance attendant testing and certification, and ambulance personnel and vehicle-registry. These functions apply to both routine and disaster situations. State **disaster plans** are sometimes coordinated under this functional unit.

Maternal and child health. Established jointly by the U.S. state and federal governments under Title V of the Social Security Act, the Maternal and Child Health Services program identifies the health needs of children and women of childbearing age and addresses those needs through a broad range of programs with a diversity of services. Family health services include maternity clinics for prenatal and postpartum care, child health clinics, and diagnostic and evaluation centers for handicapped children. Speech and hearing programs train individuals in screening techniques, check audiometers for correct calibration, and maintain a statewide registry of all audiometers, all firms that calibrate audiometers, and all persons who use audiometers for screening or diagnostic purposes.

Other programs include family planning, nutrition education and consultation, the Supplemental Food Program for Women, Infants and Children (WIC), projects for children and youth, intensive-care nursery projects for high-risk infants, and vision care programs. WIC funds from the U.S. Department of Agriculture make up the largest contribution to state health agency funds from federal agencies other than health, amounting to as much as 20% for some state health agencies.

Handicapped children's programs. If a handicapped child's parents are unable to afford adequate medical care, the Crippled Children's Services program (also under Title V of the Social Security Act) provides the necessary hospital care and specialized medical services to treat the malady. Handicapping conditions included are bone, joint, muscle, or nerve defects or deformities, congenital heart defects, and cystic fibrosis.

Chronic diseases. State or provincial cancer and heart disease programs provide communities with service, consultative, and educational resources. For example, cancer information services and tumor registry programs augment community activities with centralized computer capabilities. Ongoing care of the cancer patient is encouraged through a systematic follow-up system. Morbidity and survival data are supplied for use in continuing education programs. Workshops are held to promote the development of community cancer programs and to coordinate follow-up for cancer patients. Many diverse educational services are provided to teach individuals about the warning signs of cancer and

the hazards of smoking. The SHA usually coordinates an interagency council on smoking and health.

Another program within the chronic diseases division is kidney dialysis. The state program's primary function is to assist citizens who have end-stage renal disease and require life-sustaining dialysis treatments or a kidney transplant. This is usually a state rather than local program because many communities cannot afford the high cost of dialysis.

Chronic disease screening programs include services for cholesterol, hypertension, and diabetes detection and multiphasic screening. The object of screening activities is early recognition and treatment of persons with preventable conditions. Individuals identified as possibly having an abnormal condition are referred to the physician of their choice for medical evaluation and treatment (Figure 19-6).

Public health nursing. The state or province provides leadership to public health nurses through consultation, teaching, and demonstration. Emphasis is placed on providing a high quality of health care that accommodates a variety of cultural patterns and individual health needs. Public health nursing services are offered in community settings such as homes, schools, industrial plants, clinics, and public health centers. These services may include bedside care in the home, teaching health maintenance and prevention of illness, providing for early detection of illness, and obtaining appropriate medical care for citizens.

Provincial or state professional nursing staff help local public health nurses to keep their knowledge and practical skills current with scientific developments and progress in the medical and nursing fields. This assistance is partially accomplished through the development of continuing education courses and in-service education for nurses. Planning and helping to implement new and improved methods of delivering nursing care in collaboration

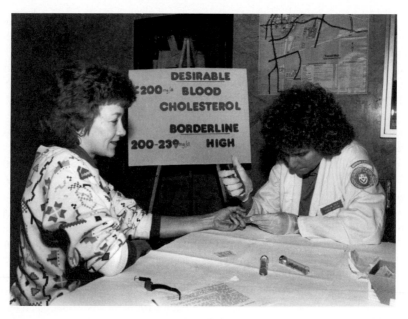

FIGURE 19-6
Screening programs for chronic diseases have been given increasing attention and support by state health departments in recent years. Some remain controversial as to their cost-effectiveness for younger age adults.
Source: Courtesy University of Texas Health Science Center at Houston. Photo by Marsha Burkes.

with other members of the health care team is another function of the state. Nursing consultation is provided to public health regional offices, local health departments, public schools, schools of nursing, and other professional workers and interested individuals as requested.

Local health services. On-the-job training to local personnel maintains and updates such skills as budget preparation, general recordkeeping, and maintenance of tuberculosis registers, birth and death records, and morbidity statistics. Financial aid also is given to help local departments provide the vital services required by their communities. Some small or sparsely populated counties even contract with the state for direct state provision of local health services, especially those that require more specialized skills or equipment.

Communicable disease services. The agency coordinates statewide disease control activities and is responsible for conducting the routine morbidity surveillance of specified reportable diseases occurring in the state. This function includes collecting and tabulating reported data and preparing graphic representation and written interpretation of communicable disease morbidity occurrence and trends. In addition, appropriate educational support for the control of infectious diseases is given by developing and distributing booklets, pamphlets, technical literature, and manuals, presenting in-service programs to selected audiences, and providing consultation upon request. These surveillance and information services are especially helpful in facilitating interaction with and support of immunization programs and sexually transmitted disease (STD) control programs.

Intercity, intrastate, and interstate activities of local STD control programs typically include comprehensive medical, nursing, educational, epidemiological (interview contact and case follow-up), and laboratory services for public and private agencies offering medical services to STD patients; and morbidity reporting and epidemiological control systems to ensure location of contacts. The state also tries to ensure support and maintenance of convenient STD clinics or other treatment facilities; educational efforts to communicate venereal disease information to people at risk, with the dual objectives of preventing exposure to infection and motivating infected individuals to seek early medical care and to cooperate in locating contacts; and efforts to involve the private medical community in all aspects of STD control. With the AIDS epidemic, STD programs dominate the state expenditures in communicable diseases, surpassing immunization in total state expenditure.

The state immunization service develops and implements programs designed to raise immunization levels in the entire state population. The SHA maintains continuous surveillance over the proper application of day-care center and school immunization laws and provides vaccinations where no local mechanisms exist. In some states vaccines distributed free of charge to local health departments and district agencies help to maintain high immunization levels across the state. Many states operate an extensive direct-mail program in which parents of newborn children are reminded and encouraged to start immunizations soon after the child's birth and to complete them shortly after the first birthday. Some provinces in Canada routinely provide for home visits to new mothers and infants. Parents return business reply cards when immunizations are started and completed. Those parents who do not respond may be contacted by a field staff member who discusses the importance of the preventive aspects of immunizations with parents by telephone or in their homes. The aides also receive referrals each month of nonimmunized preschool children identi-

fied through the Early Periodic Screening, Detection and Treatment program.

Tuberculosis services. Tuberculosis is one of the oldest communicable diseases. Modern science has developed effective methods to prevent and treat tuberculosis. The decrease in tuberculosis cases has leveled off in the last few years. This highlights the need for state agencies to continue to monitor communicable diseases such as tuberculosis, at a time when many communities cannot justify maintaining a local staff dedicated to tuberculosis control. The U.S. Department of Health and Human Services has targeted tuberculosis for eradication; it falls to the SHA, then, to (1) find and successfully treat all infectious cases of tuberculosis, and (2) prevent disease spread by early detection and treatment of tuberculosis infections. To attain these objectives the state program seeks to ensure that more patients complete the prescribed treatment (Figure 19-7). Persons suspected of having tuberculosis and contacts of known cases are examined, and infected persons at high risk of developing tuberculosis are given preventive treatment. Services are provided directly by the state in some communities; in other areas, local health departments are given support.

Epidemiology. Epidemiology, defined as the study of the distribution of disease and the determinants of disease frequency in humans, is no longer restricted to the study of epidemics or infectious diseases. It applies today as much to the chronic diseases. Public health is grounded in epidemiology, and in turn epidemiology is grounded in three disciplines: clinical medicine, pathology, and biostatistics. The SHA's professional staff therefore must have competence in these three areas, as well as in the art of applied epidemiological investigation.

Epidemiological methods are employed daily by the staffs of the SHA for planning and evaluation of particular programs. The SHA's epidemiology division is charged with carrying out epidemiological investigations of disease problems and stands avail-

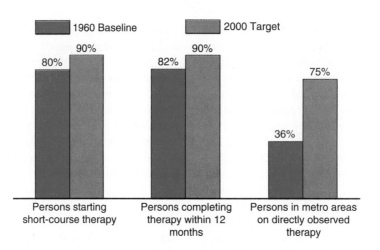

■ 1960 Baseline   ■ 2000 Target

FIGURE 19-7
Adapted from the U.S. objectives for the nation, these specific objectives for the state of Missouri reflect the commitment of the state health department to control tuberculosis not only through case finding and preventive treatment of high-risk or exposed individuals, but also through the completion of therapy by those with the disease.

Source: Missouri Department of Health: *Public health agenda for the '90s: healthy Missourians 2000,* vol 2, Jefferson City, 1992, The Department.

able to assist in investigations conducted in the state or province by other public health units.

Laboratories. One of the most essential services of the SHA is the division or bureau of laboratories—yet it remains one of the least-known agencies to people outside the health professions. **Laboratory services** are provided for communicable disease control, chronic disease detection and control, environmental protection, dental health, and many other public health activities. In addition, the laboratories serve as general diagnostic centers for private physicians, particularly for procedures that are beyond the scope or capabilities of private and local medical laboratories. Millions of samples and specimens are processed and tested in the state laboratories. As a result of these tests, hundreds of thousands of citizens are assured of prompt, accurate diagnosis and treatment by their private physician or local public health clinic.

Veterinary public health. The veterinary public health service conducts vector and zoonosis control programs responsible for the detection, investigation, and eradication of animal diseases that can be transmitted to humans. Rabies, several types of encephalitis (sleeping sickness), ornithosis (a poultry disease), and psittacosis (parrot fever) are just a few examples of such diseases, many of which can be fatal to humans as well as to animals. The veterinary public health service also conducts the state meat and poultry inspection program to ensure the health of food animals and the safety and wholesomeness of fresh meats and poultry processed or sold in the state, as described in Chapter 16. Meat-processing establishments, rendering plants, animal-food-manufacturing plants, kennels, and zoos are inspected regularly.

Hospital licensure and certification. In recent years, increasing emphasis has been placed on achieving and maintaining high standards in the quality of medical facilities (Figure 19-8). States survey and certify hospitals, home health agencies, independent laboratories, rehabilitation facilities, end-stage renal disease facilities, physical therapists in independent practice, and suppliers of portable

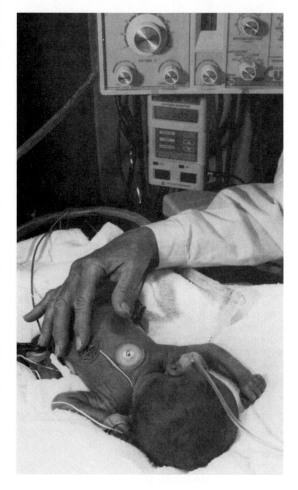

FIGURE 19-8
State and provincial health agencies have responsibility for hospital licensure and certification to ensure that high standards are maintained in medical facilities.
Source: Missouri Department of Health, photo by James Martin.

x-ray services to participants in the Medicare program. The hospital licensure and certification division usually has an intraagency agreement with the long-term care division to survey skilled nursing facilities that participate in the Medicare program. States also set and enforce standards for safety and sanitation in licensed general hospitals, state medical hospitals, state and private mental hospitals, and state schools for the retarded, deaf, and blind.

The state is also responsible for conducting appropriate United States Public Health Service proficiency examinations for selected health care personnel. The proficiency examinations provide an additional way for health care personnel to be considered qualified for Medicare purposes. States conduct proficiency examinations for clinical laboratory technicians, cytotechnologists, vocational nurses who have received licenses by waiver, and physical therapists in independent practice. These exams measure skills of selected health personnel against required standards.

Health maintenance organizations. Health maintenance organizations (HMOs) are a source of health care designed to offer the public a choice between the traditional fee-for-service system and prepaid health care. They differ from health insurance companies in that services are provided through contracts with specific providers of medical service, such as a group of doctors, a hospital, and an affiliated pharmacy. HMOs offer a broad range of health services, from routine physical exams to the most sophisticated surgical procedures. (See Chapter 21 for a more complete description of HMOs.) Similar variations on traditional medical practice such as preferred provider organizations (PPOs) and managed care have emerged more recently. States regulate and certify HMOs and PPOs. They evaluate the quality of care being provided by these groups and make recommendations for or against certification to a state board of insurance and to the federal government.

Medical disclosure panels. Some states have a medical disclosure panel composed of physicians and lawyers representing various regions of the state. The panel, often selected and staffed by the state department of health, determines what risks and hazards are involved in medical care and surgical procedures and whether these risks must be disclosed by health care providers and physicians to their patients. Informed consent procedures required by various federal and state laws have placed greater medical decision-making power in the hands of patients and families.

Vital statistics. Some of the most significant events in the lives of citizens are recorded by official state agencies, including marriage, birth of a child, and death. Maintaining such records was one of the earliest duties assigned to state and provincial health departments. Processing records of births, marriages, divorces, and deaths requires the services of skilled statisticians. Local officials forward records that provide information of great value to the state. Statistical analyses are essential in many kinds of governmental planning. For example, knowing where people are choosing to live will help determine where health facilities need to be located; knowing what diseases and injuries are occurring most often, and where, helps to plan control programs. Dozens of similar analyses enable the state government to serve its communities more effectively.

Long-term care. The state provides for facility licensing, Medicare and Medicaid certification actions, quality-of-care assurance and consultation, classifications of patient care, periodic medical reviews, and utilization reviews. The quality of care provided to the sick elderly and the physical plant safety of long-term care facilities are regulated by the state. Reviews of records and on-site visits compare a facility against established standards (Figure 19-9).

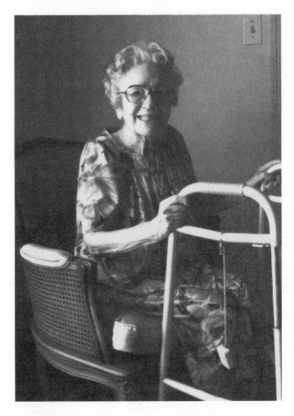

FIGURE 19-9
State and provincial agencies oversee the regulation of long-term care and the quality of services of home health care providers. With growing proportions of populations in the age groups requiring these services, this function of SHAs may be expected to grow.
Source: Missouri Department of Health photo by James Martin.

State health planning. If the department of health is the organization designated by the governor as the state health planning and resource development agency in compliance with the U.S. National Health Planning and Resources Development Act of 1974, then the department is responsible for performing all health planning and resource development functions on the state level and is charged with developing an annual state health plan and an annual state medical facilities plan. This function will be further described later in this chapter.

Consumer health protection. Most SHA product safety programs protect the public through inspection of manufacturing and distribution facilities where hazardous substances are made or handled, establishment of appropriate regulations, identification of potentially hazardous products, proper labeling, and, in some cases, the banning of products that are unnecessarily or extremely hazardous to the public. The product safety programs have directed their attention particularly toward the flammability of fabrics (especially children's clothing), aerosol sprays, cleaners, polishers, lead-based paint, and other common household products.

The state enforces laws that deal with the regulation of milk and milk products. State personnel, in cooperation with local health department regulatory officials, routinely inspect all dairies, milk and dairy product processors, milk storage and transportation facilities, single-service container manufacturers, and retail outlets where milk or milk products are sold.

The National Conference on Interstate Milk Shipments, by reciprocal agreements between states, provides assurance that all Grade ''A'' milk and milk products transferred between states are produced and processed in conformance with regulatory standards set forth in the U.S. Public Health Service Grade ''A'' Pasteurized Milk ordinance.

It is the statutory responsibility of states to administer and enforce those laws that are designed to assure the consumer of safe foods, drugs, and cosmetics. Surveillance and compliance inspections are made of the operations and premises of all food, drug, and cosmetic manufacturers (Figure 19-10), wholesalers, repackers, distributors, and retailers. Both raw materials and finished products are sampled for laboratory analysis to ensure compliance with acceptable standards.

Natural disasters impose a special responsibility

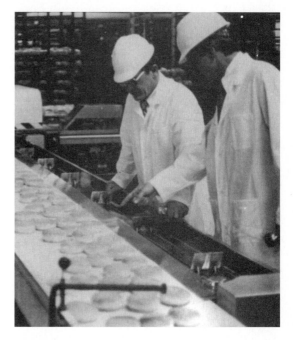

FIGURE 19-10
Food processing inspections are carried out by state or provincial health agencies because most manufacturers ship their products beyond the community.
Source: Texas Department of Health.

on the state consumer health protection program. State personnel stand ready to move into disaster areas to determine whether disaster-exposed food and drugs should be used or discarded.

Perhaps the least known of all the programs in the state department of health is the shellfish sanitation control program, which enforces state laws to ensure the wholesomeness and safety of shellfish harvested and processed in coastal states or sold in other states. Program staff perform sanitary surveys, collect samples, and evaluate the water quality in shellfish harvesting areas along the coast; inspect harvesting boats and docking areas; inspect, certify, and license processing plants; and prepare maps indicating safe harvesting areas for shellfish. Most inland states do not have such a specialized program, but for coastal states it is essential for the control of salmonellosis outbreaks.

Environmental health. The quality of the water we drink and the safety of toxic waste dumps are among the environmental health concerns of SHAs. For water, this includes the surveillance of the construction, operation, and maintenance of all public drinking water supply systems. SHAs also monitor toxic waste dumps. The state operates a certification program that assists in developing and coordinating training courses for water supply and wastewater system operators. Plans for new public water systems and for major improvements to existing systems are reviewed by the state to certify that they meet current standards. Likewise, chemical and bacteriological records of water systems are reviewed by the state to ensure compliance with standards.

Chemical and bacteriological records of water samples collected periodically from all public water systems in the state are maintained. Sanitary surveys of all public water systems conducted periodically are processed by the state, and appropriate recommendations for improvements are made to the water system officials responsible. The state or province initiates enforcement action when necessary and provides technical information and assistance to municipal officials and water system owners and operators. Public health education programs can encourage activities such as bicycle riding that help to reduce automobile air pollution while promoting cardiovascular fitness (Figure 19-11).

Administrative services. The business management functions of the SHA programs include the official fiscal and budgetary functions and controls as well as data processing, general plant supervision,

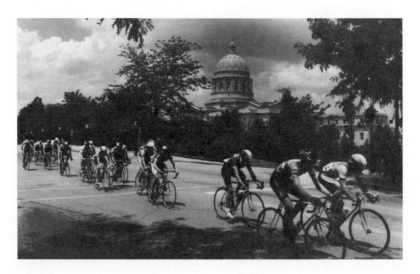

FIGURE 19-11
Environmental conditions in most state and provincial capitals and other municipal areas demand greater dependence on mass transit and other alternatives to the automobile. States and provinces now encourage regional planning to provide bicycle paths and dedicated carpool and bus lanes for commuters. The fitness benefits of bicycling are also served.
Source: Missouri Department of Health, photo by Bob Hulsey.

and sometimes public health education. All funds received and expended by the department are recorded and accounting reports prepared. Budget reports are also prepared on warehousing, shipping and receiving, property management, maintenance of buildings and grounds, utilities, equipment maintenance, the central library facilities, the department's payroll, and on-premises food services for department employees.

The SHA's data-processing services usually operate 24 hours a day, 6 days a week, with occasional Sunday shifts (Figure 19-12). Thousands of computer runs made each month draw on and feed into a library of hundreds of computer tapes. If it were not for the data-processing capabilities of the state

health department, many of today's programs would be impossible to administer, and countless other programs would be far less effective than they are. To cite an earlier example, the immunization program's use of birth certificates, recorded by the vital statistics bureau, as the source of names and addresses of families with newborn children depends on computer-printed form letters sent to the infants' parents to encourage them to have their babies immunized early. Copies of the names and addresses go to local health departments for follow-up. Most of this would not be feasible without computers.

Besides accounting for funds received and spent, the SHA must plan for future needs and translate

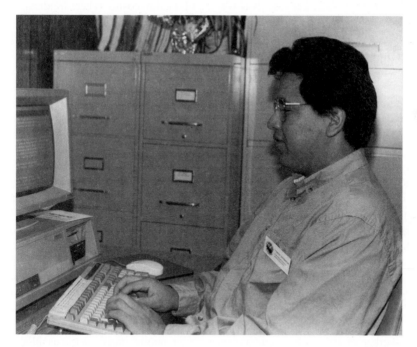

FIGURE 19-12

Computers have made possible the storage, rapid retrieval, transfer between state and local officials, and analysis of millions of records, including birth, marriage, and death certificates, communicable disease reports, chronic disease registries, behavioral risk survey questionnaires, and financial reports.

Source: Lincoln-Lancaster Department of Health.

those needs into specific budget figures. Each departmental budget is submitted to the state legislature on an annual or biennial basis.

Public health education. All SHA programs rely heavily on education to help accomplish their purpose in preventing disease and injury. The public health education division employs professional writers, editors, artists, health educators, social scientists, and other personnel to assist the other divisions in carrying out their responsibilities. With the growing emphasis on life-style causes of chronic diseases and injury, some of these units have been renamed health promotion divisions.

Most SHAs also publish dozens of new pamphlets, brochures, booklets, posters, and other pieces of literature each year. They distribute weekly newspaper columns and 5-minute radio programs, public service announcements for radio and television, and important health information to newspapers, news wire services, and magazine journalists.

Most SHAs today maintain a video and film library to supply tapes and prints to schools, clubs, and individuals, usually on a free-loan basis. Some agencies have their own printing plant to produce the millions of pieces of literature, including essential records and reporting forms, used by local health departments and private physicians.

The public health education unit also provides staff training for public health personnel at the state and local levels. Major courses or conferences are conducted each year and are supplemented by occasional 1-day training sessions.

Sources of Funds for State Health Departments

States spend an average of 20% of their budgets on health-related programs. The overall state costs for health continue to increase, the largest component of which is the medically oriented Medicaid costs. This program, primarily for the poor and disabled, now accounts for 12% of state spending; 20 years

ago it was only 3%. By 1990 the states' share of Medicaid costs were $25 billion.

Total public health expenditures by states is difficult to compare because the SHA organization and responsibilities differ, and SHA programs vary in importance and content. Total SHA expenditure in fiscal 1988 ranged from a low of $14 million (Wyoming) to a high of $793 million (California). Many states are facing decreases in services due to budget cuts. Total spending for public health across the states in 1989 was $9.7 billion, of which the state share of revenues was only slightly more than half (Figure 19-13).

With decreased contributions from the federal government, states and provinces are often faced with doing less rather than picking up a larger share of health costs. When Medicaid is added to the amounts reflected in Figure 19-13, states pay an average of 45% of health costs, the federal government 30%, and the remaining costs are supported by local government, fees, reimbursements, and other sources. At 30% the federal government picks up a larger percentage of health costs, largely because of Medicaid entitlement programs, than the average of 17% the federal government contributes to all state and local budgets.

Federal funds make up a large proportion of resources available to state health agencies. Most of these federal funds now reside in **block grants,** which give the state considerable discretion in allocating the fund to programs according to its priorities.

Funds from U.S. Department of Health and Human Services sources for public health include, in order of magnitude, the maternal and child health portion of Title V of the Social Security Act; the crippled children's portion of Title V; comprehensive public health services block grants; family-planning grants under Title X of the Public Health Service Act; and AIDS education funds from the Centers for Disease Control. The largest single federal funding source is the Supplemental Food Program for Women, Infants and Children (WIC),

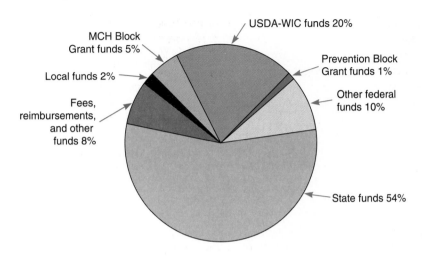

FIGURE 19-13

The distribution of state expenditures by sources of funds shows that state health agencies in the United States have depended heavily in the past on the federal government for nearly one third of their budgets. The percentages shown here apply roughly to the the 1989 total of $9.7 billion.

Source: Public Health Foundation; and National Center for Health Statistics: Health, United States, 1991. Hyattsville, Md, 1992, Public Health Service, Table 129, p. 284.

which is administered by the U.S. Department of Agriculture.

The portions of the total SHA expenditures that can be attributed to "preventive" health services vary widely, from more than 90% of immunization and health education services to less than 10% of institutional and home health care. About 30% of the total state public health expenditures are for services that are primarily preventive (Figure 19-14). The federal share of different types of prevention programs also varies. For example, the federal contribution is 9% of tuberculosis control programs, while state and local contributions amount to over 85% to the costs of such programs.

Appraisal of Official State Health Services in the United States

Activities of the typical North American SHA have been presented here to provide a sense of the different state or provincial health services and pro-

grams. The functions should provide a more complete picture of the current areas of responsibility and emphasis in U.S. state health departments than do the organizational charts in Figures 19-2 and 19-3. Organizational charts can be deceptive because the boxes are all approximately the same size, giving the illusion that the programs and services are of similar scope. The examination of budgets or expenditure figures for each program or service can help to provide additional insight into their relative magnitude and scope.

As a support service to many programs, health education funds should be set aside within the program budgets. This often is not the case, however, even though the programs require health education services. Hence certain basic functions such as health education sometimes end up with no budget, and their expenditures are from leftover funds.

As state health services have expanded and technology has advanced, the health of the public has improved, diseases have been prevented, and deaths

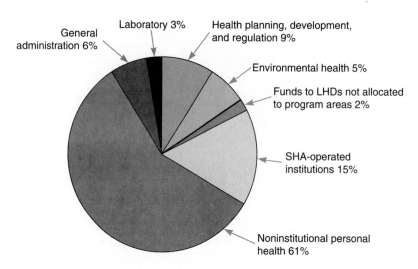

FIGURE 19-14

State expenditures by program area shows 76% of the same $9.7 billion going to personal health care. The 61% for noninstitutional personal health includes 20% for WIC (the USDA Supplemental Food Program for Women, Infants, and Children) and 41% for maternal and child health services other than WIC, handicapped children's services, communicable disease control, dental health, chronic disease control, mental health, and alcohol and drug abuse.

Source: Public Health Foundation; and National Center for Health Statistics: Health, United States, 1991. Hyattsville, Md, 1992, Public Health Service, Table 129, p. 284.

have been postponed. A full appraisal of the value and significance of the official state health services would have to consider that many of the state health services do not deal with life-and-death matters but contribute to the quality of life.

For state health services, four cardinal needs exist. The first is the need for sufficient funds to do adequately what should be done in state health promotion. A second need is to obtain better data relevant to the chronic diseases, many of which are related to life-style. A third need is to integrate or at least coordinate the health functions of all state agencies that provide health services in some form. The state health department, agriculture department, education department, labor department, and other state agencies that have health functions must work closely together to allocate responsibility for overlapping health services. They in turn must provide the fourth need by working closely with nongovern-

mental and nonhealth organizations, recognizing that many of these also receive federal health grants to complement official state and local health agency programs.

Appraisal of Provincial Health Programs in Canada

The British North American Act of 1867 and the Constitution of Canada place the mandate for health with the provinces. The federal government collects from provincial citizens personal income taxes and General Service Taxes (GST) on purchases. Then, through equalization payments favoring the poorer provinces and through transfer payments, the federal government redistributes that income to the provinces. Transfer payments provide for specific health services and hospital insurance. The provinces fund a comprehensive range of health services from their federal share and from their other sources of revenue such as sales taxes and corporate taxes. In disease prevention and health promotion the provinces build on federal policy and leadership, but each follows its own strategy, methods, and funding priorities. Examples from a few of the provinces will illustrate.

The Canadian initiatives in health promotion tend to subscribe more than those of the United States to the definitions of health and health promotion promulgated by the World Health Organization. Indeed, much of the WHO approach to health promotion owes its origins to Canadian initiatives and to the Ottawa Charter for Health Promotion from the First International Conference on Health Promotion held in Canada with WHO cosponsorship. The three functions most health promotion programs in the Canadian provinces seek to serve are to increase public awareness, to improve the capacity of individuals, families, and communities to address health issues, and to create social and physical environments that support health.

Public awareness. New Brunswick has an animated cartoon program broadcast on television to raise awareness of risk factors and their role in cardiovascular diseases. This is one of several Canadian federal-provincial initiatives in heart health, but the only one among the provinces that emphasizes a broad mass media approach to heart health. Neighboring Prince Edward Island has developed school health curriculum modules to help children understand the hazards of smoking. British Columbia has a comprehensive school health curriculum called Learning for Living required in all schools and a school-based program for alcohol and drug abuse prevention, based on the PRECEDE model, that places a prevention worker in each school to assist teachers and the community to coordinate their efforts.

Strengthening capacity. Newfoundland's AIDS prevention program combines mass media advertisements for public awareness with a specific media advocacy strategy to promote public support for preventive efforts and to mobilize key government decision makers. It also supports educational programs to provide training for youth in decision making and other social skills that would enable them to resist peer pressures. Needle-exchange programs in some 25 cities across Canada are sponsored by provincial or municipal governments, compared with only a dozen or so cities with needle-exchange programs in the United States (see Figure 11-8). The development of seniors' wellness councils in Nova Scotia is another example of strengthening community capacity, in this case to address the neglected needs of the growing population of elderly people. In the Northwest Territories more than 50 health representatives have been trained to work with the far north communities with their aboriginal populations spread over several thousand square miles and with their 10 official languages. The Healthy Schools Program of British Columbia seeks to engage school children actively in identifying their own health issues, to reach consensus, and to take collective action to deal with those issues. Similar programs for Healthy Workplaces and Healthy Communities work with employees and community residents.

Supportive environments. Beyond the actions individuals and organizations can be supported to take, policies must be developed at the provincial level and through municipal and district levels to create healthful living conditions and to make healthful personal choices the easier choices for individuals. In Manitoba, for example, a coalition of churches, food banks, and antipoverty groups work with the provincial and local governments to address problems of food security and accessibility. Alberta's injury prevention initiative uses a similar coalition approach to affect policies and to support programs for safer environments. New tobacco legislation in British Columbia, Manitoba, and Ontario has sought to tighten the accessibility of tobacco to minors and to add to the tobacco tax on cigarettes. The Healthy Community movement

("Villes et Villages" in Quebec), based on the WHO Healthy Cities model, seeks to engage community residents, policy makers, and leaders from various sectors other than health in collaborative efforts to change health-related policies, to improve living conditions, and to advocate for and with the most vulnerable populations in their communities. In British Columbia, 43,000 people in 90 communities have participated directly in Healthy Community projects affecting over 1 million people.

Finally, although Canada has not developed national and provincial objectives for disease prevention and health promotion as thoroughly as the United States and some states, a few Canadian provinces have been more aggressive than their American counterparts in going beyond objectives to set mandatory standards. The Ontario Provincial Health Act (see box) and the British Columbia *New Directions* policy are exemplary. The British Columbia

initiative includes a major emphasis on decentralizing the provincial roles to give greater decision-making authority to community health councils and regional health boards. The theme of British Columbia's provincial initiative is "bringing health closer to home."

HEALTH PLANNING IN THE UNITED STATES

The Comprehensive Health Planning Act of 1966 and the Partnership for Health Amendments of 1967 were enacted in the United States to establish comprehensive planning for health services, the health workforce, and health facilities essential at every level of government. It sought also to strengthen the leadership and capabilities of the SHAs and to broaden and make more feasible and relevant federal support of state and community health services.

The Ontario Provincial Health Act

After several years of preparation and following wide consultation, the Health Protection and Promotion Act was proclaimed in 1984 to the Ontario Legislature. The Honourable Keith Norton, Minister of Health, spoke of how the new act represented a great stride forward for public health, calling it "the most progressive public health legislation in North America." The focus of the act is "on the promotion of healthy lifestyles and the prevention of illness."

Replacing the Public Health Act, enacted more than 100 years ago, the new act was designed to prepare boards of health to exercise leadership in the era of disease prevention and health promotion. At the heart of the act is the establishment of minimum program requirements, or **mandatory programs,** which all local or district boards of health must ensure are available in health units. Programs currently offered by boards of health did not change radically as a result of the new act, but they were subject to the mandatory programs requirements. For example, the preventive dentistry mandatory program must provide preventive dental ser-

vices to the community and provide dental health education, oral hygiene instruction, and fluoride rinse programs to school children. Mandatory programs are provided in the following areas: community sanitation, communicable disease control, preventive dentistry, family health, home care services, nutrition, and public health education. Boards of health may add other services and programs to supplement those that are mandatory. Finally, public health education will be a component of all of the preceding programs.

In addition to mandatory programs, the Health Protection and Promotion Act broke new ground in several other areas of public health. For example, it formally recognizes the role boards of health play in occupational and environmental health matters. To this end, the act created the legislative ground for the close working relationship that must exist between the Ministries of Health, Environment, and Labour.

Ontario Ministry of Health: *Mandatory health programs and service guidelines,* Toronto, 1993, Queen's Printer for Ontario.

This legislation was superseded by the National Health Planning and Resources Development Act of 1974.

The federal budgets during the 1980s eliminated the support for state health planning. The state and area health planning agencies already had been weakened, and most have now been closed, by federal repeal of the Act. It is unlikely that Congress will restore funds to rebuild the planning agencies. Thus the state and local health departments once again must turn to their own devices to bring some order into the chaos of the burgeoning American medical and hospital ''nonsystem'' of care, which emphasizes high technology treatment rather than primary health care, prevention, and health promotion.

An Example of the State Planning Process

The epidemiological assessment. Recognizing that each state's problems, needs, and circumstances differ from those of other states, the state health planning process allows for the systematic assessment of those needs and circumstances within the state. This leads to an identification of the leading causes of death, illness, injury, and disability. Most states set their priorities for health action on the basis of mortality rankings rather than morbidity, injury, or disability rates. This leads to a typical set of priorities that places heart disease and cancer very high on the ratings of importance. Comparing their statistics with other states, some states also conclude that they can do much better in controlling infant mortality or congenital anomalies, even though these do not show up among the leading causes of death. Through this process of statistical analysis and comparison, different states arrive at different priorities (Figure 19-15).

Behavioral risk-factor surveys. For those health priorities for which behavioral or life-style risk factors determine most of the premature deaths, a second level of state planning draws upon the available data on the distribution of these risk factors in the population. Most states now conduct behavioral risk-factor surveys periodically to track trends in the most important behavioral risk factors. Table 19-2 shows the prevalence rates in percentages for each of four of the risk factors and the lowest and highest ranking states on the four risk factors. The more detailed tabulations allow a state like West Virginia, for example, to note that its rate of smokeless tobacco use at 8.2% is number 1 among the states. Such data enable a state to shift its priorities for purposes of primary prevention or health promotion. Depending only on mortality data would mean that the actions a state can take on chronic disease control comes 20 years too late to take preventive action. Using trends and comparisons in risk-factor data allows West Virginia to take some action on smokeless tobacco even though its mortality rates for cancer are not exceptionally high.

Setting objectives. A third phase of state planning for health is the establishment of quantitative objectives that reflect the potential for change in the mortality rates and the risk-factor prevalence rates. Such objectives can be stated for the state as a whole and for specific subpopulations such as males and females, urban and rural, teenagers and adults, whites and others. The form of the objectives, as outlined in Chapter 4, is ''how much (usually a % reduction) of what (usually a mortality rate or a risk factor) will be achieved by when (year) in which population.'' West Virginia, for example, might set its objective for smokeless tobacco control as follows: ''To reduce the use of smokeless tobacco to 2% by 1995 in 15- to 19-year-old males.'' Setting such objectives presents an opportunity to engage a wide range of professionals, experts, interest groups, and sectors other than health. Here is where the process of consensus building can be most valuable. Obtaining agreement on objectives gives all concerned parties a shared direction and commitment. Coordination of subsequent implementation plans then becomes much easier. Once objectives have been stated in

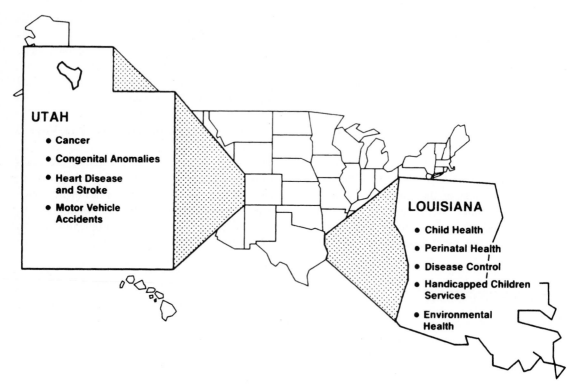

FIGURE 19-15
The assessment of vital statistics for a state will result in different priorities in the health plans of different states.
Source: Office of Disease Prevention and Health Promotion, U.S. Department of Health and Human Services.

quantified terms and with definite target dates, the allocation of resources can be made rationally.

SUMMARY

The states and provinces provide a wide variety of health-related services that touch all aspects of daily life from the sanitation of the milk poured on cereals in the morning to the quality of air inhaled during the day. The births and deaths scanned in the daily newspaper are recorded by state agencies. That information lays the basis for health services. Protection against rabid animals, surveillance of quality

health care, and inspection of food are distant and ''silent'' services that get little public attention until problems arise. When the flood of 1993 disabled the water supply to whole cities in Iowa or contaminated fast food caused the deaths of children in Washington state, the quiet daily services of state agencies move to the headlines. Public health services are vital to protect and promote health and to prevent disease.

The states play a pivotal role in achievement of the year 2000 objectives for the nation in disease prevention and health promotion. Strategies for achieving the objectives can be implemented more readily at the state level than at the national level

TABLE 19-2
The 1992 "Public Health Report Card" on the states compiled by the American Public Health Association presents the best and the worst states on each of 25 criteria. The scores for each state are contained in the book circulated by APHA to state officials and legislators to stimulate reform.

	Best	*Worst*		*Best*	*Worst*
Medical care access			*Healthy neighborhoods—cont'd*		
Population uninsured	8%	26%	Violent crime rate	63	2,142
Primary care physicians per capita	10.9	4.3	Education spending per capita	$2320.82	$708.30
Adequate prenatal care	85.2%	57.4%	Childhood poverty rate	5.8%	34.6%
Population without access to primary care	0.3%	17.2%	Graduation rate	89.3%	55.3%
Ratio of Medicaid –recipients to poor people	5.64	0.34	Unemployment rate	3.5%	11.4%
Medicaid spending per capita	$483.68	$48.55	*Healthy behaviors*		
Healthy environment			Seat belt nonuse	4.9%	59.6%
			Obesity rate	16.3%	27.4%
Pollution standard index	0	224	Smoking rate	15.3%	31.8%
Unsafe drinking water	1%	53%	Binge drinking rate	5.5%	26.8%
Fluoridated water	100.0%	2.2%	*Community health service*		
Work-related injury cases	6.4	14.3			
Healthy neighborhoods			Government health spending per capita	$188.36	$26.61
			Sanitation and sewerage spending per capita	$223.58	$34.89
Average public assistance payment per family	$620	$114	Public health workers per capita	44.4	5.6
Cigarette tax per pack	$0.45	$0.03			
Motor vehicle deaths per 100,000 miles	1.3	3.6			

Source: American Public Health Association: *America's public health report card: a state-by-state report on the health of the public,* Washington, DC, 1992, The Association, p. 57.

for several reasons. First, the breadth of authority in health matters is greater at the state level than at the national level. The opportunity through personal acquaintance or contact for cooperation between various sectors, such as education and health, is also greater at the state level. Furthermore, states now have wider latitude in their use of federal funds under the new block grants in health services. For all these reasons, state action is required for the integration of services and the cooperation of sectors necessary for effective implementation of disease

prevention and health promotion programs that address the new complexities of life-style and the environment.

In the 1990s state and provincial governments across North America are cutting back on basic services, due in part to reduced federal support and a deficit economy. They find themselves in a position of cutting services that affect health—such as education and public safety—at the same time that costs are rising for health insurance and publicly supported medical services. The typical functions of most state and provincial health departments and the progressive initiatives of some, as well as the demise of the comprehensive health planning experiment, all point ultimately to the community as the final arbiter of health needs and objectives appropriate to a population—the subject of the next chapter.

QUESTIONS FOR REVIEW

1. To what extent is the SHA the ''intermediary'' of health organization?

2. Is the state's authority over the health of the people in the United States too great or not great enough? Why?

3. What check does the public have to prevent health authorities from being too powerful and arrogant?

4. Why should citizens always have the right to appeal to a court when they believe that they have been unjustly dealt with by health officials?

5. What health functions does your state or provincial department of agriculture engage in?

6. How do you explain that local health departments were formed long before state health departments were established?

7. How frequently does your state or provincial board of health meet?

8. Should the state or provincial board of health be composed entirely of physicians?

9. Who is your health commissioner or minister of health, what has been his or her professional preparation and experience, and for how many years has he or she been in the position?

10. When was the last time you or any member of your family received direct service from personnel of your state or provincial health department?

11. What are some health problems in your area on which the state or provincial health department should be conducting research?

12. What service now required of or otherwise carried on by your state or provincial health department should not be a part of the department's activities?

13. What consolidations of official health services have taken place in your state or province in the last 10 years?

14. How has health planning affected the health of the people in your community?

15. Why did the U.S. Congress enact laws to regulate health planning in states and regions?

READINGS

Centers for Disease Control: Summary of notifiable diseases, United States, 1991, *MMWR* 40:1, 1992.
    Each week CDC's *Morbidity and Mortality Weekly Report* compiles and reports the state-by-state tabulations of important communicable diseases. This annual summary provides charts, graphs, and tables, as well as the listing of the epidemiologist and laboratory director for each state.

Centers for Disease Control: CDC surveillance summaries, *MMWR* 40:1, 1991.
    This occasional issue of *MMWR* corresponds to the previous citation with a state-by-state summary of Behavioral Risk Factor survey results for 1986 to 1990 and results of testing for intestinal parasites by state diagnostic laboratories.

Dowdle WR: The future of the public health laboratory, *Annu Rev Public Health* 14:649, 1993.
    This analysis of the functions and status of public health laboratories features the pivotal role that state laboratories play in supporting local laboratories with more specialized tests and in providing all testing for many of the smaller community health departments.

Novotny T, Romano RA, Davis RM et al: The public health practice of tobacco control: lessons learned and directions for the states in the 1990s, *Annu Rev Public Health* 13:287, 1992.
    Reviews the status of smoking by state and the ways in which states have addressed the issue through policy and program initiatives.

Tulchinsky TH, Patton MM, Randolph LA et al: Mandating vitamin K prophylaxis for newborns in New York State, *Am J Public Health* 83:1166, 1993.
    This ''Public Health Brief'' offers a concise case study of the data analysis, scientific considerations, and actions that led to the placement of a mandatory newborn-care procedure for hospitals in a state public health code.

BIBLIOGRAPHY

Access to health care: states respond to growing crisis, GAO/HRD-92-70, Washington, DC, 1992, U.S. General Accounting Office.

Advocacy Institute: *Taking initiative: the 1990 citizens' movement to raise California alcohol excise taxes to save lives,* Washington, DC, 1992, The Institute.

Alabama Department of Public Health: *Healthy Alabama 2000: health promotion and disease prevention objectives for the year 2000,* Montgomery, Ala, 1991, The Department.

Alberta Premier's Commission on Future Health Care for Albertans: *The rainbow report: our vision for health,* 4 vols, Edmunton, 1989, The Commission.

AMA Council on Scientific Affairs: Societal effects and other factors affecting health care for the elderly: report of the Council on Scientific Affairs, *Arch Intern Med* 150:1184, 1990.

American Public Health Association: *America's public health report card: a state-by-state report on the health of the public,* Washington, DC, 1992, The Association.

Australia Department of Community Services and Health, National Health Strategy Unit: *The national health strategy: a summary,* Melbourne, 1991, The Unit.

Baker F: *Coordination of alcohol, drug abuse, and mental health services,* DHHS Pub No (ADM) 91-1742, Rockville, Md, 1991, U.S. Department of Health and Human Services.

Breslow L, Johnson M: California's Proposition 99 on tobacco, and its impact, *Annu Rev Public Health* 14:585, 1993.

British Columbia Ministry of Health and Ministry Responsible for Seniors: *New directions for a healthy British Columbia,* Victoria, 1993, The Ministry.

British Columbia Ministry of Health and Ministry Responsible for Seniors: *Our new understanding of health,* Victoria, 1993, Office of Health Promotion, The Ministry.

California Conference of Local Directors of Health Education: *Standards of practice for public health education in California local health departments,* Sacramento, 1991, The Conference and California Department of Health Services.

Campbell JF, Donohue MA, Nevin-Woods C et al: The Hawaii pneumococcal disease initiative, *Am J Public Health* 83:1175, 1975.

Centers for Disease Control: *Profile of state and territorial public health systems: United States, 1990,* Atlanta, 1991, U.S. Department of Health and Human Services.

Centers for Disease Control: State tobacco prevention and control activities: results of the 1989-1990 Association of State and Territorial Health Officials (ASTHO) survey, final report, *MMWR* 40:38, 1991.

Demkovich L: *The states and the uninsured: slowly but surely, filling the gaps,* Washington, DC, 1990, National Health Policy Forum.

Goddeeris JH, Hogan AJ, editors: *Improving access to health care: what can the states do?* Kalamazoo, Mich, 1992, Upjohn.

Guide to state statistical abstracts. Appendix I in *Statistical abstract of the United States, 1992, the national data book,* Washington, DC, 1992, U.S. Department of Commerce.

Hinz RA: *Turning the tables: how to beat the tobacco industry at its own game—the New York State experience,* Atlanta, 1990, American Cancer Society.

McKenzie L, Stephenson PA: Variation in cesarean section rates among hospitals in Washington State, *Am J Public Health* 83:1109, 1993.

Missouri Department of Health: *Public health agenda for the '90s: healthy Missourians 2000,* vol 2, Jefferson City, 1992, Missouri Department of Health.

Moon RW, Males MA, Nelson DE: The 1990 Montana initiative to increase cigarette taxes: lessons for other states and localities, *J Public Health Policy* 14:19, 1993.

Ontario Minister of Health: *Mandatory health programs and services guidelines,* Toronto, 1993, Queen's Printer for Ontario.

Ontario Premier's Council on Health Strategy: *Nurturing health: a framework on the determinants of health,* Toronto, 1991, The Council.

Province of British Columbia: *Closer to home; sources for the report of the British Columbia Royal Commission on Health Care and Costs,* Victoria, 1991, The Commission.

Quebec Commission of Inquiry on Health and Social Services: *Centralization and decentralization,* Montreal, 1987, The Commission.

Saskatchewan Commission on Directions in Health Care: *Future directions for health care in Saskatchewan,* Regina, 1990, The Commission.

Scandlen G, Casey J: State benefit mandates for drug abuse, mental illness, alcoholism, *Health Benefits Lett* 2:1, 1992.

Valdiserri RO: Temples of the future: an historical overview of the laboratory's role in public health practice, *Annu Rev Public Health* 14:635, 1993.

Wolczuk P: A Canadian perspective: provincial governments. Building Cross-Border Connections in Health Education and Health Promotion: International Conference on Health Education, Toronto, August 1992.

World Health Organization, Canadian Public Health Association, and Health and Welfare Canada: *The Ottawa charter,* Ottawa, 1986, Canadian Public Health Association.

Chapter 20

Community Health
Services and Resources

❖

In the final analysis, our most basic common link is that we all inhabit this small planet. We all breathe the same air. We all cherish our children's future. And we are all mortal.

JOHN F. KENNEDY

OBJECTIVES

When you finish this chapter, you should be able to:

- Identify the sources and scope of local authority related to community health
- Describe the organization and components of community health services
- Participate in the planning and evaluation of community health services

Still closer to home than states or provinces, local communities seek some goals in the promotion of health that individuals and families cannot attain by themselves. These goals must be pursued through collective action. Some things the individual can do can be done better or more equitably on a community or cooperative basis. In today's complex society, no one is totally self-sufficient in dealing with all threats to health. To facilitate and supplement what the individual does in health promotion, and

to bring local, state, and national resources to bear on health problems, official and voluntary health organizations have been established on the local level to function both cooperatively and independently.

COMMUNITY RESPONSIBILITY

Need, demand, custom, and gradual development have led society to accept as a community responsibility certain health services on behalf of all residents and visitors. As the population grows and tends to concentrate in urban and suburban areas, new health problems develop, and most of the long-standing community health problems become more complex and more difficult to manage. With each increase in the complexity of community health problems, society has advanced its technology to cope.

Accepted responsibilities of the community include the following environmental protections: a safe, ample water supply; a safe milk supply; regulation of food establishments; waste disposal; control of air pollution, insects, and rats; and nuisance elimination. Preventive health services include screening and referral for detection of genetic and chronic diseases; collection and recording of vital statistics; communicable disease control; maternal, infant, child, adult, and senior citizen health promotion; mental health services; nutrition education; health education; laboratory service; and other services that are specific for certain communities or subpopulations.

SOURCES OF PUBLIC HEALTH LAW IN THE UNITED STATES

Woodrow Wilson defined law as "that portion of the established thought and habit which has gained distinct and formal recognition in the shape of uniform rules backed by the authority and power of government." More concisely defined, law is crystallized public opinion. Public health law applies **common law** and **statutory law** to the principles of hygiene.

Public health law in the United States is derived from several sources, each discussed in the following paragraphs. All sources of public health law have some impact on health, but the closer to a community the source of a public health law, the greater will be its enforcement by and presumably its value to the community.

Statutory Authority

The U.S. Constitution. Historically, the states came first as colonies that united and created the federal government to serve specific purposes. The Constitution is a grant of authority by the states to the federal government but with reservations as expressed in the Tenth Amendment: "The powers not delegated to the United States by the Constitution, nor prohibited by it to the States, are reserved to the States respectively, or to the people." The word *health* does not appear in the Constitution. Nor is there any reference to public health. Thus the control of public health is primarily a state function. The Constitution contains many broad provisions that affect the control of health and spell out the general responsibilities of the federal government in promoting the public well-being. These were described in Chapter 18.

State constitutions and legislation. Fundamentally promotion of public health is the function of the state. Governments have long recognized health as a basic human condition that government has an inherent obligation, right, and power to protect and promote. From colonial times states and provinces have taken measures to safeguard and promote the health of their citizens. This authority is vested in the states' **police power,** which the courts and the federal government recognize (see Chapter 19).

Delegated Authority

County and municipal ordinances and regulations. State legislatures have the authority to delegate police power to counties and cities to exercise within their own territorial boundaries. They may do this by granting **"home rule"** to counties and municipalities. A city may present a proposed city charter to the state legislature for consideration; if the legislature approves, it grants this charter and home rule to the city. This enables counties and cities to pass health ordinances and regulations to be effective within their own geographical boundaries. Community standards may be higher than state standards, but not lower. Generally counties and cities adopt the same health standards and regulations found in the state sanitary code.

The most effective governmental unit to exercise public health powers differs among the states. Those in which there is strong local control resist centralized public health authority (Figure 20-1). The state

and local authorities are under constant review in many jurisdictions.

Common law. A heritage from Great Britain, the common law derives from custom or court decision rather than from formally enacted statutes. Based on practice and experience, common law interprets a present situation in terms of past court decisions. Some health problems or controversies may be ad-

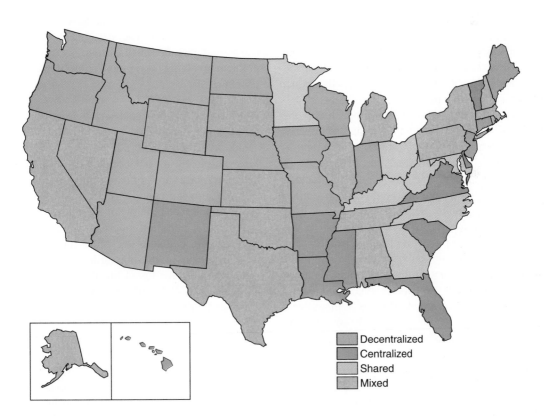

Decentralized
Centralized
Shared
Mixed

FIGURE 20-1

Relationships between state health agencies and local health departments in 1991 reflected the diversity of patterns based on history and political traditions of the various states and their degrees of home rule or local control.

Source: Centers for Disease Control: *Profile of state and territorial public health systems: United States, 1991,* Atlanta, 1991, U.S. Department of Health and Human Services.

judicated on the basis of custom or past practice. To this extent the common law represents a source of public health law.

Police Power

Police power is the authority of the people, vested in the state government, to enact laws, within constitutional limits, to promote the health, comfort, safety, order, morality, and general welfare of the people. This means the authority to promote the welfare of the public, which may sometimes necessitate restraining freedom and regulating the use of property. The police power is based on the concept of the greatest good for the greatest number of people and may operate to the inconvenience and even distress of certain individuals. All persons, business firms, and corporations must regulate their conduct subject to the police power.

Historically, the focus of public health was the protection of the public from the threats of diseases affecting large numbers of people, either communicated from infected animals or individuals or threats from identifiable environmental factors. With the increased emphasis on disease prevention and health promotion, threats to health have been identified from a wide variety of sources. The use of legal powers to protect a group of people, such as a ban on smoking in public places, can be interpreted as infringement on the individual rights of others. These kinds of debates related to public health law occur also around the use of motorcycle helmets, seat belts, emission controls on cars, and other laws intended to protect the greater good.

Limits. Any *reasonable* action taken under the shield of police power will tend to be upheld unless contrary to constitutional provisions. The First, Fourth, Sixth, and Fourteenth Amendments to the Constitution safeguard the personal rights of the citizen. Although the Constitution guarantees freedom of religious belief, such a guarantee does not invalidate a school board regulation requiring students to have a health examination or to be immunized before admission to school. Likewise it is a valid exercise of the police power for a state law to require marriage license applicants to have a physician's statement certifying that they are free from certain sexually transmitted diseases.

Jurisdiction. Any official health department has **jurisdiction** over all persons and things within its boundaries. A state law may extend the jurisdiction of a county or city health department beyond the county or city boundaries. Even in the absence of such law, a local health department may take action to correct a problem outside its territory if its own citizens are affected. The state health department can assume jurisdiction in a health dispute or health problem involving two or more cities or two or more counties.

Nuisance. A public health or environmental **nuisance** is one detrimental to the physical or mental health of one person or a large number of people. Most nuisances are not health threats, and not all health nuisances are of major importance.

The following conditions, which are nuisances, are of importance in terms of their threat to human health: water pollution, improper sewage disposal, air pollution, contaminated milk, food other than milk, lead paint in housing, rat infestation, stagnant water allowing for insect breeding, and excessive noise (see Part 4). Courts recognize three classes of nuisances: private, public, and mixed. If the nuisance cannot be corrected by negotiation, action to abate any one of these types may be taken by a private citizen or a public health official.

Health departments take all possible action to prevent nuisances by passing regulations declaring certain conditions to constitute nuisances. Such action is taken by state boards of health and local boards of health.

A nuisance that affects, injures, or damages only one individual or relatively few people, such as sewage from a septic tank flowing onto neighboring property, may be declared to be a private nuisance if the offended citizen takes court action. **Abatement** of a private nuisance may occur following a formal complaint or may require a suit for damages.

A nuisance that injures a considerable number of people, for example an industrial plant emitting objectionable fumes affecting a neighborhood, could be considered a public nuisance (Figure 20-2). A group of citizens may file court action or may request local health officials to take action in a court of equity. The court may issue an **injunction** forbidding the continuance of the condition, or may order the defendant to reduce the degree of offensiveness of the condition. Immediate action is sometimes necessary, and there is not always sufficient time to resort to court action. In this event quick abatement is the remedy.

Health Action on Nonhealth Nuisances

Some conditions declared to be health nuisances are actually of minor health significance, yet the public regards them as threats to health. Further, even though these conditions may have a minor effect on health, they can interfere with the enjoyment of life. Such conditions as the following, which have been declared to be nuisances, have slight health significance but are offensive: rubbish, untidy backyards, odors, pigsties, dead animals, garbage, and dumps. Well-defined legislation or regulations that make it an offense to cause or maintain objectionable conditions can be the basis on which health officials can proceed to correct offensive conditions. Even when a condition has been defined as a nuisance by law or regulation, diplomacy and tact should be used in taking steps to rectify the situation. It is an indication of competence in health administration when undesirable conditions can be corrected without resorting to extreme measures. However, education and diplomacy sometimes are not enough; court action may be necessary. In the absence of a regulation covering the situation, the board of health may cite a person to appear before it to answer charges of maintaining a nuisance.

LOCAL PUBLIC HEALTH ORGANIZATIONS

Multiple layers of government exist at the local level, which affect public health. Those discussed here include county government, the local board of health, and the **local public health agency** (LPHA). Depending on the size of the area served, these layers may be collapsed or highly stratified to develop public health policies and provide services. Some local areas depend for services on the state health agency (Figure 20-3).

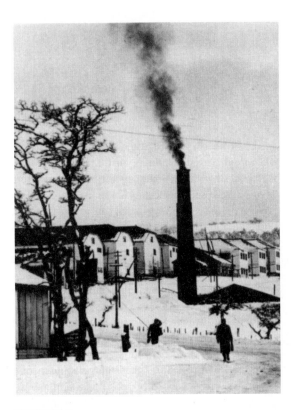

FIGURE 20-2
A public nuisance created by an industry will be tolerated more in small communities that feel dependent on that industry for jobs and economic survival than in larger cities where diversity of the economy makes the industry more expendable and therefore more accountable.

Source: WHO photo courtesy World Health Organization and International Labor Organization.

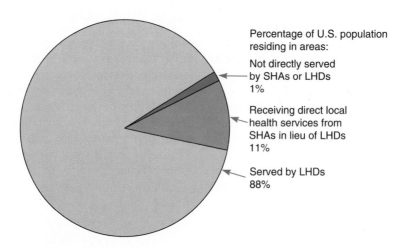

Percentage of U.S. population residing in areas:

Not directly served by SHAs or LHDs 1%

Receiving direct local health services from SHAs in lieu of LHDs 11%

Served by LHDs 88%

FIGURE 20-3
Percentages of U.S. population residing in areas served by local health departments (LHDs) or state health agencies in lieu of LHDs, or neither.
Source: Public Health Foundation and Centers for Disease Control and Prevention.

County Government

Authority to establish a LPHA in the United States is delegated by the state legislature to the legislative body of the county or parish. About 70% of counties have a county commission form of government structure. The commission consists of an elected board, ranging from 2 to over 100 members. A hallmark of the commission form of government is that commissioners share administrative responsibility with other independently elected officers such as the county clerk, auditor, assessor, treasurer, sheriff, and coroner. The commission is concerned with all matters of county government, including health.

The county commission usually appoints the county board of health. State statutes may specify how to choose the board of health and the type and number of people to serve. In some instances a county supervisor or commissioner may be appointed to the county board of health. This arrangement can promote coordination between the board of supervisors and the board of health. In other states the members of the county board of health must be

from outside the membership of the county commissioners.

The county commission has legislative powers that may include passing ordinances and adopting budgets, and administrative powers that many include supervising county departments, including health. The "home rule" option in 32 states provides counties with an opportunity to enact a "local constitution," which gives the county authority and power to levy taxes to pay for all county services and activities, including those of the local public health agency.

Local Board of Health

Local boards of health are used in most states to provide local input into or control of the operation of the LPHA. In nearly three quarters of the local public health agencies, the local board of health operates at the county level. In other areas the board may be at the city or town level or in some combined city and county combination. These local boards are concerned with the health needs of the citizens in the counties or cities they serve. Although not controlled by the state boards of health, the local boards may work with the state and other local boards on matters of health policy and services.

Appointed by the county commission, the local board of health may be composed of five, seven, nine, or any other number of members. Too small a membership may not provide adequate representation of the diverse public interests, and too large a number of members may create a debating assembly. Term of office varies from 3 to 6 years, and terms are staggered to provide for continuity as well as replacement. Many segments of the population have members on the board to assure that a cross-section of the population is represented. Usually at least one physician serves on the board, but no one profession should dominate the membership. A chairperson is elected by the board from among its own members. The county health officer usually serves as an **ex officio** member or as executive secretary of the board.

The local board of health has administrative, legislative, and quasijudicial functions. Among its administrative responsibilities, in 48 states the board appoints a health officer or director who provides leadership for the LPHA. Minnesota and Rhode Island have no local health officers. Local health officers are required to have a medical degree in 22 states; many health officers also have preparation in public health. The board may also approve professional staff appointed by the director. The local board of health votes on the budget, as recommended by the director, and then sends the budget to the county commission for approval. The commission has responsibility for the entire county budget, including that portion relating to health.

Legislative functions of the local board of health begin with the adoption of a sanitary code. This code, prepared by the professional staff, is usually the state sanitary code modified to fit the county situation. The county standards can be more rigid

than those of the state, but not less rigid. This county code has the effect of law. The board amends it from time to time as conditions require.

Quasi-judicial powers of the local board of health are inherent in the authority of the board to hold hearings preliminary to granting or revoking a license. The board has the authority to summon people to appear before it in cases where health regulations have been violated. Any decision by the board may be appealed to the courts by any citizen who believes that the decision was unjust.

Local Public Health Agency

LPHA organization. County governments are the most common type of local government structure within which the local public health agency operates. In 1991 there were nearly 3000 LPHAs across the United States. Approximately 65% of all LPHAs serve populations with fewer than 50,000 citizens. At the county level 72% of the LPHAs provide services, 11% at the town level, and the remainder have combined city and county, multicounty, or multicity arrangements. Contrasting forms of organization are found between Massachusettes and California. The former state has only one county health department (Figure 20-4). California has nearly all LPHAs organized at the county level, except two at the city level (Figure 20-5).

Some of the larger cities such as New York, Los Angeles, and Houston have a city health department that functions as the LPHA. In the early development of official health agencies in Europe and North America it was the city health department that was in most evidence. Baltimore established the first city health department in the United States in 1798. Virtually all U.S. cities had a health department of some description by the mid-twentieth century. With the spread of the population, the county became an increasingly functional level for providing public health services. In many situations smaller city health departments consolidate with county health

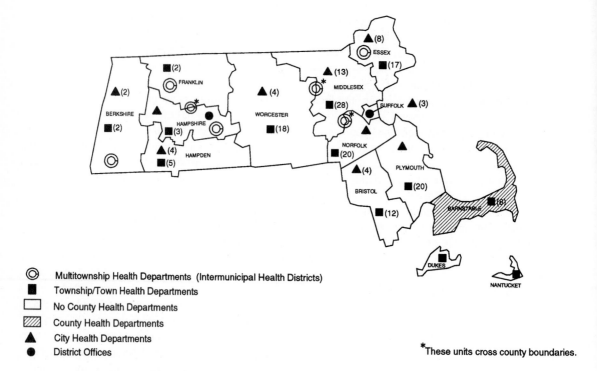

◎   Multitownship Health Departments (Intermunicipal Health Districts)
■   Township/Town Health Departments
☐   No County Health Departments
▨   County Health Departments
▲   City Health Departments
●   District Offices

*These units cross county boundaries.

FIGURE 20-4
Types of local health departments (LPHAs) by jurisdiction in Massachusetts in 1990 reflect the mixed forms of local government carried over from Colonial times.
Source: Centers for Disease Control: *Profile of state and territorial public health systems: United States, 1991,* Atlanta, 1991, U.S. Department of Health and Human Services.

departments. A city of 30,000 in a county of 70,000 will usually depend on a county health department rather than support a separate city department.

LPHA personnel. The health officer appointed by the local health board is usually the administrator for the LPHA. The health program of the LPHA is carried on by salaried professional personnel. The size of the staff depends on territorial area of the local public health area, the population, special health problems involved, resources, and the public's view of the importance of the work of the health department. In consideration of these varied criteria, the number of staff in LPHAs varies from one person to 26,000.

In the past the local health agency in smaller areas consisted of a part-time health officer, a quarantine officer, a sanitarian, and a clerk. Activities largely involved enforcing isolation and quarantine for the purpose of communicable disease control and inspection of unsanitary conditions.

Some small communities still have part-time health officers who are not trained in public health, who are political appointees, and who regard their public health duties as a side line to their medical practice. Fortunately, this situation now gives way to professionally staffed local public health agencies.

Forty-six percent of the LPHAs report a staff of nine or fewer full-time employees. Typically the

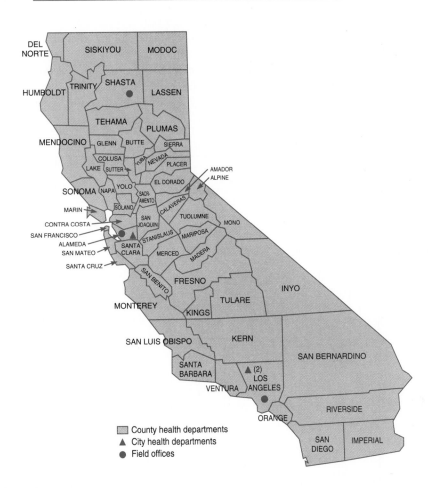

FIGURE 20-5
California has uniformly distributed county health departments. The three field offices enable the state health department to maintain field staff in three regions of the state, in addition to Sacramento. City health departments in San Jose and Los Angeles (San Francisco is a city-county combination) serve their special urban needs in large, dispersed counties.
Source: Centers for Disease Control: *Profile of state and territorial public health systems: United States, 1991,* Atlanta, 1991, U.S. Department of Health and Human Services.

majority of LPHAs serving fewer than 25,000 people employ a clerical employee (89%), a registered nurse (83%), and an engineer (65%). The employment of an clerk or administrative assistant is economically sound because it relieves the director of many routine, time-consuming tasks and increases the number of people that can be served. LPHAs serving up to 50,000 persons also report employing a physician (65%). LPHAs serving up to 100,000 persons may employ a health educator (54%) and a nutritionist or dietician (67%).

LPHA finances. Total expenditures for LPHAs are difficult to compare and interpret because of varia-

tions in their organization, responsibilities, and programs. Acceptable and adequate funding will depend on the problems of the community, the
public's perception of the importance of these problems and their causes, the efficiency of the organizations addressing them in raising local funds or obtaining state or federal grants, and the policies of the
state (SHA) in passing federal funds through to the
LPHA (Figure 20-6).

For economic reasons a population of 50,000 has

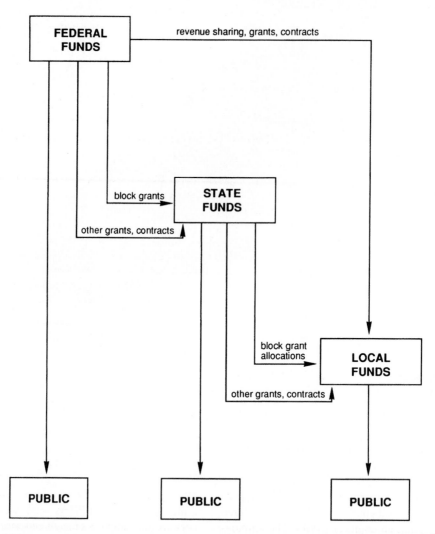

FIGURE 20-6

Block grants from federal to state and from state to local agencies have maximum flexibility for allocation to
various programs. Other grants, and especially contracts, have highly specific purposes that leave the recipient
agency little discretion in their allocation.

Source: Office of Disease Prevention and Health Promotion, U.S. Department of Health and Human Services.

long been regarded as the minimum unit for which a health department should be established. Smaller populations can either contract for services from the state or unite two or more sparsely populated areas into an LPHA with at least 50,000 people. Recently there have been debates about the minimum LPHA population, especially as some two thirds of all LPHAs in 1991 served fewer than 50,000.

LOCAL PUBLIC HEALTH SERVICES

Direct health services to the people of the community are provided by the full-time professional staff. General and specific services vary greatly among LPHAs within a state and from one state to another. A state legislature may require LPHAs to perform special services. For example, one state requires the LPHA to make medical investigations of death and child abuse while another state may require neither service. In many instances LPHAs may be providing the same service, but under different titles. For example, a service may be called family health in one LPHA and maternal and child health in another. To cite all types of service given by LPHAs would be to list unusual, rare, and minor services, along with those considered essential. The core functions and services discussed in the following pages are provided by virtually all full-time LPHAs (see box).

Vital Statistics

Biostatistics, public health statistics, human biometrics, and other terms designate public health recordkeeping. Vital statistics concern the vital facts of human existence, such as births, marriages, disease incidence, and deaths. For the health staff, vital statistics point out the health needs of the city or county as well as the strengths and weaknesses of the health program. Health data accrue from registration and enumeration.

Registration of certain health information is required by law and health regulations. Physicians

---

Ten Organizational Practices or Processes that Must Be Carried Out by a Component of the Public Health System in each Locality

Assessment

1. *Assess* the health needs of the community.
2. *Investigate* the occurrence of health effects and health hazards in the community.
3. *Analyze* the determinants of identified health needs.

Policy Development

4. *Advocate for public health, build constituencies,* and identify resources in the community.
5. *Set priorities* among health needs.
6. *Develop plans* and policies to address priority health needs.

Assurance

7. *Manage* resources and develop organizational structure.
8. *Implement* programs.
9. *Evaluate* programs and provide quality assurance.
10. *Inform and educate* the public.

---

must report to the LPHA cases of certain communicable diseases. To make reporting easy, all physicians are provided with a simple form on which the physician can quickly record pertinent data and can mail postage-free. Birth, death, and marriage records usually come from the county clerk.

Enumeration of health data usually requires that the health staff actively collect information. Health examinations, dental examinations, and water samples provide important information. Special surveys and studies also yield data regarded as important by the health staff, especially in relation to life-styles that influence chronic disease and injury rates.

Health statistics, not an end in themselves but a means to an end, can reveal health conditions, health levels, health needs, and health problems. Certain rates per year are of particular health significance. (See Chapter 3.)

Communicable Disease Control

Constant vigilance is necessary for communicable disease control. Programs can be planned and effectively administered so that epidemics do not occur and so that the number of outbreaks of communicable disease is held to a minimum (Figure 20-7). Such a control program requires certain preventive measures: (1) immunization, (2) public health education, (3) protection of water, milk, and other food supplies, (4) promotion of sanitation, and (5) control of carriers of disease. Control measures must concentrate on infected persons and their environment and entail (1) recognition of the disease, (2) prompt

reporting of all cases, (3) isolation procedures, (4) quarantine when warranted, and (5) decontamination.

In a recent national survey more LPHAs reported the provision of immunizations than any other public health service (Figure 20-8). Other communicable disease control measures rank among the most frequently provided services of LPHAs.

Maternal and Child Health

In maternal health promotion certain direct measures are taken to safeguard the health of the expectant mother, fetus, and later the newborn infant. These include promotion of prenatal care, postnatal care, and adequate delivery facilities. Indirect means of promoting maternal health include education for

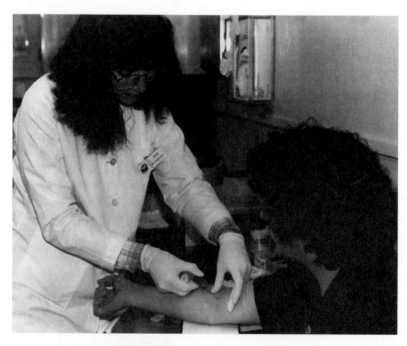

FIGURE 20-7
Immunization is the most frequently provided service of local public health agencies.
Source: Lincoln-Lancaster County Health Department, Lincoln, Nebraska.

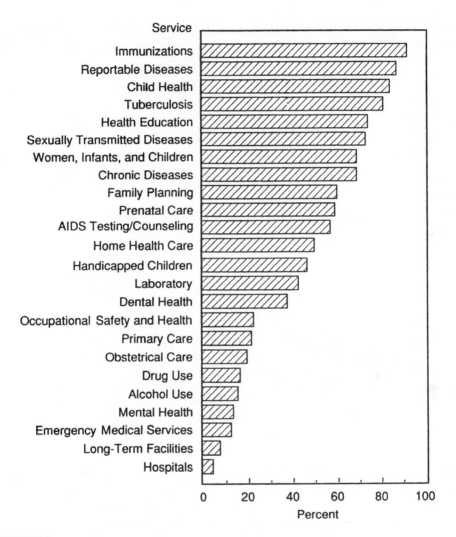

FIGURE 20-8

Percent distribution of selected services reported by 2263 local health departments (LPHAs).

Source: National Association of County Health Officials: *Selected characteristics of local health departments—United States,* 1989, *MMWR* 39:609, 1990.

family members, maternity benefits, day care, and family planning.

The LPHA provides education and some direct services for women and children. Direct services may include family planning, immunization, and well-baby clinics. In some communities the current organization of health service in the US places tension between public health agencies providing these services free to women and children and medical practitioners who charge for these services. The pre-

---

Family Planning

Guidelines for family planning, a high-priority program area for most local health departments, include the following:

- Family planning services offered through hospitals, health department clinics, private physicians, welfare agencies, and Planned Parenthood and other voluntary agencies should be monitored to assure that poor women who need these services have access.
- Services should be incorporated in existing health facilities in big cities and satellite clinics added to serve outlying neighborhoods, and rural areas, with priority given to services in or near officially designated "poverty" neighborhoods.
- Services should not be directed exclusively to any ethnic or racial group. Such restricted services would fail to reach the entire population in need and could foster suspicion among the targeted group that family planning advocates were seeking to reduce their numbers rather than to meet essential health needs.
- Overemphasis on welfare referral and reimbursement programs, including Medicaid, diverts attention from needed changes in the health system to make family planning available to all poor people.
- Clinics should be open evenings and weekends to serve working women. Transportation and baby-

sitting services are needed for mothers who otherwise must remain home to care for young children.
- Some of the women in need can be informed through newspapers, magazines, television, radio, and other traditional media. More personalized educational methods must be used for some.
- Humiliating marital-status restrictions on provision of services ignore the needs of women who are separated, widowed, divorced, or single.
- Good follow-up and outreach procedures will have long-term benefits for families in need of help.
- Services should seek to reach couples and individuals in their early twenties or even their teens, and should emphasize child spacing. By delaying and spacing pregnancies, young people have a greater opportunity to get more education, increase family income, and enjoy better health.

How do these recommendations illustrate the general approach to maternal and child health and preventive health delivery that should characterize all components of community health services? How would similar recommendations apply to other specific programs such as mental health services, hypertension control, adolescent health care, and geriatric care?

---

ventive nature of the services and the low income of most recipients enables such services to be provided.

Public health nurses are the key person in maternal and infant health. Prenatal visits may be made to high-risk mothers to provide education and counseling (Figure 20-9). Liaisons with hospitals identify new mothers in need of follow-up services. The public health nurse may do follow-up visits in homes to teach families about infant care and well-being. Families are assisted to understand the particular health needs and health problems of the infant, encouraged to have the infant examined at regular intervals by a physician, helped to secure medical diagnosis and treatment for the infant when

such needs are indicated, and taught about good nutrition, feeding, and parenting practices.

The LPHA receives most of its funding for maternal and child health services from the WIC program of the U.S. Department of Agriculture and the MCH block grants. The LPHA has an obligation to cooperate with all recognized agencies, including schools, that contribute to child health.

Chronic Disease Control

Many if not most of the organic diseases of the late years have their genesis in middle age or even early adulthood. Accordingly, adult health promotion gives emphasis to the middle years of life as well as

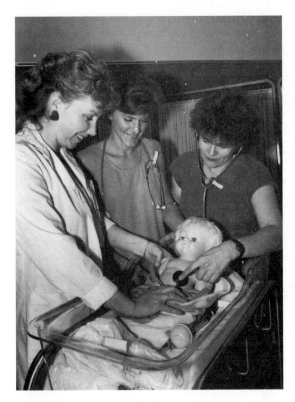

FIGURE 20-9
Public health nurses provide instruction in prenatal care and infant care to parents in classes and in home visits.
Source: University of Texas Health Science Center at Houston. Photo by Marsha Burkes.

to the elderly years. Indeed, preventive efforts directed toward the younger age groups can yield the most productive dividends. A constructive adult health promotional program ideally concentrates on the following three health factors:

1. Periodic screening and examination (Figure 20-10).
2. Correction of all remediable disorders
3. Health education that emphasizes moderation in use of alcohol, avoiding infection, diagnosis and treatment of infection and other symptoms immediately when they occur, nonsmok-

ing, exercise, proper diet, coping with stress, and checking with a physician when any abnormal condition persists

Community organization on the part of the health department is called for in getting adults examined and assuring proper follow-up of those screened. Cooperation with the medical society, industry, labor unions, and service organizations backed by a good promotional program through various media is required (see Chapters 4, 6, 7, and 12).

Mental Health Promotion

Major emphasis in mental health promotion is placed on the mental health of the normal individual. The modern mental health program offers individual and group counseling, seminars, institutes, hot lines, demonstrations, lectures, and other services. Psychiatric, psychological, and social work services are available to normal individuals, families, people with minor disturbances, delinquents, people with serious emotional problems, the disordered, people with alcohol- or drug-related problems, and those in the process of rehabilitation (see Chapter 9). The mere fact that a city, county, or district health department provides a mental health center where a person may go for consultation is extremely significant for citizens in the community. Some LPHAs integrate their drug and alcohol abuse education and substance abuse treatment programs into their mental health programs and services. They are supported by mass media and hotline services directly from the federal government and voluntary agencies (Figure 20-11).

Environmental Health Protection

Sanitarians are primarily occupied with public sanitation but provide consulting services when requested by householders. Home sanitation is encouraged through continuous educational measures. Most of the sanitarian's time and attention is directed to the inspection and appraisal of public water

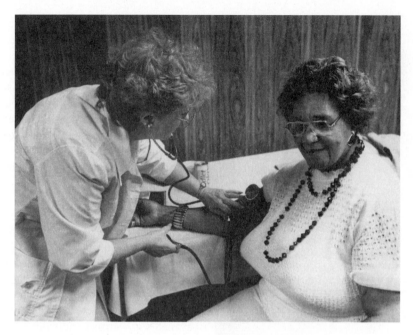

FIGURE 20-10
Blood pressure screening, referral and follow-up by local health department staff reaches high-risk groups who might not have regular access to medical care.
Source: Missouri Department of Health.

supplies, food services, milk and milk products, sewage disposal, public buildings, swimming pools, insect infestation, and industrial operations. Preventing disease is the primary goal of the sanitation program, but promotion of an esthetic environment is usually a secondary benefit. (See Chapters 13 to 16).

Laboratory Service

Most LPHAs in sparsely populated counties do not have their own laboratories but depend on the centralized laboratory of the state health department (see Chapter 19) or a local laboratory in a hospital or a clinic. Water plant operators are usually competent to run bacteriological and chlorine examinations of water. Even without its own laboratory a county health department can improvise sufficiently to provide limited laboratory service.

Having a local health department laboratory has many advantages in convenience and reduced time for running laboratory tests. Communicable disease control by means of laboratory tests requires promptness. Diagnostic tests, water and milk examinations, and food contamination tests can be done promptly in the local health department laboratory.

Dental Public Health

The most effective strategy for reducing dental caries and lost teeth is fluoridation of community water supplies. At an estimated cost of $1 per child per year, fluoridation remains the least expensive caries

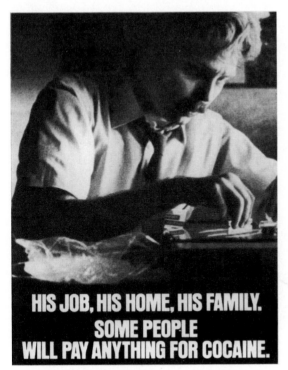

HIS JOB, HIS HOME, HIS FAMILY.
SOME PEOPLE
WILL PAY ANYTHING FOR COCAINE.

Cocaine really is expensive. Look what it almost cost this man.

He's getting help at a Drug Rehabilitation Center. They got help from the United Way. All because the United Way got help from you.

Your single contribution helps provide therapy for a child with a learning disability, a program that sends a volunteer to do the shopping for a 79 year-old woman, and a place for a 12 year-old to toss a basketball around after school.

Or, in this case, rehabilitation for a cocaine abuser. A man who, without your help, could very well have ended up paying the ultimate price.

United Way

It brings out the best in all of us.

FIGURE 20-11
United Way and other community agencies have formed coalitions to fight substance abuse.
Source: United Way of America and Advertising Council.

prevention measure. Every dollar spent for fluoridation will save $50 in dental bills. The benefits accrue to adults as well as children. Fluoride occurs naturally in most water, but usually at less than optimum levels. Since the introduction in 1945 of the practice of fluoridating community water supplies, there has been a steady increase in the number of people using water with levels of fluoride high enough to be significant for dental health. The national objective for 2000 is to assure that "at least 75% of the population on community water systems should be receiving the benefits of optimally fluoridated water." This is an example of a year 2000 objective that is lower than the previous objective set for 1990. Because of increasing amounts of fluoride consumed by the public in soft drinks and other processed foods, the target for community water supplies was lowered.

In addition to working on the fluoridation issue, some local health departments provide direct dental care to indigent populations, many conduct fluoride rinse programs for schoolchildren, and most support dental health education in the schools (Figure 20-12).

Health Education

The base of the pyramid called community health is public health education, and the breadth and stability of the base largely determines the height to which the pyramid can rise. Health education is effective to the extent that it constructively affects people's health knowledge, health attitudes, and health practices. To be effective, public health education must win public *acceptance* of a program or practice, arouse a *desire* in people to benefit from it, obtain the *involvement* of the people and support maintenance of changes in public health practice.

Public health education targets different segments of the population for different purposes. Direct communications with people whose health behavior places them at risk seek to inform them about and gain their acceptance of a program or practice

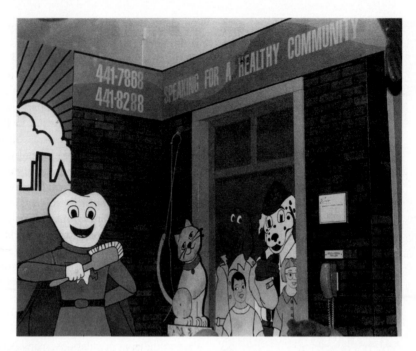

FIGURE 20-12
In 1992 the Dental Division of Lincoln-Lancaster County Health Department in Nebraska made 144 presentations to a total of 4245 elementary, junior high, and high school students on smokeless tobacco, conducted a school-based fluoride rinse program for rural schools, and placed this exhibit with the department's mascot, Mighty Molar, in the Children's Museum.
Source: Lincoln-Lancaster County Health Department.

and to increase their motivation to benefit from it. Indirect communications through parents, teachers, officials, employers, membership organizations, and peers are designed to provide a supportive social environment and reinforcement for behavior conducive to health. Additional communications directed to organizations such as service clubs, church groups, parent-teacher organizations, labor unions, health agencies, insurance companies, child study organizations, parent groups, and neighborhood organizations are designed to enable and facilitate good health habits by organizing community resources required for the health behavior to occur.

Public health education is beset by many obstacles, particularly false advertising, quackery, cult-

ism, superstition, professional and public indifference, and the human tendency to seek the easiest solution to every health problem. Yet a well-organized and effectively administered community health education program can have a substantial influence on the health of the community's population.

The head of the community health education or health promotion program has professional preparation as a community health education specialist. This person may supervise a number of organized units and individuals who have contributions to make. All members of the local health department staff engage in health education as part of their professional activities. The health educator coordinates the educational efforts of the staff, provides consultation, and initiates action that will involve other staff members of the department as well as other agencies in the community and lay self-help groups.

Voluntary health agencies, child health councils, schools, the medical society, the dental society, and a number of other organizations in the city, county, or district each contribute to health education. Imaginative, sensitive, and persistent leadership from the health department is required to get all of these organizations and individuals contributing in a coordinated way.

Numerous services and materials constitute the methods used in community health education. Each medium makes its own contribution, but it is the composite effect of a coordinated program that achieves the goal of a health-educated public (see Chapters 4 and 11).

Other Local Public Health Services

Through legislative requirement, local pressure, custom, or even coincidence, a local health agency may be engaged in one or more unique services not included in the usual list of responsibilities. Some local health agencies are responsible for the medical investigation of deaths of unknown cause. Child abuse cases and inspection of foster care homes may be referred to the health agency. Speech therapy, occupational and physical therapy, rehabilitation, and answering medical questions relating to commitment to nursing homes and mental hospitals are but some of the unique activities of different LPHAs. Someone must perform these services, but if these activities interfere with the effective performance of the basic public health functions, the public may lose more in health protection than it gains in social services.

Coalitions for Community Health

On the city, metropolitan, county, or district level, health coalitions have been valuable in coordinating the health activities of various agencies and individuals. Coalitions usually have no official status but are voluntary and composed of representatives from various organizations and groups having common health interests or goals. Coalitions usually have from 10 to 30 members, with representatives from such groups as voluntary health agencies, the medical profession, the dental profession, parent-teacher organizations, labor unions, chambers of commerce, women's clubs, church groups, social agencies, universities, and various other groups. The coalition usually represents a cross section of the organizations serving various population groups and can make known the health needs of the people. It can make recommendations to the LPHA and can be called on to support certain of its activities. It is sometimes the function of the United Way, but more often has an office in one of the participating organizations.

A community coalition can provide a valuable community service so long as it considers the overall health needs of the people and strives to assist, support, and supplement the health department. It serves as a health promoting force in the community and provides for citizen involvement in public health.

COMMUNITY HEALTH PROFESSIONALS

Health programs offered by local public health agencies are often provided by professionals specially trained in the field of public health. The core functions of public health are assessment, assurance, and policy development focused on health promotion and disease prevention at the community level, which may include environmental, physical, and mental health, and primary care. Appendix *A* identifies and describes areas of community health specialization. Appendix *B* lists common job titles in public and community health.

Community health professionals differ from those trained in personal health services by their emphasis on prevention over cure, populations over individuals, and community rather than clinical settings. A nurse, for example, working in the neonatal intensive care unit of a hospital is highly trained to work with the special equipment needed to save the life of a premature infant and to support the family in time of crisis. A community health nurse works to assure that mothers receive adequate prenatal care and education to reduce the chances of premature birth and low-birthweight babies. Both nurses are concerned about maternal and child health; the emphasis is different.

As the nation turns toward health care reform in the 1990s, greater emphasis on disease prevention and health promotion is universally acknowledged. The application of community health values, principles, knowledge, and technologies is essential to realize the benefits of effective health care reform. Many of the national goals adopted as part of Healthy People 2000 will depend on an adequate supply of those trained in community health. A 1993 report by the Bureau of Health Profession in the U.S. Department of Health and Human Services determined that there is currently a severe shortage of well-trained community health professionals, especially in the disciplines of epidemiology, biostatistics, environmental health, nutrition, and nursing (Table 20-1).

Much of the preparation of today's community health professionals focuses on schools of public health, preventive medicine programs in medical schools, public health nursing programs, and specialty public health or community health programs in a variety of disciplines. The community health emphasis is already seen in the preparation of some health professionals (Figure 20-13). For example, the University of Texas Health Sciences Center at Houston, which includes medical, dental, nursing, public health, and allied health schools, has recently adopted disease prevention and health promotion as its mission in training all health professionals.

TABLE 20-1

Projected supply of economically active public health graduates for selected categories of the professional health workforce for community health, United States, 1990-2000

	Estimated number of graduates economically active in the speciality†	
Area of specialization*	*1990*	*2000*
Biomedical and laboratory sciences	1,673	2,164
Biostatistics	2,787	3,606
Environmental sciences	7,247	9,377
Epidemiology	5,575	7,213
Health education	3,902	5,049
Health services administration	15,609	20,196
Nutrition	2,787	3,606
Occupational safety and health	1,115	1,443
Public health practice and program management	6,690	8,655
Other	8,362	10,819
TOTAL	55,747	72,128

Based on estimates and assumptions in Hall TL, Jackson RS, Parsons WB: *Schools of public health, trends in graduate education,* DHHS Pub. No. (HRA) 80-45, Washington, DC, May 1980, Division of Associated Health Professions, Public Health Service.

*See Appendix A of this text for description of the areas of specialization with illustrative jobs and job settings.

†Based on adjustments that eliminate most Canadian and other foreign graduates as well as the double counting that might result from persons with two or more degrees from schools of public health.

FEDERAL SUPPORT FOR COMMUNITY HEALTH SERVICES

Most countries subsidize local health services from state or national revenues. In the United States, the first major subsidies were federal grants-in-aid to states for maternal and child health programs and to state and local governments for the establishment and development of health departments (Titles V

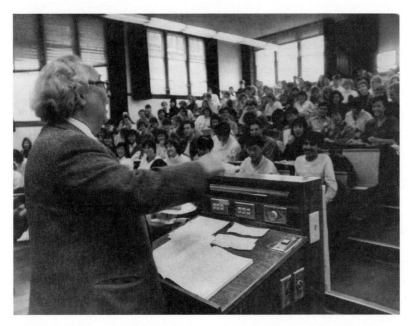

FIGURE 20-13
Students in the health professions today seek more emphasis on disease prevention and health promotion, humanities, and ethics. Allied health professionals and dental students are getting more of these subjects than are medical students.
Source: Photo courtesy University of British Columbia Community Relations Office.

and VI of the 1935 Social Security Act). Then came the Hill-Burton Hospital Survey and Construction Act of 1946, which assisted more than 3800 communities to build hospitals, extended care and rehabilitation facilities, and public health centers. The National Institutes of Health was also developed during this postwar period of federal investment, contributing over $14 billion toward the development and support of biomedical and health related research. Support for health manpower development also began during this period, providing traineeships for public health specialists, most of whom were already employed in community health agencies but without formal training in public health.

Politics and the Redistribution of Health Resources

By the early 1960s there was considerable disillusionment with the results of these massive investments in the three major areas of national health resources—facilities, knowledge, and personnel. The United States had reached the highest level of per capita expenditures for health in the world, but American health services and health statistics rated poorly among those of developed nations—in infant death rates; in the percentage of mothers who died in childbirth; in life expectancy; and in the death rate of males in their middle years.

The previous investment period had succeeded in building a massive health and medical care complex, but this complex had failed to adjust its structure appropriately to trends in the distribution of illness, demands for services, specialization of practitioners, development of more sophisticated medical equipment, and demands of office and hospital personnel for competitive wages. Physicians and hospitals clung tenaciously to traditions of individualism, endeavoring to be all things to their patients despite the obvious need to pool specialized facilities and services. Rural areas most notably were still without community health services. By the mid-1960s the United States had entered a period of ferment in the evolution of national health policy. New emphasis was placed on community health services and consumer participation in health planning.

Community mental health centers. In 1963 President Kennedy signed the Community Mental Health Centers Act. This act differed from earlier construction assistance acts in that it required centers to provide comprehensive services including outpatient care, consultation, and education. Approximately 400 community mental health centers had been established by 1970. The comprehensive approach required and the consequent innovations in delivery systems marked a new direction in organizational arrangements, with a citizen participation and community education orientation. Today, community mental health centers form a network of comprehensive services and provide continuity of care for patients discharged from state psychiatric facilities, and provide preventive services for the general population (see Chapter 9).

Maternal and Child Health, Mental Retardation, and Economic Opportunity Acts of 1963-1964. Also in 1963 the Maternal and Child Health and Mental Retardation Acts provided for similarly comprehensive, community-based approaches to prenatal and postnatal services for high-risk, low-income groups. These were combined into MCH Block grants in the 1980s. Maternity and Infant Care projects have been funded by grants from the U.S.

Department of Agriculture to many state and local health departments. (See Chapter 5.)

The Economic Opportunity Act of 1964 supported research, demonstration, and training for Neighborhood Health Centers. These grants resulted in widespread use of health care teams, indigenous community workers, and community health aides and, most significant from an educational perspective, serious attention to participation of the poor in the planning and evaluation of services. By mid-1969 about 50 projects had been funded, a drop in the bucket in relation to the needs and legitimate demands of the poor, but again significant in terms of the concepts demonstrated. Federal support for Neighborhood Health Centers declined in the 1970s.

Community action programs. The Economic Opportunity Act of 1964 created Community Action Programs, which moved consumer participation from a matter of voluntary action to a matter of public policy. Community action was suddenly defined in legal terms, which carried both new opportunities and new obligations for the poor. "Maximum feasible participation" was further mandated by PL 89-749 in 1965 (authorizing the establishment of Comprehensive Health Planning Agencies) and in the Model Cities Demonstration Act of 1966.

For all the good intentions behind the consumer participation movement, its legislated implementation was misunderstood or misused by many professionals. The "maximum feasible misunderstanding," as characterized by Daniel Patrick Moynihan a few years later, was the co-optation of consumer participants into managerial functions. This undermined the intent of the legislation and left many volunteer participants feeling exploited and suspicious of governmental purposes.

Regional medical programs. The purposes of the Regional Medical Program Act of 1965 were (1) to provide federal grants to establish regional cooperative arrangements among medical schools, research institutions, and hospitals for research and training (including continuing education) and for related demonstrations of prevention and patient care in the fields of heart disease, cancer, and stroke; (2) to afford the medical profession the opportunity of making available to patients the latest advances in diagnosis and treatment; and (3) by these means to improve generally the health manpower and facilities available in the nation, "without interfering with the patterns, or the methods of financing, of patient care or professional practice, or with the administration of hospitals, and in cooperation with practicing physicians, medical center officials, hospital administrators, and representatives from appropriate voluntary health agencies."

Note particularly the hesitation in this legislation to offend or challenge the medical establishment. This crippling clause made no mention of official (state or local) health agencies and no mention of health professionals or paraprofessionals other than those of the hospital "establishment." The Regional Medical Programs were phased out in 1976 with the advent of regional Health Systems Agencies (HSAs).

National Health Planning and Resources Development Act of 1974. Under a later federal health planning program, consumers participated in local and state efforts to correct many deficiencies and inequities in the delivery of health care. The National Health Planning and Resources Development Act of 1974 provided for a majority of consumers (51% to 60%) to serve on two major planning bodies—the more than 200 Health Services Agencies (HSAs), and the Statewide Health Coordinating Councils. These bodies, together with the State Health Planning and Resources Development Agencies, had broad authority over the allocation and development of health resources, including manpower, facilities, and services. Congress repealed this Act ten years later, after the Reagan administration systematically eliminated its budget support for the state and area health planning agencies (see Chapter 19).

Healthy Communities 2000: Model Standards

The Model Standards were developed by the American Public Health Association and the Centers for Disease Control and Prevention to help local and state agencies determine their own public health priorities and to establish objectives compatible with the national objectives for the year 2000. While many local communities share the vision of national objectives for disease prevention and health promotion, they lack blueprints to translate and implement these ideas in their own situations. The Model Standards help with this translation by the use of planning tools such as APEXPH (Assessment Protocol for Excellence in Public Health) and PATCH (Planned Approach to Community Health). The planning process for Model Standards differs from some community planning efforts in the past by linking communities nationally in a structured process to achieve identifiable local and national health goals.

11 Steps for Model Standards
Assess and determine the role of the public health agency within the community
Assess the lead health agency's organizational capacity
Develop an agency plan to build the necessary organizational capacity
Assess the community's organizational and power structures
Organize the community to build a stronger constituency for public health and establish a partnership for public health
Assess the health needs and available resources
Determine local priorities and available resources
Select outcome and process objectives that are compatible with local priorities and the *Healthy People 2000* objectives
Develop community-wide intervention strategies
Develop and implement a plan of action
Monitor and evaluate the effort on a continuing basis

The future of participatory planning. Remnants of the health-planning program survived the phase-out of the HSAs. Through the Model Standard and other planning processes, consumers continue to contribute to decisions that will help produce a more rational, responsive, effective, and equitable health care system. Good planning can, for example, help strike a better balance between the emphasis in health care from crisis intervention for the treatment of sick patients and the needs for prevention and health maintenance. Consumers can help restrain hospitals in acquiring expensive equipment—the community may not need all the available technology. Other problems also can be alleviated through more effective planning for the production and use of community health resources and services. Consider, for example, the following facts concerning the present U.S. system of health care.

- In general inner-city areas and remote rural sections are served by too few physicians.
- Primary care is often available only after the patient endures a long wait in a crowded waiting room or drives long distances to see a physician.
- The affluent areas of cities have built more hospitals than needed.
- The costs of medical care have been rising rapidly. Part of this increase is attributable to the poor location of health care facilities and the costs of staffing and equipping these facilities.

Active consumer leadership in health planning can help produce a more immediate and tangible impact on patients through improved service and staffing patterns, more equitable fees, a mechanism to respond to patient grievances, improved physical facilities, and, above all, care that protects the dignity and well-being of the individual patient. These and other issues of personal health care will be addressed in Chapter 21.

For the individual consumer participating in health planning, there are also benefits beyond promoting improvements in the health care system. Many consumers who have served on planning boards in the past report a deep sense of community involvement that has enriched their lives. Others found they had increased their effectiveness in other community activities.

In one respect, health planning is an educational process for the community. It is a way of making citizens, public officials, and health care providers aware of community needs, perceptions, and better ways of allocating health resources. By adding a nonprovider perspective, consumers can help create a climate in which community interests take precedence over special interests of dominant professions and institutions (Figure 20-14).

VOLUNTARY HEALTH AGENCIES

Non-tax-supported, voluntary health agencies provide opportunities for communities to fulfill needs beyond the scope or resources of official agencies. These voluntary health organizations have pioneered in promoting health programs and in demonstrating the contributions to health improvement that can be made. Frequently, when a voluntary health organization or a foundation demonstrates what can be done, the official agencies then enter the field and supplement the functions or services of the voluntary organization.

Two types of nongovernmental health organizations—professional health organizations and health foundations—were discussed in Chapter 18 because these tend to function at the national rather than local level and have relatively fewer local affiliates to provide direct support to community health programs. Foundations tend to identify neither with the voluntary, private sector, nor with the official, public sector, but refer to their niche as the "independent sector."

Background

In the late nineteenth and early twentieth centuries, governmental agencies took action reluctantly on

Public Policy Education Process In Context Of County Health Councils

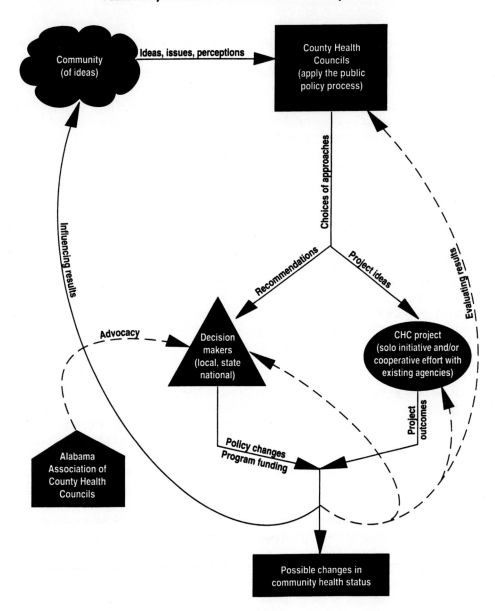

FIGURE 20-14

Alabama's county health councils and statewide Association of County Health Councils have taken the place of HSAs as a focal point for consumer and citizen participation in the planning and advocacy for health programs and reforms.

Source: Hooten EG, Raftery SR, Stalker V et al: *Alabama county health councils handbook,* Auburn University, 1992, Alabama Cooperative Extension Service, Alabama Department of Public Health, and University of Alabama at Birmingham School of Public Health.

existing health problems. They were slow to use available means for dealing with these problems and to develop new measures for disease prevention and control. Voluntary groups organized in response to the clear need to take progressive action to solve problems of disease prevention and control. Many such organizations have been formed, several of which will be discussed as representative of the types of voluntary health agencies that have served the public over the past half century or more at both national and community levels.

Examples

Lung association. Founded in 1904 as the National Association for the Study and Prevention of Tuberculosis, the American Lung Association was the first voluntary agency of the educational, promotional type. From the outset, education was the foundation of this association's program, based on the premise that, while it is essential to extend knowledge through scientific research, such knowledge serves few unless it is available to the public, medical practitioners, health personnel, and patients on the widest possible basis.

With the tuberculosis problem largely under control, in 1973 the American Lung Association turned much of its attention and efforts to the problem of emphysema and other disorders of the chest. The American Thoracic Society is a subsidiary of the American Lung Association composed of physicians and researchers who are specialists in **thoracic** diseases.

The association's program operates primarily on the community level. This emphasis has been responsible for much of the success of the program. The state association or affiliate has supervision over the local units. Financing of the association's program is primarily through Christmas Seal campaigns. The American Lung Association has an intensive and extensive research program, which is not limited to tuberculosis but includes various diseases of the chest, including those associated with smoking, occupational hazards and air pollution.

Cancer associations. The American Cancer Society, Inc, was founded in 1913 "to disseminate knowledge concerning the symptoms, diagnosis, treatment, and prevention of cancer; to investigate the conditions under which cancer is found; and to compile statistics in regard thereto." The society was established largely through the efforts of medical professionals, although the work of the organization has been carried on largely by lay people. Australia and other countries have counterpart associations called Cancer Foundations.

The leadoff educational program was designed to acquaint the public with the fact that cancer in its early stage can be cured, that early diagnosis is of primary importance, and that prompt, scientific treatment is the acknowledged method of cure. The educational campaign used an impersonal approach in an effort to avoid arousing fear of cancer.

In addition to public health education, the society has encouraged health departments to expand their cancer programs, stimulated medical schools to extend their work in cancer research, helped to organize a National Advisory Cancer Council, which influenced the passage of the National Cancer Act and the creation of the National Cancer Institute as a part of the U.S. Public Health Service. Together with the American Lung Association and the American Heart Association, the American Cancer Society joined forces to create the National Interagency Council on Smoking.

The state affiliate of the society is called a "division" and, to use Michigan as an example, is titled American Cancer Society, Inc., Michigan Division. Operation of the program is basically on the county level and enlists the active participation of lay people in a program of health education.

Income of the American Cancer Society is derived from donations, dues, endowments, and legacies. In many instances citizens losing a family member because of cancer assign life insurance benefits to the society. The official publications of the society are *Cancer—A Journal of the American Cancer Society, CA—A Cancer Journal for Clinicians,* and *Cancer News.*

The March of Dimes Birth Defects Foundation. Founded in 1938 as the National Foundation for Infantile Paralysis, the March of Dimes Birth Defects Foundation has made substantial contributions to the health field. President Franklin D. Roosevelt, stricken by poliomyelitis, gave his personal support to the foundation and thereby gave great impetus to the organization. From its start, the foundation was financed through the March of Dimes Program. Children saved allowances and contributed their own dimes during community drives. Now it sponsors ''Walkathons'' and other community fund-raising events. Several state chapters and more than 900 local chapters reach into virtually every county in the United States with programs now concentrated on birth defects prevention, including prenatal care, teenage pregnancy prevention, and reduction of smoking, drug use, and alcohol use by pregnant women. The present program also includes investigation into birth defects (congenital defects) and genetic and nutritional disorders of the newborn.

Local chapters that are branches of the national organization give direct medical assistance and raise funds to maintain national and local activities. A considerable part of the funds raised locally remains in the community to promote the local program.

Financial assistance from the March of Dimes was instrumental in demonstrating the effectiveness of the Salk vaccine in the 1954 poliomyelitis vaccine field trial. This assistance resulted in the shortest elapsed time between the discovery of a preventive measure and its widespread use.

Heart associations. Originally formed as a scientific and professional organization of physicians interested in heart disease, the American Heart Association was reorganized in 1948 as a voluntary health agency with thousands of nonprofessional members affiliated with their state associations. The objective of the association is to prevent and control heart disease through research, professional education, public education, and community service. Canada and other countries have counterpart organizations called Heart Foundations.

State and local heart associations have a large corps of volunteers who work together to plan and execute the associations' programs. The state heart association has a professional staff, which provides consultation services and works with the professional and lay volunteers in planning and implementing both the education and fund-raising aspects of the program.

Through community service the associations train volunteers in blood pressure measurement. They provide rheumatic fever control programs to prevent secondary attacks in individuals who have had a first attack. They also provide smoking cessation, nutrition, and weight control programs; speakers' bureaus; school health programs; and work simplification programs that demonstrate methods to help people who have had heart attacks organize their housework in a manner that will prevent unnecessary fatigue. The associations also maintain information and referral services that include directories of cardiac services.

Funds are raised by state drives and come from voluntary contributions, endowments, and legacies. Most of the American Heart Association funds go into heart research or an allied activity.

The Red Cross. The international Red Cross and Red Crescent societies have been most notable for their disaster relief and wartime care of casualties. The Red Cross was founded in 1881 in accordance with the Geneva Treaty of 1864, which was ratified by the United States in 1882, thanks to the efforts of Clara Barton.

The American Red Cross has a quasi-governmental status because it is incorporated under a charter granted by Congress in 1900. The president of the United States is president of the American Red Cross, an affiliate of the international organization, which has 127 national Red Cross societies. In times of peace the American affiliate has established health centers, helped to conduct public health surveys, sponsored health demonstration projects and first aid and water safety programs, and provided public health nursing service for rural areas that were not otherwise served. In 1981 the American Red Cross adopted a new set of priorities emphasizing health promotion and disease prevention. Its blood banking program has been most salient in recent years because of the AIDS epidemic. During natural disasters such as the San Francisco earthquake in 1989, Hurricane Andrew in 1992, and the great Midwest floods of 1993, the Red Cross provided relief efforts and organized volunteers to help the local victims (Figure 20-15).

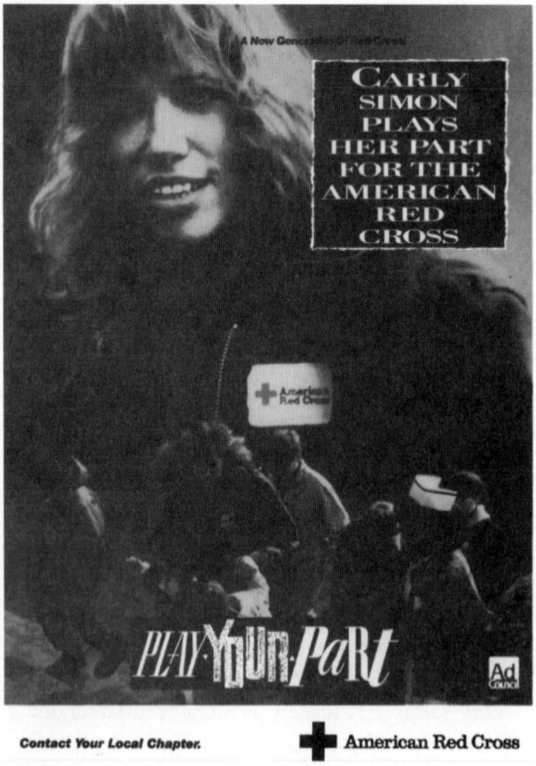

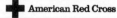

FIGURE 20-15
The Red Cross, like most of the voluntary health agencies, depends heavily on volunteers. Recruitment and fund-raising occupy a good deal of staff time.
Source: American Red Cross and Advertising Council.

The Red Cross works closely with private and governmental agencies at all levels—national, state, and community, as a matter of policy. County chapters are formed but operate under the supervision of the national office, which establishes policies and must approve all local projects.

The National Urban League. Health has been a core program activity of the National Urban League since 1910. During its early years the National Urban League published a monthly health education bulletin, and for more than 20 years it stimulated local efforts such as dental clinics, immunization programs, tuberculosis screening, well-baby clinics, and a variety of convalescent care programs through its Annual Health Education Week.

Frustrated in its attempt to eliminate discrimination in employment in the health professions and in health facilities, the National Urban League, led by Dr. Montague Cobb, joined forces with the National Medical Association, the National Association for the Advancement of Colored People (NAACP), and the Medico-Chirurgical Society. This coalition spearheaded a vigorous attack on hospital discrimination between the late 1950s and the mid-1960s.

In 1962 the National Urban League adopted a policy statement supportive of family planning in the interest of strengthening family life and reducing individual and family dependency on welfare. This was a courageous move at a time when family planning was viewed by some black activists as **genocide.**

The league has administered a number of federally funded research and demonstration programs in the health field. These projects have included evaluations of consumer health education and training programs, a study of health manpower resources and facilities in 30 cities, a poison control project, the development of allied health careers curricula in traditionally black colleges, dental services for preschool children, and a sickle-cell education/screening program.

The National Urban League firmly supports legislation for comprehensive and universal national health insurance and improvement of health services in local communities. The league continues to address these crucial issues through public testimony and participation in organized, broad-based coalitions.

The Preparing Adolescents for Responsible Parenthood Project has been the centerpiece to the national office's concern with the increase of pregnancies among black and other minority teenagers. Its importance has been increased by the Supreme Court's ruling that neither the Medicaid statute nor the Constitution requires the federal government or states to provide funding for all medically necessary abortions. It has been estimated that 35% of women receiving Aid to Families with Dependent Children (AFDC) who would have had abortions financed by Medicaid will now go full term with their pregnancies. Many of these will be young teenagers, ages 12 to 16, who are least capable emotionally, physically, or economically to be parents. The National Urban League project seeks to increase the quality and quantity of information and services, both preventive and supportive, available to minority youth.

The National Urban League has identified health promotion and disease prevention as the area in which nonmedical community-based organizations can play a significant and strategic role in improving the health status of black Americans. Organized programs for health advocacy and health promotion activities are kept realistic for National Urban League affiliates with limited health personnel and financial resources.

Other nonprofit organizations. The national offices of these and other voluntary health agencies have attempted to ensure that new health legislation and special federal initiatives addressing community health provide for the participation of nonmedical community-based organizations. (See, for example, the discussion of coalitions on p. 621). Thus future

health programs in such areas as high blood pressure education, cancer education and screening, physical fitness, and nutrition will be more likely to provide for local outreach information and education activity. Community-based organizations such as heart associations and National Urban League affiliates can qualify to operate funded programs in these health care areas. Funding, for the most part, must be obtained at the state level. This makes it particularly important for local affiliates of voluntary health agencies to stay abreast of statewide planning and the allocation of health funds to the local level from block grants at the state level.

SCHOOL HEALTH PROGRAM

The school health program, although dedicated to and supported by the education sector, should be considered as part of the community health program and thus be integrated with it. The health of the children and the health of the other members of the community should be the concern of the school, because the school can contribute to both and can benefit in its educational mission from both.

School health programs include health services, health instruction, and a healthful environment. Health services provide appraisal and remediation of existing health related conditions and prevention of future health problems. Health instruction addresses the future health of children through planned and incidental instruction. Healthful school environments include a sanitary and safe physical environment. It also incorporates consideration of the mental health of students and teachers. Administrators, teachers, parents, cafeteria workers, and the custodial staff are all potential contributors to a healthful school environment.

Schools play a role in communicable and chronic disease control. Schools have the legal authority and the responsibility to take reasonable measures for promoting of immunization. Courts have upheld the right of local boards of education to require immu-

---

> ### Case Study of a "Know Your Body" Program
>
> A systematic application of the planning principles outlined in Chapter 4 were applied in Washington, DC with Black children in grades 4 to 6 who were attending 9 District of Columbia elementary schools. The social problems of Black children in these schools were those associated with poverty, as shown in Figure 20-16. This schematic diagram also shows how the diagnostic planning model outlined in Chapter 4 was applied to identify the epidemiological relationships, the behavioral risk factors and preventive behaviors determining the health problems, the health skills that could influence the preventive behaviors, and the educational factors that a coordinated school program could influence to improve health skills (reading from right to left in Figure 20-16). At the end of two years of intervention, results indicated that the program significantly reduced blood pressures, postexercise pulse recovery rates, cholesterol levels, and smoking. Significant improvements were found also for health knowledge and attitudes toward smoking.
>
> Schools need not develop their own health curriculum and teaching materials from scratch. Numerous model curricula and media are produced by organizations such as the American Health Foundation ("Know Your Body"), the voluntary health associations, and various state and federal health agencies.

nization as a condition for school admission. Early recognition of infectious disease in schools depends on recognition by the teacher and confirmation by the school nurse. During an epidemic schools work cooperatively with the local public health agency and are governed by the regulation and recommendations of the LPHA. Although schools would seem to have a lesser role in chronic disease control, the most important risk factors for such diseases develop at young ages and track into adult life. Comprehensive school health education plays an important role in preventing these risk factors (see box and Figure 20-16).

WORKSITE HEALTH PROMOTION PROGRAMS

Employers have specific responsibilities by law for the protection of workers from illness or injury that could result from the work environment. These were outlined in Chapter 15. As a member of the community, the employer also has an opportunity to promote the health of workers, their families, and the community through policies and provisions that enable employees to have greater access to health services and health enhancing facilities. Specifically, screening programs and employee wellness programs have become increasingly common in large worksites around the United States. As an adjunct to community health programs, these sites provide the equivalent opportunity for adult health that schools provide for child health.

Scope of Worksite Health Promotion Programs

A national survey of worksites with 50 or more employees found that two thirds had one or more health promotion programs, facilities, or services. More than half of these had been started within the past five years. The types of programs ranged from health risk assessment (30%) to smoking cessation (36%), blood pressure control and treatment (16%), exercise and fitness (22%), weight control (15%), nutrition education (17%), stress management (27%), back problem prevention and care (28%), and off-the-job injury prevention education (20%).

Issues in Worksite Health Promotion

Despite their popularity with employees and their growing acceptance as a responsibility by employers, many health professionals have expressed concerns about the worksite wellness programs. The rapid development and diffusion of these programs have taken on the features of a social movement. Professionals who have devoted their careers to

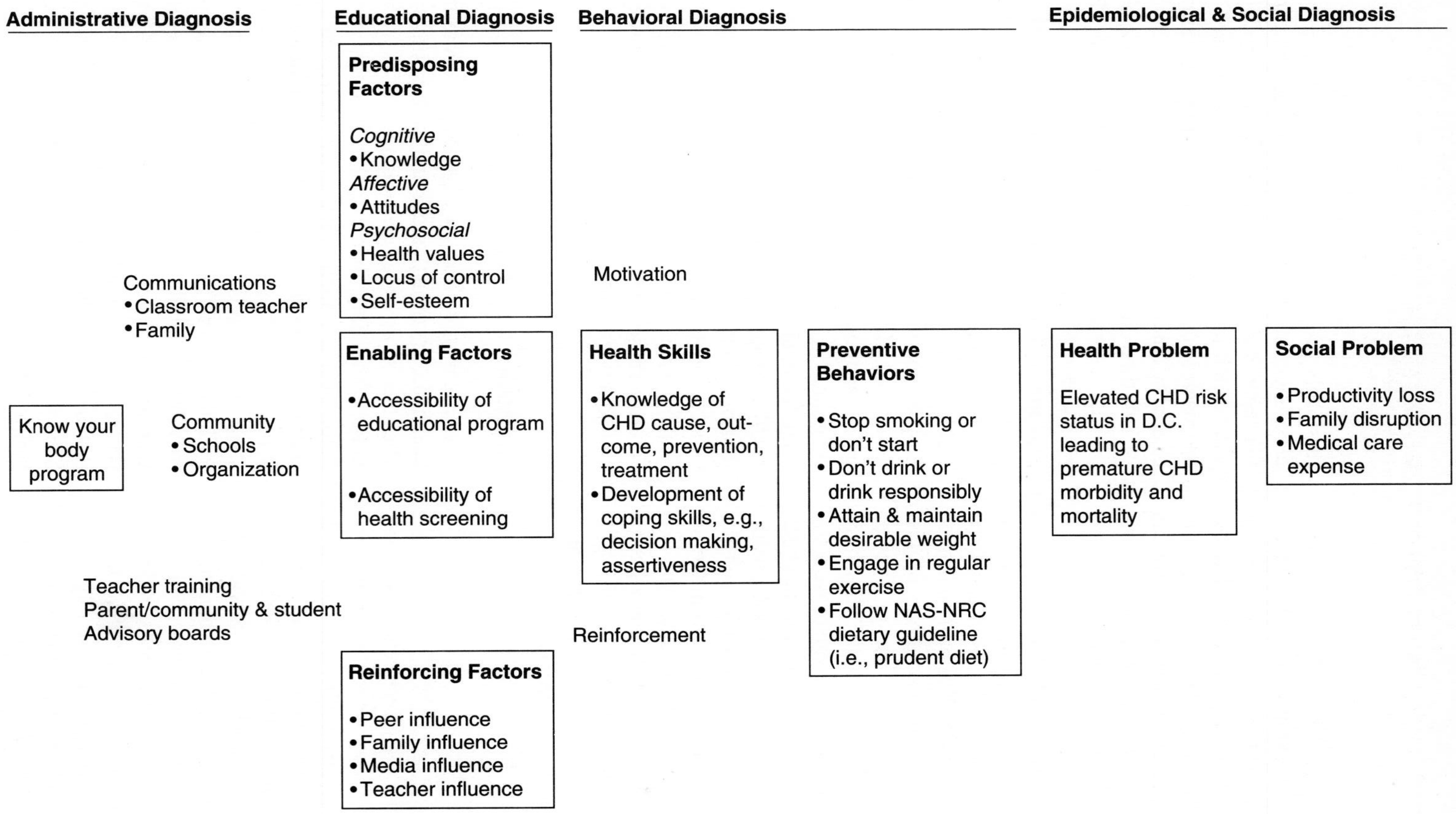

Administrative Diagnosis | **Educational Diagnosis** | **Behavioral Diagnosis** | **Epidemiological & Social Diagnosis**

Predisposing Factors

Cognitive
- Knowledge

Affective
- Attitudes

Psychosocial
- Health values
- Locus of control
- Self-esteem

Social Problem
- Productivity loss
- Family disruption
- Medical care expense

Health Problem

Elevated CHD risk status in D.C. leading to premature CHD morbidity and mortality

Preventive Behaviors
- Stop smoking or don't start
- Don't drink or drink responsibly
- Attain & maintain desirable weight
- Engage in regular exercise
- Follow NAS-NRC dietary guideline (i.e., prudent diet)

Motivation

Health Skills
- Knowledge of CHD cause, out-come, prevention, treatment
- Development of coping skills, e.g., decision making, assertiveness

Enabling Factors
- Accessibility of educational program
- Accessibility of health screening

Reinforcement

Communications
- Classroom teacher
- Family

Reinforcing Factors
- Peer influence
- Family influence
- Media influence
- Teacher influence

Community
- Schools
- Organization

Know your body program

Teacher training
Parent/community & student
Advisory boards

FIGURE 20-16
The planning model similar to that outlined in Chapters 4 and 12 was applied in a school-based community project to reduce heart disease risk factors in children. It produced significant improvements in several behavioral and physical measures of risk.

Source: From Bush PJ: *Am J Epidemiol* 129:466, 1989. Reproduced with permission.

worker protection through the regulatory and collective bargaining routes express concern that the worksite health promotion programs could divert resources and attention from the prevention of occupational hazards in the work environment or the working conditions. Other health professionals worry that the scientific bases for promoting some of the life-style modifications in these programs have not been sufficiently validated.

Another issue that must be addressed in the further development of the worksite health promotion movement is the extent to which the programs reach the people who need them most. The programs have generally served white collar (executive, professional, and managerial) personnel and to a lesser extent ''pink collar'' workers (clerical). They have barely penetrated the blue collar stratum of workers. Furthermore, the intensity of the programs has been limited by the problem of release time from work, hours of availability during the workday, and the cost of maintaining the programs. These limitations have resulted in variable participation rates and low maintenance rates. These problems plague all community health promotion programs, but the presumed advantage of the worksite in overcoming some of these problems has been less than complete.

EVALUATION

It is difficult to measure the effectiveness or value of community, school, and worksite health programs in terms of lives saved, illnesses prevented, and health improved. Inferential means of appraising a health program are based on the assumption that if certain activities or services are provided by a health or teaching staff, certain health benefits accrue to the public. This inference is based on independent studies, which have shown that certain services and activities produce certain public health results. This approach to evaluation is simply an accounting of services rendered, however. A considerable number of public health and education professionals prefer to specify the services a health department in a school should provide and contend that appraisal *should* be based on the proficiency with which the staff performs these services. This approach to evaluation is called **quality assurance** or quality control.

Full-time city, county, or district health agencies provide a direct health service available to all citizens within the area. This service provides the various means for reducing the incidence of disease, lowering the death rate, reducing invalidism and dependency, preventing disabilities, correcting remediable defects, decreasing wage losses, reducing hospital and medical costs, and reducing hazards to health and life. Some agencies attempt to get periodic measures of these outcomes to appraise their programs.

In the final analysis the evaluation of community health services is greatly complicated by the relationship of health outcomes with aspects of poverty, culture, and the environment over which community health agencies, schools, and worksites have limited control. These relationships must be acknowledged and addressed by the community.

SUMMARY

The community derives most of its authority in health matters from the state and from common law. The state or province delegates much of its authority to the community, then exercises its rights of regulation over the quality of services delivered by the community health agency. The community establishes a health board at the municipal, county, or (in some states and Canada) district level to look after its interests. In 1974 the U.S. federal government introduced additional levels of planning authority with the establishment of Health Systems Agencies (HSAs), but most of these have not survived the cuts in federal subsidies for their funding in the 1980s. Model Standards for communities provides opportunities for local public health agencies to link local areas with national objectives in disease prevention and health promotion.

Community health agencies include the official local public health agency, other official agencies having health responsibilities, private organizations with proprietary interests in health, and a variety of voluntary agencies that address health concerns. Coordination of these entities is accomplished through United Way agencies or other health councils, sometimes staffed by official health department personnel.

The minimum services provided by the official community health agency include vital statistics recordkeeping, maternal and child health care, communicable and chronic disease control, mental health services, laboratory services, and health education.

Consumers have an obviously deep and primary interest in community health services. The health professions alone cannot be the sufficient guardians of that interest. Consumers must have effective representation—wherever possible, a majority—in the policy-making processes of major health facilities and organizations. This representation must reflect all aspects of the community, including cultural, racial, and linguistic diversity. Special emphasis should be placed on meaningful representation of the poor and minority groups.

QUESTIONS FOR REVIEW

1. About one fourth of the counties (and parishes) in the United States are without full-time professional health service. What is the explanation for this situation?
2. If you lived in a county or parish without a full-time health department, what measures would you take to obtain full-time public health service?
3. Why do people in the low-income groups benefit most from the county health department program?
4. Is it just or unjust that some people get more service than others from the county health department?
5. Which health department in the United States—federal, state, or local—is most likely to give service to the individual citizen?
6. What are some regulations the state has established through the exercise of the police power in the United States?
7. Why aren't laws and regulations passed identifying as nuisances all conditions and practices that might cause hurt, injury, or inconvenience to people?
8. If a local health department refuses to take action to stop a condition that citizens regard as a nuisance, what action can the citizens take?
9. Why should there not be only medical doctors on the county board of health?
10. Why should decisions by the county board of health be subject to appeal to a court?
11. Why is it not logical to say that one position on the county health staff is more important to the public than is another?
12. Why should public health education employ a variety of media and methods of communication?
13. In matters of health, why should schools be concerned with more than just health education in the classroom?
14. What evidence can you present that people in the United States and Canada have better health today than those who lived there at the turn of the century, and what has been the contribution of official and voluntary health agencies?
15. Why must the development of worksite health promotion involve blue collar workers in the planning?

READINGS

Dabbagh L, Green LW, Walker GM: Case study: application of PRECEDE and PROCEED as a framework for designing culturally sensitive diarrhea prevention programs and policy in Arab countries, *Int Q Community Health Educ* 12:293, 1991-92.

Intensive interviews with women in their homes where direct observation of behavior and environmental conditions of living could verify their understanding and perception of home and community threats to the health of their infants. This produced recommendations for a community health program and policy, which were developed out of the application of the planning model introduced in this book.

Hancock T: The evolution, impact and significance of the Healthy Cities/Healthy Communities movement, *J Public Health Policy* 14:5, 1993.

Describes the evolution of the concept and plans of Healthy Cities from the inspiration of Toronto in 1984, through the planning of European Healthy Cities by the World Health Organization Regional Office, to the 18 national networks in Europe and North America and hundreds of towns and cities actively involved in attempting to bring about local policy changes for health, sustainability, equity, housing, and safety.

MacDougall H: *Activists and advocates. Toronto's health department, 1883-1983,* Toronto and Oxford, 1990, Dundurn Press.

This chronicle of the history of the City of Toronto Department of Public Health during its first hundred years captures the spirit of the public health movement during the latter nineteenth and early twentieth centuries, and how local citizens and health professionals advocated and worked for better community living conditions and life-styles.

BIBLIOGRAPHY

Braddy BA, Orenstein D, Brownstein JN et al: "PATCH: an example of community empowerment for health, *J Health Educ* 23:179, 1992.

British Columbia Ministry of Health and Ministry Responsible for Seniors: *New directions for a healthy British Columbia: a guide for developing community health councils and regional health boards,* Victoria, 1993, The Ministry.

Brunk SE, Goeppinger J: Process evaluation: assessing reinvention of community-based interventions, *Eval Health Professions* 13:186, 1990.

Bush PJ, Zuckerman AE, Theiss PK et al: Cardiovascular risk factor prevention in black school children—2-year results of the Know Your Body Program, *Am J Epidemiol* 129:466, 1989.

Byrd T: Project Verdad: a community development approach to health, *Hygie: Int J Health Educ* 11:15, 1992.

California Conference of Local Directors of Health Education: *Standards of practice for public health education in California local health departments,* Sacramento, 1993, The Conference.

Chavis DM, Wandersman A: Sense of community in the urban environment: a catalyst for participation and community development, *Am J Community Psychol* 18:55, 1990.

Dignan MB, Pheon EB, Michielutte R et al: Development of a direct education workshop for cervical cancer prevention in high risk women: the Forsyth County Project, *J Cancer Educ* 5:217, 1990.

Farquhar JW, Fortmann SP, Flora JA et al: Effects of community-wide education on cardiovascular disease risk factors—the Stanford 5-city Project, *JAMA* 264:359, 1990.

Floyd JD, Lawson JD: Look before you leap: guidelines and caveats for schoolsite health promotion, *J Health Educ* 23:74, 1992.

Flynn BS, Worden JK, Secker-Walker RH et al: Prevention of cigarette smoking through mass media intervention and school programs, *Am J Public Health* 82:827, 1992.

Freyens P, Mbakuliyemo N, Martin M: How do health workers see community participation? *World Health Forum* 14:253, 1993.

Gottlieb NH, Lovato CY, Weinstein R et al: The implementation of a restrictive worksite smoking policy in a large decentralized organization, *Health Educ Q* 19:77, 1992.

Gorman M, Mallon D: The role of a community-based health education program in the prevention of AIDS, *Med Anthro* 10:159, 1989.

Green LW, Kreuter MW: CDC's Planned Approach to Community Health as an application of PRECEDE and an inspiration for PROCEED, *J Health Educ* 23:140, 1992.

Hunnicutt DM, Perry-Hunnicutt C, Newman IM et al: Use of the Delphi technique to support a comprehensive campus alcohol abuse initiative, *J Health Educ* 24:88, 1993.

Jones CS, Macrina D: Using the PRECEDE model to design and implement a bicycle helmet campaign, *Wellness Persp* 9:68, 1993.

Kreuter MW: PATCH: its origin, basic concepts, and links to contemporary public health policy, *J Health Educ* 23:135, 1992.

Kroger F: Preventing HIV infection: educating the general public, *J Primary Prev* 12:7, 1991.

Levine DM, Becker DM, Bone LR: Narrowing the gap in health status of minority populations: a community-academic medical center partnership, *Am J Prev Med* 8:319, 1992.

Michielutte R, Beal P: Identification of community leadership in the development of public health education programs, *J Community Health* 15:59, 1990.

Miller CA, Moore KS, Richards TB et al: Longitudinal observations on a selected group of local health departments: a preliminary report, *J Public Health Policy* 14:19, 1993.

Monekosso GL: African universities as partners in community health development, *J Community Health* 18:127, 1993.

Orenstein D, Nelson C, Speers M, et al: Synthesis of the four PATCH evaluations, *J Health Educ* 23:187, 1992.

Potvin L, Paradis G, Laurier D et al: Le cadre d'intervention du Projet Québécois de Démonstration en Santé du Coeur, *Hygie: Int J Health Educ* 11:17, 1992.

Silverfine E, Brieger W, Churchill W: Community-based initiatives to eradicate guinea worm: a manual for Peace Corps volunteers, Washington, DC, 1990, U.S. Peace Corps and Agency for International Development.

Simons-Morton BG, Brink SG, Parcel GS et al: *Preventing alcohol-related health problems among adolescents and young adults: a CDC community intervention handbook,* Atlanta, 1989, Centers for Disease Control.

Simons-Morton DG, Parcel GS, Brink SG et al: Smoking control among women: needs assessment and intervention strategies. In Ward WB, Lewis FM, editors: *Advances in health education and promotion,* vol 3, London, 1991, Jessica Kingsley.

Steckler A, Orville K, Eng E et al: Summary of a formative evaluation of PATCH, *J Health Educ* 23:174, 1992.

Steckler AB, Israel BA, Dawson L et al, editors: Community health development: an anthology of the works of Guy W. Steuart, *Health Educ Q* Suppl 1, 1993.

Swannell R, Steele J, Harvey P et al: PATCH in Australia: elements of a successful implementation, *J Health Educ* 23:171, 1992.

Worden JK, Solomon LJ, Flynn BS et al: A community-wide program in breast self-examination training and maintenance, *Prev Med* 19:254, 1990.

World Health Organization Collaborating Center for Research, Training, and Eradication of Dracunculiasis: *Guidelines for health education and community mobilization in dracunculiasis eradication programs,* Atlanta, 1991, Centers for Disease Control and Global 2000, Carter Center, Inc.

Chapter 21

Health Care Services and Resources

❖

One of the first duties of the physician is to educate the masses not to take medicine.
SIR WILLIAM OSLER, M.D.

The greatest medications are those that are swallowed by the mind.
MOHAN SINGH

OBJECTIVES

When you finish this chapter, you should be able to:

- Identify the various types of quackery and the sources of protection for consumers of health services and health products
- Analyze major trends in personal health care resources, including types of personnel and facilities available in a community
- Describe the major features of the personal health care systems of at least two other countries

---

Those nations with the highest per capita investments in training for physicians and other health care personnel, and in hospitals and other medical facilities, do not necessarily have the greatest life expectancy or the highest level of health. This paradox can be attributed to two factors. The first is the tendency of people and communities to expose themselves to unnecessary risks in life-style and in the environment, as outlined in Parts 2, 3, and 4 of this book. The second has been the difficulty in bringing the citizen who needs medical, dental, and other health care services together with the necessary service. The people who need help the most are not getting enough help.

Previous chapters analyzed health promotion, protection, and services at the community level. This chapter focuses on health and medical care at the individual level. A common bond between the health of the community and the individual is **primary health care.** As understood in the Alma-Ata declaration introduced in Chapter 18, health of the individual and community are interwoven. Primary health care acknowledges health as a fundamental human right requiring support from all sectors of society. It is concerned with the health of the whole person, including the environment, and is not limited to the illness of isolated body parts. Primary health care includes self-care education, health pro-

---

The Hippocratic Oath

I swear by Apollo the physician, by Aesculapius, Hygeia and Panacea, and all the gods and goddesses, to keep to the best of my ability and judgment the following Oath: To reckon him who taught me this Art (of medicine) as dear to me as my own parents; to share my goods with him; to look upon his children as my own brothers; to teach them this Art if they so desire without fee or written promise; to impart a knowledge of the Art to my sons and the sons of the master who taught me, and to such disciples as have bound themselves to the rules of the profession—but to no others. I will prescribe regimen for the good of my patients to the best of my ability and judgment, and do harm to nobody. I will give no deadly medicine to anyone, even if it is requested, nor give advice that might result in death. Nor will I give a woman a pessary to produce abortion.

With purity and holiness will I practice my Art. I will not cut persons suffering from kidney stone but will leave this to be done by specialists in that Art. Whatever houses I visit, I shall enter only for the good of my patients, abstaining from any wilful evil-doing and corruption, and especially from the seduction of women or men, whether they be free or slaves. All that may come to my knowledge in the exercise of my profession or in daily commerce with men, which ought not to be spread abroad, I will keep secret and never reveal. If I keep this. Oath faithfully, may I long enjoy life and the practice of my Art, respected by all men in all times. But should I swerve from it or violate it, may the reverse be my lot!

---

motion, health resources and services directed toward the whole person in the community context, and health protection from fraudulent practices that rob the most vulnerable of their money and time in dealing with their own health.

CONSUMER HEALTH PROTECTION

When and how to use medical, dental, and other services and products is invaluable knowledge, but millions of people are victims of ignorance in matters relating to self-care and the use of health products and services. Health superstitions, fads, hopelessness, recklessness, and the gullible acceptance of extravagant claims and outright quackery must be replaced by confidence in scientific fact and personal responsibility. A primary requirement is a recognition that health does not come in a package or in a clinic. It comes with a style of life, with protective measures in the environment, and with the appropriate use of self-care products and health services.

Health Fraud

Defrauding and robbing the healthy as well as the sick, quacks are parasites of society. **Quackery** connotes a worthless treatment; **health fraud** implies an intent to deceive. The terms are used interchangeably here (Figure 21-1). Some promoters of quackery are sincere people who are, nevertheless, mistaken about their products. Others are cynical manipulators intent on fame and a fast buck. Quacks may use worthless, unorthodox, or unproven treatments to cure or prevent disease by ineffective procedures, nostrums, and diagnostic and therapeutic devices. A **nostrum** is an unauthorized, secret, or patented substance or device for which false therapeutic claims are made.

Where a certain segment of the population is inadequately educated in matters of health protection, and where scientific medicine has lost touch with

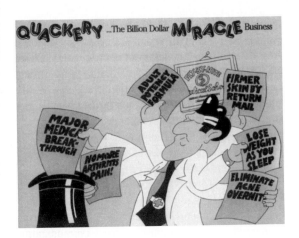

FIGURE 21-1

Quackery preys on those aspects of health and medical needs for which people seek simpler solutions than those offered by conventional medicine or "official" health advice. Particular targets include arthritis, fitness, weight loss, cancer, HIV/AIDS, and beauty or sexual attractiveness.

Source: Brochure jointly published by the Federal Trade Commission, the Pharmaceutical Advertising Council, the U.S. Food and Drug Administration, and the U.S. Postal Service.

people's needs, quacks are able to operate because many people have emotional needs not adequately met by physicians and clinics.

For generations vulnerable Americans have responded to promotions whose appeal has changed little since pitchmen in the frontier sold "golden elixir" from the back of a horse-drawn wagon. Today the U.S. Food and Drug Administration (FDA) has identified nine categories in which medical fraud is most frequent: figure enhancers, arthritis and pain relievers, sleeping aids, hair and scalp treatments, youth prolongers, sex aids, pure air and water devices, disease diagnosers, and cure-alls. The fitness movement and AIDS have brought out a whole new generation of health fraud.

Some excuse quackery as justifiable because it makes people feel good or gives them options in hopeless situations. Quackery poses many problems. Some people lose important time in seeking treatment, especially early diagnosis. Others may experience dangerous treatments. Still others lose hope when they realize they have been duped or experience guilt that their illness was caused by a lack of "natural harmony" with their body. All lose money. In 1960 Americans spent $1 billion on worthless cures; today that amount has increased to more than $25 billion. Those who purchase quack products often are least able to afford them. Individuals past age 65 spend an estimated $10 billion each year on quackery. It is estimated that most victims of quackery spend between $500 and $1000 a year.

Types of health fraud include drug and cosmetic, food and nutrition, and electrical and mechanical. Some quacks use all three, but others operate only one form so long as it is profitable.

Drug and cosmetic quackery. Many proprietary drugs mask pain and distress and thus delay the point at which the person finally seeks medical diagnosis (Figure 21-2). This delay can be critical. Drug quackery exists in many forms—rejuvenation nostrums, blood purifiers, cancer cures, hay fever remedies, cold cures, breast developers, sex vitalizers, nerve tonics, kidney cures, liver cures, and concoctions that "cure" the whole spectrum of ailments. Cosmetic quackery appears as skin "foods," hormone creams, skin restorers, geriatric cosmetics, salves, tablets, and every conceivable potion. These nostrums usually do nothing. They sometimes do harm.

Nutrition and weight-loss quackery. For more than half a century in the United States, "health foods" have been sold in the form of natural foods, organic foods, exotic foods, miracle foods, bee products, and other dietary cure-alls. "Nutrition experts" and "health lecturers" write books on food fads that find ready sales. Somewhere nutrition education has failed when food and nutrition quackery finds a clientele ever eager to pay exorbitant prices for foods that can be purchased at regular food markets at one half to one fourth the cost. Those in the

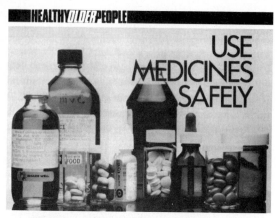

■■■**HEALTHY**▨▨▨**PEOPLE**▨

USE MEDICINES SAFELY

*M*edicines can ease pain and discomfort and improve the way you feel. And can help speed recovery when you're ill. But medicines work only when used as directed and coordinated with what you eat and drink and the other drugs you're taking. Make sure you, your doctor and pharmacist know as much as possible about the medicines you take.

FIGURE 21-2
The Healthy Older People campaign sponsored by the U.S. Department of Health and Human Services puts particular emphasis on using medicines safely. Older adults are at greater risk than other age groups of becoming victims not only of quackery and misuse of nonprescription drugs, but also of the mixing of prescription drugs that should not be taken together.
Source: U.S. Department of Health and Human Services.

multibillion-dollar weight loss industry who promise quick and painless weight loss while eating all one wants without exercise, have a ready audience in the increasingly overweight population, who want their weight loss as fast as their foods.

Electrical and mechanical nostrums. Fraudulent devices are frequently only leased rather than sold. This can be a clever bit of strategy from the legal standpoint as well as from the sales angle. Charms, crystals, "galvanic" belts, amulets, "radionized" water, water purifiers, radioactive ore, and other devices with equally mysterious designations are offered to the public and readily purchased or rented by desperate patients and hypochondriacs. The term *electronic* is to devices as the term *organic* is to foods and *secret formula* is to cosmetics. Many people assume these features make the product inherently superior.

Advertising. Most quacks use advertising and testimonials, but not in reputable scientific journals. The basis of most quack treatment is "secret," the name of a high-sounding foundation is used, and supporters may be actors, writers, athletes, politicians, or look-alikes for any of these. Quacks generally refuse inspection, contend that "the medical trust" is persecuting them, and, when challenged, promise to make their methods or drugs available to health authorities—but they seldom follow through on such a promise. Cultists, hypnotists, arthritis "specialists," and purveyors of devices use dramatic "health lectures," "clinics," late night "infomercials," and demonstrations. Communication media permit the advertising of products without sufficient regard for consumer interests, especially those of children too young to distinguish between a dramatic and a commercial message.

Protection of Consumers

All citizens are entitled to protection by their governmental agencies so that they are not victims of the fraudulent claims of health charlatans. This protection is afforded by legal agencies and by professional organizations that help set standards and offer mechanisms of "quality control."

To be protected, the consumer needs two kinds of information: information for **"informed consent"** (whether or not to use a product, submit to a medical or surgical procedure, or take a medication), and information for safe and effective use of a product or service after the initial decision to use it has been made. At the very minimum, a consumer has the right to information about risks and benefits associated with any product or procedure. It is appropriate for governments and institutions to establish some core, or "floor," of information that should be available to their citizens or members. What that information is, how it might be relayed, and what the government's responsibility is regarding that information are issues to be resolved on a case-by-case basis (Figure 21-3).

Proposed Pediatric Regulations

The U.S. Food and Drug Administration (FDA) has proposed to amend labeling regulations for prescription drugs, including biological products, to promote their safe and effective use in children. The proposed regulation would provide for the labeling to contain more complete data on pediatric use of a prescription drug and any hazards associated with its use in children.

A 1990 survey conducted by the American Academy of Pediatrics determined that the labeling of 80% of new drugs approved between 1984 and 1989 had no information on pediatric use. Other surveys have shown that for many prescription drugs commonly prescribed for children, the labeling stated that the safety and effectiveness in children had not been established. Without adequate information, physicians may be reluctant to prescribe certain drugs for their pediatric patients, or they may prescribe them inappropriately. As a result, children may be exposed to an increased risk of adverse reactions or decreased effectiveness of the drugs, or they may be denied access to valuable therapeutic agents.

FDA press release Oct. 27, 1992

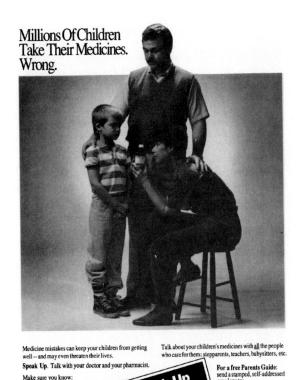

FIGURE 21-3
The best protection against the misuse of prescription drugs is patient education. This campaign appeals to physicians to talk to their patients about medications and to parents to talk to their physician, their pharmacist and their children.
Source: National Council on Patient Information and Education.

Nutritional labeling of food. Consumer protection laws saw their best times in the U.S. Congress in the 1970s. Food labeling laws in the 1970s represented a fundamental shift in regulatory philosophy and put more information and power in the hands of consumers. By the 1990s, however, these laws are only partially implemented and in need of revisions. While more than half of all packaged foods sold in the U.S. carry nutrition labeling, the information is often incomplete and may be confusing to the average consumer. When a product is described as "lite" or "light," does it have fewer calories, lower fat, less sodium, a fluffy texture, scant seasoning, or less breading than similar products? While trying to understand current products, consumers face an average of 12,000 new food products

annually. Information about food contents also needs extension to the 46 million people who eat in fast food restaurants daily.

With the Nutrition and Labeling and Education Act of 1990, consumers will be able to find complete nutrition information on most packaged foods, raw produce, and fish. The rules will make it possible to compare serving sizes for similar items; descriptor claims will be clearly defined; health messages will be regulated to ensure that they are supported by

What Is a Food Additive?

In its broadest sense, a food additive is any substance added to food. Legally, the term refers to "any substance the intended use of which results or may reasonably be expected to result—directly or indirectly—in its becoming a component or otherwise affecting the characteristics of any food." This definition includes any substance used in the production, processing, treatment, packaging, transportation, or storage of food.

If a substance is added to a food for a specific purpose in that food, it is referred to as a *direct additive*. For example, the low-calorie sweetener aspartame, which is used in beverages, puddings, yogurt, chewing gum, and other foods, is considered a direct additive. Many direct additives are identified on the ingredient label of foods.

Indirect food additives are those that become part of the food in trace amounts due to its packaging, storage, or other handling. For instance, minute amounts of packaging substances may find their way into foods during storage. Food packaging manufacturers must prove to the U.S. Food and Drug Administration (FDA) that all materials coming in contact with food are safe, before they are permitted for use in such a manner.

scientific evidence; ingredient statements will be more informative.

Labels are needed to convey information, but it is impossible to list in the space of a label everything that consumers might need to know. It is generally agreed that the effect of a labeling program depends on information made available to consumers in other ways. A foundation of knowledge from schooling and general consumer education is needed for a consumer to be able to use labels effectively and to comprehend other messages available at point of use or point of purchase.

Generic drugs. Compilation in 1980 of an Approved Drug Products List by the FDA gave American consumers another protection in relation to

drugs. Generic drug products are those sold under their established chemical name. They often sell for less than brand-name products. Consumers pay higher prices when they buy prescription drugs under their brand names when therapeutically equivalent drugs are available at lower prices.

The Approved Drug Products List includes over 5000 prescription drug products approved by the FDA for marketing in the United States. It identifies those that the FDA believes to be therapeutically equivalent to others within a therapeutic category based on criteria proposed for evaluation of therapeutic equivalency. Consumers can save when the pharmacist dispenses an available lower-cost drug product. For example, a patient who needs ampicillin, a common antibiotic, can save money if the pharmacist dispenses a lower-cost generic ampicillin product, knowing that the FDA has approved it as being therapeutically equivalent to higher-priced brand-name versions. Prescription drugs also cost more in the U.S. than in Canada (Figure 21-4).

Protective Agencies in the United States

The Food and Drug Administration. The FDA, described in Chapters 16 and 18, conducts over 50,000 inspections and about 1500 court actions per year in the United States in connection with seizure of harmful products and requests for injunctions restraining persons from continuing a practice or selling products hazardous to public health. This agency also tests products, sets standards, passes on claims, investigates imports, and cooperates with state and local officials in matters of food and drug production, marketing, adulteration, and contamination.

The Federal Trade Commission. The Federal Trade Commission (FTC) has authority over false advertising and deceptive practices in the United States. Following complaints, the commission investigates and may issue orders to the offending person or firm to cease and desist from continuing the practice. Many Americans accept the validity of advertisements for health products on the belief that

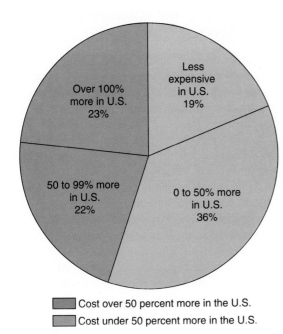

Cost over 50 percent more in the U.S.

Cost under 50 percent more in the U.S.

FIGURE 21-4

As a result of more restraint on drug prices by Canada's federal and provincial governments, many drugs (some 45%) cost over 50% more in the United States than in Canada.

Source: U.S. General Accounting Office: *Prescription drugs: companies typically charge more in the United States than in Canada,* Washington, DC, 1992, General Accounting Office Report to the House of Representatives.

they must be factually correct or such agencies as the FDA and FTC would not permit them to appear.

The U.S. Postal Service. Post office officials in the United States and some other countries prevent the use of the mail service for the shipment and sale of deceptive, adulterated, contaminated, or fraudulent foods, drugs, cosmetics, or devices. A citizen complaint is sufficient to initiate an investigation, followed by legal action when warranted.

The U.S. Consumer Product Safety Commission. The U.S. Consumer Product Safety Commission (CPSC) evaluates the safety of consumer goods. The box at right illustrates the frequency and types of *Safety Alerts* issued by the CPSC in two

---

Consumer Product SAFETY ALERT

These Consumer Product Safety Alerts about some hazards to children were published during 1991 and 1992:

Child-Resistant Packaging (December 1992)
Toy Guitar Strap Strangulations (November 1992)
Art Materials (November 1992)
Movable Soccer Goals Can Tip Over (October 1992)
Mesh Playpens (September 1992)
Child-Resistant Cigarette Lighters (August 1992)
Playground Cargo Net Strangulations (August 1992)
Baby Walkers (July 1992)
Caps for Toy Guns (June 1992)
Infant Cushion Ban (June 1992)
Infant Carrier Seats (June 1992)
Stroller Entrapment (May 1992)
Bucket Drownings (April 1992)
Baby Bath Rings—Drowning Hazard (April 1992)
Crib Toys (March 1992)
Strangulation on Wall Decorations (March 1992)
All Terrain Vehicles (March 1992)
Burns on Hot Metal Playground Equipment (March 1992)
Poisonings with Iron-Containing Medicine (February 1992)
Automatic Garage Door Openers (December 1991)
Child Drownings in the Home (November 1991)
New Hair Dryers Prevent Electrocutions (October 1991)
Strings and Cords Can Strangle Children on Playground Equipment (September 1991)
Safety Devices (November 1991)
In-Line Roller Skates (August 1991)
Crib Cornerposts (August 1991)
Strings and Cords Can Strangle Infants (July 1990)
Bed Entrapment/Suffocation (January 1991)

From the U.S. Consumer Product Safety Commission, Washington, D.C.

recent years. Some systems that assist the CPSC in assessing injury rates include a computerized compilation of emergency room records, coroners' reports, and consumer hotlines. Depending on the degree of hazard assessed, actions taken by the CPSC include (1) working through voluntary standards organizations, (2) information and education campaigns, (3) mandatory labeling, (4) banning, and (5) recall. The first two approaches involve some costs and may meet with industry resistance, but the last three are the most expensive and generally meet with the most significant resistance. These last three approaches are reserved for situations that pose the most potentially serious risks to consumers.

Nongovernmental professional and voluntary agencies. The American Medical Association (AMA) has had a Bureau of Investigation, a Council on Foods and Nutrition, and a Committee on Cosmetics. Such units work through state medical associations and together carry out measures in the public interest such as interviewing study participants and reviewing their backgrounds, examining clinical or experimental evidence, examining biopsy or autopsy data, securing drug samples for analysis, and summarizing findings.

The American Cancer Society and the Arthritis Foundation are examples of other agencies that alert the U.S. public to fraudulent health claims. Patients with cancer or arthritis are prime targets of quacks, and special vigilance is essential to protect these patients because of their greater desperation and vulnerability to deceptive claims. The Council of Better Business Bureaus also is alert to health frauds and provides protection to the public.

All such official and voluntary agencies help protect against quackery, but individuals remain vulnerable without self-protection. Education concerning recognition of symptoms requiring diagnosis is the first measure. The second need is education to select and to use wisely the available medical, dental, and hospital services when necessary, and safe forms of self-care at other times.

PRIMARY CARE: THE COMMUNITY AND INDIVIDUAL HEALTH LINK

One of the reasons quackery and health fraud can have such a toehold in the United States is the disconnection many have from a health and medical care system that they cannot afford or that denies them access or insurance. Measured against feelings of hopelessness, an annual insurance premium, or a day's hospital stay, a ''quick cure'' seems like a bargain to the vulnerable.

To include everyone in health and medical care requires reform of the current system. Such reform is a top political priority for the 1990s. The health care system in the United States has gradually become dominated by costly, specialized medical care providers, driving up health care costs and limiting the access of millions of Americans to basic health care services (see Figure 21-5).

Primary health care is seen as one key to health care reform. It is a community-based concept of health care in which an individual's first contact with the system is with broadly trained, generalist physicians, nurses, and other professionals. These providers consider not only medical needs of individuals, but their broader health needs and living situations. Primary care providers offer continuous, comprehensive care at lower costs than do health specialists. A system of health care firmly built on a foundation of interdisciplinary, preventive, community-based, primary health care may be the most effective way to provide high-quality, broad-based services at reasonable cost to the entire population—especially the elderly, people residing in rural areas, and other populations with special needs.

In trying to balance the seemingly incompatible goals of access to health care and escalating health care costs, little attention has been given to those who provide health care services. Because health care depends so heavily on personnel, any discussion about primary health care and health care reform needs to engage the community recipients of services as well as the health care personnel who provide them.

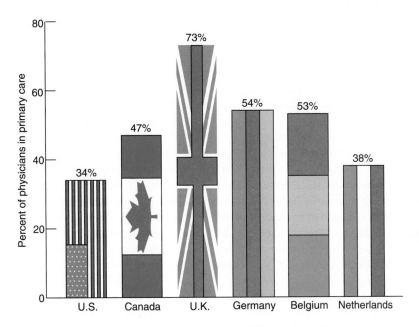

FIGURE 21-5
Of countries with comparable standards of living, the United States has the lowest percentage of primary care physicians among all physicians. This means that more American physicians are specialists, which accounts in part for the higher cost of medical care in the United States.

Source: Based on Asch DA, Ende J: The downsizing of internal medicine residency programs, *Ann Intern Med* 117:839, 1992.

Even with all the current agreement on the importance of primary health care, many systems, traditions, and attitudes will need to change if it is to be implemented. The education of all health professions needs to be redirected toward health needs of the population, not only the medical needs. Health care financing policies need to favor primary care. Health personnel need to find reward in disease prevention. Television crews rush in for the medical miracles. No one shows the successful outcome of prevention when something did not happen. Interdisciplinary efforts may mean sharing of responsibilities and power that individuals and regulatory agencies need to confirm. For health care reform to succeed, issues of health personnel availability, employment, and training must be considered.

PROFESSIONAL PERSONNEL
Supply and Demand

One of the considerations in providing primary health care is the number of health care workers to be involved. The terms *supply* and *requirements* are used in discussions about the health work force. In addition, the terms *demand* and *need* are used in discussions of requirements. *Supply* and *demand* are well-defined concepts in economics. **Supply** is the number of individuals in a specific occupational category who are seeking employment at the current pay level. **Demand** is the number of individuals in a specific occupational category that employers will employ at various wages. This is sometimes referred to as "economic demand" or "effective economic demand." Therefore supply and demand are different theoretical concepts. What actually happens when demand draws on supply is described in economic theory.

Need and **requirements** are less well and more variously defined terms. They are both value judgments separate in concept from supply and demand. The "need for a specific health occupation" is defined as an adequate minimum quantity and quality of persons in that health occupation that widespread consensus holds ought to be available to the citizens of a country or community for the purpose of their remaining or becoming reasonably healthy. The requirement for a health occupation is implied in the match between the number of workers needed and the assumed level of their contribution to health goals. *Requirements* contains value judgments that reflect many considerations including economics, health priorities, traditional organization of health services, and political clout.

Rarely are the data and methods available for a complete analysis of all four concepts of supply, demand, requirement, and need. In the next sections a summary of the supply and requirements for the health occupations in the United States will be given as an illustration of health resource analysis applicable to communities and other countries.

Health Care Services Work Force

The supply and requirements for the health care services work force change over time. Adjustments to shortages or oversupply of health care workers at one point in time sets off decades of chain responses in multiple sectors. The 1970s saw a time of rapid expansion in the number of physicians, nurses, pharmacists, and dentists. Between 1970 and 1980, the number of those graduating in medicine increased by 81%, nursing by 75%, pharmacy by 56%, and dentistry by 40%. The nation was in a resource-building mode, until the cost containment concerns of the late 1970s slowed this rapid expansion. As federal support was withdrawn, most of these pro-

fessions peaked in the number of graduates by the mid-1980s.

A comparison of 1989 and 1980 graduates shows that the number of nursing and dental graduates dropped by 18% and pharmacy graduates dropped by 12%. Only medical schools showed an increase of 3% in 1989 of the number of graduates over that in 1980. Whether these graduates represent an over- or undersupply is a matter of some debate, depending on assumptions about the organization of the health care system and understanding roles and responsibilities of health care providers. For example, projections by the Health Resources and Services Administration in 1988 were that supply would exceed requirements in selected health professions by the years 1990 and 2000 (Table 21-1). A 1993 report by the U.S. Bureau of Health Professions, however, cites a current and future shortage of primary health care providers. The later report endorses primary care as a key to health care reform.

Physicians. In the United States in 1989 there were 560,000 active medical doctors. This represents an 88% increase in the number of physicians since 1970. In 1970 there were 139 active doctors per

TABLE 21-1

Requirements for selected health occupations: projections to 2000

	2000	
	Supply	*Requirements*
Medicine	708,600	637,000
Optometry	30,100	29,500
Pharmacy	198,600	193,000
Nursing*		
RN	1,799,000	1,743,000
LPN/LVN	630,200	585,400

Source: Health Resources and Services Administration, 1988.
*Full-time equivalents.

100,000 population. By 1989 the number of medical doctors increased to 215 for the same population unit.

Just as important as the relative number of physicians is their distribution in practice and population. Today approximately one third of physicians practice primary care. This percent is in stark contrast to the 80% who were in primary care in 1931. In 1992 only 15% of medical school graduates chose primary health care. The financial incentives for specializing are tempting. At an annual income of $95,000 in 1989, general/family practice physicians have annual incomes that are 50% to 60% less than those of medical specialists (Figure 21-6).

Physicians, like other North Americans, tend to congregate in metropolitan areas. Rural and inner city areas are not favored practice sites. The result

is uneven distribution of health care services to the population. Medical schools have admitted a more ethnically diverse population and more women, although graduates do not reflect broader social diversity. In 1991 minorities constituted 22% of the U.S. population, but only 8% of practicing physicians.

How to make general practice attractive is the problem that must be resolved or the cry will continue that there is a shortage of physicians, when in fact it is merely a shortage of general practitioners. To increase the availability of community-based primary care practitioners, a variety of strategies are considered that involve admission requirements to medical school, financial incentives for primary practice, curriculum changes that include community settings, and retraining current specialists.

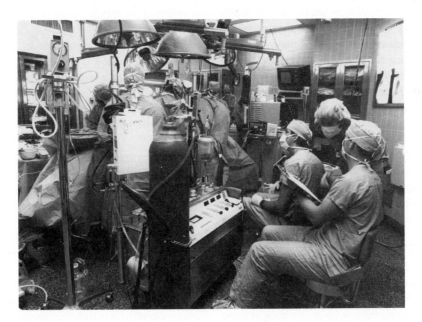

FIGURE 21-6
Besides the economic incentives, the prestige and glamor that attaches to medical and surgical specialties as a result of two decades of hospital dramas on television have made the family doctor and the primary care physician seem a throwback to another era.
Source: University of Texas Health Science Center at Houston, photo by Masha Burkes.

Some communities have been able to attract general practitioners by building a small but adequate hospital, providing office facilities, and guaranteeing a minimum salary.

Inefficient use of physician services also drives up the cost of their services. Too many physicians are taking too much valuable time doing tasks that others could do or should be trained to do. Others can be and are trained to take family and personal histories and to perform further duties. Examples are physicians' assistants, nurse practitioners, accredited record technicians, medical secretaries, medical transcriptionists, physical therapy aides, inhalation therapists, surgical technicians, darkroom technicians, dietitians, and patient counselors.

Nurses. As discussed in the previous chapter on community health, nurses play an important role in the health care system. Nurses are the largest health care profession; they outnumber physicians by nearly 3 to 1. Nurses and other allied personnel have assumed expanded roles in health services. Nurses have taken increased responsibility for patient education to help patients cope with emotional and learning aspects of self-care and rehabilitation. The potential for nurses and other allied health workers to bring a humanizing and preventive orientation back into a highly technological health care system gives them a most promising and central role in the future of community health and health promotion.

As with physicians, the number of nurses has been subject to debates about shortages and oversupply. There was a 122% increase in the number of nurses from 1970 to 1.6 million in 1989. Such overall dramatic increases fail to show the rapid decrease in the number of nursing graduates in recent years, a 25% decrease from 1985 to 1989 (Figure 21-7). Baccalaureate nursing levels are back to those of the early 1970s.

These decreases come at a time when health care providers report continuing and emerging shortages and maldistribution in key basic disciplines in nursing and allied health. Hospitals and nursing homes in particular report nursing shortages. Increasing controls over rising health care costs are creating a demand for more community-based services provided by professionals other than physicians.

Other health care practitioners. Primary care engages all health practitioners in education about health at some level. Certified health education specialists are those whose primary training is in health education. Their role in community and individual health education provides direction, support, and coordination to the health educational efforts of other health practitioners. The health education role is an important one in primary care.

The U.S. Bureau of Health Professions has set as its goal for the year 2000 the development of an ''appropriate'' mix of personnel to support the expansion of access to primary and preventive care services. That mix includes primary care providers, for example, family physicians, general internists, pediatricians, nurse practitioners, physician assistants, and certified nurse midwives. Other health professionals have important primary care roles, including pharmacists, dentists, dental hygienists, respiratory technicians and therapists (Figure 21-8), optometrists, dieticians/nutritionists, therapists, and social workers. All of these professionals need community ties that make primary health care the community-based effort it is intended to be, not the medical care bureaucracy the current health care system seems to have become.

Accessibility. An adequate total supply of personnel, however, does not guarantee **accessibility** for all people; other barriers—money, education, geography, or language—still keep too many people from needed health care. Many rural and inner city areas are still experiencing shortages of all health personnel despite the increases in supply. The designations of specific areas with shortages of health personnel encompass a broad range of different types of areas, and although a majority of those areas designated are rural (nonmetropolitan) areas, ur-

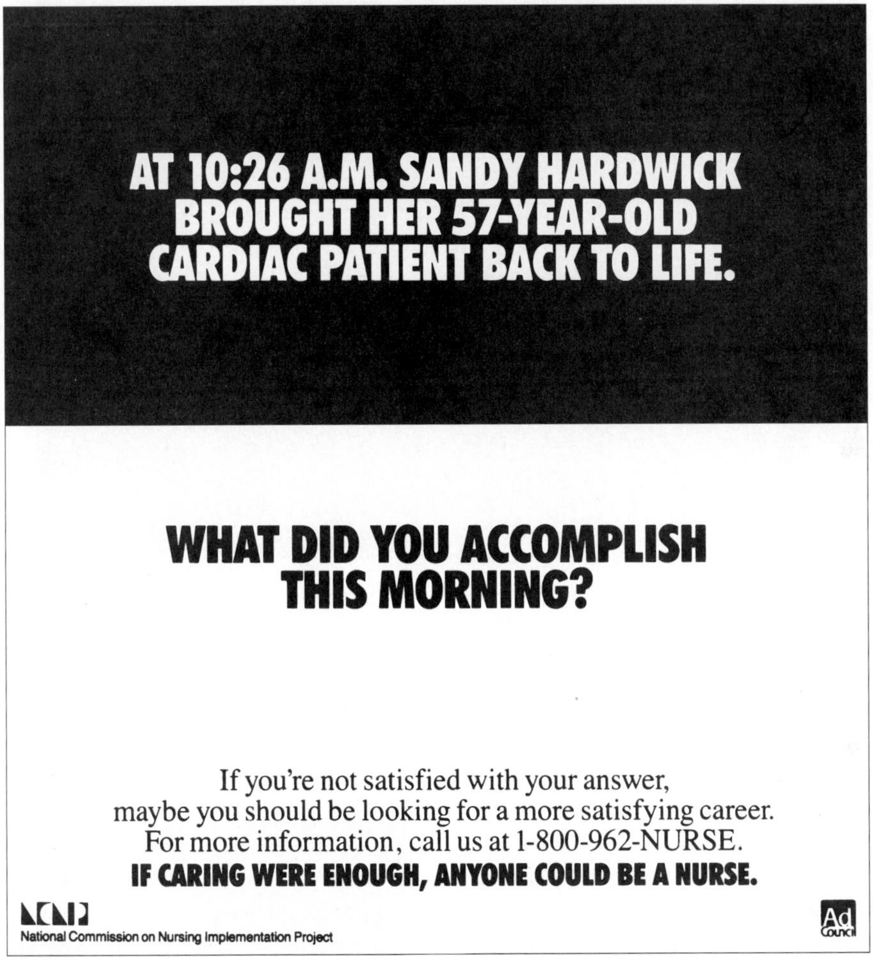

AT 10:26 A.M. SANDY HARDWICK BROUGHT HER 57-YEAR-OLD CARDIAC PATIENT BACK TO LIFE.

WHAT DID YOU ACCOMPLISH THIS MORNING?

If you're not satisfied with your answer,
maybe you should be looking for a more satisfying career.
For more information, call us at 1-800-962-NURSE.
IF CARING WERE ENOUGH, ANYONE COULD BE A NURSE.

National Commission on Nursing Implementation Project

FIGURE 21-7
In an effort to reverse the trend in declining nursing school enrollments, a nurse recruiting campaign featured public service ads that tried to capture the same hospital high drama and heroics that have become synonomous with health care in the minds of large segments of the American population.
Source: National Commission on Nursing Implementation Project and the Advertising Council.

ban areas contain about half of the population who live in shortage areas. Efforts to identify these areas and a number of federal programs, including especially the National Health Service Corps, have attempted to correct the problems of access. Special population groups, such as American Indians, those who are Spanish-speaking, blacks, and the medically indigent, have been designated as having health manpower shortages, as have special facilities such as state and county jails. Currently, approximately 30 million people in the United States live in designated health manpower shortage areas.

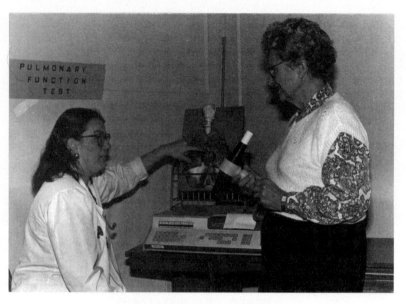

FIGURE 21-8
Respiratory technicians conduct pulmonary function tests as one of the many contributions of allied health professionals to a wider range of services and supports offered to patients, some with potential for patient education to increase self-care and prevention.
Source: Franklin Regional Hospital, Franklin, New Hampshire.

HOSPITAL FACILITIES
Overall Supply

Consideration of the adequacy of community hospital facilities must be centered on short-term general and special hospitals and their bed capacity. It is the bed capacity that is the key factor. Actually, the number of short-term general and special hospitals in many countries was greater 50 years ago than it is today. Half a century ago, because of limited transportation, almost every little hamlet in the United States, for example, had its 15- or 20-bed hospital, poorly equipped, poorly serviced, and poorly administered, but accessible. With modern transportation it is altogether logical to have fewer hospitals and maintain only those hospitals with a large enough bed capacity to warrant extensive equipment and highly specialized personnel. There is no longer a need for every town to have a hospital.

Social Work with a Hospice

Medical and nursing staffs of hospices cooperate closely with social workers to help patients and their families to adjust in a homelike atmosphere to terminal illness and to overcome their particular difficulties at a time that is potentially overwhelmingly stressful. For those facing death, feelings emerge that are bewildering and can be contradictory. A patient who is able to return home may need a variety of financial and visiting services to modify the home environment. The social worker can arrange such services as well as help the patients to feel more secure outside the protective care of the hospice or the family to feel more secure with the patient in the hospice.

Wheatfields—A Sue Ryder Home for Cancer Patients, Leeds, England. The Sue Ryder Foundation.

As a result, large, well-equipped, well-staffed, and well-administered hospitals are erected in the large centers of population.

The old standard of four general hospital beds for every 1000 inhabitants is attained in most Western countries. Australia, Canada, England, Wales, Scotland, and the United States all have close to four beds per 1000 population, as an average; however, many communities and countries have but half this number. The uneven distribution of hospital beds in the United States was partially corrected by the Hill-Burton Hospital Survey and Construction Act of 1946, which instituted a federal program that made more than $4.1 billion in grants to hospitals in all of the states during the 29 years of its existence and added 496,000 beds to the nation's hospital system. These grants were made to local government hospitals, church hospitals, and nonprofit hospitals.

Characteristics

General hospitals. In 1948, at the time the Hill-Burton program was becoming operational, there were 3.4 hospital beds per 1000 population. As result of Hill-Burton, nearly 4000 communities were aided in the construction of 6549 public and nonprofit medical facilities. Following the buildup of hospitals, there has been a steady decrease since 1970. By 1990 there were 3.9 beds per 1000 population, dropping back closer to the pre–Hill-Burton ratio. The average occupancy rate for all general hospitals was about 67% in 1990. Occupancy tends to be higher in the winter months and lower in the summer.

In the intervening years there has been a redistribution in the location of hospitals and a change in some kinds of hospitals. The Hill-Burton program more evenly distributed hospitals across the United States, within states, and among less and more affluent areas. Between 1970 and 1990 tuberculosis hospitals decreased the most dramatically (94%) as this disease was being reduced in the overall population and drugs permitted outpatient treatment. As

large state-run "warehouses" for the mentally ill were closed down over the last two decades, there has been an increase in small, private psychiatric hospitals (43%). It has not been an even trade of populations, since many from state institutions were left to the streets and were not the concern of privately run facilities. Many hospital emergency rooms continue to be used as a primary source of care by those without insurance or other means of care. Emergency room visits have increased by over 50% in the last 20 years.

Hospital costs approached $204 billion in 1990, with an average patient to staff ratio of 2 to 1. The highly technological services offered by hospitals continue to increase. Such facilities as intensive care, open-heart surgery, radioisotope, and renal dialysis units have proliferated. This addition of special facilities to a hospital's capacity has been one of the factors in rising hospital costs and the general inflation of the medical care dollar. By 1990 the average cost per day in a hospital was $687; the average cost per stay was $4947 (Table 21-2).

Nursing homes. The number of beds in U.S. nursing homes nearly doubled between 1963 and 1983. This increase resulted in part from the coverage of the charges for certain types of nursing home care under the Medicare and Medicaid programs, which began in 1967. Some of the growth in nursing home use appears to be the result of placement in nursing homes of older patients who in earlier years would have been residents in state and county mental hospitals. With the aging of the population and an increasing life span, a greater need to care for the frail elderly is expected. Some of this need may be met through better home care service.

Home Health

The availability of home health services is often a factor in determining hospital staffing requirements and whether a patient must be hospitalized or can remain at home.

TABLE 21-2
Costs of treatment for preventable conditions in the United States

Condition	Overall magnitude	Avoidable intervention*	Cost per patient†
Heart disease	7 million with coronary artery disease 500,000 deaths/yr 284,000 bypass procedures/yr	Coronary bypass surgery	$30,000
Cancer	1 million new cases/yr 510,000 deaths/yr	Lung cancer treatment Cervical cancer treatment	$29,000 $28,000
Stroke	600,000 strokes/yr 150,000 deaths/yr	Hemiplegia treatment and rehabilitation	$22,000
Injuries	2.3 million hospitalizations/yr 142,500 deaths/yr 177,000 persons with spinal cord injuries in the United States	Quadriplegia treatment and rehabilitation Hip fracture treatment and rehabilitation Severe head injury treatment and rehabilitation	$570,000 (lifetime) $40,000 $310,000
HIV infection	1-1.5 million infected 118,000 AIDS cases (as of Jan 1990)	AIDS treatment	$75,000 (lifetime)
Alcoholism	18.5 million abuse alcohol 105,000 alcohol-related deaths/yr	Liver transplant	$250,000

Drug abuse	Regular users:
	  1-3 million, cocaine
	  900,000, IV drugs
	  500,000, heroin
	Drug-exposed babies: 375,000
		Treatment of cocaine-exposed baby	$66,000 (5 years)

Low-birthweight baby	260,000 LBWB born/yr 23,000 deaths/yr	Neonatal intensive care for LBWB	$10,000

Inadequate immunization	Lacking basic immunization series:
	  20-30%, aged 2 and younger
	  3%, aged 6 and older
		Congenital rubella syndrome treatment	$354,000 (lifetime)

Source: Office of Disease Prevention and Health Promotion: *Healthy people 2000: national health promotion and disease prevention objectives,* Washington, DC, 1990, U.S. Department of Health and Human Services.
*Examples (other interventions may apply).
†Representative first-year costs, except as noted. Not indicated are nonmedical costs, such as lost productivity to society. Most of the costs tend to be concentrated in hospital care and rehabilitation. The costs shown here are only those for the first year of medical treatment, not the other social and rehabilitation costs. These data have drawn greater public and Congressional attention to the potential for prevention to help contain the escalating costs of medical care.

Staffing for a home health agency or a Visiting Nurse Association usually includes the following personnel:

Nurses provide skilled nursing, specialized nursing, and liaison services.

- Skilled nursing includes general nursing services and technical procedures, such as intravenous (IV) therapy, catheterization, and dressing wounds, as well as management of a physician-prescribed medical regime and in-

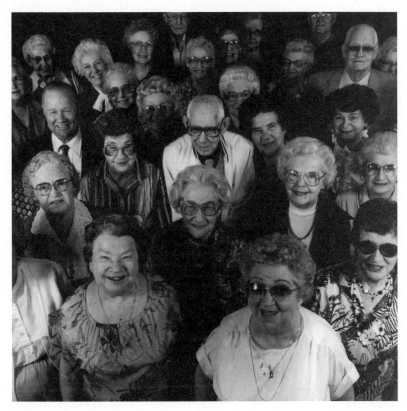

FIGURE 21-9
Demographic trends alone will dominate many of the health care reforms seeking to control costs of medical and nursing home care in the years ahead. Today's well elderly and the aging baby boomers will require larger government outlays for medical, nursing, and home care even as the older population enjoys better health than in the past.
Source: Missouri Department of Health. Photo by Bob Hulsey.

struction in patient care for the patient and family.

- Specialized nursing includes services of oncology clinical specialists, a psychiatric mental health nurse, an enterostomal therapist, and pediatric nurse practitioners.
- A liaison nurse consults with local hospitals and nursing homes, provides information concerning VNA's services, and helps process the transition from the hospital to home.

Therapists provide restorative physical therapy care for patients with stroke, fractures, and birth defects; occupational therapy for activities of daily living; and speech therapy for clients with communication problems related to speech, language, or hearing.

Home health aides, certified paraprofessionals, provide personal care, such as bathing, grooming, bed changing, and grocery shopping.

Social workers provide services that include evaluation, short-term counseling, and referral to community agencies.

The number of home health agencies approved for participation in the Medicare program increased appreciably between 1966 and 1970, the first four years of the program. After that the number of approved agencies remained stable at about 2200 until 1985, when renewed growth occurred as a result of the new hospital discharge policies. Most of the earlier agencies were governmental health agencies or visiting nurse associations, but now proprietary home health agencies are developing in response to the demand created by earlier discharges of patients from hospitals (Figure 21-9).

HEALTH CARE SYSTEM COSTS

Growth in U.S. health care expenditure has been faster than growth of the total GNP for 27 of the last 30 years. Table 21-3 shows the increase in overall costs, in percentage of Gross National Product (GNP), and the public share of all costs. The government now pays over 40% of all health care costs. As of April 1993, the United States spent $838.5 billion annually on health care, double what it was in 1985. This amount approaches 14% of the GNP. The average amount spent per individual was $3160. Despite paying the highest costs in the world, the United States lags behind other developed countries in vital health statistics such as infant mortality and immunization rates. The high-tech medical care system we have created is not a system that has extended health care as a right to all American citizens.

Unchecked, health care costs are estimated to exceed $1 trillion by 1995 and consume 25% of the GNP (Figure 21-10). Because the government pays such a large amount of the total health care bill through Medicaid and Medicare, it has an interest in controlling costs. The Clinton administration has put top priority on health care reform to bring costs under control, at the same time extending care to the 37 million uninsured Americans. While most agree on the need for such reform, competing proposals and vested interests will make this the political debate of the decade.

Changing Costs

Hospital costs, physicians' fees, and other medical care services will continue to rise, despite the decline in the average length of hospital stay resulting from incentives, regulation, and advances in medication, surgery, and other procedures. Nursing homes, rest homes, hospices, and home care as adjuncts to the general hospital have reduced the cost of hospitalization during the period of convalescence or dying. Patients who do not require the extensive care available in hospitals can recover as rapidly or die as peacefully in these homes at a lower cost, and at even lower costs with good home health care services and self-care education for patients and families.

The medical profession is the only industry in the United States that is free of both market controls and governmental regulations. It has a virtual monopoly in the American economy, but physicians are sensitive to the image of their profession and attempt to exercise supervision and discipline over members of the profession through professional organizations. Instances of exorbitant medical charges have been substantiated. At the other extreme are the instances in which physicians have donated their professional services. It is not the extremes of overcharging or charity where the problem of the cost of medical care rests, but in the general inflation of prices in this relatively uncontrolled sector of the economy.

The economics of these trends were introduced in Chapter 2. Their further analysis would be beyond the scope of this text, but three major causes of cost increases (principally runaway hospital prices) and the national policy initiatives to remedy or check these causes are central to community health (see box).

TABLE 21-3
National health expenditures in the United States from 1960 to 1990

	1960	*1970*	*1980*	*1988*	*1989*	*1990*
			% distribution			
National health costs	100.0	100.0	100.0	100.0	100.0	100.0
Private	75.5	62.8	58.0	58.4	58.1	57.6
Public	24.5	37.2	42.0	41.6	41.9	42.4
Federal	10.7	23.9	28.8	28.7	29.0	29.3
State and local	13.8	13.3	13.3	12.9	12.9	13.1
		Percentage of gross national product				
National health costs	5.3	7.3	9.2	11.2	11.6	12.2
			Amount in billions			
National health costs	$27.1	74.4	250.1	546.0	602.8	666.2

Source: Health Care Financing Administration, Office of Actuary: Data from National Center for Health Statistics. The current rate of increase is running at twice that of the overall economy. The health percentage of GNP continues to grow, especially the federal share, even as the percentages devoted to education and defense have declined.

Containing Personal Health Service Costs

Source of Cost Increases	**Recommended Policies**
Physician salaries or fees	Increasing use of paraprofessional, allied health, and ''physician-extender'' personnel
Unnecessary hospitalization, laboratory tests, length of stay, and elective surgery	Increased incentives for keeping patients out of hospitals by requiring outpatient surgery and allowing physicians to share in the profits of prepaid medical plans, preferred provider organizations, and health maintenance organizations; also, peer review of medical practice, utilization review of hospital practice, and second opinions regarding suggested surgery.
Increased use of medical services for conditions that might have been prevented, and readmissions for chronic conditions not adequately controlled by patients	Increased emphasis on preventive medicine and health education, including occupational health, patient education, self-care education, health promotion, and environmental health

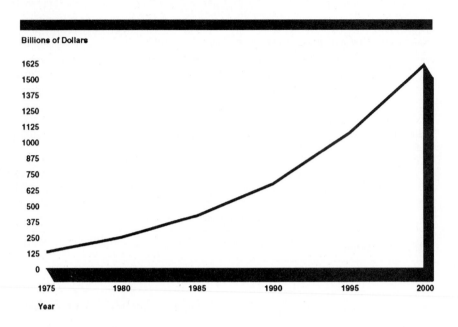

Billions of Dollars

1625	
1500	
1375	
1250	
1125	
1000	
875	
750	
625	
500	
375	
250	
125	
0	

1975   1980   1985   1990   1995   2000

Year

Note: Values after 1990 are estimates.

FIGURE 21-10
National health expenditures will top $1 trillion by 1995 and the rate of increase will likely continue to escalate with the growth of the aging population and technology.

Source: Health Care Financing Administration, Office of the Actuary; and U.S. General Accounting Office: *Access to health care: states respond,* Washington, DC, 1992, General Accounting Office.

A Community Health Perspective on Health Costs

Education in use of health services. The proper use of health services and health insurance mechanisms requires an informed and motivated public. If the *ideal* health care system for some countries were installed tomorrow, it would be highly subject to disuse, misuse, and abuse by an unprepared public operating under the control of habits, attitudes, and expectations inculcated by a lifetime of coping with their traditional system. Many of the failures or temporary breakdowns in the implementation of new programs in various countries have been traced to problems of communication, knowledge, attitudes, and habits. Consumers need to understand how health care organization and escalating costs affect

them. Consumers are indifferent to costs when private insurance companies or the government pays the bill. These problems would be more readily addressed in the planning of health care services if those who use the services are involved in planning them. Unless planning and implementation of services are closely tied, the best ideas of policy will not be expressed in practice.

Disease prevention and health maintenance. Any new plan that makes health care more accessible and more acceptable to more people will place pressure on existing resources unless it is accompanied by a new orientation to prevention and health maintenance. A major criticism of the traditional fee-for-service structure of American medicine is that it of-

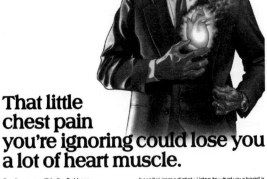

That little chest pain you're ignoring could lose you a lot of heart muscle.

Cardiac care within the first hour could save your active life.

It can certainly increase your chances of saving heart muscle. And heart muscle sustains not only life...but the quality of life. It could mean the difference between living an active healthy life, or spending the majority of your life inactive.

Chance of saving heart muscle

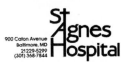

good treated within 1 hour

fair treated within 2-4 hours

poor treated after 4 hours

Act to survive with early cardiac intervention treatment.

Chest pain could mean a heart attack. Be prepared. At the first sign of heart pain, go to your hospital immediately. Listen to what your heart is trying to tell you. It could save your life.

Check on the availability of early cardiac care at your community hospital.
For more information and a free brochure, write Raymond D. Bahr, M.D., CCU Medical Director.

The Paul Dudley White Coronary Care System ...20 years of promoting concepts in community cardiac care.
The Chest Pain Emergency Room...6 years experience in cardiac intervention.

St Agnes Hospital

900 Caton Avenue
Baltimore, MD
21229-5299
(301) 368-7844

A Daughters of Charity Hospital Serving the Community Since 1862. A Tradition of Caring for 125 years

This information made possible by a grant from the National Emergency Medicine Association through its National Heart Research Project. 11 West Pennsylvania Avenue, Towson, MD 21204.

FIGURE 21-11
Hospitals have taken more active community health education and health promotion roles in recent years, in part to improve their image in the face of growing public cynicism about organized medicine, but in part because they see much of the preventable damage that arrives in their emergency rooms and beds with problems that could have been avoided with better understanding and more timely action.
Source: St. Agnes Hospital, Baltimore.

fers little incentive for the providers of services to give attention to prevention, health promotion, and health education. The rewards are tied almost entirely to treatment of the sick. When Americans speak of health care, they usually mean medical treatment.

Continuing education of professionals. All health care professionals must become better trained to communicate effectively with patients and consumers, and to place greater emphasis on disease prevention and health promotion with their patients (Figure 21-11). This will call for expansion and reorientation of training programs for medical, nursing, and allied health professionals.

The community health perspective on health services personal, then, emphasizes consumer participation in planning, issues of distribution and education for appropriate use of health care resources, preventive health maintenance, communication with patients, and reorientation of health professional training. The remainder of this chapter comments specifically on national health plans from the community health perspective.

SOCIALIZED MEDICAL SERVICES

A medical program is socialized when it is administered by the government. More than 50 nations have national medical service programs, and virtually all of these are socialized programs. For generations the federal and local governments in the United States have socialized various services—mail service, education, and police and fire protection—but only parts of their medical systems. A city that sells water or electricity to its residents is engaged in the socialization of an economic enterprise.

Personal health services vary from one nation to the next. The first national medical program was the German Sickness Insurance Plan, but the Swedish and Canadian programs have been of special interest to Americans. These programs have similarities and dissimilarities and represent basic types of national medical programs.

Sweden

Medical economists generally agree that Sweden has the best structured and administered national health program. Sweden's experience in pension programs, maternal and infant care programs, geriatrics programs, and welfare programs was excellent preparation for establishing the System of Medical Care and Sickness Benefit insurance, which the Riksdag instituted on January 1, 1955.

Access. The national health insurance program covers all Swedish citizens and alien residents. The national health insurance system is a principal means of creating socioeconomic equality while also functioning as a financing instrument and one

of state control and supervision. The system is based on the fundamental principle that all citizens are entitled to good health and equal access to health and medical care, regardless of where they live and their economic circumstances.

Organization. Sweden's program is administered by the Ministry of Health and the National Board of Health and Welfare (Figure 21-12). but is highly decentralized. On the local level each county has a

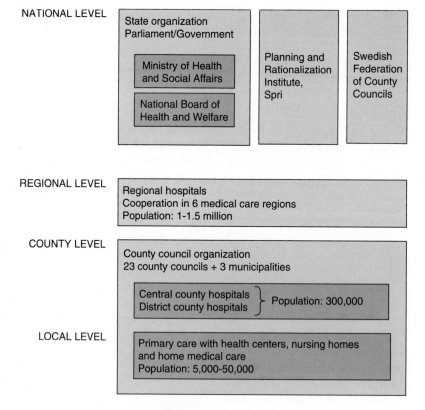

FIGURE 21-12

The organization of health care in Sweden features an integrated distribution of facilities such that areas of small population concentration have adequate primary care resources, but can access more specialized hospital services at more centralized levels. The system provides universal care at less cost per person than the United States, and Sweden enjoys better health statistics by most indicators.

Source: The Swedish Institute: *Fact sheet prepared for Swedish information service abroad,* Stockholm, 1991, The Institute.

county council elected by the local people responsible for local problems. A managing committee composed of a delegate from the county council, a physician, and a supervisory official conducts necessary business between meetings of the county council. Physicians who are government employees receive a straight salary dependent on rank but irrespective of specialty. Hospitals are operated by the government.

Financing. Under the national health insurance system, payments are made when a person seeks medical and dental care and hospital treatment. These payments are normally paid by the social insurance office to the health care administration or the individual practitioner concerned, with the patient usually paying a fee at consultation. The patient pays a standard charge set by the county council for public outpatient services. Costs covered by the national system include consultation with a physician, birth control counseling, x-rays, lab tests, and referrals. Costs not covered include physical, occupational, and speech therapy. A ceiling caps costs for those with catastrophic illness. Dental coverage up to 60% is included in the system.

Health and medical care costs have increased in recent decades. During the last few years increases have not exceeded 1.5% in fixed prices and today amount to 8.8% of the GNP. This compares with 14% of GNP for the United States. The system is financed primarily by income taxes levied by the county councils. General state subsidies level out differences in income between the county councils. The remainder comes from state funds for education, research, and psychiatry, reimbursements from the national health insurance system, and patient fees (4%).

The Swedish system enjoys a high level of public confidence, and its universality contrasts with the current U.S. system. The main weaknesses of the current Swedish system are the lack of integration between services, high proportion of direct referrals to hospitals, long waiting lists for some types of treatment, some limited choice, and insufficient incentives for health personnel to improve the productivity and efficiency of the health sector.

Canada

On the surface there are many similarities between Canada and the United States, including the health care systems. But while Americans have been concerned about having the best health care system in the world, Canadians have been concerned about building an equitable and universally accessible system, with portability of rights to care from one province to another. Surface similarities between the two systems need to be understood in light of the underlying value differences between the United States and Canada.

Organization. As with any system of health care, the Canadian system must be understood in the context of political structure and philosophy. Canadians are traditionally more accepting than their American neighbors of the role of government in social and human services. Canada considers health a right and a national responsibility. Canadian patients have freedom of choice in selecting their health care providers. They are obliged to see a primary care provider before they can expect to use the services of specialists, which must be by referral. The medical profession is independent and self-regulating. Physicians are not salaried, but instead are reimbursed on a fee-for-service basis, with fee schedules established independently by each province. Hospitals are not government owned, but are locally controlled, nonprofit organizations.

Financing. Although the federal government has provided approximately half the funding in the past, the 10 provinces are covering an increased share, administer their own programs, and have the final say about how much is spent and how resources are allocated. Many of the key features of the Canadian system such as access, affordability, and comprehensiveness have long been policy goals in the United States with bipartisan appeal. Furthermore, in most respects the program does not violate the traditional practice of medicine. The system is decentralized, with considerable autonomy given local governments regarding the scope and provision of health care services. Providers of care are reimbursed in a manner similar to that of the United States and, while some incentives to affect distribution of physicians have been adopted, there are few real restraints on specialization or location of practice. The provinces agreed in 1993 to a 10% reduction in medical school enrollments to control the escalation of cost now understood to be driven by oversupply of physicians.

Access. Public access to personal health services improves with the removal of economic barriers to care. Canada has seen some shift in resource allocation from rich to poor. Poor people have increased their use of physicians, as have the middle- and upper-income groups. Not all problems related to access can be solved merely through changes in financing, however, and certain inequities persist. For example, the poor still use hospital emergency rooms more for primary health care problems than other income groups, indicating that physician maldistribution may be a persistent problem in primary care.

Use of services. Use of services has not increased at the alarming rate originally projected in some quarters. If Canada's experience is any guide, a national health insurance scheme does not necessarily create a "flood" of people seeking medical care.

Cost containment. In 1992 Canadians spent $71 billion on health care, which is more than $2550 per person. Health care costs were almost 10% of the GNP. This compares with U.S. figures at $3160 per person and nearly 14% of the GNP. Escalating costs present critical problems. Hospital cost inflation in Canada has less to do with higher use than with increases in earnings of hospital workers and

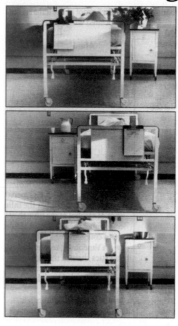

A sickening fact:
1 in 3 hospital cases is alcohol or drug related.

Alcohol and drug abuse isn't something you think about when you look at the cost of health care in B.C.

But you should.

Because a third of all our hospital beds, space that's needed to treat injuries and illnesses, is taken up by people who got there because of alcohol and drugs.

The problem is province-wide and we all pay the price. In hospital overcrowding. Taxes. Higher insurance rates.

So if you don't think alcohol and drug abuse affects you, think again.

The Responsibility is Yours.

1-800-663-1441

Alcohol and Drug Programs
Ministry of Labour and Consumer Services
The Honourable Lyall Hanson, Minister

FIGURE 21-13
Even though Canadians do not pay most of their medical and hospital costs directly, Canadian government agencies know the public is sensitive to the collective costs of their cherished health care system. They are reminded of how some preventable costs can be avoided, in this case the social burden associated with alcohol and drugs.

Source: Alcohol and Drug Programs, now in the Ministry of Health, Government of British Columbia.

intensity of care. The structure of reimbursement and the organization of medical practice are further contributing to the cost crisis. Because hospital insurance was passed 10 years before the physician reimbursement portion, incentives were put in place to hospitalize patients rather than to treat them in more cost-effective ambulatory settings. Global budgets are negotiated in advance for each hospital. There is a substantial degree of freedom of expenditures within the budget. If at the end of a fiscal year an institution has an operating surplus, the surplus is not necessarily reclaimed by the government. This provides the hospitals with an incentive to economize.

Health care as a right. Canadians discovered that granting health care as a "right" has been costly, but Canada now spends a lower percentage of its gross national product on health care than does the United States, and its rate of increase has been lower than that of the United States. Consumers have virtually no out-of-pocket expenses for regular hospital and medical care. Some provincial plans have imposed cost-sharing provisions for hospital stays, but the amounts are nominal. At the same time, Canada has an active supplementary insurance market, primarily for drugs, dental care, private rooms in hospitals, and other services not covered by the program.

Health education. In recent years Canada has educated the health care consumer about overuse of services and how to use the system more effectively (Figure 21-13). Great emphasis is being put on health promotion to support better health habits and conditions of living. Community health promotion has greater support in some Canadian provinces than in most states of the U.S.

U.S. PROGRAMS

Throughout U.S. history, Americans have attempted in various ways to make medical care available. Industrial firms and other employers have provided medical and hospital services for employees and their dependents. For generations the medical profession has used a sliding scale of fees based on the ability of the patient to pay. Socialized medicine was selectively in existence in the United States before the turn of the century. The federal government has provided medical and hospital care for members of the Armed Services and their dependents, war vet-

erans, American Indians on reservations, foreign service personnel, and various categories of government employees. The federal government, together with the state and local governments, has provided medical and hospital services for families on welfare. A universal program to ensure access and equity in health services, however, has never materialized. Although there are many different names for health insurance plans used currently, three main types include: private insurance, Health Maintenance Organizations (HMOs), and Preferred Provider Organizations (PPOs).

Private Insurance

Private or fee-for-service health insurance is the traditional health care policy in the United States. Commercial insurance companies were once reluctant to initiate health insurance but began with hospital insurance where **actuarial data** were available and costs were reasonably stable and predictable (see box). Success with hospital insurance encouraged the companies to expand to medical insurance and, finally, insurance for physician visits. Voluntary, noncommercial organizations have developed insurance programs for both groups and individuals.

Insurance is a financial contract that exchanges average costs for variable costs. It is not possible to predict the medical and hospital expenses for one person for the next year, but it is possible to predict total medical and hospital expenses for a million people. From such data, insurance premiums are determined and medical and hospital costs are spread among many rather than falling heavily on a few.

Extent of coverage. In 1990, approximately 86% of all Americans had some form of health insurance. Approximately 75% of those covered had private health insurance and 8% were covered by Medicaid. Loss of jobs during the recent recession and cutbacks on benefits to employees have meant an increase in the number of those without health cov-

1798   U.S. Marine Hospital Service established by U.S. Congress. Compulsory deductions for hospital service were made from seamen's wages.

1847   The first insurer to issue sickness insurance was organized: The Massachusetts Health Insurance Company of Boston.

1849   New York State passed the first general insurance law.

1850s   The first insurance supervisory boards were created in New Hampshire, Massachusetts, Rhode Island, and Vermont.

1850   Individual accident insurance became available in the United States with the chartering of the Franklin Health Assurance Company in Massachusetts.

1851   One of the earliest voluntary mutual protection associations, *La Societe Francaise de Bienfaisance Mutuelle,* was organized in San Francisco. It is noteworthy for having established a hospital in 1852 to provide care for its members.

1855   The first separate insurance department, independent of any established agency, was created in Massachusetts.

1859   The first full-time insurance commissioner was appointed in New York.

1863   The Travelers Insurance Company of Hartford, Connecticut, offered accident insurance for railway mishaps, then all forms of accident protection. It was the first company to issue insurance on a basis resembling its present form.

1875   A number of mutual benefit associations, called "establishment funds," were formed for employees of a single employer. The benefits provided usually included small payments for death and disability.

1890   Policies providing benefits for disability from specified diseases were first offered.

1890s   This period brought the promotion of many fraternal associations, assessment mutuals, and industrial insurers. Because many of these companies and associations were inadequately financed and poorly managed, many states passed legislation against them.

1900   Shortly after the turn of the century, disability benefits became available for substantially all diseases.

1910   Montgomery Ward & Co., Inc, replaced its "employee establishment fund" with an insured contract. This plan is generally regarded as the first group health insurance policy.

1912   The Standard Provisions Law drafted by the National Convention of Insurance Commissioners (now the NAIC) was enacted by most states. This model law sought to provide uniformity and fairness in the "operating conditions" of the health insurance contract.

1916   First noncancellable disability income contract was offered.

1917   Group accidental death and dismemberment insurance was first written.

1920s   Early in this decade individual hospitals began offering hospital expense benefits on an individual prepaid basis.

1920s   First partial disability benefits for sickness and accidents became available.

1929   The first health maintenance organization, the Ross-Loos Clinic, was established in Los Angeles, California.

1929   A group of school teachers arranged for Baylor Hospital in Dallas, Texas, to provide room and board and specified ancillary services at a predetermined monthly cost. This plan is considered the forerunner of what later became known as the Blue Cross plans.

1929   With the depression, many companies entered a period of retrenchment in their disability income product line, particularly in the area of maintaining reasonable indemnity limits in order to avoid overinsurance.

1930s   The depression stimulated the expansion of insurance coverages through both public demand and hospitals' encouragement.

1932   First citywide Blue Cross plan was tried out with a group of hospitals in Sacramento, California.

1935   The Social Security Act (P.L. 74-241) provided for the first time federal grant-in-aid to states for such public health activities as maternal and child care, aid to crippled children, blind persons, the aged, and other health-impaired persons.

erage. In 1993 it was estimated that 37 million Americans have no health insurance. Among those uninsured, 60% were working but at low-paying service or retail industries that did not offer insurance benefits.

Health insurance coverage varies among sectors of the population. The people least likely to have coverage are those between 16 and 24 years of age. Twenty-two percent of this age group lacked insurance in 1990, compared to the nearly complete coverage by medicare or private supplemental insurance of the over-65 age group. People in the Northeast and Midwest are more likely to have health insurance than those in the South and West. Nearly a third of those of Hispanic origin lack insurance coverage (Figure 21-14).

Kind of coverage. Fee-for-service insurance provides the most choice of doctors and hospitals. While such plans usually pay some doctor and most hospital expenses, most do not cover preventive services such as physical checkups or immunizations and limit well-child care. Of the 670 million visits made to doctors' offices in 1991, 36% were paid for by private insurance. In addition to medical care, about 40% of the population now have plans that include dental insurance of varying generosity.

There are two basic kinds of fee-for-service coverage: basic and major medical. Basic protection pays toward the costs of a hospital room and care received in the hospital. It covers some hospital services and supplies, such as x-rays and prescribed medicine. Basic coverage also pays toward the cost of surgery and/or some doctor visits. Major medical insurance takes over where basic coverage leaves off. It covers the cost of long, high-cost illness or injuries. Some policies combine both types of insurance into a "comprehensive plan."

The insured person pays three different kinds of costs: a monthly premium, an annual deductible, and coinsurance toward costs. The deductible, which might be $250 in a typical plan, must be paid each year before the insurance payments begin. After the deductible amount for the year is paid, the policy

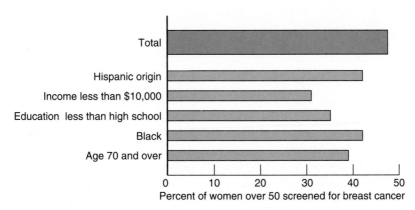

FIGURE 21-14

The absence of adequate insurance coverage in some population groups and for some preventive services shows up in the low rates of screening and preventive examinations in those population groups at highest risk. Here the rates are for women 50 years and over in the United States in 1990 who had received a clinical breast examination and a mammogram within the past 2 years.

Source: National Center for Health Statistics, data from the National Health Interview Survey of 1990.

Significant Events in Development of Access to Health Care between World War II and the Medicare-Medicaid Act	
1948 The National Labor Relations Board ruled, in a dispute between the United Steel-workers' Union and the Inland Steel Company, that the term ''wages'' be construed to include pension and insurance benefits. The U.S. Supreme Court upheld this ruling in a 1949 decision.	1961 First state enrollment plan was made available by Connecticut to persons 65 and over on a state basis and under special enabling legislation allowing the pooling of risks by a group of insurance companies (Associated Connecticut Health Insurance Companies).
1949 Major medical expense benefits were introduced by Liberty Mutual Insurance Company to supplement basic medical care expenses.	1963 The Health Professions Educational Assistance Act (P.L. 88-129) aided training of physicians, dentists, and public health personnel.
1954 Congress introduced the disability ''freeze'' that stated that the quarters during which a worker is disabled are not counted in determining the number of quarters needed to be fully or currently insured under Old Age and Survivors Insurance (OASI).	1964 Prescription drug expense benefits were introduced.
	1964 The Nurse Training Act (P.L. 88-581) provided special Federal effort for training professional nursing personnel.
1956 Disability insurance was added to the Social Security System, providing monthly cash benefits for insured persons who are totally disabled.	1965 Social Security Amendments of 1965 (P.L. 88-97) established a Social Security hospital insurance program for the aged and voluntary supplementary medical insurance program (Medicare) and grants to states for medical assistance programs (Medicaid).
1957 Vision care expense benefits were introduced by private insurers, followed in 1959 by extended care facility expense benefits.	
1959 Continental Casualty Company issued the first comprehensive group dental insurance plan written by an insurance company.	1966 Program of governmental health insurance, Medicare, for people aged 65 and over, became effective July 1.
1960s Eligibility for disability benefits under Social Security was expanded.	1967 The Age Discrimination in Employment Act (ADEA) guaranteed employees between the ages of 40 and 65 the same benefits under employee benefit plans as younger employees.

holder shares the remaining bill with the insurance company. In a typical arrangement the policy holder's **coinsurance** portion of the shared bill may be 20% and the insurer pays 80%. Most fee-for-service plans have a ''cap''—the highest amount an individual will have to pay for medical bills in a given year. A cap is reached when deductible and coinsurance payments exceed a certain amount, which may be as low as $1000 or as high as $5000. The insurance company pays the full amount in excess of the cap for items it covers.

Health Maintenance Organizations (HMOs)

HMOs, which are prepaid health plans, have experienced substantial growth over the last two decades, from 175 in 1976 to 556 in 1991. Today over 34 million people are served by HMOs.

Between the passage of the Social Security Act in 1934 and the amendments in 1965 that created Medicare and Medicaid, most of the significant advances in ensuring greater access to medical care were made by private insurance companies and states. Then came the 1960s, discussed in the previous chapter as a period of ferment in the health care system. Some of the more significant events during the postwar years and up to Medicare and Medicaid are summarized in the box on the preceding page. Of particular note during this period was the evolution of the health maintenance organization concept.

The most momentous American initiative in providing prepaid medical care has been the development of health maintenance organizations (HMOs), sometimes identified merely as prepaid group practice. In recent instances the programs have been subsidized, at least at the outset, but in the main, these have been self-sustaining enterprises. Four principles characterize an HMO. It is (1) an *organized system* of health care that accepts the responsibility to provide or otherwise ensure the delivery of (2) an agreed-upon set of *comprehensive health maintenance and treatment services* for (3) a voluntarily *enrolled group* of people in a geographical area and (4) is reimbursed through a *prenegotiated and fixed periodic payment* made by or on behalf of each person or family enrolled in the plan. These four principles of HMO development are further defined and described by Congress in the Health Maintenance Organization Assistance Act of 1973.

An organized system. An HMO must be capable of bringing together directly, or arranging for, the services of physicians and other health professionals with the services of inpatient and outpatient facilities for preventive, acute, and other care, as well as any other health services that a defined population might reasonably require. The system is organized in such a way as to ensure for the enrollee the most efficient and effective entry into the health care system. It also promises continuity of care for the enrolled population through linkages between the components of organization.

In nearly all HMOs, members are assigned or choose one doctor to serve as a primary care doctor. This doctor monitors the member's health and pro-

vides most of the medical care, as in the Canadian and Swedish systems, referring to specialists and other health care professionals as needed. In some HMOs doctors are salaried and have offices all in the same location. In other arrangements, independent doctors contract with the HMO to take care of patients. These are called individual practice associations (IPAs), and doctors are located in scattered locations in their own private offices.

Comprehensive health maintenance and treatment services. The HMO must be capable of providing or arranging for the provision of the health services that a population might require, including primary care, emergency care, acute inpatient hospital care, and inpatient and outpatient care and rehabilitation for chronic and disabling conditions. Primary care, one of the keystones of the HMO, emphasizes those services aimed at preventing the onset of illness or disability, at the maintenance of good health, and at the continuing evaluation and management of early complaints, symptoms, problems, and the chronic aspects of disease. Typical services include doctor visits, hospital stays, emergency care, surgery, lab tests, x-rays, and therapy. HMOs typically provide preventive care such as office visits, immunizations, well-baby checkups, mammograms, and physicals.

An agreed-upon set of services. The consumers and the HMO agree on which services will be purchased from the HMO in return for the prepayment figure. Because some HMOs may have groups or enrollees paid for by Medicare, Medicaid, or employer-employee arrangements, the benefit schedule for population groups may differ.

An enrolled group. Members of an HMO are those people who voluntarily join the HMO through a contract arrangement in which the enrollee (or head of household) agrees to pay the fixed monthly or other periodic payment (or have it paid on his or her behalf) to the HMO. Enrollees agree to use the HMO as their principal source of health care if they become ill or need care.

Type of coverage. Those enrolled in an HMO pay a monthly premium. This is a fixed fee that covers the agreed-on set of services. There may be a small copayment for each office visit, such as a $5 fee for a doctor visit or $25 fee for hospital emergency room treatment. Rather than completing multiple forms usually required by fee-for-service insurance, members present a card, like a credit card, at the doctor's office or hospital.

Preferred Provider Organizations (PPOs)

This type of organization is a combination of the traditional fee-for-service plan and an HMO. Like the HMO, the consumer-member has a limited number of doctors and hospitals to choose from. When members use one of the "preferred" providers, most of the medical bills are covered. Usually there is a small copayment for each visit. Some services require a deductible and coinsurance. PPOs also use a primary care doctor to monitor members' health. Most cover preventive care such as doctor visits, well-baby care, immunizations, and mammograms. PPOs also allow members to use doctors who are not part of the plan and still receive some coverage. Usually the member will pay a larger portion of the bill when using someone other than a preferred provider.

Medicare

The United States launched its first widespread program of socialized medicine in 1965, when the Medicare program went into operation. Medicare was established as a federal health insurance program for Americans age 65 and older, for certain disabled Americans under age 65, and people of any age who have permanent kidney failure. It is not necessary to have Social Security or government

work credits to be eligible for Medicare. In 1991 Medicare covered approximately 35 million people, of whom about 3 million were disabled and some 150,000 were kidney disease patients.

Medicare is administered by the Health Care Financing Administration of the U.S. Department of Health and Human Services. Commercial insurance companies serve as agents or intermediaries for the program. Claimants under the program fill out a form and mail it to the designated insurance company serving as agent for the government.

Medicare has two basic forms of coverage—Part A provides hospital insurance, and Part B provides supplemental medical insurance for costs such as payments for doctors and related services and supplies ordered by a doctor. All who meet the eligibility requirements can participate in Part A of Medicare free. Part B requires payment of a premium.

Medicare hospital insurance, Part A, is financed mainly from a portion of the Social Security payroll tax (the FICA) deduction. The Medicare part of the payroll tax is 1.45% from the employee and 1.45% from the employer on wages up to $125,000 in 1991. The optional Medicare medical insurance, Part B, is financed by the monthly premiums paid by enrollees and from general federal revenues. The monthly premium in 1991 was $29.00. The premium pays about 25% of the cost of the Part B program, and general tax revenues pay about 25%.

Part A: Hospital insurance. Medicare hospital insurance pays for up to 90 days of inpatient care per benefit period. For the first 60 days, Medicare pays for all covered services, except for a deductible. In 1991 the deductible was $628 per benefit period. Those services include a semi-private room, regular nursing service, operating room, drugs, lab tests, x-rays, medical supplies, and rehabilitation services. From days 61 to 90, Medicare continues to pay for these services, but the beneficiary must pay a daily coinsurance amount. In 1991 coinsurance was $157 per day.

Medicare also pays for skilled nursing or rehabilitation services up to 100 days. Hospital insurance pays for all covered services for the first 20 days. For the next 80 it pays for all covered services except for a daily coinsurance amount of $78.50 per day in 1991. Medicare makes a careful distinction between skilled nursing care and "custodial care." The former is provided by those who are medically trained, and Medicare pays for such services. The latter type of care includes help with dressing, walking, or eating, which does not required skilled care; therefore, Medicare does not pay for such services.

Medicare pays the full approved cost of home health visits by an approved agency. There is no limit to the number of covered visits for intermittent skilled nursing care and physical or speech therapy. A 20% copayment does apply to medical equipment such as wheelchairs or hospital beds. Medicare can help pay for hospice care for terminally ill beneficiaries up to a maximum of two 90-day periods and one 30-day period and one extension.

Part B: Medical insurance. This supplemental insurance pays for doctor services and many other medical services and supplies that are not covered by the hospital insurance part of Medicare. Each year before Medicare medical insurance begins paying for covered services, beneficiaries must meet the annual medical insurance deductible, which was $100 in 1991. After the deductible is met, Medicare will generally pay 80% of the approved charges for covered services during the rest of the year.

The Medicare law specifically prohibits federal interference in the physician-patient relationship, but this also precludes monitoring of quality. Freedom of choice is guaranteed—there is no "preferred" group of physician providers (see box).

Services not covered. Medicare does not pay for custodial care, most nursing home care, most care outside the United States, dental care, routine checkups, prescription drugs, routine foot care, hearing aids, and eyeglasses. Many private insurance com-

Coordinated Care Plans

The preceding sections explain how Medicare Part B works if you receive your benefits through the traditional fee-for-service (pay-as-you-go) delivery system. As a Medicare beneficiary, you also have the option of receiving physician and other health care services through coordinated care plans that have contracts with Medicare, such as health maintenance organizations (HMOs), and competitive medical plans (CMPs).

In a coordinated care plan, a network of health care providers (physicians, hospitals, skilled nursing facilities, etc.) generally offers medical services to plan members on a prepaid basis. Services usually must be obtained from the professionals and facilities that are part of the plan. If you enroll in a plan that has a contract with Medicare, a Medicare claim will seldom need to be submitted on your behalf. Medicare pays the plan a set amount and the plan provides your medical care. Additionally, instead of paying Medicare's deductible and coinsurance as you would under fee-for-service care, most coordinated care plans charge enrollees a monthly premium and nominal copayments.

Most plans serving Medicare beneficiaries are required to provide all Medicare hospital and medical benefits available in the plan's service area. Some plans also provide benefits beyond what Medicare pays for, such as preventive care, prescription drugs, dental care, hearing aids, and eyeglasses.

HCFA, 1992.

panies sell insurance to pay for costs not covered by Medicare. Such "Medigap" coverage varies among states and was standardized in 1992 to a core package of benefits.

Medicaid

Title XIX of the Social Security Act, also called the Kerr-Mills medical assistance plan (Medicaid), provides medical care not only for indigents 65 years of age and older but for those of any age who are defined as medically indigent (Figure 21-15). This program is a joint enterprise of the federal and state governments, which subsidize all of the costs.

Like Medicare, the Medicaid "Grants to States for Medical Assistance Programs" was addressed exclusively to the problem of purchasing power and made little or no effort to deviate from "usual and customary fees" to hospitals and physicians or from the prevailing organization of delivery systems. Both programs under PL 89-97 were established on the assumption that the existing delivery systems would respond to the needs and demands of the population if sufficient fees for services were provided. The increased demand contributed to increased prices. The two programs rose from $5 billion in their initial year to over $129 billion in 1992 for Medicare and nearly $68 billion for Medicaid.

Federal requirements. The purpose of Medicaid was to provide medical assistance for the "medically indigent" families with dependent children, the aged, the blind, and the disabled. The law extended coverage to rehabilitation and other services to help such families attain independence and self-care. The distinguishing mechanism of this plan is that it authorizes appropriations on a fiscal-year basis for payments to states that submit approved plans. The act required that state plans must (1) cover the entire state, (2) contribute at least 40% of the nonfederal share, (3) provide for a fair hearing to any individual whose claim is denied or delayed, (4) provide for administration of the state program or supervision of locally administered plans, (5) designate a single state agency for administration or supervision of the plan, (6) provide reports to the Secretary of Health and Human Services, (7) pro-

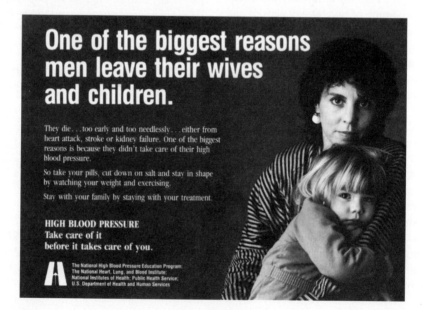

FIGURE 21-15
Medically indigent families with dependent children (particularly prevalent in single-parent families) are eligible for Social Security payments to the dependents of disabled or deceased beneficiaries, and for Medicaid for their medical care requirements.

Source: National High Blood Pressure Education Program, National Institutes of Health, U.S. Department of Health and Human Services.

TABLE 21-4
Preventive care services in various countries

Country	Newborn care	Infant and preschool-age care	School-age care
England	First exam performed in the hospital; all mothers seen in the home by health visitors about 10 days after birth	General practitioners provide most care; public clinics also provide care in urban areas	School nurses and physicians provide exams to children with special needs or on demand
France	First exam performed in the hospital; clinic nurses then visit the homes of all children at medical or social risk	Private physicians provide about 70% of care; the remainder is provided in clinics, crèches, and preschools	Education authorities provide one or two exams in school, with optional exams on demand, and student counseling sessions
Germany	First two exams performed in the hospital; public health office nurses sometimes visit socially disadvantaged families	Private pediatricians or general practitioners provide about 90% of care; the remainder is provided by public health offices	Public health offices generally offer three exams in school, but significant variation exists by region
Japan	Initial screening is performed in the hospital; public health nurses then visit homes with low birth weight babies and others as needed	Public health centers deliver most care, with the rest rendered by private clinics and hospitals	Health and education authorities provide annual exams in school and health education
The Netherlands	Initial exam done by a physician at home or in a hospital; public health nurses then visit new mothers within 2 weeks of birth to perform other screening tests	Public infant and toddler clinics provide about 95% of care, with the rest done privately	Municipal or district health authorities provide between four and six exams in school or in health centers

vide safeguards for confidentiality of records, (8) provide that all individuals wishing to make application for medical assistance under the plan have an opportunity to do so, and (9) designate an authority for establishing and maintaining standards for participating institutions.

Assessment. Consider some of the implications of these first nine requirements. Numbers 1 and 2 clearly distinguish Medicaid from Medicare as a *state* plan. Number 3 places emphasis on repairing damage that should be prevented by requirements 8 and 9. From an educational perspective, number 8 should require states to include coordinated pro-

grams to ensure that all eligible beneficiaries know of their eligibility and that all applicants know of and have access to sources of assistance in maneuvering the application process. According to a survey in California, 95% of the potential beneficiaries and many of the community workers interviewed confused Medi-Cal (the California name for Medicaid) with *welfare* and with Medicare. (Some thought it was a soft drink.) Even among those using the program, 90% thought Medi-Cal was the same as welfare. The welfare stigma is found to be highly unsettling for most users, a cause of misuse, and a clear deterrent to use by potential beneficiaries.

The coverage of preventive services by Medicaid

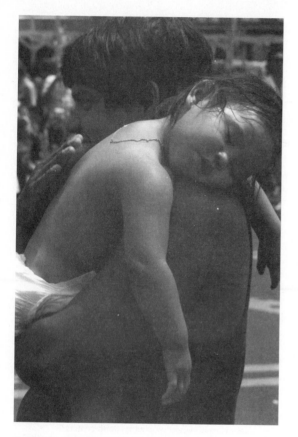

FIGURE 21-16
Health insurance and Medicaid provisions for children vary widely across the states. Children, therefore, are at great risk of having no coverage or at best uneven coverage with no continuity of care.

Source: Center for Substance Abuse Prevention, U.S. Department of Health and Human Services.

varies widely from state to state. New federal requirements for states to cover prenatal and infant care services have been implemented by states at considerable cost but still without the systematic coverage provided in other countries (Table 21-4).

Cost containment. Of high concern to both state and federal governments are uncontrolled growth of health care costs and the lack of physicians and other providers willing to treat Medicaid patients. Under traditional fee-for-service arrangements neither the state nor any other entity monitors the physician's provision of services. These arrangements are inadequate in terms of controlling costs and ensuring quality care.

During most of the 1980s, Medicaid costs grew up to 10% a year, and, in 1989, began to rise even more rapidly. As the federal contribution to Medicaid has declined, states have picked up a larger share. In 1970 Medicaid took 3% of state spending; in 1990 it took 12% of state spending. In 1992 federal and state spending on Medicaid totaled $119 billion, a 29% increase over the previous year's total. In addition, the number of beneficiaries from 1991 to 1992 increased an estimated 10% to about 31 million.

The distribution of costs with the Medicaid system varies by population group. For example, while 27% of Medicaid recipients are on Supplemental Security Income, these mostly elderly recipients account for nearly 70% of Medicaid expenditures. Aid to Families with Dependent Children (AFDC) recipients constitute about 70% of those eligible for Medicaid, but only account for 29% of Medicaid costs (Figure 21-16).

Managed care. To deal with the costs, access problems, and aging of the overall population, states have increasingly turned to managed care delivery systems. These systems are a continuum of models that share a common approach. At one end of the continuum are prepaid models that pay organizations a per capita amount each month to provide or arrange for all covered services. At the other end of the spectrum are primary care case management models similar to traditional fee-for-service arrangements. The difference with managed care is that providers receive a per capita management fee to coordinate a patient's care in addition to reimbursement for the services they provide. Common to all managed care models in the Medicaid program is the use of a primary care physician to control and coordinate the delivery of health services in a cost-conscious manner.

By 1994 nearly all states expect to have at least one managed care program in place. Four key issues to resolve in managed care systems include planning for implementation, making enrollment mandatory, setting capitation rates, and educating beneficiaries about the program.

HEALTH CARE REFORM

With escalating costs, a huge deficit, an aging population, the role of life-style and community in health, a new administration in the White House,

and bipartisan support, the United States is poised for major health care reform. What reform will look like after it runs the gauntlet of economic, political, social, and philosophical considerations is not clear at this time (Figure 21-17).

Proposals for reform have come from all sectors of society. The more than 30 health care proposals currently being considered by Congress divide into three main groups: (1) market-based proposals to assist some people now without insurance to purchase it, (2) "pay-or-play" plans in which employers either provide insurance to employees or pay taxes to finance an alternate public system, and (3) proposals for a single-payer health care system like Canada's. Most plans aim to hold down the soaring costs of health care and to enable those without health insurance to have access to the health care

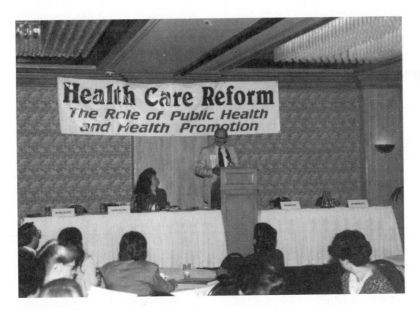

FIGURE 21-17
Health care reform and how it will affect community health services, especially disease prevention and health promotion, have been widely debated and discussed in professional meetings during the early years of the 1990s. The answers are not yet in as this text goes to press.
Source: California Conference of Local Directors of Health Education, San Diego.

system. A smaller number of proposals would insure the costs of long-term care. Almost all proposals require new financing to meet start-up expenses or shifting of costs from the private to the public sector.

While Washington moves cautiously toward health care reform, various states have taken creative steps toward reform at home. Through community participation, Oregon has established priorities for health care services for which it will pay. Preventive services lead the list. While the proposed rationing of services stirs strong emotional debate, it acknowledges limits to services the state can afford to pay. Under the Hawaii health plan called QUEST, Medicaid, State General Assistance, and the State Health Insurance Program are joined to form a large purchasing pool that will buy health care coverage for 150,000 individuals. Through a process of competitive bidding among managed care plans Hawaii hopes to hold costs down. Minnesota has several current proposals for reform to extend coverage to the uninsured.

Health care reform will be difficult. Most fundamentally, health care reform will not only mean looking at our wallets, it will mean looking at our values. Do we really concur with the principles of Alma-Ata that health is a fundamental human right? If we believe health is a right, how do we express and pay for that value in a system that provides liberty, justice—and health care—for all?

SUMMARY

Community health is concerned with the health of the whole person and the context within which people live. The current health care system is one primarily concerned with treating sickness, not enhancing health. While Americans are rightfully proud of advances in medical care, the United States lags behind other developed countries in some health care indicators and matches some less developed countries in infant mortality. Americans spend

> ## To Ensure Clinical Preventive Services Objective
>
> Objectives target increasing quality years of life, increasing receipt of recommended services, increasing access to primary care, removing financial barriers to receipt of services, ensuring clinical preventive services for publicly funded programs, ensuring provision of recommended preventive services by clinicians, ensuring access to clinical preventive services by local public health departments, and increasing the representation of racial and ethnic minority groups among health professionals.

billions on "miracle" cures and quick weight loss, while 37 million Americans have no health insurance. The increased specialization of medical services, the aging of the population, and uncontrolled health care costs have forced health care reform as a priority on the national agenda. How the system is reformed will depend as much on fundamental values as on current circumstances.

Most of the countries that rank higher than the United States in life expectancy statistics have a national health program (either financing or providing services) and most have lower per capita costs for health care than does the United States. Comparison with Canada has been most instructive for policy development in the United States.

Most health insurance is not prevention-oriented. It is *sickness* rather than *health* insurance. It gives partial rather than comprehensive benefits, and fails to control either costs or quality.

Numerous proposals for restructuring the health care system have been introduced recently by public and private groups recognizing the inadequacy of the Social Security amendments on Medicare and Medicaid to provide health insurance for the elderly and the medically indigent. Cost containment remains a compelling consideration in all proposals, and this led to an emphasis on competitive and free-market mechanisms in the political climate of the 1980s. The outcome of the health care reform initiatives of the Clinton Administration and the reorganized Health Canada were unknown as this book went to press.

QUESTIONS FOR REVIEW

1. Why is it paradoxical that of the developed countries, the United States has neither the highest level of health nor the greatest life expectancy?

2. Why is health education of the poor an urgent need in the United States?

3. Why does health fraud tend to flourish?

4. Why might an adult citizen wear a charm around his or her neck to keep sickness away?

5. What should the communications media do to protect the public from health fraud?

6. Is the U.S. hospital admissions rate too high or too low? Why?

7. What is the ratio of physicians to population in your community or country, and what is your appraisal of the situation?

8. How does your country measure up to the standard of four hospital beds per 1000 people?

9. Why is the average length of stay in a hospital of limited value in the analysis of medical and hospital costs to citizens?

10. To what extent should the number of nursing homes and personal care homes in your community be increased in the next 10 years?

11. Why are medical and hospital costs increasing at a greater rate than the cost-of-living index?

12. What would be your proposal for paying hospital and medical care for low-income families not on welfare?

13. Why are people often slow in paying their medical and hospital bills?

14. What is the case for and against the federal government totally subsidizing education in the medical, dental, and other health professions?

15. Why should the consumer of medical services have a voice in how the costs of these services are to be paid?

READINGS

Donovan CL: Factors predisposing, enabling and reinforcing routine screening of patients for preventing fetal alcohol syndrome: a survey of New Jersey physicians, *J Drug Educ* 21:35, 1991.
This application of the PRECEDE model, which was introduced in Chapter 4 of this book, illustrates how physicians are influenced in their decisions to screen women for alcohol use during pregnancy or to employ other procedures in the clinical setting to prevent fetal alcohol syndrome.

Rodwin MA: *Medicine, money and morals: physicians' conflicts of interest,* Oxford, 1993, Oxford University Press.
Documents the commercialization of medicine and how medical ethics are replaced in many settings by business ethics; challenges the public and the professions to confront financial conflicts of interest that harm patients and society.

Scherl DJ, Noren J, Osterweis M, editors: *Promoting health and preventing disease,* Washington, DC, 1993, Association of Academic Health Centers, Health Policy Annual 2.
Reviews experience of various academic health centers in tackling the issues of university and hospital relationships with the communities in which they are located, especially in disease prevention and health promotion.

Shugars DA, O'Neil EH, Bader JD, editors: *Healthy America: Practitioners for 2005, an agenda for action for U.S. health professional schools,* Durham, NC, 1991, The Pew Health Professions Commission.
The commission study presents the data and the issues on the training of future health professionals, giving special emphasis to the need for stronger prevention training.

BIBLIOGRAPHY

Allegrante JP, Kovar PT, MacKenzie CR et al: A walking education program for patients with osteoarthritis of the knee: theory and intervention strategies, *Health Educ Q* 20:63, 1993.

Anderson LA, Zimmerman MA: Patient and physician perceptions of their relationship and patient satisfaction: a study of chronic disease management, *Pat Educ Counsel* 20:27, 1993.

Barer ML, Evans RG: Interpreting Canada: models, mindsets, and myths, *Health Aff* 11:44, 1992.

Boelen C: The challenge of changing medical education and medical practice, *World Health Forum* 14:213, 1993.

Bruhn JG, Levine HG, Levine PL: *Managing boundaries in the health professions,* Springfield, Ill, 1993, Charles C Thomas.

Costanza ME: Physician compliance with mammography guidelines: barriers and enhancers, *J Am Board Fam Pract* 5:1, 1992.

Council on Scientific Affairs: A role for physicians and the efficacy of health education efforts, *JAMA* 263: 1816, 1990.

Cummins RO: Emergency medical services and sudden cardiac arrest: the "chain of survival" concept, *Annu Rev Public Health* 14:313, 1993.

Davis DA, Thomson MA, Oxman A et al: Evidence for the effectiveness of CME: a review of 50 randomized controlled trials, *JAMA* 268:1111, 1992.

Dignan MB, Michielutte R, Sharp P et al: The role of focus groups in health education for cervical cancer among minority women, *J Community Health* 15:369, 1990.

Enthoven AC: The history and principles of managed competition, *Health Aff* 12(suppl):24, 1993.

Frankle RT, Owen AL: *Nutrition in the community: the art of delivering services,* ed 3, St Louis, 1993, Mosby.

Gaucher EJ, Coffey RJ: *Total quality in healthcare: from theory to practice,* San Francisco, 1993, Jossey-Bass.

Green LW: The revival of community and the obligation of academic health centers to the public. In Bulger RE, Reiser SJ, editors: *Integrity in health care institutions: humane environments for teaching, inquiry and practice,* Des Moines, 1990, University of Iowa Press.

Green LW, Mullen PD, Friedman RB: Epidemiological and community approaches to patient compliance. In Cramer JA, Spilker B, editors: *Patient compliance in medical practice and clinical trials,* New York, 1991, Raven Press.

Hellinger F: Forecasting the medical care costs of the HIV epidemic: 1991-1994, *Inquiry* 28:213, 1991.

Levine DM, Becker DM, Bone LR: Narrowing the gap in health status of minority populations: a community-academic medical center partnership, *Am J Prev Med* 8:319, 1992.

Macklin R: *Enemies of patients,* Oxford, 1993, Oxford University Press.

Matzen RN, Lang RS: *Clinical preventive medicine,* St Louis, 1993, Mosby.

Mesters I, Meertens R, Crebolder H et al: Development of a health education program for parents of preschool children with asthma, *Health Educ Res* 8:53, 1993.

Mullen F: Missing: a national medical manpower policy, *Milbank Q* 70:381, 1992.

Mullen PM, Green LW: Educating and counseling for prevention: from theory and research to principles. In Goldbloom MD, Lawrence RB, editors: *Preventing disease: beyond the rhetoric,* Cambridge, 1990, Springer-Verlag.

Mansour AA, Al-Osimy MH: A study of satisfaction among primary health care patients in Saudi Arabia, *J Community Health* 18:163, 1993.

Murray RB, Zentner JP: Nursing assessment and health promotion: strategies through the life span, ed 5, Norwalk, Conn, 1993, Appleton & Lange.

Rachlis M, Kushner C: *Second opinion: what's wrong with Canada's health-care system and how to fix it,* Toronto, 1989, Collins.

Roemer MI: National health systems throughout the world, *Annu Rev Public Health* 14:335, 1993.

Shapiro DW, Lasker RD, Bindman AB et al: Containing costs while improving quality of care: the role of profiling and practice guidelines, *Annu Rev Public Health* 14:219, 1993.

Simons-Morton DG, Mullen PD, Mains DA et al: Characteristics of controlled studies of patient education and counseling for preventive health behaviors, *Patient Educ Counsel* 19:175, 1992.

Tabak ER, Mullen PD, Simons-Morton DG et al: Definition and yield of inclusion criteria for a meta-analysis of studies of patient education in clinical preventive services, *Eval Health Professions* 14:388, 1991.

U.S. Consumer Product Safety Commission: *Consumer product safety alert,* Washington, DC, 1993, The Commission.

Vogel DE: *Family physicians and managed care: a view to the 90s,* Kansas City, Mo, 1993, American Academy of Family Physicians.

Walsh J, McPhee S: A systems model of clinical preventive care: an analysis of factors influencing patient and physician, *Health Educ Q* 19:157, 1992.

Weissman JS, Epstein AM: The insurance gap: does it make a difference? *Annu Rev Public Health* 14:243, 1993.

Zapka JG, Chasan L, Barth R et al: Emphasizing screening activities in a community health center: a case study of a breast cancer screening project, *J Ambulatory Care Manage* 15:38, 1992.

Zapka JG, Hosmer D, Costanza ME et al: Changes in mammography use: economic, need, and service factors, *Am J Public Health* 82:1345, 1992.

APPENDIXES

APPENDIXES

Areas of Community
Health Specialization

❖

Area of specialization	Differentiating characteristics (pertaining to the area of specialization and illustrative ways it contributes to improved health)	Illustrative jobs and job settings (for graduates of the area of specialization)
Biostatistics *The application of statistical procedures, techniques, and methodology to characterize or investigate health problems and programs*	Biostatistics is concerned with such activities as the collection, organization, retrieval, and analysis of data; design of experiments; and application of techniques of inference and probability to the examination of biological, social, and environmental data. Biostatistics closely interacts with the field of epidemiology, while also extending into the congruent areas of vital statistics and demography, computer systems programming and analysis, and program planning and evaluation. The specialty helps to anticipate needs and improve decision making with regard to health problems, programs, and technologies through (1) the development and operation of ongoing statistical information systems concerned with vital events, health status, and program operations and (2) the proper design and carrying out of studies, and the analysis and interpretation of data obtained from such studies.	In local and state agencies employment includes the collection, tabulation, and analysis of statistics bearing on all aspects of health problems and programs. In state, provincial, federal, and academic settings employment includes providing assistance to investigators in the design, performance, and data analysis of research on health problems and programs. In academic institutions employment includes training health workers in the use and interpretation of statistics and carrying out research to discover improved ways of using statistical measures and procedures.
Epidemiology *The science devoted to the systematic study of the distribution and determinants of disease or disability*	Epidemiology determines disease frequencies and trends in populations, and those factors that increase or reduce disease and disability. Epidemiology has both a	In health agencies at all levels epidemiologists are employed in the design and execution of studies or information systems concerned with ascertaining the distribu-

Based on Hall TL, Jackson RS, Parsons WB: Schools of public health, trends in graduate education, DHHS Pub No (HRA) 80-45, Washington, DC, May 1980, Division of Associated Health Professions, Public Health Service; American College of Preventive Medicine: *What is preventive medicine?* Washington, DC, 1993, The College.

Area of specialization	Differentiating characteristics (pertaining to the area of specialization and illustrative ways it contributes to improved health)	Illustrative jobs and job settings (for graduates of the area of specialization)
Epidemiology—cont'd	descriptive and an analytical role. In the former, and in conjunction with the field of biostatistics, it makes use of statistical methods to determine morbidity, mortality, prevalence, incidence and case fatality rates, and estimates of risk of developing specific diseases in a given population. In its analytical role, epidemiology uses a variety of techniques to examine and evaluate data that seek to identify predisposing, precipitating, and prolonging factors bearing on disease and disability. By developing new or improved information on the distribution and determinants of disease, epidemiology helps the health care system design better ways to prevent, detect, and treat disease and disability.	tion and determinants of disease or disability. In academic settings epidemiologists teach, do research, and assist clinical investigators in the study of disease and in the evaluation of new or improved measures for disease prevention, therapy, and rehabilitation.
Health services administration *The application of skills in resource management to accomplish the effective and efficient delivery of health services*	Areas of expertise relevant to this specialization include those of planning, organizing, directing, controlling, policy formulation and analysis, financial management, economics, accounting, and operations research. While persons with prior professional degrees are not uncommon, students in specialized programs of health services administration tend to have recent bachelor's degrees or to have been practicing administrators without other advanced training. Health services administrators seek to ensure that the resources available for the promotion, protection, and restoration of health are applied as effectively and efficiently as possible, consistent with the scientific knowledge base that exists about health and disease.	Health services administrators are employed at all levels of government and in the private sector to plan, implement, manage, coordinate, and evaluate programs for the delivery of health care and to design administrative systems appropriate to the needs of the population being served.
Public health practice and program management *The application of specialized knowledge and skills to the planning, implementation, management, and evaluation of activities carried out relevant to selected types of*	This area of specialization encompasses many of the identifiable public health programs and activities, some of which are organized according to the demographic characteristics of the target population (maternal and child health, gerontology), others according to a health	Employed at all levels of government and in the private and educational sectors, these specialists assume leadership roles in community-based health care, health promotion and disease prevention programs and systems; apply technical expertise to planning, implementation, and evaluation of technical programs within a defined

Area of specialization	Differentiating characteristics (pertaining to the area of specialization and illustrative ways it contributes to improved health)	Illustrative jobs and job settings (for graduates of the area of specialization)
Public health practice and program management—cont'd health professional disciplines and health problems or target populations	problem or organ system (mental health, dental public health), and still others according to professional discipline (nursing, social work). Specialists in each of these programmatic areas usually have a prior professional degree in one or more health disciplines in addition to specialty training relevant to their field of choice. They seek to integrate the body of knowledge of the basic discipline (medicine, nursing, etc.) with skills relevant to public health practice (planning, program development, etc.) to design and implement programs appropriate to specific health needs.	organizational framework; and carry out training and research activities.
Health education The process of influencing health-related social and behavioral change in human populations by predisposing, enabling, and reinforcing voluntary decisions and actions conducive to health	Health education specialists use specific methods, skills, and program strategies to help people change to healthful lifestyles, make more efficient use of health services, adopt self-care practices wherever possible, and participate actively in the design and implementation of programs that affect their health. Skills in the social and behavioral sciences, communication dynamics, educational theory, and community organization are relevant to this specialty, which has given leadership to health promotion.	Employment is available in many different types of agencies in both the public and private sectors to identify social and health needs of population groups, adapt the health care delivery system to the needs of individuals and communities, develop and implement patient education in health care and community settings, and use the media effectively as a means of achieving the above. Health education and health promotion programs in schools, companies, and clinical and other community settings employ health educators.
Environmental sciences Those specialties concerned with the identification and control of factors in the natural environment that affect health	Environmental sciences specialists are concerned with the relationships between the characteristics of the natural environment (air, water, soil, chemicals, etc.) and mental and physical health. This information is used to establish limits on pollutants that the environment can absorb without detrimental effects, to develop control technology, and to implement controls as necessary for the benefit of human and animal populations. The educational background of most environmental scientists usually includes disciplinary training in one or more of the natural sciences plus advanced courses in those aspects of environmental health relevant to their primary discipline.	Employment is available at all levels of government, public and private organizations, and industry to provide technical knowledge and methods in the investigation, planning, controlling, and regulation of matters pertaining to environmental health hazards. In addition, employees carry out basic and operational environmental research procedures and provide training to community workers and interest groups in methods and techniques of environmental protection.

Area of specialization	*Differentiating characteristics (pertaining to the area of specialization and illustrative ways it contributes to improved health)*	*Illustrative jobs and job settings (for graduates of the area of specialization)*
Occupational safety and health *The identification of health and safety hazards related to work and the work environment, and prevention and control of these hazards*	In collaboration with many disciplines such as medicine, nursing, statistics, engineering, and psychology, this area of specialization seeks to minimize ill health, injury, and maladjustments to work that may occur as a result of a person's association with work and the work environment.	In industry, occupational safety and health specialists are concerned with establishing the causes and effects of industrial health problems and the implementation of acceptable control methods. In government they are involved with monitoring morbidity and mortality associated with the work environment, formulating and enforcing safety standards, investigating specific health and safety problems, and planning and implementing appropriate health programs. Those employed by academic institutions are involved with the training of specialists in this field and with research.
Nutrition *The study of the interaction between nutrients, nutrition, and health; and the application of sound nutritional principles to improve or maintain health*	One specialty in nutrition is concerned primarily with the scientific study in laboratory and clinical settings of the effects of nutrients on growth, development, and health; the other specialty is concerned with the application of specialized nutrition knowledge and skills to improve or maintain the health of target population groups. In the former category are found persons with basic preparation in biochemistry, medicine, and related sciences; in the latter are persons with training in dietetics, clinical nutrition, and related fields.	Employment opportunities for specialists in nutrition exist at all levels of government and in private agencies, institutions, and industry. Examples of typical job activities include the assessment of nutritional problems in individuals and population groups, development and implementation of programs to change patterns of food consumption, and fundamental research into human and animal nutrition.
Biomedical and laboratory practice *Various specialty disciplines that use laboratory techniques for the diagnosis and treatment of disease, and for the investigtion of conditions affecting health status*	The two main defining characteristics of this broad area of specialization are (1) the type of facilities and equipment used and (2) the fact that it is concerned with the scientific investigation in individuals of biological and biochemical processes that affect or reflect health status. Specialists working in this area may be primarily concerned with the development of new knowledge or with the application of existing laboratory-based techniques for the maintenance of health and for the prevention, early detection, and treatment of disease, on an individual-case basis and in mass screening and prevention programs.	Those trained in this specialty are employed at all levels of government, in medical and academic institutions, and in public and privte laboratories. Illustrative job opportunities include laboratory research for the detection and treatment of disease, and the planning and operation of training programs concerned both with the basic training of laboratory personnel and with their needs for continuing education.

Area of specialization	Differentiating characteristics (pertaining to the area of specialization and illustrative ways it contributes to improved health)	Illustrative jobs and job settings (for graduates of the area of specialization)
Preventive medicine and community medicine *The application of clinical medicine and public health skills to understand and reduce risks of disease, disability, and death in both individuals and populations*	Preventive medicine (in the United States) and community medicine (in Canada) specialists manage programs in public or community health and conduct research to prevent and control disease; provide direct patient care; use scientific methods to identify health and safety hazards in the workplace and work to prevent occupational illness and injury; work to improve preventive and primary care services to underserved and high-risk populations; assess and eliminate environmental health hazards.	Preventive medicine and community medicine specialists work in varied community settings. Examples of activities include revival of an inactive tuberculosis control program, management of an inner-city clinic for sexually transmitted diseases, development of a statewide breast cancer screening initiative, development of a community health center in an underserved urban area, identification of drinking water safety problems, and development of a program to evaluate the health of a population living near a hazardous waste site.
Public health nursing *The application of nursing and public health principles to promote the physical, mental, and social well-being of people and communities*	Public health nurses provide health counseling and education to individuals, families, and communities. They are concerned with individual health in the broader community context, which may include: being the liaison with multiple community agencies to meet health needs; staff public health clinics; demonstrate patient care to family caregivers, but not generally provide direct patient care; serve on community boards and committees to affect health policy and services; organize and implement educational programs.	PH nurses play a key role in many community programs. For example, they promote maternal and infant health through such activities as counseling parents on health matters; assisting parents in developing skills to deal with health needs of their children; urge regular health exams and immunization; help parents secure screening services; teach home nursing and parenting skills; assist in improving social conditions that affect health; recognize and report child abuse.
Other *Although they do not fit within any of the preceding categories, various other specialties nevertheless make important contributions to community health. These specialties are defined in different ways, such as by disciplinary background (e.g., behavioral and social sciences) or by the kinds of phenomena under consideration (e.g., the study and treatment of health problems in an international setting).*		Employment opportunities exist primarily at the federal and state levels, in academic institutions, and in some private agencies and foundations. Skills of particular relevance to this broad area of specialization include the collection and analysis of data pertinent to the health status of defined populations, and the planning, development, and operation or evaluation of programs designed to deal with particular health needs.

Common Job Titles— Public and Community Health

Administrator

Director (of a specific service or program)
Health administrator
Health care administrator
Health officer
Health services administrator
Hospital administrator
Nursing home administrator

Analyst

Computer specialist
Demographer
Epidemiologist
Systems analyst

Dentist

Public health dentist

Engineer

Air pollution engineer
Environmental engineer
Product safety engineer
Waterworks engineer

Health Educator

Community health educator
Health promotion specialist
Public health educator
School health educator

Hygienist

Dental hygienist
Industrial hygienist

Inspector

Food and drug inspector
Hospital inspector
Milk and food inspector
Nursing home inspector

Laboratory Technician/Technologist

Biochemical technologist
Food technologist
Laboratory technician
Microbiology technologist
Radiological technologist
Veterinary lab technician

Nurse

Industrial health nurse
Mental health nurse
Nurse practitioner
Occupational health nurse
Public health nurse
School nurse
Visiting nurse

Nutritionist

Community nutritionist
Public health nutritionist
School nutritionist

Physician

Industrial health physician
Occupational health physician
Public health physician
School health physician
Aerospace physician
Medical officer of health
District health officer
Health officer

Planner

Facilities planner
Health planner
Manpower planner
Services planner
Program planner

Sanitarian

Environmental technician
Sanitarian

Scientist

Anthropologist
Bacteriologist
Behavioral scientist
Biologist
Chemist
Dairy scientist
Ecologist

Entomologist
Microbiologist
Parasitologist
Psychologist
Social scientist
Sociologist
Soil scientist
Zoologist

Social Worker

Medical social worker
Mental health counselor
Public health social worker
Psychiatric social worker

Statistician

Analyst
Biometrician
Biostatistician
Survey statistician
Vital statistician

Therapist

Occupational therapist
Physical rehabilitation therapist
Physical therapist
Recreation therapist
Speech therapist
Vocational rehabilitation therapist

Veterinarian

Public health veterinarian
Vector control technician

U.S. Schools of Public Health and Graduate Public Health Programs*

Schools of Public Health

University of Alabama at Birmingham School of Public Health, 720 South 20th Street, Birmingham, AL 35294-0008 (Dean—O. Dale Williams, MPH, PhD) (1978)

Boston University School of Public Health, School of Medicine, 80 East Concord Street, A-407, Boston, MA 02118-2394 (Director—Robert F. Meenan, MD, MPH) (1981)

University of California at Berkeley School of Public Health, 19 Earl Warren Hall, Berkeley, CA 94720 (Dean—Patricia A. Buffler, PhD, MPH) (1946)

University of California at Los Angeles School of Public Health, Center for the Health Sciences, Los Angeles, CA 90024-1772 (Dean—A.A. Afifi, PhD) (1960)

Columbia University School of Public Health, 600 West 168th Street, New York, NY 10032 (Dean—Allan Rosenfield, MD) (1946)

Emory University School of Public Health, 1599 Clifton Road, Atlanta, GA 30329 (Dean—Raymond Greenberg, MD, PhD) (1978)

Harvard University School of Public Health, 677 Huntington Avenue, Boston, MA 02115 (Dean—Harvey V. Fineberg, MD, PhD) (1946)

University of Hawaii School of Public Health, 1960 East-West Road, Honolulu, HI 96822 (Interim Dean—Barbara Z. Siegel, PhD) (1965)

University of Illinois at Chicago School of Public Health,

M/C 922, Box 6998, Chicago, IL 60680 (Acting Dean—Bernard Turnock, MD, MPH) (1972)

The Johns Hopkins University School of Hygiene and Public Health, 615 North Wolfe Street, Baltimore, MD 21205-2179 (Dean—Alfred Sommer, MD, MHS) (1946)

Loma Linda University School of Public Health, Loma Linda, CA 92350 (Dean—Richard H. Hart, MD, DrPH) (1967)

University of Massachusetts School of Public Health School of Health Sciences, 108 Arnold House, Amherst, MA 01003-0037 (Dean—Stephen H. Gehlbach, MD, MPH) (1971)

University of Michigan School of Public Health, 109 South Observatory Street, Ann Arbor, MI 48109-2029 (Dean—June E. Osborn, MD) (1946)

University of Minnesota School of Public Health, Box 197, Mayo Memorial Building, 420 Delaware Street, S.E., Minneapolis, MN 55455-0318 (Dean—Stephen C. Joseph, MD, MPH) (1946)

University of North Carolina School of Public Health, CB 7400 Rosenau Hall, Chapel Hill, NC 27599-7400 (Dean Michel A. Ibrahim, MD, MPH, PhD) (1946)

University of Oklahoma College of Public Health, Health Sciences Center, 801 Northeast 13th Street, Oklahoma City, OK 73104-5072 (Dean—Bailus Walker, Jr., PhD, MPH) (1967)

University of Pittsburgh Graduate School of Public Health, 111 Parran Hall, 130 DeSoto Street, Pittsburgh, PA 15261 (Dean—Donald R. Mattison, MD) (1950)

University of Puerto Rico School of Public Health, Medical Sciences Campus, GPO Box 5067, San Juan, Puerto Rico 00936 (Dean—Juan Silva-Parra, PhD) (1956)

Saint Louis University School of Public Health, O'Donnell Building, Fourth Floor, 3663 Lindell Avenue, Saint Louis, MO 63108 (Dean—James R. Kimmey, MD, MPH) (1983)

---

*Accredited by the Council on Education for Public Health as of May 1993.

The date in parentheses noted for each school or program represents the year first accredited or preaccredited.

San Diego State University Graduate School of Public
Health, San Diego, CA 92182-0405 (Director—F. Douglas
Scutchfield, MD) (1982)
University of South Carolina School of Public Health, Co-
lumbia, SC 29208 (Dean—Winona B. Vernberg, PhD) (1977)
University of South Florida College of Public Health, 13201
Bruce B. Downs Boulevard, (MDC-56), Tampa, FL 33612-
3805 (Dean—Peter J. Levin, ScD) (1987)
University of Texas School of Public Health, Health Science
Center at Houston, P.O. Box 20186, Houston, TX 77225
(Dean—R. Palmer Beasley, MD, MS) (1969)
Tulane University School of Public Health and Tropical
Medicine, 1430 Tulane Avenue, New Orleans, LA 70112
(Dean—Harrison C. Spencer, MD, MPH, DMH) (1947)
University of Washington School of Public Health and
Community Medicine, Mail Drop SC-30 Seattle, WA 98195
(Dean—Gilbert S. Omenn, MD, PhD) (1970)
Yale University Department of Epidemiology and Public
Health, School of Medicine, PO Box 3333, 60 College Street,
New Haven, CT 06510 (Chair—Burton H. Singer, PhD) (1946)

Graduate Programs in Community Health Education

California State University-Long Beach MPH and MS Programs in Community Health Education, Health Science Department, College of Health and Human Services, 1250 Bell-
flower Boulevard, Long Beach, CA 90840 (Chair—Alan C.
Henderson, DrPH) (1990)
California State University-Northridge MPH Program in
Community Health Education, Department of Health Science, School of Communication, Health and Human Services,
18111 Nordhoff Street, Northridge, CA 91330 (Director—Robert Huff, MPH, PhD) (1971)
East Stroudsburg State University MPH Program in Community Health Education, Health Department, East Stroudsburg, PA 18201 (Chair—William C. Livingood, PhD) (1990)
Hunter College MPH Program in Community Health Education, School of Health Sciences, CUNY, 425 East 25th
Street, New York, NY 10010 (Director—Stephen R. Zoloth,
PhD, MPH) (1972)
University of Illinois at Urbana—Champaign MSPH Program in Community Health Education, Department of Com-
munity Health, 1206 South Fourth Street, Champaign, IL
61820 (Head—R. Warwick Armstrong, PhD, MPH) (1983)
New York University MPH Program in Community Health
Education, Department of Health Education, School of Educa-
tion, Health, Nursing and Arts Professions, 35 West Fourth
Street, Suite 1200, New York, NY 10003 (Chair—Vivian P.J.
Clarke, EdD) (1971)
University of Northern Colorado MPH Program in Community Health Education, Department of Community Health

and Nutrition, College of Health and Human Sciences, Greeley,
CO 80639 (Chair—James Robinson, III, EdD) (1989)
San Jose State University MPH Program in Community
Health Education, Department of Health Science, School of
Applied Sciences and Arts, San Jose, CA 95192 (Chair—Helen
S. Ross, EdD, MPH) (1974)
Temple University MPH Program in Community Health
Education, Department of Health Education, College of
Health, Physical Education, Recreation & Dance, 304 Seltzer
Hall, Philadelphia, PA 19122 (Coordinator—Sheryl Rusek,
PhD, MPH) (1985)
University of Wisconsin at LaCrosse MPH Program in
Community Health Education, Health Education Department,
203 Mitchell Hall, LaCrosse, WI 54601 (Director—Gary D.
Gilmore, MPH, PhD) (1992)

Graduate Programs in Community Health/Preventive Medicine

University of Colorado MSPH Program, Department of Pre-
ventive Medicine and Biometrics, School of Medicine, Health
Sciences Center, 4200 East Ninth Avenue, Box C-245, Denver,
CO 80262 (Director—Phoebe A. Lindsey Barton, MPH, PhD)
(1985)
University of Connecticut MPH Program, Department of
Community Medicine and Health Care, School of Medicine,
Farmington, CT 06030-1910 (Director—Holger Hansen, MD,
DrPH, FACE) (1984)
George Washington University MPH Program, School of
Medicine and Health Sciences, 2150 Pennsylvania Avenue,
NW, Washington, DC 20037 (Director of Public Health Pro-
grams—Richard Riegelman, MD, PhD) (1990)
University of Miami MPH Program, Department of Epidemi-
ology and Public Health, School of Medicine, PO Box 016069,
Miami, FL 33101 (Director—Richard Donahue, PhD) (1982)
University of Medicine and Dentistry of New Jersey—Rob-
ert Wood Johnson Medical School and Rutgers, The State
University of New Jersey Graduate Program in Public
Health, Environmental and Occupational Health Sciences Insti-
tute (EOHSI), 681 Frelinghuysen Road, Piscataway, NJ 08855-
1179 (Director—George G. Rhoads, MD, MPH) (1986)
Ohio State University Graduate Programs in Preventive
Medicine, Department of Preventive Medicine, College of
Medicine, B-201 Starling Loving Hall, 320 West 10th Avenue,
Columbus, OH 43210-1228 (Graduate Studies Chair—Richard
Lanese, PhD) (1985)
University of Rochester MPH Program, School of Medicine
and Dentistry, 601 Elmwood Avenue, Rochester, NY 14642
(Director—James G. Zimmer, MD) (1978)
University of Tennessee at Knoxville MPH Program, De-
partment of Health, Leisure and Safety, College of Education,
1914 Andy Holt Avenue, Knoxville, TN 37996-2700 (Chair—
Charles B. Hamilton, MPH, DrPH) (1969)

Tufts University School of Medicine Combined MD/MPH Program, Department of Community Health, 136 Harrison Avenue, Boston, MA 02111 (Director—Markley H. Boyer, MD, MPH) (1992)

Uniformed Services University of the Health Sciences MPH and MTM&H Graduate Programs, Department of Preventive Medicine and Biometrics, School of Medicine, 4301 Jones Bridge Road, Bethesda, MD 20814-4799 (Director—Kenneth E. Dixon, MD, MPH) (1985)

University of Utah MPH and MSPH Programs, Department of Family and Preventive Medicine, School of Medicine, 50 North Medical Drive, Salt Lake City, UT 84132 (Director—Charles C. Hughes, PhD) (1978)

Medical College of Wisconsin MPH Program, Department of Preventive Medicine, 8701 Watertown Plank Road, Milwaukee, WI 53226 (Director—William W. Greaves, MD, MSPH) (1991)

Glossary

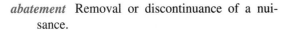

abatement Removal or discontinuance of a nuisance.

abortion Termination of a pregnancy before it is carried to full term, either by induced means (legal and illegal abortions) or by involuntary means (spontaneous abortion).

accessibility The distribution of health resources (for example, personnel and facilities) such that people in need are able to avail themselves of the resources with reasonable convenience and at reasonable cost.

accident An occurrence in a sequence of events that produces unintentional injury, death, or property damage.

accidental death Official classification of a death caused by unintentional injury.

acid rain Sulfur oxide pollutants carried in rain clouds.

acquired immunity Resistance to disease resulting from previous exposures that produced the disease and the antibodies against subsequent exposures.

active immunity Resistance to disease resulting from the host's body producing its own antibodies, either from exposure to the disease or from artificial introduction of the antigenic substance by vaccination or immunization.

active life expectancy Years before death in which individuals are able to perform activities of daily living and to function relatively independently.

actuarial data Information used to predict the average risks of deaths or other vital events, based on population experience in a recent period.

adaptation The process by which an organism or person makes a successful change to accommodate new circumstances. Some scholars argue that adaptation is the most generalizable measure of health.

addiction A derangement in cellular metabolism causing physiological and psychological dependence on a substance.

adolescence The years between childhood and adulthood, defined biologically by the advent of reproductive sex characteristics.

adulthood The years following adolescence, beginning with any age defined by the community, by custom, or by legal responsibilities and rights.

Aedes aegypti The mosquito found to be the transmitter of yellow fever by Walter Reed and colleagues in 1900.

age-adjusted rate The total rate for a population, adjusted to ignore the age distribution of specific population by multiplying each of its age-specific rates by the proportion of a standard (for example, national) population in that age group, then adding up the products.

ageism The stereotyped perceptions resulting in prejudice or discrimination against elderly people.

agent An epidemiological term referring to the organism or object that transmits a disease from the environment to the host.

age-specific rate The incidence (number of events during a specified period of time) for a specific age group, divided by the total number of people in that age group.

aging The process of growing older, especially referring to the period in which body functioning declines.

air exchange rate The frequency with which inside air is replaced with outside air.

ALARA As low as is reasonably achievable, a principle applied to control some pollutants where an absolute standard (MPC) or a cost-benefit analysis cannot be applied to set a permissible limit on emissions or concentrations.

allocation A distribution of resources to specific categories of expenditure.

Alzheimer's disease A syndrome characterized by symptoms associated with loss of mental capacities and functioning; often equated with senility.

ambient Surrounding condition of environment, usually referring to air quality or noise.

ambulatory care services Those health services provided to patients who are not placed in beds, usually performed in outpatient clinics.

amniocentesis A procedure for extracting fluid from the uterus of a pregnant women to use for screening and diagnosis, especially in relation to birth defect possibilities.

anaerobic Without oxygen, referring in this book to pathogenic organisms, such as *Clostridium botulinum,* that do not produce toxin in free air.

Anopheles The mosquito found to be responsible for transmitting malaria by Ronald Ross in India and Battista Grassi in Italy in 1898.

anorexia nervosa A compulsive nutritional disorder in which the obsession to lose weight leads to self-starvation.

antenatal care Care of the expectant mother, ideally begun during the first trimester of pregnancy; more commonly called prenatal care.

antibiosis Antagonism to specific organisms.

antibodies Protein molecules formed in the blood stream by exposure to a foreign substance such as an invading organism, later they are available to bind to the same substance and prevent its growth and reproduction.

antigen A substance that causes the production of antibodies when introduced into the body.

antiseptic Any substance used to kill or retard the growth of potentially harmful microorganisms, first discovered by Lister.

appropriation The placement of funds in a budget category previously authorized; the final step in the legislative process of initiating action in the administrative branch.

aquifers Large underground rock formations containing water that has percolated down from the earth's surface via cracks and faults.

arthritis A range of diseases afflicting the joints, including rheumatoid arthritis—an inflammatory disease with onset usually between the ages of 20 and 45—and osteoarthritis, which affects only older persons and weight-bearing joints, notably hips and knees.

asbestos A flameproof product used widely in the past as insulation material in buildings, now known to produce a toxic dust that causes lung diseases.

atherosclerosis A thickening and hardening of arteries in which the blood vessels are less elastic and narrower so that blood flow is impeded or clots may block the flow of blood.

atrophy The loss of strength or functioning of a muscle or skill from nonuse.

attributable risk The proportion of a specific disease or cause of death that can be blamed on a particular risk factor.

authority The power to take action legally or constitutionally.

authorization The step in legislative action in which resource allocations are made possible.

automatic-protective strategies Those preventive methods that bypass the motivation and decisions of people by structuring the environment in such a way that choices of action are minimized.

bacteriology The branch of science concerned with the study of microorganisms, the contributions of which were critical to the control of communicable diseases at the turn of the twentieth century.

bacteriostasis An arrest in the multiplication of bacteria, enabling the host's natural defenses to destroy the invading organism.

barriers The obstacles to performing a prescribed action or to carrying out a program.

behavioral diagnosis Delineation of the specific health actions most likely to effect a health outcome.

behavioral objective A statement of a desired outcome that specifies who is to demonstrate how much of what actions by when.

bereavement The loss of loved ones—one of the transitions most commonly experienced by elderly people, requiring adaptation and coping by the individual and the community.

bioassay Assessment of chemical substances in animal or plant tissue.

biotic potential The highest possible birthrate for a population, thought to be around 50 per 1000 in human population.

Black Death The common name for bubonic plague, a disease transmitted by fleas that became pandemic in past centuries.

block grants Funds transferred from one level of government to another with minimal earmarking of how they must be spent.

BOD Biochemical oxygen demand, an indicator of the amount of organic waste in water based on the amount of oxygen required to decompose it.

botulism A disease caused by a toxin produced by a spore-forming organism that is found in soils and that contaminates vegetables and other foods.

building codes Ordinances restricting the materials and standards of construction to assure safe habitation of indoor spaces.

bulimia A compulsive eating disorder in which the dual obsessions to eat and to lose weight lead to bingeing on large quantities of food, then purging or vomiting.

Byzantine Referring to the Eastern Roman Empire; connoting bureaucracy, luxury, and decadence.

carcinogen A cancer-causing substance.

cardiorespiratory fitness The combination of health benefits associated with aerobic exercise, including a more efficient heart, a stronger diaphragm, a slower resting heart rate, and lower levels of cholesterol and fibrin in the blood and arteries.

cardiovascular disease A group of conditions including heart disease, hypertension, atherosclerosis, stroke, rheumatic heart disease, and other disorders of the heart or blood vessels.

cardiovascular fitness The combination of heart rate (resting pulse), circulation, and other physiological signs resulting from adequate functioning and conditioning of the heart and circulatory system.

carriers Those hosts that continue to harbor the infectious agents even after their own recovery, making them a risk to the health of others.

cause-specific rate A death rate for a given disease or cause of death, such as the heart disease death rate, based on the number of deaths attributed to a specific cause divided by the total population at the midpoint of the period of measurement.

CDC Centers for Disease Control, a part of the United States Public Health Service.

cerebrovascular disease Atherosclerosis specifically in the arteries of the brain, often resulting in stroke.

chemotherapy The treatment of an illness or condition with chemical substances. In the case of mental illness, the use of alkaloids has reduced the need to keep patients in hospitals.

chlorination Treatment of water with chlorine, which kills all bacteria pathogenic to man at concentrations above 0.2 ppm.

Clean Air Act The legislation passed by the U.S. Congress in 1965, renewable every 5 years, providing for federal assistance and standards for air pollution control.

coalition A group of individuals, usually representing organizations or agencies in a community, working together on an issue of mutual concern.

coercive strategies Preventive methods that bypass the motivation and decisions of people by dictating or precluding choices.

coinsurance The portion of medical care costs required by an insurance plan to be paid by the insured.

coliform test A standard bacteriological examination of drinking water safety, using *E. coli* organisms as an indicator of fecal contamination.

common law The unwritten rules of society honored by courts because they have been established by custom or by previous court decisions.

communicable disease A potentially harmful organism or its toxic products that can be transmitted from one human host, reservoir, or lower animals to susceptible human hosts.

community For most purposes in this book, the term is applied to a group of inhabitants living in a somewhat localized area under the same general regulations and having common norms, values, and organizations.

community health A field of practice encompassing and coordinating at the local level the overlapping aspects of school health, public health, employee health, maternal and child health, environmental health protection, and the personal health practices of individuals and families.

community health education Any combination of learning experiences designed to facilitate voluntary actions in individuals or groups that will be conducive to health.

community health events High-visibility activities such as marathon races or health fairs that provide both recreation and health information and involve a broad spectrum of the community.

community health promotion Any combination of educational, social, and environmental actions conducive to the health of the population of a geographically defined area.

conservation The wise use of resources; the most effective use of the environmental resources necessary for survival and quality of life.

contamination The presence of toxins or pathogenic organisms on inanimate objects such as food, soil, water, or fomites.

convalescence The period following the acute phases of an illness during which some symptoms and potential infectiousness continue to exist, so continuing rest or isolation is needed.

coping The process of adjusting to stress in a constructive manner.

coronary artery disease Narrowing of the heart vessels due to deposits of cholesterol and fat, thus weakening the function of the heart and increasing the risk of myocardial infarction.

coronary heart disease Atherosclerosis specifically in the arteries of the heart muscle.

corrosivity The potential of a substance to oxidize or rust metals and other surfaces with which it comes in contact.

cost-benefit analysis A procedure for policy decisions, based on a comparison of the expense of a program with its expected monetary yield or savings.

crude death rate The total number of deaths divided by the total population, usually multiplied by 1000 so that the result can be expressed as deaths per 1000 population.

decibel A measure of noise intensity, based on just noticeable differences in sound.

decontamination The killing or removing of pathogens or toxins in or on inanimate objects.

defection The period during or following convalescence from an infectious disease during which organisms are still being cast off by the body, so isolation may continue to be necessary.

defervescence The period following the most acute phase of an infectious illness during which symptoms subside but relapse remains probable without continuing treatment or rest.

deinstitutionalization The policy or practice of placing mentally ill patients back in the community, made possible by drugs that control the symptoms of illness.

demand The economic concept of consumer desire for a product or service resulting in greater tendency to purchase it and thereby to affect its supply or price.

demography The study of human population growth, decline, and movement, using measures of fertility, mortality, and migration.

deregulation An administrative strategy to reduce governmental responsibility for surveillance and enforcement.

diabetes A metabolic disease that affects the arteries as a result of failure to metabolize carbohydrates.

disabling injury An injury that results in death, permanent disability, or any duration of temporary total disability.

disaster plans The detailed procedures to be followed in the event of a catastrophe such as a tornado, flood, of nuclear accident.

disease A harmful departure from the normal state of a person or other organism.

disinfection The killing or removing of organisms capable of causing infection.

disintegration of personality The process of failing to cope with stress constructively; the opposite of coping.

DPT The trivalent vaccine, given in a single inoculation, that inoculates against diphtheria, pertussis, and tetanus.

diffusion The process by which an idea, innovation, behavior, disease, or other transmissible thing spreads in a population, described over time by an S-shaped growth curve showing the cumulative number of people reached or changed.

early adopters The segment of the population accepting a new idea or practice soon after the innovators but before the middle majority, and who tend to be opinion leaders for the middle majority.

E-codes Classification of injuries according to the International Classification of Disease (ICD) coding for emergency medical care.

ecology The study of the interaction of life-forms with their environment.

economy of scale The point in the growth of a program or service at which each additional element of service costs less to produce.

educational diagnosis The delineation of factors that predispose, enable, and reinforce a specific health behavior.

educational strategies Preventive methods that seek to assure that people are able to take voluntary action based on informed decisions.

efficiency The ability to function as needed with a minimum of energy expenditure, and to meet emergencies or special demands.

emergency medical services system The coordinated resources responsible for urgent medical care, including ambulance service, communications, and medical facilities and personnel.

Employee Assistance Program A fairly standardized offering of counseling and referral to troubled employees with the intent of improving their performance by reducing or eliminating their dependence on or misuse of alcohol or drugs.

enabling factor Any characteristic of the environment that facilitates health behavior, and any skill or resource required to attain the behavior.

endemic Epidemiological term referring to a disease or condition that persists within a geographical area.

enforcement Action taken to assure compliance with the law or legislative intent.

environment All factors external to the organism that may impinge on its behavior or well-being.

EPA Environmental Protection Agency, a U.S. federal agency responsible for air and water quality standards.

epidemic Widely and rapidly spreading disease, more than an outbreak but less than a pandemic.

epidemiological diagnosis The delineation of the extent, distribution, and causes of a health problem in a defined population.

epidemiology The study of disease transmission, development, and consequences in populations to identify causes and distributions of diseases.

etiology The origins or causes of a disease or condition under study; the first steps in the natural history of a disease.

evaluation The comparison of an object of interest against a standard of acceptability.

excise tax A tax on the manufacture, sale, or use of certain products such as alcohol or tobacco to generate revenue for a government or to control consumption, or both.

ex officio Serving as a member of a committee or board because of one's official position rather than by election.

extramural Activities such as research conducted outside the agency.

facilitators Those enabling factors helping to overcome barriers.

family A group of two or more people related by birth, marriage, or adoption and residing together in a household.

family planning The process of establishing the preferred number and spacing of children in one's family and selecting the means by which this objective is achieved.

family violence Spouse abuse, child abuse by parents, child-to-parent abuse, sexual abuse of family members, and most common of all, child-to-child abuse.

farm safety survey A procedure for the assessment of hazardous conditions on a farm.

fastigium The period during which a disease is at its most acute or intense expression of symptoms.

fatal accident Official classification of an event producing injuries resulting in one or more deaths within 1 year.

fecundity The state and degree of being capable of conceiving and giving birth to offspring.

federal The level of government representing the collective interests of states.

federalism That system of governance emphasizing the powers retained by states making up a federation.

fetal death rate The number of deaths of fetuses with gestations of 20 weeks or more per 1000 total births (i.e., live births plus fetal deaths).

filtration Removal of particulate matter in water by percolation through a layer of sand or other porous material.

fitness The condition of being physically, mentally, and socially at a high level of efficiency.

flash mix The first step in rapid sand filtration method of water treatment, in which aluminum sulfate is added to the water to congeal suspended matter as a floc that can be trapped or filtered.

flocculation Trapping particles suspended in water by adsorption and settling.

fluorocarbon propellants Inert gases used in some pressurized containers to propel other gases because they do not react with other gases, but they do release chlorine in the upper atmosphere when exposed to ultraviolet rays.

fomites Inanimate objects other than water, milk, food, air, and soil that might be contaminated and provide vehicles of disease transfer; examples include plates, glasses, clothing, bed linen, and handrails.

food poisoning The common term for either of two reactions: (1) a toxic reaction to a food that is itself poisonous, or (2) a reaction to food that has transmitted a pathogen or toxin.

formative evaluation Steps taken to assess the circumstances and performance of a program before it is fully launched, with the specific purpose of improving its form and delivery.

frank cases Those individuals whose disease becomes known through symptoms.

full-time equivalent A measure of staffing or personnel requirements based on counting each full-time employee as 1 and each part-time employee as a fraction of 1.

functional health That state of health enabling one to carry out social responsibilities and to be a productive member of the community.

greenhouse effect The accumulation of carbon dioxide in the atmosphere around the earth, which results in the gradual heating of the atmosphere.

genocide The systematic killing (elimination) of a race or nation of people.

geriatrics The field of professional practice addressed to the health needs of the elderly.

gerontology The field of research devoted to the processes and problems of old age.

groundwater Naturally occurring underground reservoirs used by many small communities and a few large cities as their source of water.

habituation The incorporation of a pattern of behavior into one's life-style to the degree that it is performed virtually without thought, but does not necessarily entail physical or psychological dependence.

health A state of complete physical, mental, and social well-being, not merely the absence of disease (WHO), or the ability of an organism to adapt to its environment and circumstances.

health care organization The pattern of arrangements for access to medical, dental, nursing, and related facilities, resources, and services in a community.

health education Any combination of learning experiences designed to facilitate voluntary actions conducive to the health of individuals, groups, or communities.

health field concept The notion that the factors influencing health can be subsumed under four categories: environment, human biology, behavior, and health care organization.

health fraud Promotion of a health or medical product or service with an intent to deceive.

health promotion Any combination of educational, organizational, economic, and environmental supports for conditions of living and behavior of individuals, groups, or communities conducive to health.

Health Systems Agency A federally mandated, state-approved organization to carry out systematic assessments of a region's health needs and to develop health service goals and implementation plans for that geographical area.

heart attack Insufficient supply of blood to the heart muscle, causing the failure of the muscle to function.

high-pressure food processing A method of preserving certain foods by using water pressure instead of heat, thereby preserving vitamins and minerals while killing bacteria.

homeless Any person who routinely sleeps in bus, railway, airport, or subway terminals, in abandoned buildings, or outside.

home rule A grant of authority from the state to counties through statutes or constitutions allowing local self-determination and ability to levy local taxes for specific purposes.

home safety survey A procedure for the assessment of hazardous conditions in a home.

host A concept in epidemiology referring to an individual who harbors or is at risk of harboring a disease or condition.

hypercholesterolemia Elevated cholesterol levels in the blood, resulting from high percentages of saturated animal fats in the diet and leading to increased risk of heart and vascular diseases.

hypertension A vascular disease associated with increased risk of stroke, the cause of which is unknown but which is easily diagnosed, treated, and controlled. Also called high blood pressure.

hypothermia A drop in deep body temperature under 95°F (35°C), which typically develops in isolated elderly people over a period of days.

immunity Resistance to a specific disease.

immunization The process of producing antibodies that protect the individual from a disease by introducing an antigenic substance into the body.

incidence A measure of frequency of occurrence based on the number of new cases appearing over a given period of time.

industrial safety Injury control in a branch of trade or production on a broad geographic scale.

infant mortality The number of deaths of live-born children under 1 year of age per 1000 live births.

infection The successful invasion of a host by pathogens under such conditions as will permit them to multiply and harm the host.

infectious disease A communicable disease that results in a reaction of the host to the invading organism, producing abnormalities in the host and usually killing the invading pathogen.

informed consent A medical-legal doctrine that holds providers responsible for ensuring that consumers or patients understand the risks and benefits of a procedure or medicine before it is administered.

injunction An official order restraining a person or organization from continuing an action or maintaining a condition that is deemed a nuisance.

injuries Bodily damage caused by trauma.

injury control The prevention or limitation of harm to health either through prevention of, or through the protection of, victims of accidents, natural disasters, or intentional violence.

innovators The segment of the population first to adopt a new idea or practice, usually based on information from sources outside the community.

incubation The period and process during which organisms are growing within their host, within an egg, womb, or artificial incubator.

insurance A financial contract by which a company collects average costs (premiums) from the insured in exchange for guaranteed payment of variable costs in the event of certain types of loss.

intentional injury Homicide, suicide, assault, battery, rape, and most instances of family violence.

irradiation A method for decontaminating food by damaging the genetic material of bacteria so they cannot survive or multiply, without making the food radioactive or increasing human exposure to radiation.

isolation Segregation of an infected person or lower animal until the danger of conveying infection has passed.

jurisdiction The boundaries within which an agency or official has authority.

laboratory services Analytical bioassays for clinical, environmental, toxicological, forensic, and related assessments.

latchkey syndrome Pattern of problems associated with children who come home from school and have no guardian to supervise them.

late adopters That portion of a population who are among the last to accept an innovation.

late majority The segment of the population most difficult to reach through mass communication channels or to convince of the need to adopt a new idea or practice, sometimes because they cannot afford it or cannot get to the source, or because of cultural or language differences or other difficulty.

lead paint Any paint containing more than 0.06% lead.

leisure The use of time not devoted to work.

life expectancy The average number of years that an individual of a given age can expect to live, based on the longevity experience of the population.

life span A biological estimate of the maximum number of years a species is expected to live, based on the longest living cases observed and inherited characteristics.

life-style A complex pattern of habituated behavior that is socially and culturally conditioned and may be health-related but not necessarily health-directed.

local public health agency The officially designated authority for the planning and execution of facilities, programs, and services to protect and promote a community's health.

longevity The expected duration of life, based on life-table analyses of age-specific death rates.

mandatory programs Programs required by law, usually for one level of government regulated by the next higher level.

market testing The placement of a message or product in a commercial context to determine how it influences consumer behavior.

maternal mortality The number of women dying from complications of pregnancy or childbirth per 100,000 live births.

Medicaid A state-operated program of medical reimbursement for the medically indigent in the United States.

Medicare A federal program of health insurance for the elderly.

mental health The emotional and social well-being and psychological resources of the individual.

metastasis The spread of cancerous cells from the site of the original development of the cancer.

miasma phase A period of the nineteenth century in which disease transmission was thought to be through "bad air." Though scientifically unsound, this assumption led to many of the environmental and sanitary reforms that resulted in some of the greatest health improvements in history.

middle majority The segment of the population who adopt a new idea or practice after the innovators and early adopters but before the late adopters, usually influenced by a combination of mass media, interpersonal communication, and endorsements by famous personalities or organizations of which they are members.

MPC Maximum permissible concentration, a standard applied to radiation.

mutation The adaptation of a species or strain of organism from one generation to another as a result of the survivors of the previous generation reproducing themselves, the effect being that an organism originally susceptible to a germicide or antibiotic can become resistant to it.

natural history of health The theoretical cycle describing what would maintain health in the absence of any social organization.

natural immunity Resistance to disease conferred by genetic inheritance.

natural increase The growth (or decline) of population attributable to births minus deaths.

need The assessed problem or aspiration requiring intervention or fulfillment.

neonatal mortality The number of deaths of infants under 28 days of age per 1000 live births.

NIH National Institutes of Health, a part of the U.S. Public Health Service.

NIOSH National Institute for Occupational Safety and Health, a component of the U.S. Centers for Disease Control and Prevention.

nitrogen cycle The continuous natural process of organic waste decomposition.

nitrogen oxides Air pollutants arising from all combustion.

normal That which is expected and tolerated by the community. What is considered normal in one community may be considered abnormal in other communities.

norms A sociological concept describing the expected patterns of behavior in a population, based on the prevalence of the behavior.

nosocomial infection Disease incurred in a hospital environment, especially threatening because the extensive use of antibiotics and antiseptics in hospitals has produced resistant strains of pathogens there.

nostrum A secret or patented substance or device for which false therapeutic claims are made.

nuclear winter The series of expected consequences of the massive cloud of dust and smoke that would be produced by extensive nuclear explosions.

nuisance A condition that adversely affects or injures one or more persons. A **public nuisance** is one that affects many people.

obesity The condition of being significantly overweight, as determined by skinfold measurements, body mass, or ratio of weight to height. Obesity is usually defined as 120% or more of ideal weight for height and age, based on statistical tables.

occupational injury Injury arising out of and in the course of gainful employment, regardless of where the accident occurs.

occupational safety Injury control in specific worksite.

official agency A tax-supported or governmental authority.

official health agency A governmental organization designated as having authority in some sphere of health.

OSHA Abbreviation referring either to the Occupational Safety and Health Act of 1970 or to the Occupational Safety and Health Administration, a federal agency of the United States.

outbreak Two or more illnesses linked to a common source.

outcome evaluation The comparison of the results of a program or intervention against ultimate objectives of the program or against some other standard of acceptability.

ozone One of the gases contributing to pollution in the lower atmosphere and to protection against ultraviolet radiation in the upper atmosphere.

PAHO Pan American Health Organization, which also serves as the WHO Regional Office for the Americas.

pandemic A widespread epidemic, usually affecting several countries and sometimes the entire globe.

passive immunity Protection against disease conferred at least temporarily by the mother's antibodies in the infant or by serum from another person.

pasteurization Heating a medium to a certain temperature for a given time period required to kill pathogenic organisms.

pathogenic Disease-producing.

perinatal Stillborn and early neonatal deaths covering the period from 28 weeks of pregnancy to 1 week following birth.

permanent disability Any degree of permanent impairment of the body, such as amputation, loss of vision, and other crippling nonfatal injuries.

physiological efficiency The ability of an organ or system to carry out its biological function with a minimum of stress.

planning The process of establishing priorities, diagnosing causes of problems, and allocating resources to achieve objectives.

poison control center An emergency information source for the diagnosis and management of injuries caused by poisonous substances.

poisoning Damage caused by the chemical effect of a toxic substance ingested, injected, or on the skin.

police power The authority of the people, vested in their government, to promote and protect their general welfare.

postneonatal mortality The number of deaths of infants from 28 days to 365 days of age per 1000 live births.

predisposing factor Any characteristic of a patient, consumer, student, or community that motivates behavior related to health.

prematurity rate The percentage of babies born who weigh 2500 grams (5½ pounds) or less.

prenatal care Medical services and counseling, combined with the personal protective and health promotion actions of the pregnant woman and her family, on behalf of the unborn fetus.

preretirement counseling Preparation of older employees for the transition from working to nonworking status.

prevalence A measure of frequency of occurrence based on the number of cases (old and new) existing at a given time.

primary health care As used in North America, refers to medical diagnosis and treatment of most symptoms not requiring specialist or hospital care; as used by WHO, refers to an approach to community health encompassing principles of the Alma Ata Declaration.

process evaluation Assessment of the ongoing delivery or conduct of the program or method to determine its appropriateness and acceptability, short of assessing its outcomes.

prodrome That stage of the disease process in the individual that precedes the acute manifestation of symtoms.

Professional Standards Review Organizations Peer review groups created by federal legislation in 1972 to assure the maintenance of standards in medical and hospital practices and to restrain cost increases. *psychiatry* Discipline or medical specialty that concerns itself with the diagnosis, treatment, and cure of mental disorders.

puberty The period of development during which the child develops adult sexual characteristics.

public nuisance A condition sufficiently objectionable to invoke police power of the health department or other local authority.

public pool A swimming facility used by people other than the owners or their families.

puerperium Following birth.

pumice Small bits of light, expanded lava found in volcanic ash.

quackery False medical or health claim for a worthless product or procedure.

quality assurance An approach to evaluation based on measure of the proficiency or quality of services rendered rather than on health outcomes achieved.

quarantine The segregation or detention of susceptible individuals who have been exposed to a communicable disease.

rate Any ratio that contains an element of time.

recreation The act or process of refreshing or recovering after work or stress.

rehabilitation The restoration to the fullest degree of physical, mental, social, vocational, and economic usefulness of which an individual is capable.

reinforcing factor Rewards or punishments following or anticipated as a consequence of a health behavior.

relative risk The ratio of deaths or cases of a disease in those who have a particular characteristic (e.g., age, sex, or a risk factor) to those deaths or cases not having that characteristic.

relative-risk ratio The rate in the exposed population divided by the rate in the unexposed population.

Renaissance Literally, rebirth; referring to a period following the Dark Ages in Europe when the arts and sciences flowered again after having been denigrated as unworthy and ungodly pursuits.

requirements The assessed resources needed to implement a program, to overcome barriers, and to accomplish its objectives.

reservoir The natural habitat of an infectious agent, where it lives and multiplies until it can be transmitted to a susceptible host.

rhinitis A respiratory condition characterized by nasal congestion and inflammation, associated with allergic reactions to food and other substances.

risk factors Those characteristics of the individual that predispose him or her to greater probability of developing a disease.

salmonella A pathogenic organism sometimes present in uncooked meat or unpasteurized milk and producing acute gastrointestinal distress after being ingested.

scholasticism Philosophical systems of thought based on assumptions about God, truth, and ideology rather than on observable realities. This approach ruled human affairs during the Dark Ages and was displaced by realism and science during the Renaissance.

school health education Any combination of learning experiences conducted in the school setting to predispose students to and enable them to carry out future decision making and behavior conducive to health.

school health program The main channel of health promotion, health services, and health protection for children, consisting of health education, school health services, and a healthful school environment.

sedentary living A pattern of physical activity insufficient in vigor, duration, or frequency of movement to maintain fitness.

sediment Material that settles on the bottom of a body of water.

sedimentation The removal of floc in the treatment of water by collecting it at the bottom of settling tanks.

skinfold measures Measurement of subcutaneous fat by means of calipers on areas such as biceps, triceps, trunk, thighs, or calves.

slum An area in which any four of the criteria of substandard housing are met.

smog The atmospheric result of the photochemical reaction of hydrocarbons and sulfur oxides produced by sunlight.

social diagnosis Assessment of the factors influencing the quality of life.

social health The capacity of individuals to work productively and to participate actively in the life of their community.

social history of health A theoretical cycle describing what happens to the natural history of health when social organization is imposed on it.

social pathology Failures of adjustment leading to antisocial acts that are destructive to other individuals or to community property.

socialization A process of developing behavioral patterns or life-style through modeling or imitating socially important persons.

society The larger community of people who share a common government, cultural heritage, territory, or some combination of these; a community of communities; sometimes synonymous with nation.

sphygomanometer A device using an inflatable cuff, a stethoscope, and a mercury meter to measure blood pressure.

spontaneous generation An early theory of how maggots and other larvae (''worms'') appeared on rotted food and infested flesh, disproved when scientists observed the laying of eggs by flies and lice.

statutory law Those rules of society established by legislation.

stroke Cerebrovascular disease caused by a thrombus (blood clot) in an artery of the brain.

subclinical infection The existence of disease that does not manifest itself as a frank case.

subcutaneous fat Nonmuscular tissues beneath the skin.

substandard housing House or apartments failing to meet criteria established by city ordinances or building codes, based usually on national standards.

sulfur oxide A pollutant of air, arising primarily from burning of sulfur-containing coal and fuel oil.

summative evaluation The assessment of outcomes or impact of a program, service, intervention, or method.

superfund A special-purpose budget, set aside for a large task that is limited in time, such as cleaning toxic waste sites.

supply The available resource, service, or product in response to need or demand.

supply and demand The economic factors determining the price of a consumable product or service.

surface water Water above ground in runoff sources such as streams. Surface water used to supply a community is usually stored in a reservoir, treated, and piped to homes and other use sites.

synergistic When two or more factors combine to produce an effect that is greater than the sum of their individual effects.

temperature inversion A layer of warm air above a layer of cooler air that prevents surface air from carrying pollutants from the lower atmosphere.

thoracic Of or pertaining to the chest and lungs.

turbidity A cloudy state of otherwise clear liquid, caused by particulate matter suspended in the liquid.

unintentional injury Term currently preferred by public health experts in place of the term *accident* to emphasize health consequences and to avoid the implication that the injury-causing event was necessarily uncontrollable.

vector Any animal that harbors and transfers disease from one human host to another, or from intermediate animal hosts to human hosts.

vehicle An inanimate object or a living thing that can act as a vector or as an intermediate host or reservoir for transmission of disease.

ventilation The transfer of outside air and inside air and the control of temperature, humidity, and movement of air.

vital index The difference between births per 1000 population and deaths per 1000 population, reflecting the rate of natural increase.

voluntary health agency A nongovernmental organization devoted usually to a particular set of health problems, operating on funds donated by the public.

well-being A good or satisfactory condition of existence.

WHO World Health Organization.

YPLL Years of potential life lost, a measure of the longevity of a population giving greater weight to premature deaths proportionate to the years before age 65 or age 75 that the deaths occurred.

zoning The restriction on types of buildings or facilities that can be constructed or operated in specific areas of a community.

zoonoses Diseases transmitted to man by vertebrate animals rather than by arthropods (insects, spiders, ticks, etc.) or other invertebrates.

Index

Abortions
 "gag rule," 127
 pro-choice and pro-life controversy, 127
 Roe v. Wade, 126-127
 spontaneous or artificial, 126
 strategies to provide abortion services, 127
 "undue burden," 126
Acid rain, 443
Acquired immunodeficiency syndrome (AIDS), 3, 161, 181, 306, 317
Active life expectancy approach, 212-218
Activity, specific forms and levels of, 279-280
Adaptation, 33
Adaptation and conservation, 32
Administration of Aging, 554-555
Administrative diagnosis, 103-104
Adolescence, early
 adult guidance and understanding, 150
 health consequences, 151
 momentous changes, 150
 other transitions, 151
 potential health problems, 151
 stress and coping, 151
 transitions in the life span, 151
Adolescent abuse and neglect, U.S. objectives for, 168
Adolescent awareness, 173-174
Adolescent health, 149-175
Adolescent health behavior, 158-175
Adolescent health, demography and epidemiology of, 153-156
Adolescent suicide rates, U.S. objectives for, 168

Adult deaths, principal causes of, 183-184
Adult health, 179-199
Adult-onset diabetes, 359-360
Advocacy groups, 51
Aedes aegypti, 13, 327
Age-based organizations, 225
Age-specific rates, 74-76
Agency for Toxic Substances and Disease Registry, 550-551
Aggregating educational targets, principle of, 95-96
Aging, as a concern of political systems, 225
Aging, religion and, 224
Aging, specific health priorities of, 218-220
Aging, transitions in, 214-217
Agricultural and technological factors, 48-49
Aid to Families with Dependent Children (AFDC), 161, 554
AIDS. *See* Acquired immunodeficiency syndrome
AIDS-related complex (ARC), 317
AIDS virus, 317
Air pollution
 aerosol shaving cream, 518
 asbestos, 518-519
 asbestosis, 518
 and asthma, 510
 capital investment, 514
 carcinogenic pollutants, 517
 Clean Air Act, 511, 513
 coal, 511
 community programs, 516

Air pollution—cont'd
 control, 511
 cost-benefit analysis, 515-516
 current issues, 514-515
 double edge of public policy, 513
 economic and aesthetic aspects, 510
 Environmental Protection Agency (EPA), 515
 environmental tobacco smoke, 519
 epidemiology, 508-510
 health aspects, 508-509
 indoor air pollutants, 517
 methyl isocyanate, 509
 mineral fibers, 518
 nitrogen oxides, 511
 pumice, 510
 second-hand smoke, 519
 smog, 508
 standards, 516-517
 state programs, 516
 sulfur oxide, 511
 U.S. legislation, 511, 513
 volcanic ash, 510-511
 volcanic winter, 510
 1990 amendments, 513-514
Alcohol, 163-164, 388
Alcohol misuse
 epidemiology, 353-354
 fetal alcohol syndrome, 354
 hepatic cirrhosis, 354
Alcohol misuse, prevention of
 advertising and counter-advertising, 356
 agent, 354-355
 American Heart Association, 355
 economic supports, 357
 environment, 355